NURSE'S PROBLEM SOLVER

Springhouse Corporation
Springhouse, Pennsylvania

Staff

Executive Director, Editorial
Stanley Loeb

Senior Publisher
Matthew Cahill

Clinical Manager
Cindy Tryniszewski, RN, MSN

Art Director
John Hubbard

Senior Editor
H. Nancy Holmes

Clinical Project Manager
Patricia Dwyer Schull, RN, MSN

Clinical Editors
Judith Schilling McCann, RN, BSN;
Beverly A. Tscheschlog, RN

Editors
Marylou Ambrose, Neal Fandek,
Elizabeth L. Mauro, Maureen N. Pross,
Gale A. Sloan, Elizabeth Weinstein

Copy Editors
Cynthia C. Breuninger (manager),
Lynette D. High, Jennifer George Mintzer,
Nancy Papsin, Doris Weinstock

Designers
Stephanie Peters (associate art
director), Linda Jovinelly Franklin (senior
designer), Susan Hopkins Rodzewich
(book designer), Laurie Mirijanian, Anet
Oakes, Ann Raphun

Photographers
Gary Donnelly, John Gallagher

Illustrators
Michael Adams, Jackie Facciola, Jean
Gardner, Linda Gist, Frank Grobelny, Bob
Jackson, Mark Mancini, Robert
Neumann, Judy Newhouse, Mary Stangl,
Jim Story, Larry Ward

Typographers
Diane Paluba (manager), Elizabeth
Bergman, Joyce Rossi Biletz, Phyllis
Marron, Robin Mayer, Valerie
Rosenberger

Manufacturing
Deborah Meiris (director), Anna Brindisi,
T.A. Landis

Production Coordinator
Patricia McCloskey

Editorial Assistants
Maree DeRosa, Beverly Lane, Mary
Madden, Dianne Tolbert

Printed in the United States of America.
NPS-011094

Ⓡ A member of the Reed Elsevier plc group

Library of Congress Cataloging-in-Publication Data		
Nurse's problem solver.		
p. cm.		
Includes index.		
1. Nursing assessment.	2. Nursing.	
I. Springhouse Corporation.		
[DNLM: 1. Nursing Care.	2. Nursing.	
WY 100 N97418 1994]		
RT48.N85 1994		
610.73—dc20		94-21374
DNLM/DLC		CIP
ISBN 0-87434-727-0		

Foreword

With a changing health care system, your patient care has become more complex than ever before. Patients stay in the hospital for hours and days rather than weeks and months, and they seldom have diseases involving only one organ system. They worry about the cost of their health care and want to participate in decisions about managing their conditions. And, after discharge, they may require a range of home care services.

In a time of such rapid and significant change, how can you provide skilled and compassionate care? How can you assess chest pain in one patient, teach another about a cholesterol-lowering diet, comfort and counsel a patient with newly diagnosed liver cancer, and deal with his distraught family?

The key to solving complex problems like these lies in your ability to tap the right resources and use them well. Fortunately, *Nurse's Problem Solver* provides practical, on-target solutions to the multiple problems that arise in nursing today.

Chapter 1 helps you obtain an effective history—even when you're pressed for time. It also provides tips on dealing with patients who have special needs, such as physical or cognitive impairments or a specific cultural or religious background.

Chapters 2 offers strategies for interpreting ominous, confusing, or subtle clinical signs, such as nonpalpable pulses or a rapid heart rate. Chapter 3 explains how to interpret puzzling laboratory findings, ranging from arterial blood gases to cardiac enzymes.

Chapters 4 through 6 provide solutions for difficult problems involving the care of acutely ill patients, medication administration, drug interactions and dosage errors, and complex procedures. Each chapter gives you specific directions on how to solve or sidestep problems.

Chapter 7 provides useful information about the increasingly complex technology used in hospitals today. When you're faced with unexpected difficulties with ventilators, cardiac monitors, and other devices, this chapter will tell you how to detect and correct the problem. Chapter 8 deals with patient teaching—how to get your point across and how to tell if you've succeeded.

Chapters 9 through 11 explore professional problems. When doctors, colleagues, or patients present interpersonal difficulties, Chapter 9 offers solutions. Chapter 10 steers you away from perilous documentation practices, and Chapter 11 provides insight on handling legal and ethical problems in nursing care.

Throughout this handbook, you'll find logos, or special graphic devices, that highlight important information for you. One logo, *Rule of Thumb,* offers guidelines to follow when nursing actions aren't clear-cut or could cause complications. Another logo, *Stat Care,* spells out the immediate nursing actions to take in a crisis. The *Preventive Practice* logo shows you how to avoid recurrence of a problem. *Clinical Close-up* clarifies pathophysiology through detailed illustrations, and *60-Second Solution* identifies problems you can solve in 1 minute or less.

In all, *Nurse's Problem Solver* covers over 600 clinical and professional topics and provides solutions to thousands of troublesome problems. It will help you respond to sudden emergencies, handle "people problems," and avoid legal obstacles. In short, *Nurse's Problem Solver* will help you successfully address just about any clinical or professional problem in your practice.

Marilyn Sawyer Sommers, RN, PhD, CCRN
Associate Professor
College of Nursing and Health
University of Cincinnati

1 Handling History-Taking Problems

Health history basics

History-taking skills

Data collection

Health history basics

You probably know there are two types of health histories: a doctor's health history and a nurse's. What you might not realize is that the main difference between the two lies not in the type of information obtained but in the reason for collecting it and the way it's used. A doctor takes a medical history to guide diagnosis and direct treatment. A nurse focuses on the patient's response to his illness.

During the interview, you'll gain essential information that will help you develop an individualized plan of care. You'll also have the opportunity to teach the patient techniques to promote wellness.

❖

History-taking skills

For a health history to be of value, it must be accurate and complete. Obtaining the necessary information requires effective interviewing skills.

Recording and using information

Most hospitals and other health care facilities use a standard format for taking health histories. These formats provide a logical sequence for the interview and an organized record of the patient's responses.

Most health histories contain four major sections: biographical data, health and illness, health promotion, and role and relationship. (See *Contents of the nursing health history.*)

Using the information

As a nurse, you'll use your health history to provide care, of course. But you'll also use it to assess the impact of the patient's condition on himself and his family. The information will also help you evaluate the patient's health education needs and start discharge planning.

Sharpening your interview technique

You should treat the interview as an open exchange, not as a question-and-answer session. (See *Asking the right questions,* page 4.)

To conduct a productive interview, you'll need a working knowledge of pathophysiology and psychosocial principles, along with sharply honed interpersonal and communication skills. Below are some guidelines for improving your interviewing skills.

Learning to accept yourself

Being self-aware—that is, recognizing and accepting your own feelings and values as well as your personal biases—will allow you to communicate more effectively with patients who have different values.

Contents of the nursing health history

Listed below are the categories that a thorough nursing health history should include.

Biographical data
• Name, address, and telephone number
• Social Security number
• Sex
• Age, birth date, and birthplace
• Race, nationality, and cultural background
• Marital status and names of persons living with the patient
• Contact person
• Occupation, education, and religion

Health and illness
• Reason for seeking health care
• Current health status
• Past health status

• Family health history
• Body system appraisal
• Developmental history

Health promotion
• Health beliefs
• Personal habits
• Sleep
• Exercise and recreation
• Nutrition
• Stress and coping ability
• Socioeconomic concerns
• Environmental health issues
• Occupational health issues

Role and relationship
• Self-image
• Family role and relationships
• Sexuality and reproduction
• Cultural and religious influences
• Social support
• Emotional health

If you accept your own values but respect another person's right to hold his own views, you can respond therapeutically to your patient, allowing him to express feelings that may be negative without taking the anger personally or acting judgmentally. This is vital to gathering accurate, unbiased information.

Your own health experiences and life encounters can influence the effectiveness of your relationship with your patient.

Reading body language

Effective interviewing skills hinge on picking up nonverbal cues. Throughout the interview, be alert for such nonverbal communication from the patient. Body movements, gestures, touch, and tone of voice convey important messages. Discrepancies between what the patient is saying and the way he's acting may give you important insights.

Be aware that your own nonverbal cues can add to or relieve a patient's anxiety. Your eye movements, posture, and use of touch and space influence your

Asking the right questions

By strengthening your interviewing skills, you can make your patient feel comfortable, respected, and trusting. You can also help him identify resources and improve his problem-solving skills.

Direct your questions
Begin with a question such as "What brought you here today?" This will direct the patient to discuss his most significant concerns. Comments like "What happened next?" foster open communication.

Restate concerns
Repeat the gist of your patient's comments. For example, if he says he takes digoxin twice a day, respond with "I see, once in the morning and once at night." Then if he says, "No, I take it at 8 a.m. and noon," you've opened the door to a patient-teaching opportunity.

Promote introspection
Encourage the patient to think about his answers. For instance, if he says he's told you what he considers important about his meals, such as their timing, ask about the nutritionally significant aspects, such as fat and calorie content.

Explore concerns
Gain additional insights into your patient's concerns by delving into his unspoken meaning. For example, if he complains that the demands of his new job complicate his relationship with his wife, ask how he feels about the amount of time he spends with her.

Stay with the issues
Help your patient identify significant health concerns by sticking to the point. When he tells you his occupation, ask if he's aware of any health hazards connected with that line of work.

Use a logical approach
Place each problem in proper sequence so you can better identify it and draw a conclusion. Ask such questions as "What events led to this?"

Encourage participation
Invite your patient to express his opinions or concerns by asking such questions as "What do you think about the exercise plan we've discussed?" Also ask your patient to comment on implementation strategies. Making him a participant promotes compliance.

Explore nonverbal cues
Ask your patient about significant nonverbal behavior, which could lead to new areas for discussion. For instance, by saying "I see you're rubbing your eyes a lot. Do they bother you?" you could uncover problems with allergies, vision, or insomnia.

interactions, especially during an initial interview, so be sure to convey your interest and concern about your patient's problems.

Using silence

Talking with another person involves silence as well as speech. Learn how and when to be silent during the interview. Listen carefully to what the patient says in response to your questions, and make eye contact with him as much as possible. Don't rush him or attempt to figure out what he's going to say before he says it. If you're thinking of your next question while the patient is speaking, you may need to ask him to repeat himself, giving him the impression that what he's saying isn't worthwhile.

Sometimes accepting a few moments of silence until the patient feels like talking again can be therapeutic. He may just not be a talkative person. Or his lapse into silence may indicate that he's thinking carefully about how to answer your question. Give him time.

Demonstrating acceptance

For the interview to succeed, you'll need to demonstrate acceptance of your patient's verbal and nonverbal communication. But this doesn't mean you must agree with him—only that you should remain neutral and nonjudgmental. You can do this verbally by saying "I see" or "Okay" as the patient speaks. Or you can do it nonverbally by nodding or making eye contact. These techniques reassure the patient without showing agreement or disagreement on your part.

Staying calm

The same nonthreatening techniques can help you handle a hostile or angry patient. By not arguing or acting insulted, you can keep control of the interview. Instead, show that you accept his emotional response as an expression of important feelings. Then try to help him figure out why he's angry. Anxiety, frustration, and helplessness are the most common causes.

Speak in a firm, quiet voice and use short sentences. If you stay composed, unobtrusive, and nonthreatening, your manner will probably soothe your patient. If you can't stay calm, postpone the interview and call for help if needed.

If the patient appears very nervous, first make sure that his awareness of your own nervousness isn't the cause. Then, with a reassuring approach, ask why he seems anxious. Knowing the cause will help you determine how to put the patient at ease.

Appreciating cultural diversity

Your patient's cultural and ethnic background can affect the health history interview in ways that are both subtle and complex. To understand this effect, consider the difference between culture and ethnicity.

Culture refers to an integrated system of learned behavior patterns that are typical of members of a society but are not biologically inherited. Ethnicity refers to membership in a group of people classified according to a common racial, national, religious, linguistic, or cultural origin or background.

Understanding the effect

Both culture and ethnicity affect beliefs, values, attitudes, and customs. They also help shape educational, occupational, and familial expectations. Culture also affects the way a person experiences health and illness.

The degree of these effects depends on whether the patient has undergone acculturation (modification caused by contact with another culture) or assimilation (loss of cultural identity when an individual becomes part of a different, dominant culture).

To communicate effectively with a patient from a different cultural group, never assume that he understands English well enough to comprehend all interview questions or medical terms. Speak clearly and carefully, avoiding jargon.

Learn the cultural practices and health beliefs of your patient's ethnic group so that you don't inadvertently offend him. For example, although a gentle touch usually conveys warmth, concern, and reassurance, some people interpret this form of nonverbal communication differently.

Recognizing your biases

Try to avoid assuming that your own culture is superior and judging others by your cultural standards. Instead, develop an attitude that acknowledges others' cultural standards, and judge a patient's actions by his own cultural standards. Above all, don't stereotype a patient based on your idea of his cultural background. Instead, respect the cultural factors and individual differences that have influenced the patient's habits, beliefs, and attitudes about health care. Concentrate on developing the patient's trust in and rapport with you.

❖

Avoiding interview pitfalls

Some interviewing techniques create communication problems between you and your patient. (See *Communication do's and don'ts*.) Here are techniques to avoid.

Asking "why" or "how" questions

Your patient could perceive a question that begins with "why" or "how" as a threat or a challenge because it forces him to justify feelings and thoughts. Some patients invent an answer if they don't have one. "Why" questions may also be difficult for patients who lack specific knowledge or are unaware of a crucial fact. For example, if a patient says he feels awful, don't ask why. A better response would be simple acknowledgment or a question such as "What do you think is making you feel awful?"

Being too persistent

Excessive persistence in asking a particular question usually increases patient discomfort, creates defensive feelings, and makes the patient feel manipulated. Try once or twice to ob-

Communication do's and don'ts

During your first interview — and in later conversations with the patient — effective communication is essential. To gain accurate information from a patient, listen to what he has to say and respond appropriately. Below are some communication techniques that will help you learn more about the patient and avoid inappropriate responses.

TECHNIQUE	PURPOSE OR EFFECT	EXAMPLE
Do's		
Using open-ended questions	Allows the patient to clarify and elaborate on his thoughts	PATIENT: I haven't felt comfortable since I went on this new treatment schedule. NURSE: How is your new treatment affecting you?
Using closed-ended questions	Directs the patient to provide specific information	PATIENT: I had a battery of tests done at my last doctor's appointment. NURSE: When was your last doctor's appointment?
Restating	Clarifies meaning for you and the patient	PATIENT: The day after New Year's, I went in for tests, and they found the cause of my stomach pain right away. I took my medication very carefully, but I had to go back to the hospital again last month because the gastritis had started up again. NURSE: So this is your third visit this year? You were admitted in January and again in May, each time for gastritis?

(continued)

Communication do's and don'ts *(continued)*

TECHNIQUE	PURPOSE OR EFFECT	EXAMPLE
Do's *(continued)*		
Communicating support (empathy)	Encourages the patient to continue his thoughts and shows your concern	PATIENT: My folks have gone out of their way recently to care for me, and I'm grateful to them. But I find myself thinking back to just a month ago when I was all on my own. NURSE: It must be hard to rely on your parents after being independent for so long.
Reflecting (echoing)	Allows the patient to evaluate his thoughts and feelings through your restatement of them	PATIENT: I don't know. My family is so upset by my illness that I guess I've tried to ignore other treatment possibilities. NURSE: So your family has been so upset by your illness that you haven't explored other treatments.
Using silence	Allows the patient to collect his thoughts and to reflect on the conversation	PATIENT: I guess what it comes down to is that I felt too guilty about being a burden. NURSE: (Remains silent)
Don'ts		
Changing the topic	Makes the patient think you don't care or aren't listening	PATIENT: I think I'm doing all right today. NURSE: What time does your doctor usually come in?
Giving false reassurances	Misleads the patient	PATIENT: I'm afraid the test results will be bad news. NURSE: Oh, I bet they'll be fine.

Communication do's and don'ts *(continued)*

TECHNIQUE	PURPOSE OR EFFECT	EXAMPLE
Don'ts *(continued)*		
Interrupting	Forces the patient to reinitiate the conversation	PATIENT: You know, the thing I've been— NURSE: Would you hold your arm straight, please?
Making assumptions	Fails to clarify and creates confusion	PATIENT: I haven't felt this way for days. NURSE: I know what you mean.
Trivializing feelings	Ignores the patient's feelings	PATIENT: I'm not sure I'm doing the right thing, asking my sister to come here. NURSE: Well, you know what they say: 'Nothing ventured, nothing gained.'
Giving advice	Makes the patient more dependent	PATIENT: How do you think I should explain this to my children? NURSE: Tell them the truth.
Being defensive	Interferes with getting at the root of the problem	PATIENT: This hospital isn't very clean. NURSE: It's as clean as any hospital you'll find.

tain information about a particular topic, and then move on.

Using jargon

Don't use technical jargon or medical terms that your patient might not understand. He could see this as an unwillingness to share information or an attempt to hide something from him.

Giving advice

Refrain from sharing personal experiences and giving opinions or advice. Seeming to know what's best for your patient blocks the chance to collaborate with and encourage him to participate in health care decisions.

Giving false reassurance

Don't try to reassure your patient with comments such as "Everything will be fine." You only devalue his feelings and impart a lack of sensitivity. If you're unable to help your patient, avoid offering false reassurances to make yourself feel better.

Changing the subject or interrupting

Both of these tactics keep your patient from completing a thought, shift the conversation's focus, and convey a lack of empathy. They may also confuse your patient. Wait until he finishes speaking before you clarify a point.

Asking leading questions

By its phrasing, a leading question suggests the "right" answer. This type of question may force your patient to supply a socially acceptable response rather than an honest one. For example, the question "You've never had a venereal disease, have you?" may prompt him to answer "No." ❖

Creating a conducive setting

The interview's setting, its components, and the way you question the patient can all affect the course of the interview. To be an effective interviewer, you'll have to fit your communication style to each patient and create a mood that encourages the patient to share the information you need to know.

Creating a comfortable environment

Both you and the patient must be comfortable to communicate with each other effectively. Make an effort to create a private environment for your talk. A private room with the door closed will help you avoid interruptions. If the patient is in a semiprivate room but ambulatory, you can take him to a quiet area outside the room. If he isn't ambulatory but his roommate is, you might ask the roommate to leave you alone with the patient for the length of time you need for the interview. If you can't achieve privacy with your patient in or outside of his room, draw the curtains around the bed and speak in a low tone to convey respect for his privacy.

Make sure you and the patient agree on the temperature and lighting in the room. If the room is too warm or too cool, ask the patient's permission to adjust the temperature, if possible, or provide the patient with extra blankets or ventilation as necessary. If the room is too dark, you may have trouble maintaining eye contact with your patient and observing his gestures and facial expressions. If the room is too bright or glare from a window is distracting, the patient may be too uncomfortable to provide a good history. Before changing the lighting, ask for the patient's permission. He may want the room dark because he has a headache or irritated eyes or because he feels depressed.

By creating a comfortable, private, and quiet environment for the health history interview, you let your patient know that you're interested in what he tells you and that you respect the confidentiality of the information he shares with you.

Setting the proper mood

In addition to providing comfortable surroundings, you should create a pleasant mood that puts your patient at ease. Speaking in a moderate tone and maintaining a calm, unhurried manner will help you achieve this goal.

Accommodate your methods to your patient's needs. For example, sit facing your patient to foster a friendly feeling and to facilitate eye contact and hearing.

If your patient is a child, stoop to his level or sit in a low chair. If your patient is accompanied by small children, provide toys and books to occupy the children during the interview.

If your patient is confined to bed, reduce any feelings of intimidation or powerlessness by sitting in a bedside chair rather than standing. If an elderly patient seems to have difficulty hearing the questions, move closer so that he can see your facial expressions and lip movements. Also, speak louder, more slowly, and in a lower pitch.

Timing the interview

The health history interview should take 45 to 60 minutes. However, you might have to spend additional time with some patients, such as an elderly patient with an extensive health history. You can also obtain a history in stages while performing other tasks, such as patient baths or dressing changes.

To avoid tiring a patient who is seriously ill, plan to take the

When to shorten the interview

A patient who is acutely ill, in pain, or sedated may have difficulty providing the information you need for a complete health history. Start by eliciting essential information pertaining to the patient's immediate problem, and ask questions that minimize his requirement to respond. Pause now and then to give the patient a rest. Obtain noncritical parts of the history in subsequent interviews.

history in several sessions. Or ask the patient if a relative or close friend can supply essential information. (See *When to shorten the interview*.) If your patient is acutely ill, collect pertinent medical information first. Do the less urgent phases of the interview last, or wait until the patient feels better.

Other ways to make the most of your interview time include asking the patient to complete a written form before the interview. Then, during the interview, you can focus on the most significant information. In addition, some of the information you need can come from other sources, such as admission forms or the medical history. Not only does this shorten the interview time, but it also helps avoid duplication of effort.

Above all, don't appear rushed or preoccupied, because this will work against the trust and rapport you're trying to build with your patient.

Structuring the interview

Your interview will have a mood-setting introductory phase, a data-gathering phase, and a summary (or wrap-up) phase.

Begin by introducing yourself to the patient and explaining that you need to take a history to identify his problem and formulate a plan of care best suited to his needs. Address the patient respectfully, using "Mr.," "Mrs.," or "Ms." and the patient's surname. Don't use the patient's first name until he gives you permission to do so.

Explain the interview's goal to help allay the patient's fears and avoid any misconceptions. You should also discuss the duration of the first interview; the time, place, and duration of any subsequent visits; and the number of visits that will be required. Ask the patient about his expectations, and assure him of the confidentiality of all information. (See *Starting off right.*)

Phrasing your questions

Straightforward questioning usually succeeds in eliciting most of the information you need about your patient's past and present health status. At times, however, you'll want to examine a response further or explore your patient's concerns about his condition, which can call for more subtle interviewing skills. Using both open-ended and closed-ended questions can help you meet your goals.

Asking open-ended questions lets the patient explain the problem in his own words. This usually provides the most useful information in terms of quantity and quality. Also, open-ended questions give the patient the feeling that he's actively participating in the interview and has some control over it. (See *Using open-ended questions,* page 14.)

Asking closed-ended questions, which require only a yes or no response, can be useful at certain times and for certain types of information. Such questions are useful when you need information quickly—for example, when a patient reports severe pain. They're also appropriate for confirming biographical information and for refocusing a patient who tends to digress. However, closed-ended questions may affect the patient's word choice, discourage him from elaborating on a reply, and prevent you from obtaining valuable information.

Benefits of the health history

Taking a comprehensive health history helps you plan individualized, patient-centered care. You'll discover what you need to teach the patient and whether he has any health-related beliefs that may hinder compliance with treatment. Also, what you learn about his family and social support systems can help focus your discharge planning—an important consideration because of the trend toward shorter hospital stays.

Contributing to the success of your care planning is the care you take during the interview itself. Your personal interaction with the patient can help him see the health care facility as a less impersonal place and promote his compliance with the treatment regimen.

Starting off right

The following sample dialogue shows how to set the proper mood at the outset of the interview, clarify the interview goals, establish a time frame, and make a verbal contract. Experience will show you the communication style that works best for you and how to adapt it to each patient's needs.

NURSE: Good morning, Mrs. Gregg. My name is Barbara Janka. I'm a registered nurse, and I'd like to spend about an hour with you this morning to obtain a comprehensive nursing history. Let's sit down and I'll explain what that means.
PATIENT: Okay.
NURSE: Would you like something to drink before we start? Coffee, tea, or juice?
PATIENT: No, thanks. I just had lunch.
NURSE: I hope this isn't an inconvenient appointment time. Did you have to rush to get here?
PATIENT: A little bit – the bus was late.

NURSE: Would you like to rest a few minutes?
PATIENT: No, thanks. I'm fine.
NURSE: Then let's get started. The health history has several parts. The first is about your current and past health and the history of illness in your family. The next is about your daily lifestyle, your family, and your job; and the last is about diet and exercise.
PATIENT: No one ever asked me all that before.
NURSE: We'll use this information to understand you better so that we can provide better care. This is the only time we ask you all these questions, and some of them are personal, but all of the information is confidential. The information becomes part of your permanent record, which is seen only by other health care professionals. It can't be given to anyone else without your written permission. Feel free to tell me if there's a question you don't want to answer.

Data collection

After verifying biographical data, you'll begin your history taking with an exploration of the patient's chief complaint or concern. Then you'll cover his medical history, family history, psychosocial history, and activities of daily living. The personal information you uncover about the patient – such as his cultural background, his religious beliefs, and his socioeconomic standing – can significantly influence his health and the way he perceives health care. A thorough

Using open-ended questions

Review the following examples of closed- and open-ended questions. Note how closed-ended questions suggest a yes or no response and can limit the scope and accuracy of your evaluation. But open-ended questions encourage a detailed response.

CLOSED-ENDED QUESTIONS	OPEN-ENDED QUESTIONS
Are you physically active during the day?	What sort of activities do you perform during a typical day?
Do you have episodes of pain during the day?	What type of activity makes the pain start?
Do you eat a lot of foods that are high in cholesterol?	Tell me about your eating patterns. When do you usually eat and what sorts of foods do you usually have?
Do you shovel snow?	How often do you shovel snow in the winter?
Have you quit smoking?	How much are you smoking now? When do you usually smoke?
Do you know how you got this disease?	What do you know about your disease?
Do you know how to give yourself an insulin injection?	Would you show me how you give yourself an insulin injection?

history may also uncover overlooked medical or social problems. If your patient is a child or an elderly person, you'll need to make some slight modifications when taking the health history. Naturally, the more complete you can make the history, the better you'll be able to understand your patient's health problems.

Conducting a thorough interview

Begin your data collection by determining your patient's current health status. (See *Guarding against disease.*)

Current health
Ask your patient why he's seeking health care. Then record his exact words, using quotation marks.

PREVENTIVE PRACTICE

 Guarding against disease

When asking about the patient's current health status, be sure to find out whether he has any communicable disease, such as herpes, hepatitis B, or acquired immunodeficiency syndrome. This information will alert you to follow the necessary precautions.

A patient may not have a chief complaint; he may be feeling fine and simply seeking a complete physical checkup. If so, ask if he has any particular health needs or issues he wants to discuss, and record his response. Then proceed with a comprehensive history.

If the patient has specific symptoms, record that information in his words—for example, "I've had a headache for 3 days." Then explore the symptom's history in detail.

Ask the patient to describe the symptom, including how and when it developed and any suspected cause. (See *Tips for analyzing symptoms*, pages 16 and 17.) The patient's response may help you assess his ability to cope with illness.

If the patient's chief complaint relates to his work, record occupational information, such as length of time on the job, number of hours worked, and job responsibilities and satisfaction. Ask, too, about health hazards at the workplace, such as exposure to chemicals, heavy metals, or excessive dust or noise levels.

Health history
Questions about the patient's health history provide you with information about his previous major health problems, his experiences with the health care system, and his attitude toward it. They also usually yield important clues about his present condition, help determine the treatment plan, and suggest his prognosis.

Ask your patient about childhood and infectious diseases, especially those with sequelae. For example, if the patient reports having had rheumatic fever, determine his age when he contracted it, whether he was diagnosed by a doctor, and whether he's now taking prophylactic drugs. Ask about immunizations, especially for poliomyelitis and rubella, which can affect unvaccinated adults. Also ask about foreign travel and military service to uncover recent immunizations and assess potential exposure to such health hazards as malaria or parasitic infections.

Ask about the patient's history of accidents, specifically childhood fractures. A good way to elicit this information is to ask the patient if he was ever treated in an emergency department. Continue with questions about past surgical procedures

Tips for analyzing symptoms

When assessing a patient with a symptom or health concern, use a symptom analysis to help him describe the problem fully. A method for obtaining a systematic and thorough assessment, the symptom analysis is easy to remember with the mnemonic device PQRST. Use the questions that follow as a guide to effective symptom analysis.

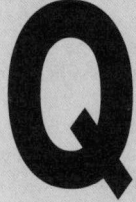

Provocative or palliative
What causes the symptom? What makes it better or worse?
• What were you doing when you first experienced or noticed the symptom? What seems to trigger it: stress? Certain positions or activities? What makes the symptom worse? What relieves it?

Quality or quantity
How does the symptom feel, look, or sound? How much of it are you experiencing now?
• How would you describe the symptom? How does it feel, look, or sound?
• How severe is the symptom now? Is it so severe that it prevents you from performing any activities? Is it more or less severe than at any other time?

and hospitalizations, because his current illness may relate to a previous illness. Include mention of common procedures such as tonsillectomy and appendectomy. Record the information chronologically, listing events by date or by the patient's age at the time.

Ask the patient about any allergies to foods, medications, substances such as soap, and textiles. Specifically cite allergies to antibiotics, such as penicillin, and to sulfa drugs.

Ask which medications he's currently taking—over-the-counter as well as prescription drugs, and especially aspirin, laxatives, antacids, vitamins, and cold remedies. Find out his reasons for taking them and any reactions he's had to them. This may alert you to possible drug interactions, help you distinguish drug adverse effects from allergies and toxic reactions, and identify teaching opportunities. Also find out if the patient uses any recreational drugs.

R

Region or radiation?
Where is the symptom located? Does it spread?
• Where does the symptom occur?
• Does it travel down your back or arms, up your neck, or down your legs?

S

Severity scale
How does the symptom rate on a severity scale of 1 to 10, with 10 being the most extreme?
• Does the symptom force you to lie down, sit down, or slow down?
• Does it seem to be getting better, getting worse, or staying about the same?

T

Timing
When did the symptom begin? How often does it occur? Does it develop suddenly or gradually?
• On what date did the symptom first occur?
• Did the symptom start suddenly or gradually?
• How often do you experience the symptom: hourly? Daily? Weekly? Monthly? Seasonally? When do you usually experience it: during the day? At night? In the early morning? Does it awaken you? Does it occur before, during, or after meals?
• How long does an episode last?

Specifically, assess tobacco and alcohol use. Because caffeine may harm the cardiovascular and other systems, ask the patient how many caffeine-containing products (coffee, tea, cola, chocolate) he consumes regularly and how long he's been consuming them. Ask if he notices any caffeine-related physiologic effects, such as palpitations, nervousness, or sleeplessness.

Finally, assess the patient's diet and elimination habits, exercise and recreational activities, and sleep and rest patterns.

Family health history

A brief description of the medical history of the patient's family helps to identify hereditary patterns common to some illnesses. Ask your patient if anyone in his family had allergies, asthma, tuberculosis, hypertension, heart disease, or a stroke. Inquire about anemia, hemophilia, arthritis, migraine headaches, diabetes, cancer, and emotional problems.

As in the section of the history dealing with current and past health, record negative findings as well as positive ones.

Psychosocial history

To formulate an effective nursing diagnosis, you often have to evaluate the patient in terms of his place in society, relationships with others, and satisfaction with himself. Assessing the patient's family ties can provide insight into family stressors, coping mechanisms, and values and beliefs about health care. A patient's family may be a source of strength and support or a source of stress, which may underlie the chief complaint.

To establish how family members interact, ask the patient how family members treat each other. How do they handle one another's needs and wants? Can family members openly express both positive and negative feelings? When family members disagree, how do they handle conflict?

To gain information about family responsibilities and role flexibility, which may help in planning the patient's discharge, ask what the family roles are and who performs each role. If the patient has children, who is responsible for their care? Are family roles negotiable within the limits of age and ability? Does the patient share cultural values and beliefs with his children?

Determine who performs the health care function in the family so that you can use this information when planning care. Ask the patient who takes care of sick family members. Who makes the doctor's appointments? How does the family adjust when a member is sick?

To assess how well the family will be able to meet the patient's needs, ask how far away extended family members live and how important they are to the patient as sources of physical, emotional, and economic support. Find out who makes up the immediate family and if anyone other than the immediate family lives with him. Does the patient have friends whom he considers part of his family?

Because financial problems often lead to family conflict, ask questions to determine financial concerns and how money issues relate to power roles within the family. Does family income meet the family's basic needs? Who makes the decisions about money allocation? Are family and individual needs considered when money is being allocated?

Cultural background

A patient's culture or ethnic group can profoundly affect his health beliefs and expectations, dietary and other health habits, and family roles and dynamics. For example, patients from cultures that consider illness a fate to be accepted or a punishment for some wrongdoing may resist seeking health care or taking responsibility for changing behaviors that cause health problems because they feel powerless to control their illness. Assessing cultural influences will help you evaluate these health-related factors and identify culture-related strengths such as a strong family unit.

To learn how culture and ethnicity affect a patient, begin by identifying his cultural group and asking how closely he associates with that group. Find out how his lifestyle or belief system resembles or differs from that of most people in his ethnic group.

To evaluate the cultural impact on health promotion and protection patterns, ask the patient what types of food he usually eats. Ask if his family follows any special nutritional practices or dietary restrictions, especially during illness. In your assessment of his cultural role and relationship patterns, determine which aspects could be vital to his health. For example, a fatalistic view of illness may make family members feel incapable of learning to care for the patient, a complicating factor in discharge planning.

Throughout the cultural assessment, also note any beliefs or practices that may affect the patient's health, such as whether pain is openly expressed or never voiced.

Spiritual influences

A patient may consider his religious or spiritual beliefs to be the central aspect of his life.

Spirituality is a person's definition of the purpose and meaning of his life, the world, and the cosmos. It may guide his daily behavior, lifestyle, and community activities, and it may define his attitude toward death. It may also define acceptable health care.

Religion is the component of spirituality that includes a belief in a divine power or being. It usually includes more specific beliefs, including codified and prescribed behaviors, rituals, or practices that express the person's faith in those beliefs.

A patient's health beliefs and practices may be linked closely to his religion. For example, for Muslims, Hindus, and Buddhists, self-disclosure is difficult, a factor that may complicate your history taking. A Jehovah's Witness may refuse to accept blood transfusions or blood products for himself or family members, even if the situation is life-threatening. A Jewish patient may want a mohel (ritual circumciser) rather than an obstetrician to perform infant circumcision, a religious rite.

In some religions, such as Roman Catholicism, family members may insist on having the patient receive the Sacrament of the Sick (annointing the critically ill or injured). Many religions also require baptism of a sick infant.

Religious beliefs may also affect how comfortable your patient feels completing certain parts of the health history, such as questions about his family life, sexuality, or elimination patterns. By recognizing such sensitivities, you can modify your questions to promote patient cooperation.

————————————— ❖

Interviewing patients with special needs

Your standard health history format should work with little modification for most patients. But you might want to adapt it somewhat for a pediatric, elderly, or disabled patient. The guidelines that follow will help you do just that.

Interviewing pediatric patients

In taking a pediatric health history, the child's age and personality should influence the way you phrase your questions as well as the information you expect to obtain. Substitute questions about school for occupational questions. Assess safety hazards by focusing on parent and staff efforts to prevent accidents.

In exploring the child's family role and relationships, concentrate on interactions with parents, siblings, and peers. Ask the parents to describe the child's temperament and ability to get along with siblings and peers, the activities the child performs well, any behavioral problems, and the disciplinary measures that the parents use.

If the parents cannot describe many positive aspects about the child or indicate that the child is aggressive, withdrawn, or having school problems, perform an in-depth assessment of the family relationship patterns.

Address the child

In most cases, you'll obtain information about a child's present health from one of his parents, another relative, or a guardian. When a parent is present, take advantage of the opportunity to observe parent-child interactions. However, don't direct all of your questions to the adult. Even a young child can discuss symptoms and confirm the information a parent is giving you. An older child can participate more fully. As much as possible, get the information directly from the child, rather than talking to others about him in his presence.

The way you approach a child and phrase your questions can determine the success of the interview. Avoid a condescending manner; a child can sense this easily.

Young children

When interviewing a young child, base your questions on his developmental age so that he can understand and answer them. Obviously, a child who hasn't mastered language skills can't describe his problem in detail, if at all. But you can ask him to *draw* how he feels.

Place yourself physically at the child's level by sitting or stooping to his eye level.

Adolescents

An adolescent may not wish to have a parent present during the interview for reasons of privacy. Also, you may want to ask questions about sexual development; in this situation, a parent's presence might inhibit your patient's responses.

Be particularly sensitive to an adolescent's request for confidentiality. If you must share an adolescent's history information with a parent, obtain the patient's permission first.

Interviewing elderly patients

When interviewing an elderly patient, make sure you avoid stereotypical misconceptions that may interfere with your interaction. For example, not all elderly people are frail, slow moving, confused, and sensory impaired. Many lead active, healthy, and productive lives.

Modify the health history interview for an elderly person

only if he shows age-related cognitive or sensory impairment or a specific physiologic problem, such as aphasia from a cerebrovascular accident. Be alert for common age-related visual difficulties, and stand or sit where the patient can see you as you speak to him. Speak clearly, distinctly, and slowly, in a well-modulated voice. If the patient has difficulty hearing you, you might consider turning your stethoscope around, placing the earpieces in the patient's ears, and talking into the diaphragm. If the patient has an extensive medical history and difficulty relating it chronologically, you might ask if he had a particular illness, injury, or operation before or after a life milestone, such as his 80th birthday or the birth of a grandchild.

Otherwise, focus the history on the same areas you would for any adult—but place special emphasis on use of medications, including over-the-counter drugs. In many cases, an elderly patient's chief complaint may result from noncompliance with a prescribed medication regimen, a drug interaction, or an overdose of medication, such as digitalis glycosides or antiarrhythmic drugs.

When exploring the chief complaint, be aware that your patient may hesitate to report symptoms because he attributes them to "old age" and feels that nothing can be done to ease them. The patient also may have adjusted to gradual changes and thus simply may not have noticed his symptoms.

If your patient tires easily or cannot concentrate, try scheduling two or more sessions to complete a comprehensive history. If he appears confused, skip over most assessment areas and concentrate on specific, current symptoms (pain, nausea, depression, or impaired sight). Ask a relative or close friend of the patient to supply missing information.

Focusing on current ills

Because of advanced age, an elderly patient is more likely to have chronic illnesses causing various symptoms and requiring several medications. Therefore, focus on current problems instead of past ones. Asking an elderly patient about childhood immunizations or childbirth experiences isn't necessary.

Also, if possible, ask the patient to bring in all medications he's taking and a dated list of hospitalizations to speed the history taking and clarify or verify information.

Assessing lifestyle

To assess support systems and coping mechanisms, you'll want to evaluate the elderly patient's role and relationship patterns. You'll also want to analyze health behaviors, safety precautions, and self-image.

For example, how is the patient dealing with changes in physical appearance or in the ability to perform activities of daily living? Ask him to describe a typical day at home, including activities, sleep patterns, and eating habits. Because questions about food may suggest other significant lines of questioning, find out how much of an appetite he usually has, how he prepares his food (including how much salt he uses), and how much fluid he normally consumes. Can he move around at home easily and safely? Can he supply his basic needs—food, clothing, and shelter? Does he drive to the supermarket, ride with a friend or relative, or use public transportation? Ask if he expects to be able to continue his routine after being discharged from the hospital.

Interviewing patients with disabilities

Any modifications you make in the health history interview for a patient with a disability depends on the individual patient and the impairment. Take your lead from the patient. If he seems comfortable, continue with the interview. However, if you pick up verbal or nonverbal cues that something is making the patient feel stressed, adapt the interview to fit the patient.

Visually impaired patients
You'll need to orient a visually impaired patient to his surroundings. During the interview, remember to respond to him by speaking rather than gesturing or nodding.

Hearing-impaired patients
If the patient is severely hearing impaired or mute, use a written health history questionnaire. After he completes the questionnaire, concentrate on the identified problem areas. Write down any additional questions you have, and pass notes back and forth with the patient.

If the patient has severe hearing and vision impairments, ask him to bring a relative or friend to help with the interview. You might also want to request the services of a sign language interpreter.

Patients with other disabilities
For a patient who is physically disabled, you don't need to modify the health history format unless he can't tolerate the length of time required to complete the history.

For a patient with a mild or moderate intellectual impairment, use simple phrases and schedule brief sessions to accommodate a short attention span.

For a severely impaired or intellectually disabled patient, you'll probably need a close relative or friend to provide information.

2 Assessing Ominous Signs and Symptoms

Systemic sign

A common sign, fever arises from disorders that affect virtually every body system. Alone, it has little diagnostic significance. However, a persistently high fever is a medical emergency.

Fever

An elevation of body temperature above 98.6° F (37° C), fever (or pyrexia) is classified as low (an oral reading of 99° to 100.4° F [37.2° to 38° C]), moderate (100.5° to 104° F [38° to 40° C]), or high (above 104° F). Fever above 108° F (42.2° C) causes unconsciousness and, if prolonged, brain damage.

Fever can also be classified as intermittent or sustained. Intermittent fever, the most common type, refers to the daily fluctuations between normal and above-normal temperatures. Sustained fever refers to a persistent elevation with little fluctuation.

History

Explore your patient's problem by asking appropriate questions.
• When did the fever begin? How high did it reach?
• Is the fever constant, or does it disappear and then reappear later?
• Does the patient also have chills, fatigue, or pain?
• Has he had any immunodeficiency disorders or treatments, infections, recent trauma or surgery, or diagnostic tests? Has he traveled recently?
• Has the patient been overexposed to environmental extremes, such as to very hot weather?
• Which medications is he taking? Has he recently had anesthesia?

Physical examination

Use your history findings to determine the extent of the physical examination. Because fever can accompany many disorders, your physical examination may include a brief evaluation of one body system or a comprehensive review of all systems.

Causes

Your assessment may lead you to suspect one of the conditions or causes that follow.

Infectious and inflammatory disorders

Fever may be low, as in Crohn's disease and ulcerative colitis, or extremely high, as in bacterial pneumonia. It may be remittent, as in infectious mononucleosis; sustained, as in meningitis; or relapsing, as in malaria. Fever may arise abruptly, as in Rocky Mountain spotted fever, or insidiously, as in mycoplasmal pneumonia. Typically, it accompanies a self-limiting disorder such as the common cold.

Medications

Fever and rash often result from hypersensitivity to quinidine, methyldopa, procainamide hydrochloride, phenytoin, anti-infectives, barbiturates, iodides, and some antitoxins. Fever can also result from the use of chemotherapeutic agents and medications that decrease sweating, such as anticholinergics. Plus, toxic doses of salicylates, amphetamines, and tricyclic antidepressants can cause fever.

Other causes
Fever may result from dehydration, an injection of contrast medium used in diagnostic tests, surgery, and blood transfusion reactions.

———————————————❖

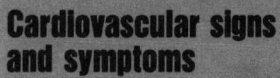

Cardiovascular signs and symptoms

To perform swift, accurate cardiovascular assessments, you must be able to distinguish normal from abnormal heart sounds, rates, and rhythms. Because some signs and symptoms such as bradycardia are nonspecific and others such as chest pain have both benign and life-threatening causes, you must also be able to interpret them in light of the patient's other complaints.

Abnormal heart sounds

The abnormalities you hear during auscultation are among the most significant signs of cardiovascular disease. Be prepared to recognize and interpret them. If you don't do cardiac assessment regularly, periodically review your knowledge of normal heart structure and function.

Two sets of valves—the atrioventricular and the semilunar valves—connect the four chambers of the heart. The atrioventricular valves are the mitral valve (between the left atrium and left ventricle) and the tricuspid valve (between the right atrium and the right ventricle). The semilunar valves are the aortic and pulmonic valves. The aortic valve connects the left ventricle to the aorta; the pulmonic valve connects the right ventricle to the pulmonary artery.

Each time these valves close during the normal cardiac cycle, they produce vibrations, called heart sounds. You can hear these sounds on auscultation, but you won't hear them directly over the four valves. That's because the vibrations are transmitted away from the valves in the direction of blood flow. (See *Heart sounds: Where to listen*, pages 26 and 27.)

History
Explore your patient's problem by asking appropriate questions.
• Does he have a history of cardiovascular disease, such as cardiomyopathy, or previous valve surgery or bypass surgery? Does he have a history of pulmonary disease, such as pulmonary hypertension?
• Has he had any recent trauma such as an auto accident?
• Does he have a history of rheumatic fever, recent fever, or unexplained illness?
• Were heart murmurs noted on previous physical examinations?
• Has the patient recently undergone dental procedures or GI or genitourinary surgery that may have resulted in endocarditis?
• Does he have a recent history of chest pain, which might indi-

(Text continues on page 28.)

Heart sounds: Where to listen

To hear heart sounds best, auscultate at these four cardiac "listening posts" (see the illustration below):
• *mitral valve (M):* fifth intercostal space (ICS) on the midclavicular line

• *tricuspid valve (T):* fourth or fifth ICS at the left sternal border (LSB)
• *aortic valve (A):* second ICS at the right sternal border
• *pulmonic valve (P):* second or third ICS at the LSB.

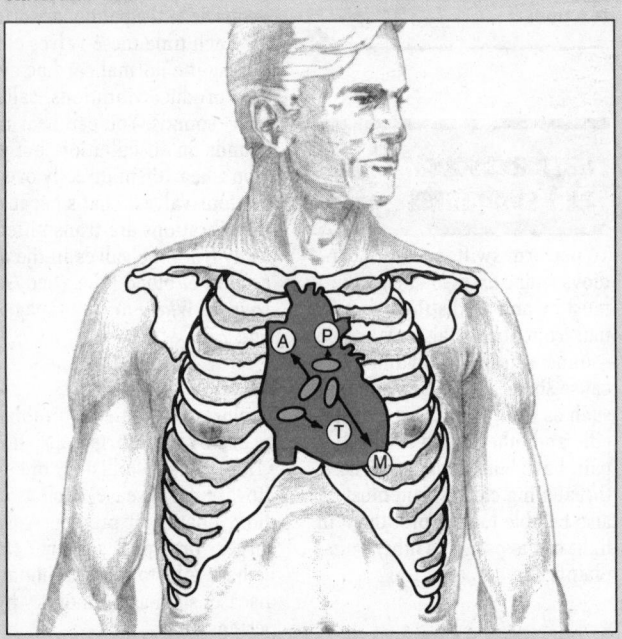

What you hear

The cardiac cycle consists of two phases—diastole (or relaxation) and systole (or contraction). After blood is ejected into the aorta and pulmonary artery, ventricular pressure falls below the aortic and pulmonary artery pressures. This drop in pressure causes the aortic and pulmonic valves to close, and diastole begins. At this point, ventricular pressure is lower than atrial pressure, causing the mitral and tricuspid valves to open and allowing for ventricular filling. When ventricular volume and pressure exceed atrial pressure, the mitral and tricuspid valves close. Then, pressure begins building in the ventricles, causing the aortic and pulmonic valves to open. This is the start of systole.

The closures of the mitral and tricuspid valves produce the heart sound S_1 — commonly referred to as the *lub* of the *lub-dub* sound made by the first of two heart sounds. Because the mitral valve closure is louder than that of the tricuspid, S_1 can be heard best at the mitral valve area (see the illustration below).

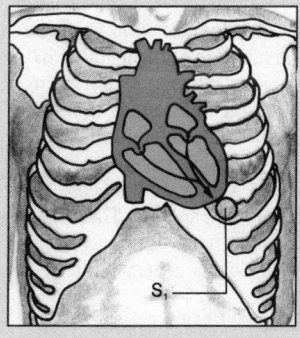

Pressure continues building in the ventricles. When it exceeds the pressure in the aorta and the pulmonary artery, the semilunar valves open and blood is ejected from the ventricles. As the ventricles relax, ventricular pressure falls below the pressure in the aorta and the pulmonary artery. Then the aortic and pulmonic valves snap shut and ventricular diastole begins again. This causes the second heart sound (S_2) — the *dub* of the *lub-dub*. The closure of the aortic valve is

louder than that of the pulmonic, so S_2 is heard best at the aortic valve area (see the illustration below).

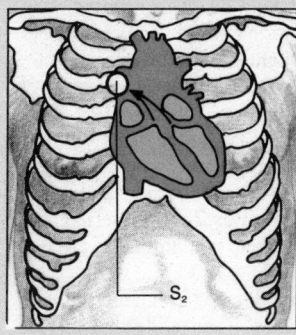

When you listen to heart sounds, you may actually hear a splitting of both S_1 and S_2. That's because events in the left side of the heart occur just before those in the right side. So the mitral valve closes before the tricuspid valve, causing a physiologic splitting of S_1, and the aortic valve closes before the pulmonic valve, producing a similar splitting of S_2.

During diastole, you may also hear two other heart sounds, S_3 and S_4, considered normal variants in children and young adults. A low-pitched sound, S_3 results from early rapid ventricular filling. You'll hear this sound right after S_2 in early diastole. Then, just before S_1, you may hear S_4, which is caused by increased resistance to ventricular filling after atrial contraction.

cate an undetected myocardial infarction (MI) followed by papillary muscle rupture?

Physical examination

Before examining the patient, make sure the room is quiet and well lit. Have the patient lie supine with his chest exposed. Stand to his right (unless you're left-handed) and briefly inspect the chest for general size and symmetry.

Now locate the heart's four "listening posts," corresponding to the atrioventricular and semilunar valves. Use the sternal angle to help you find these areas.

First, palpate the sternal notch, located at the top of the sternum. Then, slide your fingers down to the sternal angle, the elevated ridge two to three fingerbreadths below. When you move your fingers directly to the left of this landmark, you'll feel the second rib. From here, you can count up or down to find other ribs and intercostal spaces and thus locate the four listening posts.

Before auscultating your patient's heart sounds, warm the diaphragm of the stethoscope with your hands. Then place the diaphragm on the mitral valve area and listen to the patient's heart rate and rhythm. Next, concentrate on hearing S_1 and S_2.

Normal heart sounds

At the mitral valve area, S_1 will be louder than S_2; you should expect to hear the *lub* sound more distinctly than the *dub* sound. After you hear S_1 and S_2 at this area, move on to the other three sites. You'll be able to hear the distinctive *dub* sound more easily than the *lub* at the aortic and pulmonic valve areas.

If you have difficulty distinguishing S_1 from S_2, try palpating the carotid pulse as you auscultate. The *lub* sound of S_1 will occur at almost the same time as the beat of the carotid pulse.

Once you've auscultated S_1 and S_2 at all four valve areas, listen for the splittings of S_1 and S_2. Again, start at the mitral valve area, and move on to the tricuspid, aortic, and pulmonic areas. Hearing these splittings of S_1 and S_2 will take more concentration than hearing just S_1 and S_2. A normal split S_1 can be best heard at the tricuspid valve area. The familiar *lub* will sound like a broken syllable. A split S_2, in which the *dub* sounds broken, is best heard at the pulmonic valve area during inspiration. Typically, a split S_2 will be easier to hear than a split S_1. That's because the sound of the tricuspid valve closing is very faint.

Abnormal heart sounds

Abnormal heart sounds you may hear during chest auscultation include three types of pathologic split S_2 sounds, an S_3, an S_4, a summation gallop, pleural and pericardial friction rubs, ejection clicks, and an opening snap. Heart murmurs are covered in the next entry.

Split S_2, S_3, and S_4. There are three types of pathologic split S_2 sounds: wide split, fixed split, and paradoxical split. The *wide split S_2* is heard on both inspiration and expiration, but the split sound is wider on inspiration. The *fixed split S_2* is present during both inspiration and expiration, and the length of the split is equal in both phases. The *paradoxical split S₂* is present on expiration but not on inspiration.

The S₃ sound (known as ventricular gallop) and the S₄ sound (known as atrial gallop) are low pitched. To detect them, have the patient lie supine or on his left side. Then auscultate at the mitral valve area with the bell of your stethoscope. You'll hear S₃ in early diastole, right after you hear the *lub-dub*. It may sound like *lub-dub-dee*. S₄ comes late in diastole or presystole, just before the *lub-dub*.

Summation gallop is the cumulative effect of S₃ and S₄.

Pleural and pericardial friction rubs. Heard best with the diaphragm, friction rubs are high-frequency sounds. Often described as scratchy, squeaky, or leathery, these sustained noises are often mistaken for murmurs.

You'll usually hear pleural friction rub during inspiration; on expiration the sound may be audible or absent.

The sound is easy to reproduce: Press the palm of one hand over your ear and rub the back of it with the fingers of your other hand. The rub is commonly heard in the lower anterolateral chest wall, the most mobile part of the chest. You'll seldom hear it over the lung apices alone. The sound is superficial—unmistakably close to the surface—and decreased respirations will cause it to grow fainter.

To hear pericardial friction rubs, listen for one systolic rub, occurring at any point during systole, and two diastolic sounds. The sound may be mimicked as—*lub-sh-dub-sh-sh—lub-sh-dub-sh-sh*. You may hear it

anywhere on the precordium, but it's usually loudest along the left sternal border (LSB) and heard most often during forced expiration, with the patient leaning forward.

A simple way of distinguishing pleural from pericardial rubs is to have the patient hold his breath. If the rub disappears when the patient holds his breath, it's a pleural rub; if the rub doesn't change, it's pericardial.

Ejection click. A click is a short, high-frequency sound, best heard with the diaphragm firmly pressed against the chest. In aortic stenosis, the click doesn't change with respiration and is best heard at the apex. In pulmonic stenosis, the click is best heard during expiration at the upper LSB. You may hear a single click or multiple clicks.

Opening snap. An opening snap is another short, high-frequency sound. But unlike the click of mitral valve prolapse and an ejection sound, an opening snap occurs during diastole, right after S₂. The sound, usually produced by the opening of a stenotic mitral valve, is heard best with the diaphragm placed between the apex and the LSB. The higher the left atrial pressure, the shorter the interval between S₂ and the opening snap.

Causes
Your assessment may lead you to suspect one of the conditions that follow. (See *Implications of abnormal heart sounds*, pages 30 and 31.)

A wide split S₂ sound indicates pulmonic stenosis or right

Implications of abnormal heart sounds

To find the cause of an abnormal heart sound, make sure you can identify the sound as well as its timing in the cardiac cycle.

ABNORMAL HEART SOUND	TIMING	POSSIBLE CAUSES
Accentuated S_1	Beginning of systole	Mitral stenosis; fever
Diminished S_1	Beginning of systole	Mitral insufficiency; severe mitral insufficiency with calcified immobile valve; heart block
Split S_1	Beginning of systole	Right bundle-branch block
Accentuated S_2	End of systole	Pulmonary or systemic hypertension
Diminished or inaudible S_2	End of systole	Aortic or pulmonic stenosis
Persistent S_2 split	End of systole	Delayed closure of the pulmonic valve, usually from overfilling of the right ventricle, causing prolonged systolic ejection time
Reversed or paradoxical S_2 split that appears in expiration and disappears in inspiration	End of systole	Delayed ventricular stimulation; left bundle-branch block or prolonged left ventricular ejection time
S_3 (ventricular gallop)	Early diastole	Normal in children and young adults; overdistention of ventricles in rapid-filling segment of diastole; mitral insufficiency; pulmonary hypertension; ventricular failure

Implications of abnormal heart sounds *(continued)*

ABNORMAL HEART SOUND	TIMING	POSSIBLE CAUSES
S₄ (atrial gallop or presystolic extra sound)	Late diastole	Forceful atrial contraction from resistance to ventricular filling late in diastole; left ventricular hypertrophy, pulmonic stenosis, hypertension, coronary artery disease, and aortic stenosis
Pericardial friction rub (grating or leathery sound at left sternal border; usually muffled, high pitched, and transient)	Throughout systole and diastole	Pericardial inflammation

bundle-branch block. The fixed split S₂ sound may be caused by atrial septal defects and right ventricular failure. Intensity of the split S₂ provides key diagnostic information. A louder aortic component of the split may indicate systemic hypertension or aortic dilation. A softer aortic component may signal aortic stenosis. A louder pulmonary component may be associated with pulmonary hypertension, but it may also be normal in a patient with a thin chest wall. A softer pulmonary component suggests pulmonic stenosis.

The S₃, or ventricular gallop, results from vibrations during ventricular filling with abnormal left ventricular filling pressure and signals congestive heart failure or cardiomyopathy. Movements that increase venous return may strengthen S₃. The sound usually disappears when the rapid-filling disorder resolves.

S₃ may also be associated with acute MI, pulmonary edema, ventricular or atrial septal defect, and either mitral or aortic insufficiency.

S₄, or atrial gallop, may be a sign of cardiovascular problems, such as hypertension, aortic stenosis, mitral insufficiency, acute MI, systemic or pulmonary hypertension, and coronary artery disease.

Summation gallop may be audible in adult patients with severe myocardial disease and tachycardia.

Pleural friction rubs indicate pleural inflammation, which may result from pneumonia, viral infection, tuberculosis, cardiac surgery, or pulmonary embolism. Pericardial friction rubs indicate pericardial inflammation, which may result from MI, pericarditis, or uremia.

Ejection click is often associated with stenotic aortic or pulmonic valves. The sound may also be produced as a result of hypertension and a dilated aorta or pulmonary artery.

Bradycardia

A heart rate that is less than 60 beats/minute, bradycardia may occur normally in young adults, athletes, and elderly people. It's also a normal response to vagal stimulation triggered by coughing, vomiting, or straining during a bowel movement. In such cases, the heart rate rarely falls below 40 beats/minute. But when bradycardia results from a pathologic cause—a cardiovascular disorder, for example—the heart rate may plummet to below 40 beats/minute.

By itself, bradycardia is nonspecific. When accompanied by chest pain, hypotension, dizziness, shortness of breath, or a decreased level of consciousness, it may indicate a life-threatening disorder.

History
Explore your patient's problem by asking appropriate questions.
• Does he have chest pain, dyspnea, hypotension, headaches, or palpitations? Is he dizzy or fatigued? Does he feel weak, especially in the legs? What was he doing when the bradycardia began?
• Ask your patient if he's had bradycardia before. If so, what relieved it? Does he have a family history of it?
• Was the patient exposed to cold for a prolonged period? An elderly person with a low income may have inadequate heat in his home. An alcoholic or homeless person may have slept outside in cold weather.
• Does he routinely engage in strenuous aerobic activity? If so, what kind and for how long? Has he had a recent episode of head, neck, or spinal cord trauma? Did he recently undergo cardiac catheterization, electrophysiologic studies, cardiac surgery, or suctioning?
• Find out if he has a congenital heart defect, systemic infection, brain tumor, cardiomyopathy, or cirrhosis of the liver. Has he ever had a cerebrovascular accident or a cardiac disorder, such as myocardial ischemia, myocardial infarction (MI), or heart block? Does he have a history of endocrine or metabolic disorders?
• Is the patient taking any drugs that slow the heart rate, such as digoxin, pilocarpine, beta blockers, calcium channel blockers, or quinidine? Has he taken a drug that may cause MI, such as dextrothyroxine? Has he taken a large dose of phenothiazines or drunk a lot of alcohol?

Physical examination
Base your examination of the patient on the health history information you've collected.

RULE OF THUMB

 Bradycardia and pulse deficit: How to tell them apart

Sometimes, when you detect a low peripheral pulse rate, the problem isn't bradycardia—it's a pulse deficit. To determine which one is causing the low pulse rate, you need to take the patient's apical-radial pulse. Here's how:

Auscultate the patient's heart rate while palpating his radial pulse. If you hear beats that you can't palpate, the patient has a pulse deficit, not bradycardia. The difference between the number of apical beats and the number of radial beats is the pulse deficit.

Inspection

Observe the patient's respiratory rate and depth. Does he have difficulty breathing or an abnormal respiratory pattern? Then check his skin for signs of dehydration and temperature changes. Inspect his nail beds and mucous membranes for peripheral and central cyanosis—late signs of inadequate cardiac output.

Look for pupillary changes and assess the patient's level of consciousness. Then check for edema or neck vein distention. To determine if the patient has experienced trauma, look for bruising and lacerations.

Palpation

Palpate the radial pulse while auscultating the apical pulse, comparing the pulses for a full minute. (See *Bradycardia and pulse deficit: How to tell them apart.*) As you palpate the muscles of the arms and legs, note decreased muscle tone or rigidity. Then test the strength of each limb, comparing one side to the other. Also, palpate the upper abdomen for an enlarged liver.

To check for abdominal pain or tenderness, lightly palpate the entire abdomen. Also, note any abnormal percussion sounds. Then assess the brachial, patellar, and Achilles tendon reflexes, noting any abnormal responses.

Auscultation

Listen to the patient's heart rate and rhythm, and note any abnormal heart sounds. Auscultate each lung field for diminished or absent breath sounds and adventitious sounds such as crackles. Also monitor the patient's blood pressure and pulse pressure.

Causes

Your assessment may lead you to suspect one of these conditions or causes, some of which are life-threatening.

Cervical spine injury. Transient or sustained bradycardia will be associated with sympathetic denervation in this life-threatening disorder. The more severe the spinal injury, the longer the bradycardia. Associated signs and symptoms may include hypotension, hypothermia, slowed peristalsis, leg or partial arm paralysis, and respiratory muscle paralysis. The history may include a spinal cord injury or tumor.

Hypothermia. When the body's core temperature drops below 89.6° F (32° C), bradycardia – a marker of this life-threatening disorder – occurs. You may also note hypotension, bradypnea, shivering, peripheral cyanosis, confusion leading to stupor and coma, muscle rigidity, joint stiffness, and cardiac arrhythmias. The patient has probably been exposed to the cold for a few hours. He may also have ingested a large dose of phenothiazines or a large amount of alcohol.

Increased intracranial pressure. Occurring late in this life-threatening disorder, bradycardia follows hypertension, tachycardia, altered mental status, headache, and perhaps projectile vomiting. The bradycardia will be accompanied by tachypnea or apneustic respirations and a widening pulse pressure. The patient may complain of a persistent headache. You may note progressive loss of consciousness, seizures, and pupillary changes. Cheyne-Stokes respirations indicate deteriorating brain function.

MI. Mild or severe bradycardia, which results from vagal stimulation or inadequate perfusion of the conduction system, may accompany the cardinal signs of life-threatening MI. These include crushing chest pain that may radiate to the jaw, shoulder, arm, or epigastrium; dyspnea;

anxiety; nausea or vomiting; diaphoresis; cool, pale, or cyanotic skin; and a feeling of impending doom. The patient may be hypotensive or hypertensive. You may auscultate an atrial gallop, a murmur and, occasionally, an irregular pulse. The patient may have a history or a family history of cardiac disease. He may have recently experienced extreme stress. His lifestyle may include excessive sodium and fat intake, little or no exercise, and smoking.

Other disorders. Bradycardia appears in patients with cardiomyopathy, congenital heart disease, or hypothyroidism. Fetal bradycardia – a heart rate of less than 120 beats/minute – may develop from prolonged labor or complications of delivery, including compressions of the umbilicus, partial abruptio placentae, and placenta previa.

Drugs. Transient bradycardia may result from use of diazepam, I.V. nitroglycerin, protamine sulfate, quinidine, beta blockers, calcium channel blockers, digitalis glycosides, narcotics, sympatholytics, and topical miotics such as pilocarpine.

Procedures. Cardiac catheterization and electrophysiologic studies may induce temporary bradycardia. Suctioning produces hypoxia and vagal stimulation, causing bradycardia. Edema or damage to conduction tissues from cardiac surgery will also trigger bradycardia. ❖

Chest pain

Patients describe chest pain in many ways: a dull ache, a sensation of heaviness or fullness, a feeling of indigestion, or a sharp, shooting pain. The pain may be constant or intermittent; it may radiate to other body parts; and it can start suddenly or gradually. Stress, anxiety, exertion, deep breathing, or certain foods may trigger the pain.

Chest pain may indicate several acute and life-threatening cardiopulmonary and GI conditions. It can also result from musculoskeletal or hematologic disorders, anxiety, and certain drugs.

History

Explore your patient's problem by asking appropriate questions.
• When did the chest pain begin? Did it begin with the patient at rest or under exertion? Did it develop suddenly or gradually? Is the pain localized or diffuse? Does it radiate to the neck, jaw, arms, or back? Is the pain sharp and stabbing or dull and aching? Is it constant or intermittent? Does breathing, changing positions, or eating certain foods exacerbate or relieve the pain?
• Has the patient had related complaints, such as coughing, dyspnea, headache, nausea, palpitations, vomiting, or weakness?
• Does the patient have a history of cardiac or respiratory disease, cardiac surgery, chest trauma, or intestinal disease? Does he have a family history of cardiac disease?
• Does the patient drink alcohol or use any illicit drugs? Which medications is he taking?

Physical examination

Assess the patient's skin temperature, color, and general appearance. Note any coolness, cyanosis, diaphoresis, mottling below the waist, pallor, peripheral edema, or prolonged capillary refill time. Look for facial edema, jugular vein distention, and tracheal deviation. And note any signs of altered level of consciousness, anxiety, dizziness, or restlessness.

Observe the rate and depth of the patient's respirations, noting any abnormal patterns or breathing difficulty. If the patient has a productive cough, examine the sputum.

Palpate the patient's neck, chest, and abdomen. Note any asymmetrical chest expansion, masses, subcutaneous crepitation, tender areas, tracheal deviation, or tactile fremitus. Also, palpate his peripheral pulses; record the rate, rhythm, and intensity.

As you percuss over an affected lung, note any dullness. Then auscultate the lungs to identify crackles, diminished or absent breath sounds, pleural friction rubs, rhonchi, or wheezes. Auscultate the heart for clicks, gallops, murmurs, and pericardial friction rub. To check for abdominal bruits, apply the bell of the stethoscope over the abdominal aorta. Be sure to monitor the patient's blood pressure closely.

Causes

Your assessment may lead you to suspect one of these conditions and causes, some of which are life-threatening. (See *Evaluating chest pain*, pages 36 to 41.)

(Text continues on page 40.)

Evaluating chest pain

When your patient complains of chest pain, determine what makes it better or worse. Have the patient describe the quality and quantity of the pain, its location, its severity, and its timing. As you can see from the chart below, this information can help you determine if the pain results from cardiac, pulmonary, or gastrointestinal disorders.

PROVOCATIVE FACTORS AND PALLIATIVE ACTIONS	QUALITY OR QUANTITY
Angina pectoris	
Provocative factors: emotional stress, extreme weather, heavy meal, hot bath or shower, physical exertion, sexual intercourse, spontaneous (no apparent cause) *Palliative actions:* nitroglycerin, rest, high Fowler's position, oxygen	Crushing or squeezing sensation; feeling of heaviness, pressure, or tightness; dull ache; or indigestion
Myocardial infarction	
Provocative factors: same as above *Palliative actions:* morphine, nitroglycerin	Crushing or squeezing sensation; feeling of heaviness, pressure, or tightness; dull ache; or indigestion
Postmyocardial syndrome	
Provocative factors: coughing, deep breathing, laughing, movement *Palliative actions:* aspirin, high Fowler's position, indomethacin, nitroglycerin	Knifelike, sharp, or stabbing sensation
Pericarditis	
Provocative factors: coughing, deep breathing, laughing, lying down, movement *Palliative actions:* high Fowler's position, leaning forward	Knifelike, sharp, or stabbing sensation
Dissecting aortic aneurysm	
Provocative factors: lifting heavy weight, spontaneous (no apparent cause) *Palliative actions:* narcotic analgesic, surgery	Ripping or tearing sensation, throbbing of chest with heartbeat

REGION AND RADIATION	SEVERITY	TIMING
Substernal region; radiation to left shoulder, jaw, neck, arm, elbow, or wrist	Mild to severe	Gradual or sudden onset; 5 to 15 minutes' duration
Substernal region; radiation to left shoulder, jaw, neck, arm, elbow, wrist, or fingers	Asymptomatic to severe	Gradual or sudden onset; constant duration during episode
Substernal region or at the left sternal border; radiation to shoulders (but not down arms)	Severe	Sudden onset (typically occurs 2 to 10 weeks after myocardial infarction and tends to recur); constant duration
Substernal region; radiation to back, neck, left shoulder, or arm	Mild to severe	Sudden onset; constant duration
Upper back (or upper anterior chest) region; radiation through back, abdomen, or thighs	Severe (especially at onset)	Sudden onset; few hours' to days' duration

OMINOUS SIGNS
AND SYMPTOMS

Evaluating chest pain *(continued)*

PROVOCATIVE FACTORS AND PALLIATIVE ACTIONS	QUALITY OR QUANTITY
Pulmonary artery hypertension	
Provocative factors: anemia, carbon monoxide, chronic hypoxemia (acute flare-up), high altitude *Palliative action:* oxygen	Crushing or gripping sensation
Pulmonary embolism	
Provocative factors: coughing, deep breathing, immobility *Palliative actions:* high Fowler's position, splinting of chest, position change	Gripping or stabbing sensation that worsens with deep breathing or feeling unable to take a breath
Pneumothorax	
Provocative factors: coughing, exertion, Valsalva's maneuver, spontaneous (no apparent cause) *Palliative action:* chest tube insertion	Sharp or tearing sensation
Pneumonia	
Provocative factors: aspiration, hypoventilation (from other disorders) *Palliative actions:* analgesic, rest	Burning, stabbing, or tearing sensation
Rib fracture	
Provocative factors: chest compression during cardiopulmonary resuscitation, coughing, deep breathing, laughing, movement *Palliative actions:* analgesic, heat	Sore, stabbing, or sticking sensation
Esophageal reflux	
Provocative factors: alcohol, aspirin, caffeine, constipation, spicy meal, lying down after meal, lifting heavy weight, obesity, smoking, straining, wearing clothing too tight at waist *Palliative actions:* antacid, food	Heartburn or dull, burning, or squeezing sensation

REGION AND RADIATION	SEVERITY	TIMING
Substernal region; doesn't radiate	Severe	Sudden onset; intermittent, nocturnal, or constant duration
Affected region; may radiate to neck or shoulder	Mild to severe	Sudden onset; few minutes' to days' duration
Lateral thorax; radiation to ipsilateral shoulder	Mild to severe	Sudden onset; few hours' duration
Retrosternal region; usually does not radiate	Mild to severe	Gradual or sudden onset; days' to weeks' duration
Affected area (rib, sternum, or costochondral joint); doesn't radiate	Mild to severe	Gradual or sudden onset; few weeks' duration
Epigastric and retrosternal region; mimics angina pectoris but rarely radiates to left shoulder, jaw, neck, arm, elbow, or wrist	Mild to severe	Onset during or after meal; intermittent duration (usually 10 minutes to 1 hour)

Evaluating chest pain (continued)

PROVOCATIVE FACTORS AND PALLIATIVE ACTIONS	QUALITY OR QUANTITY
Esophageal spasm	
Provocative factors: cold liquids, exercise, swallowing, spontaneous (no apparent cause) *Palliative action:* nitroglycerin	Dull, burning, crushing, gripping, or squeezing sensation or feeling of pressure
Esophageal rupture	
Provocative factors: alcohol, coughing, external trauma, heavy meal, swallowing, vomiting *Palliative action:* surgery	Tearing or crushing sensation
Gastric dysfunction	
Provocative factors: carbonated beverage, heavy meal, paralytic ileus *Palliative actions:* belching, relief of distention	Sharp, aching, burning, or bloated sensation

Angina pectoris. Pain usually begins gradually in this life-threatening disorder, builds to a peak, and then slowly subsides. The pain can last from 2 to 10 minutes. It occurs in the retrosternal region and radiates to the neck, jaw, and arms. Associated signs and symptoms include diaphoresis, dyspnea, nausea, vomiting, palpitations, and tachycardia. On auscultation, you may detect an atrial gallop (or S_4) or a murmur. Attacks may occur at rest or be provoked by exertion, emotional stress, or a heavy meal. (See *Understanding angina pectoris,* page 42.)

Aortic aneurysm (dissecting). A patient with a dissecting aortic aneurysm complains of sudden, excruciating, tearing pain in the chest and neck, radiating to the upper back, lower back, and abdomen. Other signs and symptoms of this life-threatening disorder include abdominal tenderness; heart murmurs; jugular vein distention; systolic bruits; tachycardia; weak or absent femoral or pedal pulses; and pale, cool, diaphoretic, mottled skin below the waist.

Cholecystitis. With this disorder, the patient has sudden epigastric or right upper quadrant (RUQ) pain, which may be steady or intermittent, radiate to the back, and be sharp or intense. Other signs and symptoms include chills, diaphoresis, nausea, and vomiting. Palpation of the RUQ

REGION AND RADIATION	SEVERITY	TIMING
Retrosternal region and area across chest; radiation to left arm, neck, jaw, or back	Mild to severe	Sudden onset; seconds' to minutes' duration (with lingering ache); tends to recur
Epigastric and retrosternal region; radiation to lower thoracic spine	Severe	Sudden onset; constant duration
Epigastric and lower retrosternal region; radiation to left shoulder	Mild to severe	Sudden onset; variable duration (usually worsens during day; ache lingers)

may reveal distention, rigidity, tenderness, and a mass.

MI. Usually, the patient with myocardial infarction (MI) has severe, crushing substernal pain that radiates to the left arm, jaw, or neck and lasts longer than 30 minutes. The pain of this life-threatening disorder may be accompanied by anxiety, clammy skin, diaphoresis, dyspnea, a feeling of impending doom, nausea, vomiting, pallor, and restlessness. The patient may have an atrial gallop, crackles, hypotension or hypertension, murmurs, and a pericardial friction rub. A history of heart disease, hypertension, hypercholesterolemia, or cocaine abuse is common.

Peptic ulcer. A sharp, burning pain arising in the epigastric region, usually hours after eating, characterizes peptic ulcer. Other signs and symptoms include epigastric tenderness, nausea, and vomiting. Food or antacids usually relieve the pain.

Pneumothorax. A collapsed lung produces a sudden, sharp, severe chest pain that's often unilateral and increases with chest movement. In this life-threatening disorder, you may detect decreased breath sounds, hyperresonant or tympanic percussion sounds, and subcutaneous crepitation. Other signs and symptoms include accessory muscle use, anxiety, asymmetrical chest expansion, nonproductive cough,

OMINOUS SIGNS
AND SYMPTOMS

CLINICAL CLOSE-UP

Understanding angina pectoris

Angina may be precipitated by physical or emotional stress. In a typical attack, stress activates the sympathetic nervous system, causing vasoconstriction and increased heart rate, contractility, and blood pressure. These effects raise the heart's oxygen needs. Two processes then take place.

The resulting hypoxia and ischemia increase the membrane permeability of heart cells, white blood cells, and platelets, which then release potassium, histamine, and serotonin, respectively. These substances stimulate pain

nerve endings in the heart.

Hypoxia also causes the metabolism to switch from aerobic to anaerobic. This process produces lactic acid, which also stimulates pain nerve endings in the heart.

Pain fibers from the heart synapse with sensory nerves from other areas of the body at the thoracic level of the spinal cord, as shown in the illustration below. Thus, pain is referred from the heart to areas supplied by these nerves, usually on the left side of the body. These areas include the jaw, neck, shoulder, arm, or hand.

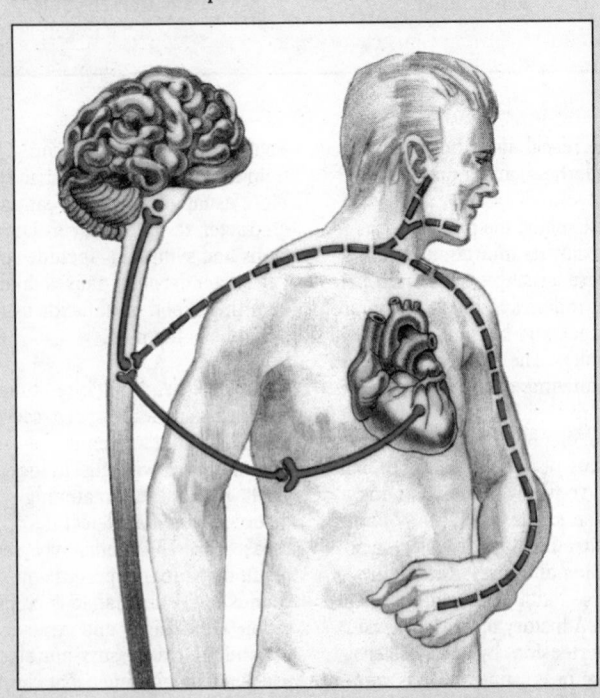

tachycardia, and tachypnea. The history may include chronic obstructive pulmonary disease, lung cancer, diagnostic or therapeutic procedures involving the thorax, or thoracic trauma.

Pulmonary embolism. Typically, the patient experiences sudden dyspnea with an intense angina-like or pleuritic ischemic pain aggravated by deep breathing and thoracic movement. Other findings in this life-threatening disorder include anxiety, cough with blood-tinged sputum, crackles, dull percussion sounds, restlessness, and tachycardia. If the embolism is large, the cardiovascular, pulmonary, and neurologic systems may be compromised. The patient's history may reveal thrombophlebitis, a hip or leg fracture, acute MI, congestive heart failure, pregnancy, or the use of oral contraceptives.

Other causes. Chest pain may also result from abrupt withdrawal of beta blockers, acute bronchitis, anxiety, esophageal spasm, lung abscess, muscle strain, pancreatitis, pneumonia, a rib fracture, or tuberculosis.

❖

Heart murmurs

One of the most common abnormal heart sounds, a heart murmur is a sustained noise that's audible during systole or diastole, or both. Although many murmurs are benign, numerous abnormal conditions can produce murmurs.

History
Because heart murmurs are often first detected during routine physical examinations, you may already have taken a general health history. If so, be sure to question your patient further about any family history of murmurs or heart disease. Also ask if the patient has a history of rheumatic fever, congenital heart abnormalities, or previous cardiac surgery.

Physical examination
To identify a heart murmur, you need to consider six characteristics of the abnormal sound you're hearing: location, loudness, frequency, quality, timing, and radiation.

Follow the same auscultatory pattern while assessing for each characteristic. Start at the right base of the heart or the second intercostal space (ICS) to the right of the sternum. Then move to the left base (second ICS to the left of the sternum), then to the left sternal border (LSB) at the fifth ICS, and finally to the apex, which is along the left midclavicular line (MCL) at the fifth ICS. Use the bell and diaphragm of your stethoscope at each of these four sites.

Location
Just as with normal heart sounds, a murmur originates near a heart valve. But the murmur's location, determined through auscultation, won't necessarily be right over the valve. The sound is referred in the direction of blood flow.

You'll usually hear mitral murmurs best at the apex of the

heart, along the left MCL at the fifth ICS. Tricuspid murmurs are best heard at the LSB over the fifth ICS; pulmonic murmurs, at the left base, along the LSB over the second ICS; aortic systolic murmurs, at the right base, along the right sternal border (RSB) over the second ICS; and aortic diastolic murmurs, at the third ICS, along the LSB.

Loudness

Because loudness is roughly related to the rate of blood flow through the heart or the amount of blood regurgitated, it's another key factor in assessing heart murmurs. The following is a common way to classify the loudness of the abnormal sound:
1. Not audible immediately on auscultation
2. Audible immediately, but faint
3. Loud but without thrust or thrill
4. Loud and possibly associated with thrust or thrill
5. Loud (audible with chestpiece only partially applied) with thrust or thrill
6. Loud (audible with chestpiece off chest entirely) with thrust or thrill.

Thrust (or heave) is a palpable (sometimes even visible) intermittent sensation at the site auscultated. *Thrill* refers to a continuous palpable sensation, like the purring of a cat.

To chart the loudness of a murmur, you can use a fraction, such as ²⁄₆. The "2" refers to the second of the categories listed above; the "6" indicates the number of categories.

Frequency

The frequency of a heart murmur refers to its pitch. Is it high or low? The faster the vibrations produced by the murmur, the higher its frequency; the slower the vibrations, the lower the frequency. You'll hear high-frequency murmurs best with the diaphragm of your stethoscope firmly pressed against the chest; low-frequency murmurs, with a lightly held bell.

Quality

The quality of the sound may be described as "blowing" (high frequency), "harsh" or "rough" (medium frequency), or "rumbling" (low frequency). Keep in mind these four patterns:
• A *crescendo* murmur starts softly and builds in intensity. Its sounds can be described as coarse, hard, or whooping.
• A *decrescendo* murmur starts loudly and drops in intensity. Its sounds are described as either blowing or whistling.
• A combination of the two, the *crescendo-decrescendo* murmur starts softly, becomes louder, and softens again. Its sound is described as harsh, grating, or coarse.
• If a murmur sounds constant throughout, its pattern is a *plateau*.

Timing

If the murmur occurs between S_1 and S_2, it's a systolic murmur; between S_2 and the next S_1, it's a diastolic murmur. A murmur is considered "early" if it peaks early in systole or diastole; "mid" if it peaks in the middle of the cycle; and "late" if it peaks late in the cycle. A pansystolic, holosystolic, or holodiastolic murmur

Understanding heart murmurs

Heart murmurs may result from three mechanisms: high rate of blood flow through a normal valve, decreased blood flow through a stenotic valve, or backflow due to an incompetent valve leaflet. The illustrations below show these three causes of murmurs.

High blood flow

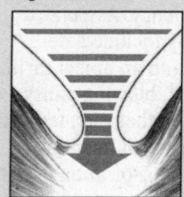

Decreased blood flow

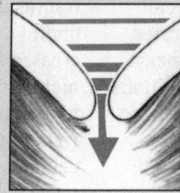

Backflow of blood

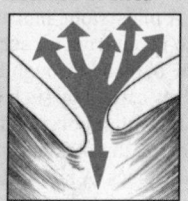

remains at the same intensity throughout the cycle and its pattern is a plateau.

Radiation

To assess for radiation, listen for the murmur in several places. Murmurs may radiate to other parts of the precordium, neck, back, and shoulder. Whether or not a murmur radiates depends on its pitch and quality. Where it radiates may help identify it. The murmur of mitral stenosis, for example, is heard best at the apex of the heart but may radiate to the axilla.

Types and their causes

Three basic mechanisms create heart murmurs. (See *Understanding heart murmurs*.) Your assessment of the murmur's characteristics may lead you to suspect a cause.

Systolic murmurs

These murmurs occur during ventricular systole and may result from turbulent blood flow through a stenotic aortic or pulmonic valve, regurgitant flow through an incompetent mitral or tricuspid valve, or flow through a ventricular septal defect.

The timing of the murmur helps you identify the cause. For instance, an early systolic murmur reflects a direct blood flow between the right and left ventricles and may indicate a small ventricular septal defect. Usually, the shunt is from left to right because of the higher pressure in the left ventricle.

A midsystolic murmur accompanied by a palpable thrill at the pulmonic valve area, a split S_2, and an ejection click suggest pulmonic stenosis. Characterized by a crescendo-decrescendo pattern, the murmur varies with respiration. It's best heard at the pulmonic valve area and radiates to the left shoulder.

A midsystolic murmur that radiates to the neck and apex may stem from aortic stenosis. Associated findings may include a palpable thrill at the aortic valve area, a softened S_2, and an ejection click. The murmur is harsh with a crescendo-decrescendo pattern.

A midsystolic murmur can also result from an accelerated flow of blood through the heart valves caused by such conditions as fever, fluid overload, exercise, anemia, thyrotoxicosis, and heart block. A late systolic murmur associated with an ejection click may indicate mitral valve prolapse.

Diastolic murmurs

These murmurs occur during ventricular diastole and may result from turbulent flow through a stenotic mitral or tricuspid valve or regurgitant flow through an incompetent aortic or pulmonic valve.

Suspect pulmonic insufficiency if you hear an early diastolic murmur that increases with respiration and is harsh, short, rough, and soft-pitched with a decrescendo pattern. An early diastolic murmur that is best heard over the aortic valve area and may radiate to the LSB may stem from aortic insufficiency. This high-pitched, blowing decrescendo murmur is often heard in conjunction with S_3 and may be caused by rheumatic fever, congenital heart disease, endocarditis, Marfan syndrome, or aortic root dissection.

Middiastolic to late diastolic murmurs are low-pitched and rumbling. These murmurs may indicate mitral or tricuspid stenosis or mitral insufficiency.

Pansystolic or holosystolic murmurs

These murmurs may reflect a significant ventricular septal defect. A loud, high-pitched pansystolic murmur in the mitral valve area that radiates toward the left axilla may stem from mitral insufficiency. Associated findings may include a decreased S_1 and an apical thrill. A high-pitched, blowing pansystolic murmur that radiates to the right of the sternum and is accentuated by inspiration over the tricuspid valve area suggests tricuspid insufficiency.

❖

Nonpalpable pulses

An absent or weak pulse may be generalized, or it may affect only one limb. When generalized, this sign usually indicates low cardiac output. A localized loss or weakness of a usually strong pulse may indicate arterial occlusion.

Sometimes, a normal pulse may be misinterpreted as absent or weak. This is because palpation can temporarily diminish or obliterate a superficial pulse, such as the posterior tibial or the dorsal pedal. Keep in mind that bilateral weakness or absence of these pulses isn't necessarily abnormal.

To avoid misinterpretation when assessing infants and small children, evaluate arterial circulation to the limbs by palpating the brachial, popliteal, or femoral pulse. In these patients, the radial, dorsal pedal, and posterior tibial pulses aren't easy to palpate. If you use them, you may mistake a hard-to-palpate pulse for an absent or weak one.

History

Even if emergency treatment is needed, ask the patient all appropriate questions.

• Does the patient have accompanying signs and symptoms, such as dyspnea, light-headedness, fatigue, anxiety, a feeling of impending doom, itching, weakness, palpitations, dizziness, nausea, vomiting, diarrhea, chills, or cool, clammy skin? Does he have a cough? If so, is it productive?

• Is the patient in pain? If so, ask him to describe it. Where is it? Did it start suddenly or gradually? Does it radiate? Does it abate or worsen with activity?

• Has the patient recently experienced trauma or undergone surgery? Has he had a systemic infection?

• Does he have a history of cardiovascular, pulmonary, or GI disease? If he has allergies, has he been exposed to allergens?

• Which medications is he taking?

Physical examination

Based on the information you've collected, conduct a physical examination.

Inspection

Examine the patient's skin for diaphoresis, lines of frank demarcation, mottling, pallor, or flushing. Also, check the skin temperature. If an arm or leg is cool and pale, elevate it slightly and observe for cadaveric pallor in the toes or feet. Then check for prolonged (longer than 2 seconds) capillary refill time.

Observe the patient's respirations, noting their rate and depth. Does he have difficulty breathing or an abnormal breathing pattern? During the respiratory cycle, listen for stridor or hoarseness. Note any blood-tinged sputum produced from coughing.

Then inspect the patient's neck for jugular vein distention. Assess his level of consciousness, noting restlessness, confusion, anxiety, or seizures. Be sure to measure his abdominal girth and monitor for any increase. To check for muscle weakness, hemiplegia, or focal neurologic deficits, observe his motor activity. Examine him for signs of trauma, such as bruising, erythema, and abrasions. Monitor his urine output for oliguria or anuria.

Palpation

As you palpate the peripheral pulses, note their rate, rhythm, and intensity. Palpate the abdomen for rigidity, pain, and tenderness. If you note any guarding, gently palpate the area for a mass or hepatomegaly. If you detect a palpable mass, does it pulsate?

Percussion

Carefully percuss the abdomen. Note any areas of tympany, hyperresonance, or dullness. Gently percuss the chest and back, listening for areas of dullness.

Auscultation

Listen to the patient's lungs for abnormal breath sounds. Especially note diminished sounds, rhonchi, wheezes, crackles, and pleural friction rubs.

Auscultate the heart for abnormal sounds, particularly faint or muffled heart sounds, murmurs, gallops, or pericardial friction rubs. Then auscultate the abdomen for aortic bruits and bowel sounds.

Monitor the patient's blood pressure and pulse pressure. Also monitor the intensity of Korotkoff's sounds. To detect orthostatic hypotension, measure his blood pressure while he's supine and while he sits.

Causes

Your assessment may lead you to suspect one of these causes, some of which are life-threatening.

Anaphylactic shock. Generalized weak pulses develop suddenly from a dramatic fall in blood pressure and a narrowed pulse pressure in this life-threatening disorder. This usually follows extreme anxiety, restlessness, feelings of impending doom, intense itching (especially of the hands and feet), and a pounding headache. Symptoms usually start within seconds or minutes of exposure to an allergen; however, delayed reactions may occur up to 24 hours after exposure. Later, anaphylactic shock may also produce flushing, cardiac arrhythmias, tachycardia, seizures, coughing, sneezing, dyspnea, nasal congestion, stridor and hoarseness from laryngeal edema, as well as nausea, abdominal cramps, involuntary defecation, and urinary incontinence. The patient may have allergies or a family history of them.

Aortic aneurysm (dissecting). A weak or absent femoral, popliteal, or pedal pulse may be unilateral in this life-threatening disorder. Associated signs and symptoms vary, depending on whether the patient has an abdominal or thoracic aneurysm. With an abdominal aneurysm, the patient may experience persistent abdominal and back pain, weakness, sweating, tachycardia, dyspnea, restlessness, and confusion. You may note mottled skin below the waist, increasing abdominal girth, abdominal rigidity, and cool, clammy skin. On auscultation, you may find a systolic bruit. And on palpation, you may detect tenderness over the area of the aneurysm and an epigastric mass that pulsates before rupturing.

With a thoracic aneurysm, the patient will feel a severe ripping or tearing pain in his chest, which radiates to the neck, shoulders, lower back, or abdomen. This may be accompanied by pallor, syncope, sweating, dyspnea, tachycardia, cyanosis, leg weakness, and a sudden onset of neurologic symptoms. Auscultation may reveal a murmur suggesting aortic insufficiency.

Aortic bifurcation occlusion (acute). With this life-threatening disorder, femoral, popliteal, and pedal pulses will be absent in both legs. These signs will be accompanied by sudden ischemic pain, sensory and motor deficits distal to the obstruction, and cadaveric pallor of the toes and feet even when they're only slightly elevated. The patient may also complain of pain in the abdomen, lumbosacral area, or perineum.

Arterial limb occlusion (acute). Pulses distal to the obstruction are weak and eventually disappear in this life-threatening disorder. A line of color and temperature demarcation develops at the level of obstruction. With a more ischemic limb, the patient will feel pain at rest, and you'll note a cadaveric pallor when the limb is elevated even slightly. Varying degrees of limb paralysis can also develop along with intense intermittent claudication.

Cardiac arrhythmias. With these life-threatening disorders, you'll note generalized weak pulses and cool, clammy skin. Other signs and symptoms reflect the type and severity of the arrhythmia. These may include hypotension, chest pain, dizziness, and a decreased level of consciousness. Low blood pressure may alternate with normal pressure and may be accompanied by lightheadedness, weakness, fatigue, and palpitations.

Cardiac tamponade. In this life-threatening disorder, as the pericardium fills with blood or fluid, weak and rapid peripheral pulses may be accompanied by these classic findings: pulsus paradoxus, jugular vein distention, hypotension, narrowed pulse pressure, and muffled heart sounds. However, some hypovolemic patients may not have jugular vein distention, and if the patient is sitting upright, his

heart sounds may not be muffled. The patient may appear anxious, restless, and cyanotic. He may also have chest pain, clammy skin, dyspnea, and tachypnea. You may note pericardial friction rubs and hepatomegaly.

Cardiogenic shock. Depending on the degree of vascular collapse in this life-threatening disorder, peripheral pulses may be absent and central pulses, weak. You may see a decrease in systolic pressure to less than 80 mm Hg or 30 mm Hg less than the patient's baseline pressure. Other signs and symptoms include anginal pain, narrowed pulse pressure, diminished Korotkoff's sounds, peripheral cyanosis, restlessness, anxiety that can progress to disorientation and confusion, and pale, cool, clammy skin. You may also detect dyspnea, jugular vein distention, and oliguria.

Hypovolemic shock. Depending on the severity of the hypovolemia in this life-threatening disorder, peripheral pulses become weak and then uniformly absent. As shock progresses, the remaining pulses become thready and more rapid. Systolic pressure falls to less than 80 mm Hg or 30 mm Hg less than the patient's baseline pressure. This drop is accompanied by orthostatic pressure changes, diminished Korotkoff's sounds, narrowed pulse pressure, and tachypnea and tachycardia, which increase as blood volume decreases. Other symptoms include angina pectoris (in patients with coronary artery disease), light-headedness, irritability, diaphoresis, extreme thirst, hypothermia, decreased capillary refill, confusion, disorientation, restlessness, and anxiety. Decreased renal perfusion causes oliguria and peripheral vasoconstriction, leading to cyanosis of the limbs and pale, cool, clammy skin.

Neurogenic shock. Uniformly weak pulses accompanying hypotension and bradycardia are the cardinal signs of life-threatening neurogenic shock. Vasodilation occurring in neurogenic shock causes the relative hypovolemia that produces the symptoms.

Pulmonary embolism. A generalized weak, rapid pulse may accompany the sudden dyspnea that's the hallmark of this life-threatening disorder. You may also find sudden angina-like or pleuritic pain aggravated by deep breathing and thoracic movement. Accompanying signs and symptoms include hypotension, apprehension, restlessness, syncope, and diaphoresis. Other findings are anxiety, tachypnea, decreased breath sounds, crackles, a nonproductive cough or one that produces blood-tinged sputum, a low-grade fever, pleural friction rubs, diffuse wheezing, dullness on percussion, signs of cerebral ischemia (transient unconsciousness, coma, seizures), and (particularly in the elderly) hemiplegia and other focal neurologic deficits. Central cyanosis occurs when a large embolus causes significant obstruction of the pulmonary circulation.

Septic shock. Depending on the degree of vascular collapse in this life-threatening disorder, pulses become weak and then may become uniformly absent. Shock is heralded by chills, sudden fever, and possibly nausea, vomiting, and diarrhea. Typically, the skin is flushed, warm, and dry. Tachycardia and tachypnea commonly occur. As shock progresses, these signs and symptoms appear: hypotension (systolic pressure less than 80 mm Hg or 50 to 80 mm Hg less than the patient's baseline pressure), thirst, anxiety, restlessness, and confusion. Pulse pressure narrows and the skin becomes cold, clammy, and cyanotic. The patient experiences oliguria or anuria, respiratory failure, and coma.

Other causes

In dialysis patients, a localized pulse absence may occur distal to arteriovenous shunts or fistulas.

❖

Tachycardia

Easily detected by assessing the apical, carotid, or radial pulse, tachycardia is a heart rate greater than 100 beats/minute in adults, and higher in children. Usually, the patient also complains of palpitations or of his heart "racing."

A common sign, tachycardia normally results from emotional or physical stress, such as excitement, exercise, pain, or fever. Stimulants such as tobacco and caffeine can also cause this sign. But tachycardia also can be an early sign of a life-threatening

CLINICAL CLOSE-UP

Understanding tachycardia

Tachycardia represents the heart's effort to deliver more oxygen to body tissues by increasing the rate at which blood passes through the vessels. This sign may result from overstimulation within the sinoatrial node, the atrium, the atrioventricular node, or the ventricles.

Cardiac output is equal to heart rate (the number of contractions per minute) times stroke volume (the ventricular output for each contraction). Thus, tachycardia can lower cardiac output by reducing ventricular filling time and stroke volume.

As cardiac output plummets, arterial pressure and peripheral perfusion decrease. Tachycardia further aggravates myocardial ischemia by increasing the heart's demand for oxygen while reducing the duration of diastole—the period of greatest coronary artery blood flow.

disorder. (See *Understanding tachycardia*.)

History
Explore your patient's problem by asking appropriate questions.
• Did the patient feel palpitations when the tachycardia began? If so, has he had palpitations before? How were they treated?
• Is the patient dizzy or short of breath? Weak or fatigued? Is he experiencing chest pain? A feeling of impending doom? Severe itching of the hands and feet? Any nausea and vomiting, diarrhea, light-headedness, cold or heat intolerance, visual disturbances, or excessive thirst, appetite, or urine output?
• Is your female patient pregnant or in the postpartum period? Is she amenorrheic? If she's pregnant, has she had a sudden weight gain?
• Has the patient been exposed to allergens or organisms known to cause respiratory infections?

• Has he recently experienced a pulmonary or systemic injury that could predispose him to adult respiratory distress syndrome (ARDS) or shock? Also, ask about recent episodes of excessive fluid intake or loss—for instance, from wound or burn drainage or diuretic therapy.
• Does the patient have a history of trauma, diabetes, or cardiac, pulmonary, or thyroid disorders? If the patient is a child, note a history of rhinitis, fever, malaise, or anorexia. Obtain a drug history.

Physical examination
Base your examination of the patient on the health history information you've collected.

Inspection
Observe the rate, rhythm, and quality of the patient's respirations. Keep in mind that respiratory rate and other vital signs will be different for children.

Note whether the patient has any difficulty breathing. Check for asymmetrical chest wall movement, accessory muscle use, stridor, hoarseness, or abnormal respiratory patterns. Note whether he has a cough. If he has a productive cough, describe the sputum.

Next, inspect the patient's skin for pallor, cyanosis, poor turgor, and evidence of trauma. Assess his nail beds for delayed capillary refill time (greater than 2 seconds) and pulsations. Be sure to observe for jugular vein distention, an enlarged thyroid, tracheal deviation, and exophthalmos.

Evaluate the patient's level of consciousness (LOC), noting decreased mental acuity, restlessness, anxiety, disorientation, or confusion. Also, note any seizures.

Monitor the patient's urine output for oliguria or anuria.

Gently palpate the eyeballs for softness and the neck for evidence of tracheal deviation or thyroid enlargement. Also, palpate over the chest and sternum for subcutaneous or bony crepitus. Check the patient's arms and legs for peripheral edema and palpate his peripheral pulses to assess rate, rhythm, and intensity.

Percussion
Percuss over the lungs, noting dullness, hyperresonance, or tympany. To help detect hepatomegaly, percuss the abdomen.

Auscultation
Listen over the heart for murmurs, gallops, and pericardial friction rubs. Then auscultate over the lungs, noting any abnormal sounds.

To detect orthostatic hypotension, check the patient's blood pressure with him supine and sitting. Monitor his blood pressure and pulse pressure.

Causes
Your examination may lead you to suspect one of these conditions or causes, some of which are life-threatening.

ARDS. In this life-threatening disorder, tachycardia typically follows acute dyspnea and tachypnea. Other common findings include restlessness, grunting respirations, accessory muscle use, cyanosis, anxiety, decreased mental acuity, crackles, and rhonchi. Severe ARDS can produce signs of shock, such as hypotension and cool, clammy skin. Typically, the patient has no history of cardiac or pulmonary disease but has sustained a recent pulmonary or systemic insult.

Anaphylactic shock. In this life-threatening disorder, tachycardia, a dramatic drop in blood pressure, and a narrowed pulse pressure develop either within minutes or within 24 hours of exposure to an allergen, such as penicillin or an insect sting. Typically, the patient appears extremely restless and has severe pruritus, perhaps with a feeling of impending doom and a pounding headache. Later, he may develop flushing, cardiac arrhythmias, seizures, coughing, sneezing, difficulty breathing, nasal congestion, stridor and hoarseness, nausea, abdominal cramps, and urinary and bowel incontinence. The patient may have allergies or a family history of them, and he may have been exposed to a known or common allergen.

Cardiac arrhythmias. In some life-threatening arrhythmias, tachycardia with a regular or irregular rhythm may be accompanied by acute or gradual dyspnea, intermittent hypotension, and palpitations. The patient also may report dizziness, lightheadedness, weakness, and fatigue. He may have a history of cardiac disease or of using drugs that can cause cardiac arrhythmias—cocaine, digitalis glycosides, certain beta blockers, calcium channel blockers, or certain antiarrhythmic drugs, for instance.

Cardiac contusion. Resulting from blunt chest trauma, life-threatening cardiac contusion can cause tachycardia accompanied by hypotension, dyspnea, and intermittent, excruciating chest pain that may radiate to the neck, the jaw, or down the arm. Inspection may reveal external bruising of the chest and abdominal area.

Cardiac tamponade. In this life-threatening disorder, tachycardia commonly occurs with hypotension, narrowed pulse pressure, neck vein distention, and muffled heart sounds. The patient may report fever and malaise. You also may detect pulsus paradoxus, dyspnea, Kussmaul's respirations, and cyanosis. The patient's history may include recent chest trauma, pericarditis, myocardial infarction (MI), or chronic tamponade.

Cardiogenic shock. In this form of shock, tachycardia typically is accompanied by a drop in systolic pressure to less than 80 mm Hg or 30 mm Hg less than the patient's baseline pressure. Other common findings in this life-threatening disorder include narrowed pulse pressure, diminished Korotkoff's sounds, peripheral cyanosis, and pale, cool, clammy skin. The patient may be restless and anxious and, later, disoriented and confused. Associated signs and symptoms may include anginal pain, dyspnea, jugular vein distention, oliguria, and a weak, rapid pulse. On auscultation, you may detect tachypnea, faint heart sounds, ventricular gallop and, possibly, a holosystolic murmur.

Congestive heart failure. In left ventricular failure, tachycardia occurs with dyspnea, which can develop suddenly but usually does so gradually or occurs as chronic paroxysmal nocturnal dyspnea. Other signs and symptoms in this life-threatening disorder include fatigue, tachypnea, low or normal blood pressure, cold intolerance, orthopnea, cough, central cyanosis, ventricular or atrial gallop, bibasilar crackles, and diffuse apical impulse. You may also note dependent edema, jugular vein distention, and prolonged capillary refill time (greater than 2 seconds).

In right ventricular failure, tachycardia is accompanied by peripheral edema, ascites, jugular vein distention, peripheral cyanosis, and hepatomegaly. The patient may have a history of cardiovascular disease or previous dyspneic episodes, fatigue, weight gain, pallor or cyanosis, diaphoresis, and anxiety. His medication history may include drugs that can cause congestive heart failure (CHF), such as angiotensin-converting enzyme inhibitors, antihypertensives, beta blockers, calcium channel blockers, corticosteroids, nonsteroidal anti-inflammatory drugs, amiodarone, carbamazepine, flecainide, recombinant interferon alfa-2a, or recombinant interleukin-2.

Diabetic ketoacidosis. Osmotic diuresis and dehydration cause tachycardia along with low blood pressure, decreased pulse pressure, and a characteristic flushed face. Accompanying signs and symptoms of this life-threatening disorder may include abdominal pain and distention, nausea and vomiting, Kussmaul's respirations, seizures, and stupor possibly progressing to coma.

Epiglottitis. In this life-threatening disorder, which occurs more commonly in children than in adolescents or adults, tachycardia is accompanied by dyspnea, inspiratory stridor, accessory muscle use, decreased breath sounds, high fever, drooling, and dysphagia. The child may be anxious and have a sore throat and a muffled voice. Later, he may develop cyanosis from hypoxemia that results when the swollen epiglottis obstructs the airway.

Flail chest. Multiple rib fractures may cause flail chest, producing tachycardia along with characteristic sudden dyspnea, paradoxical chest movement, severe chest pain, hypotension, tachypnea, and cyanosis. If this life-threatening disorder, you'll note bruising and decreased or absent breath sounds over the affected side.

Hyperosmolar nonketotic syndrome. In this life-threatening disorder, tachycardia occurs with a drop in blood pressure, which can be dramatic if the patient loses a significant amount of fluid from osmotic diuresis. A rapidly deteriorating LOC may be accompanied by polyuria, polydipsia, weight loss, fever, shallow respirations, poor skin turgor, dry flushed skin and, occasionally, focal or generalized tonic-clonic seizures.

Hypertensive encephalopathy. This life-threatening disorder is characterized by tachycardia, tachypnea, and extremely high blood pressure (systolic pressure exceeding 200 mm Hg, diastolic pressure exceeding 120 mm Hg). Typically, the patient experiences severe headache, vomiting, seizures, visual disturbances, and transient paralysis. Eventually, he develops Cheyne-Stokes respirations and a decreased LOC that may progress to coma.

Hyponatremia. This life-threatening electrolyte imbalance produces tachycardia as well as several other signs and symptoms. You may note anxiety, orthostatic hypotension, headache, muscle twitching and weakness, fatigue, oliguria or anuria, cold and clammy skin, decreased skin turgor, irritability, lethargy, a thready pulse, and a decreased LOC possibly progressing to coma. Excessive thirst, nausea, vomiting, and abdominal cramps also may occur. The patient's history may include a fluid imbalance resulting from profuse sweating, diarrhea, or vomiting; excessive water intake; excessive infusion of dextrose in water; diuretic therapy; overuse of tap water enemas; malnutrition; extensive burns or wound drainage; adrenal insufficiency; syndrome of inappropriate antidiuretic hormone secretion; or renal disease.

Hypovolemic shock. Slight tachycardia that increases as blood volume decreases is an early sign of shock from blood volume loss. In this life-threatening disorder, this sign may be accompanied by tachypnea, restlessness, thirst, and pale, cool skin. As hypovolemic shock progresses, systolic pressure falls to less than 80 mm Hg or to 30 mm Hg less than the patient's baseline level, causing orthostatic pressure changes, diminished Korotkoff's sounds, and narrowed pulse pressure. The patient's skin becomes clammy and his pulse is increasingly rapid and thready. He also may experience light-headedness, irritability, anxiety, and a decreased LOC. Other associated signs and symptoms may include anginal pain (in patients with coronary artery disease), diaphoresis, hypothermia, delayed capillary refill time (greater than 2 seconds), oliguria, and peripheral cyanosis.

Laryngotracheobronchitis. This life-threatening pediatric disorder produces tachycardia with a harsh barking cough, accessory muscle use, restlessness, anxiety, and stridor. Auscultation reveals diminished breath sounds, crackles, and rhonchi. The child may have rhinitis, fever, malaise, and anorexia for 2 to 3 days before the other symptoms appear.

MI. This life-threatening disorder may cause tachycardia or bradycardia. Its classic symptom, however, is crushing substernal chest pain that may radiate to the left arm, jaw, neck, abdomen, or shoulder blades. Unrelieved by rest or nitroglycerin, the chest pain may be accompanied by sudden dyspnea, pallor, clammy skin, diaphoresis, nausea, vomiting, anxiety, restlessness, weakness, dizziness, and a feeling of impending doom. The patient may develop hypotension or hypertension, an atrial gallop, murmurs, a pericardial friction rub, and crackles.

Pneumonia. In this life-threatening disorder, tachycardia may be accompanied by sudden dyspnea, fever, shaking chills, and pleuritic chest pain that's exacerbated by deep inspiration. Depending on the stage and type of pneumonia, the patient may have a cough that produces discolored and foul-smelling sputum. Associated signs and symptoms may include decreased breath sounds, crackles, rhonchi, dull percussion sounds, whispered pectoriloquy, tachypnea, myalgia, fatigue, headache, abdominal pain, anorexia, central cyanosis, and diaphoresis.

Pneumothorax. This life-threatening disorder produces tachycardia and other signs and symptoms of distress, such as severe dyspnea, central cyanosis, and sharp chest pain that may mimic

MI. Related findings commonly include decreased or absent breath sounds with hyperresonance or tympany, subcutaneous crepitation, and decreased vocal fremitus. You also may note asymmetrical chest expansion, accessory muscle use, a nonproductive cough, tachypnea, anxiety, and restlessness. A patient with tension pneumothorax will also have tracheal deviation.

Pulmonary edema. Tachycardia and severe dyspnea commonly follow signs and symptoms of CHF, such as jugular vein distention and orthopnea. Other findings in this life-threatening disorder may include tachypnea, crackles in both lung fields, an S_3 gallop, oliguria, a thready pulse, hypotension, diaphoresis, fatigue, recent rapid weight gain, pallor or cyanosis, and marked anxiety. The patient's cough may be dry or produce copious amounts of pink, frothy sputum.

Pulmonary embolism. In this life-threatening disorder, tachycardia typically develops after the onset of sudden dyspnea and intense angina-like or pleuritic pain that's aggravated by deep breathing and thoracic movement. You also may detect hypotension, narrowed pulse pressure, and diminished Korotkoff's sounds. Central cyanosis occurs when a large embolus obstructs pulmonary circulation. Other findings may include anxiety, tachypnea, low-grade fever, restlessness, diaphoresis, crackles, pleural friction rubs, diffuse wheezing, and dull percussion sounds. The patient's cough may be dry or may produce blood-tinged sputum. He also may have signs and symptoms of circulatory collapse (weak, rapid pulse and hypotension), cerebral ischemia (transient unconsciousness, coma, seizures), and hypoxia (restlessness).

Septic shock. Initially, life-threatening septic shock produces tachycardia, chills, sudden fever, tachypnea and, possibly, nausea, vomiting, and diarrhea. The patient's skin is flushed, warm, and dry; his blood pressure, normal or slightly decreased. Eventually, he may exhibit anxiety, restlessness, thirst, oliguria or anuria, and cool, clammy, cyanotic skin. As shock progresses, hypotension becomes severe (with systolic pressure dropping to less than 80 mm Hg or to 30 mm Hg less than the patient's baseline pressure). This may be accompanied by arrhythmias; a weak, thready pulse; decreased or absent peripheral pulses; rapid, shallow respirations; and a decreased LOC possibly progressing to coma.

Thyrotoxicosis (thyroid storm). In this acute, life-threatening metabolic disturbance, tachycardia occurs with a sudden rise in systolic blood pressure, widened pulse pressure, bounding pulse, pulsations in the capillary nail beds, and palpitations. Other common findings include exophthalmos, thyroid gland enlargement, heat intolerance, exertional dyspnea, fever exceeding 100° F (37.8° C), diarrhea, dehydration, atrial fibrillation, and warm, moist skin. The patient may appear nervous and emotionally unstable and show occasional outbursts of psychotic behavior. A female patient may experience oligomenorrhea or amenorrhea. A patient with latent hyperthyroidism may have a history of excessive dietary iodine intake; symptoms may recur following stressful conditions, such as surgery, infections, pregnancy, or diabetic ketoacidosis.

Diagnostic tests. Cardiac catheterization and electrophysiologic studies may induce transient tachycardia.

Drugs. Many drugs that affect the nervous system, circulatory system, or heart muscle can cause tachycardia. Common ones include sympathomimetics such as epinephrine; phenothiazines such as chlorpromazine; anticholinergics such as atropine; thyroid drugs; vasodilators such as hydralazine and nifedipine; nitrates such as nitroglycerin; alpha-adrenergic blockers such as phentolamine; and bronchodilators such as theophylline. Alcohol, such stimulants as caffeine and tobacco, and illicit drugs such as marijuana can also cause tachycardia.

Procedures. Tachycardia also may result from cardiac surgery or pacemaker malfunction or wire irritation.

❖

Respiratory signs and symptoms

To detect and differentiate among respiratory disorders, many of which can be life-threatening, you must know where best to auscultate breath sounds and how to distinguish between normal and abnormal sounds. The quality of your patient's respirations and the presence of additional signs and symptoms, such as cyanosis and hemoptysis, will provide a diagnostic focus.

Abnormal breath sounds

Any breath sounds that are louder or quieter than normal – or absent – are considered abnormal or *adventitious*. Such sounds occur when air passes either through narrowed airways or through moisture, or when the membranes lining the chest cavity and the lungs become inflamed. Adventitious breath sounds usually indicate pulmonary disease.

History
Explore your patient's problem by asking appropriate questions.
• Have the patient's symptoms been chronic or acute?
• Does he have dyspnea during the entire day? Does he have orthopnea or paroxysmal nocturnal dyspnea?
• If he has a cough, is it productive? What color is the sputum? Does it have an odor? Is hemoptysis present?
• Does the patient have chest pain, nasal symptoms, hoarseness, anorexia or weight loss, fever, or night sweats?
• Does he tire easily? Can he tolerate exercise?
• Has he had a recent upper respiratory infection, other illness, or contact with inhaled irritants,

such as pollutants or industrial toxins?
• Has the patient been exposed to tuberculosis (TB) recently? What was the date of his last TB test? His last chest X-ray?
• Does he smoke? Does he have any allergies?
• Does he have a family history of respiratory illness?

Physical examination
Begin auscultating over the patient's trachea. As you auscultate, have the patient take full, slow breaths through his mouth. (Nose breathing changes the pitch of the breath sounds.) Listen for one full inspiration and expiration before moving the stethoscope.

Moving on to the upper lobes, auscultate a point on one side of the anterior chest and then on the other side, following the same sequence you use for percussion.

To assess the middle lung lobes, auscultate laterally at the level of the fourth to sixth intercostal spaces, following the lateral auscultation sequence.

In the same way you auscultated your patient's anterior chest, auscultate his posterior chest, comparing sounds on both sides before moving to the next area.

As you auscultate, classify normal and abnormal breath sounds according to their location, intensity (amplitude), characteristic sound, pitch (tone), and duration. Also note the timing: Identify the inspiratory and expiratory phases of normal and abnormal breath sounds, and then determine whether the sound occurs during inspiration, expiration, or both.

Normal breath sounds
To detect abnormal breath sounds, you must first be able to readily identify normal breath sounds. You'll hear four types of normal breath sounds – tracheal, bronchial, bronchovesicular, and vesicular – in specific areas. (See *Recognizing normal breath sounds.*)

You'll hear tracheal breath sounds – harsh, discontinuous sounds – over the trachea. These sounds occur equally during inspiration and expiration. Bronchial breath sounds – high-pitched, discontinuous sounds that occur during expiration – can be heard over the manubrium. Bronchovesicular breath sounds – medium-pitched, continuous sounds that are equally audible during inspiration and expiration – occur over the upper third of the sternum anteriorly and in the interscapular area posteriorly. Vesicular breath sounds – low-pitched, continuous sounds that are prolonged during inspiration – can be heard over the peripheral lung fields.

If you hear any of these four sounds in areas other than those described, you've detected an abnormal breath sound. For instance, bronchial breath sounds over the peripheral lung fields may indicate consolidation or atelectasis.

Adventitious breath sounds
Lung auscultation can detect abnormal airway fluid, mucus, or obstruction and the sounds these conditions produce: crackles, rhonchi, wheezes, and pleural friction rubs. (See *Recognizing abnormal breath sounds,* pages 60 and 61.) Auscultation can also indicate the condition of the

Recognizing normal breath sounds

Use these illustrations to note the location of the normal breath sounds: tracheal, bronchial, bronchovesicular, and vesicular.

Anterior chest

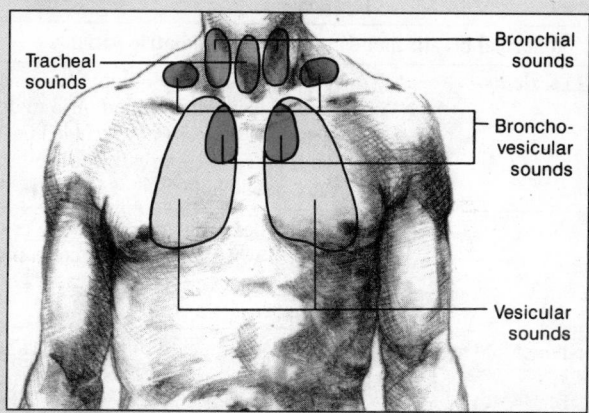

Posterior chest

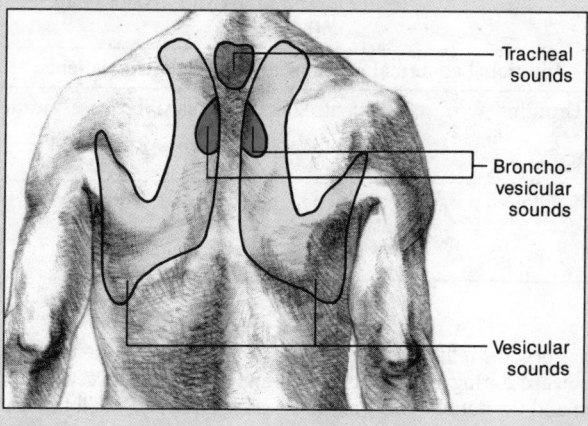

alveoli and the surrounding pleura.

Crackles. These discrete sounds occur when air passes through fluid-filled airways, causing collapsed alveoli to pop open as airway pressure equalizes. They can also occur when membranes lining the chest cavity and the

Recognizing abnormal breath sounds

Abnormal breath sounds occur when air passes through narrowed airways or through moisture, or when the membranes lining the chest cavity and the lungs become inflamed. Use this chart to help you assess abnormal auscultation findings.

TYPE	LOCATION
Abnormal breath sounds in adult and pediatric patients	
Crackles	Anywhere, but initially in lung bases; usually heard during inspiration. Also in dependent lung portions of bedridden patients. If crackles clear with coughing, they are not pathologic.
Wheezes	Anywhere; heard during inspiration or expiration. If wheezes clear with coughing, they may be coming from the trachea or larger upper airways.
Rhonchi (gurgles)	Central airways; heard during inspiration and expiration
Pleural friction rub	Lateral lung field; heard during inspiration and expiration (with patient in upright position)
Additional abnormal breath sounds in pediatric patients	
Grunting	Central airways; heard during expiration
Stridor	Trachea; heard during inspiration

lungs become inflamed. Crackles are heard during both inspiration and expiration. They vary in pitch and intensity and can be classified as fine, medium, or coarse.

Fine crackles, often called end-inspiratory crackles, are high-pitched sounds heard near the end of inspiration. To simulate this sound, hold several strands of hair close to your ear and roll them between your fingers. Typically, you'll first detect fine crackles over the lung bases.

Fine crackles result from fluid in small airways or small atelectatic areas that expand when the patient breathes deeply. You may hear fine crackles in a patient who has either pulmonary edema or pneu-

CAUSE	DESCRIPTION
Air passing through moisture, especially in the small airways and alveoli, with pulmonary edema	Light crackling, popping, non-musical sound, like hairs being rubbed together; further classified by pitch: high, medium, or low
Fluid or secretions in the large airways or airways narrowed by mucus or bronchospasm	Whistling sound; can be described as sonorous, bubbling, moaning, musical, sibilant and rumbling, crackling, groaning
Air passing through fluid-filled airways, as in upper respiratory tract infection	Bubbling sound
Inflamed parietal and visceral pleural linings rubbing together	Superficial squeaking or grating sound, like pieces of sandpaper being rubbed together
Physiologic retention of air in lungs to prevent alveolar collapse	Grunting noise
Forced movement of air through edematous upper airway	Crowing noise

monia. Usually, fine crackles won't clear when the patient breathes deeply or coughs.

Medium crackles, lower-pitched and coarser than fine crackles, result from fluid in slightly larger airways, such as the bronchioles. They occur during the middle or end of inspiration; thus, you may hear them called mid-inspiratory crackles.

Medium crackles won't clear when the patient breathes deeply or coughs.

Coarse crackles result from a large amount of fluid or exudate in the large airways, including the primary and the secondary bronchi. They produce a loud bubbling or gurgling sound on both inspiration and expiration. Coarse crackles indicate increas-

Interpreting wheezes

During auscultation, you're more likely to hear wheezing on expiration when the airways normally narrow. Hearing both inspiratory wheezes and expiratory wheezes usually indicates that your patient's condition is severe.

However, if your patient's wheezing stops, you shouldn't assume that his condition has improved. This change could mean that the affected portion of the airway has narrowed so much that no air is passing through it.

ing pulmonary congestion and usually won't clear with deep breathing or coughing.

Rhonchi. When thick secretions partially obstruct airflow through the large airways, rhonchi develop. Loud, coarse, and low-pitched, these sounds resemble snoring. You'll hear rhonchi most often on expiration and sometimes on inspiration. A patient may be able to clear rhonchi by coughing up secretions.

Wheezes. Like rhonchi, wheezes occur on expiration and sometimes on inspiration. Continuous, high-pitched, musical squeaks, wheezes result when air moves rapidly through airways narrowed by asthma or infection—or when an airway is partially obstructed by a tumor or foreign body.

In a patient with mild asthma, you'll probably hear bilateral wheezes on expiration. If his condition worsens, you'll hear wheezes on both expiration and inspiration. Unilateral, isolated wheezing usually indicates a tumor or foreign body obstruction. (See *Interpreting wheezes*.)

Pleural friction rubs. As the name suggests, these adventitious breath sounds result when inflamed visceral and parietal pleurae rub together. The distinctive grating sound resembles the sound made by rubbing leather. Pleural friction rubs may be caused by pleuritis, pneumonia, a tumor, or a pulmonary infarction extending into the pleural space. A small pleural effusion in a patient with cancer or one who is receiving hemodialysis may also cause a pleural friction rub.

Causes

Magnified breath sounds may indicate an area of consolidation. Because solid tissue transmits sound better than air or fluid, breath sounds (as well as spoken and whispered sounds) are louder than normal over an area of consolidation.

Diminished breath sounds may indicate an obstructed airway due to a foreign body or secretions, partial or total lung collapse, thickening of the pleurae, emphysema, or chronic lung disease. When pus, fluid, or air fills the pleural space, breath sounds are quieter than normal.

Absent breath sounds typically indicate loss of ventilation power. Underlying causes may include laryngospasm, bronchospasm, pneumonectomy, phrenic nerve palsy, pneumothorax, hemothorax, or a malpositioned endotracheal tube. If a foreign body or secretions obstruct a bronchus, breath sounds will be diminished or absent over distal lung tissue.

❖

Abnormal respirations

The rate, rhythm, and depth of your patient's respirations provide important clues to his respiratory status and overall condition. Abnormal respiratory patterns include tachypnea, bradypnea, apnea, hyperpnea, Kussmaul's respirations, Cheyne-Stokes respirations, and Biot's respirations. (See *Recognizing abnormal respiratory patterns*, page 64.)

History
Explore your patient's problem by asking appropriate questions.
• Did the breathing change occur suddenly or gradually? If it occurred suddenly, did anything happen just before its onset?
• Does the patient have any associated symptoms, such as seizures, headache, weakness, fatigue, nausea, vomiting, or diarrhea? Has he recently experienced flulike symptoms or upper respiratory infections?
• Does the patient have a chronic illness, such as diabetes, renal failure, chronic obstructive pulmonary disease, or thoracic cage

disorder? Has he recently been exposed to industrial toxins or pollutants? Does he have a history of head trauma, brain tumor, neurologic infection, or cerebrovascular accident?
• Has the patient used nonprescription drugs, such as laxatives and antacids, or undergone treatments, such as GI suctioning and diuretic therapy, which might predispose him to acid-base imbalance? (See *Respiratory acidosis: Recognizing predisposing conditions*, page 65.)
• Does the patient have a history of drug abuse? If so, try to determine which drugs he took, and by which route.
• Is the patient taking any prescribed medications that can affect respirations? If so, is he taking them as ordered?

Physical examination
Base your examination on the health history information you've collected.

Inspection
Observe the patient's respirations, noting rate and depth. Also, look for breathing difficulty and abnormal respiratory patterns, such as asymmetrical chest movement or paradoxical respirations. Assess for use of accessory muscles. Then assess his level of consciousness, noting belligerence, slow mental responses, restlessness, or disorientation. Does the patient have seizures, uncoordinated movements, or flapping tremors?

Check the arms and legs for needle marks, which may indicate drug abuse. Also inspect the skin for signs of dehydration, including dryness and poor turgor.

Recognizing abnormal respiratory patterns

Tachypnea
Shallow breathing with 20 or more breaths/minute

Bradypnea
Fewer than 10 breaths/minute but regular respirations; often precedes life-threatening apnea or respiratory arrest

Apnea
Absence of breathing; may be periodic, as in Biot's respirations, but more often a life-threatening emergency

Hyperpnea
Deep respirations at normal rate; also called hyperventilation

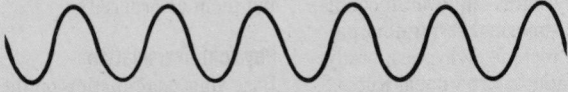

Kussmaul's respirations
Deep, rapid, sighing respirations without pauses; over 20 breaths/minute

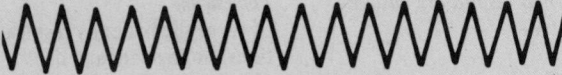

Cheyne-Stokes respirations
Respirations gradually becoming faster and deeper than normal and then slower; alternates with periods of apnea; the most common pattern of periodic breathing

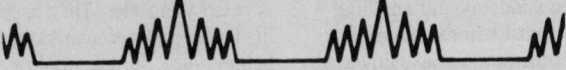

Biot's respirations
Fast, deep, equal respirations with abrupt pauses between them; a late, ominous sign of neurologic deterioration

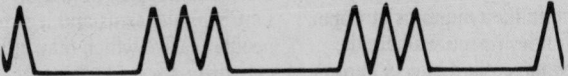

Respiratory acidosis: Recognizing predisposing conditions

The list below shows conditions that can predispose a patient to respiratory acidosis and common causes of those conditions.

Airway obstruction
- Aspiration
- Foreign bodies
- Pulmonary embolus
- Severe bronchospasm
- Pulmonary edema
- Laryngeal edema

Respiratory center depression
- Sedatives
- Chronic narcotic abuse
- Metabolic acidosis
- General anesthesia
- Increased intracranial pressure
- Medullary tumor
- Meningitis
- Vertebral artery embolus or thrombus

Muscle or nerve defects
- Myasthenia gravis
- Guillain-Barré syndrome
- Poliomyelitis
- Botulism
- Spinal cord injury
- Hypokalemia
- Hyperkalemia

Pulmonary disease
- Chronic obstructive pulmonary disease
- Smoke inhalation
- Pneumonia
- Atelectasis
- Asthma
- Interstitial lung disease
- Bronchitis
- Bronchiectasis

Thoracic cage disorders
- Flail chest
- Pneumothorax
- Pickwickian syndrome
- Ankylosing spondylitis

Palpation

Gently palpate the chest wall, sternum and, if possible, the posterior thorax for crepitus and bone pieces associated with rib or sternum fractures. Evaluate motor function, comparing the right and left sides for strength and muscle tone. Palpate the muscles for evidence of neuromuscular irritability and tetany. Palpate the peripheral pulses for rate, rhythm, and intensity.

Percussion

Test deep tendon reflexes (brachial, ulnar, patellar, Achilles). Note any abnormal responses.

Auscultation

Auscultate all lung fields for diminished or adventitious breath sounds, particularly crackles, rhonchi, and pleural friction rubs. Auscultate for heart sounds, noting any murmurs, pericardial friction rubs, or irregular rhythms. Check for hyperactive bowel sounds. Then monitor blood pressure and pulse pressure.

Causes

Tachypnea may result from pleuritic chest pain, restrictive lung disease, respiratory distress, and an elevated diaphragm.

Bradypnea may result from life-threatening metabolic alkalosis or respiratory acidosis. It can also result from such conditions as central nervous system depression, excessive sedation, diabetic coma, tumors of or trauma to the medulla, and narcotic overdose, which depress the brain's respiratory control centers.

Hyperpnea may result from anxiety, pain, metabolic acidosis, or exercise. In the comatose patient, this sign may indicate hypoxia or hypoglycemia.

Kussmaul's respirations are usually associated with metabolic acidosis.

Cheyne-Stokes respirations may result from brain damage, congestive heart failure, and uremia. This pattern may be normal in children and in elderly people during sleep.

Biot's respirations may be caused by respiratory depression and brain damage.

❖

Cyanosis

Bluish or bluish black discoloration of the skin and mucous membranes, cyanosis results from an excessive concentration of unoxygenated hemoglobin in the blood. It may develop abruptly or gradually and can be classified as central or peripheral, although the two types may exist together.

Central cyanosis reflects inadequate oxygenation of systemic arterial blood caused by right-to-left cardiac shunting, pulmonary disease, or hematologic disorders. The result is an excessive amount of unsaturated hemoglobin in the arterial blood. You may see central cyanosis anywhere on the skin, the mucous membranes of the mouth and lips, and the conjunctiva.

Peripheral cyanosis reflects sluggish peripheral circulation caused by vasoconstriction, reduced cardiac output, or vascular occlusion. This leads to reduced venous blood oxygen saturation. Peripheral cyanosis may be widespread, or it may occur just in one arm or leg. You won't see peripheral cyanosis on a patient's mucous membranes. Typically, you'll see it on the exposed areas, such as the fingers, nail beds, feet, nose, and ears.

Although cyanosis is an important sign of cardiovascular and pulmonary disorders, it isn't always an accurate gauge of oxygenation. Several factors contribute to its development, including hemoglobin concentration and oxygen saturation, cardiac output, and partial pressure of arterial oxygen. Although severe cyanosis is obvious, mild cyanosis is more difficult to detect—even in natural, bright light. In a dark-skinned patient, mild cyanosis is most apparent in the mucous membranes and nail beds.

History

Explore the patient's problem by asking appropriate questions.
• How long has the patient had the cyanosis? Does it subside and recur? Does it occur with fatigue or dyspnea? If the cyanosis is peripheral, is it aggravated by cold, smoking, or stress? Is it alleviated by massage or rewarming?
• Does the patient have a cough? Is it productive? If so, have him describe the sputum color and consistency.
• If the patient also has chest pain, how severe is it? Does it radiate? Does anything aggravate or alleviate it?
• Does he have any pain in his arms and legs – especially when he walks? Any abnormal sensations, such as numbness or tingling, coldness, weakness, or paralysis?
• Does the patient have a history of cardiac, pulmonary, or hematologic disorders, specifically rheumatic heart disease, myocardial infarction (MI), congestive heart failure (CHF), cardiogenic shock, cardiomyopathy, atherosclerosis, or prosthetic valves? Also ask about asthma, obstructive lung disease, thrombophlebitis, and varicose veins. Has the patient had an acute bleeding episode or septicemia? What about chest, hip, or leg trauma? Find out, too, about recent pregnancy, weight gain, exposure to allergens, or severe emotional stress.
• If the patient is a child, has he recently experienced a high fever, a muffled voice, a sore throat, drooling, dysphagia, restlessness, rhinitis, malaise, or anorexia?

• Which medications is the patient taking? Ask about drugs that can precipitate CHF, such as angiotensin-converting enzyme inhibitors, antihypertensives, beta blockers, calcium channel blockers, corticosteroids, nonsteroidal anti-inflammatory drugs, amiodarone, carbamazepine, flecainide, recombinant interferon alfa-2a, or recombinant interleukin-2. Has the patient recently received an ergot alkaloid injection, an intra-arterial drug injection, or mechanical ventilation under pressure? Does the patient use aspirin or indomethacin, which could precipitate asthma, or oral contraceptives, which could cause thrombophlebitis?

Physical examination

Base your examination on the health history information you've collected.

Inspection

Determine the extent of cyanosis by examining the patient's skin and mucous membranes for coolness, pallor or redness, and ulceration. Note whether the affected arm or leg blanches when elevated even slightly. Also note clubbing, edema, or neck vein distention.

Observe the patient's respirations, noting the rate and depth. Also, note any breathing difficulty or abnormal respiratory patterns. Check for nasal flaring, stridor, audible wheezes, muffled voice, barking cough, costal retraction, and use of accessory muscles. Inspect for asymmetrical chest expansion or barrel chest. Then observe the abdomen for ascites and a visible fluid wave.

Palpation

Check the rate, rhythm, and intensity of peripheral pulses, and test capillary refill time. Palpate the neck for enlarged lymph nodes, indicative of infection; the trachea for normal midline position; and the liver for enlargement and tenderness. Then palpate over the chest to detect decreased vocal or tactile fremitus, decreased diaphragmatic excursion, asymmetrical chest expansion, or subcutaneous crepitation. To evaluate muscle tone and strength, palpate the major muscles.

Percussion

Next, percuss over the liver to detect enlargement and tenderness and over the entire abdomen to detect shifting dullness. Also percuss over the lungs, noting hyperresonant or tympanic percussion notes.

Auscultation

As you auscultate for heart rate and rhythm, be alert for gallops and murmurs. Also auscultate the abdominal aorta and femoral arteries to detect any bruits. Auscultate the lungs for decreased or adventitious breath sounds, such as wheezes, crackles, or whispered pectoriloquy. Then monitor the patient's blood pressure and pulse pressure.

Causes

Your assessment may lead you to suspect one of these causes, some of which are life-threatening.

Asthma. In this life-threatening disorder, cyanosis is a late sign of hypoxemia resulting from airway obstruction. During an asthma attack, a patient typically experiences dyspnea, tachypnea, intercostal retraction during inspiration and intercostal bulging during expiration, accessory muscle use, and flaring nostrils. During a severe episode, you may note tachycardia, paradoxical pulses, wheezing, or decreased breath sounds. Associated findings may include hyperresonance, decreased vocal and tactile fremitus, and decreased diaphragmatic excursion. The patient may have a history of emotional stress, asthma, or recent exposure to an allergen. Or he may have recently taken aspirin, indomethacin, or beta blockers.

CHF. Typically, cyanosis is a late sign of this life-threatening disorder. The cyanosis may be central, peripheral, or both. In left ventricular failure, central cyanosis occurs along with tachycardia, fatigue, dyspnea, tachypnea, normal or low blood pressure, cold intolerance, orthopnea, cough, ventricular or atrial gallop, bibasilar crackles, and a diffuse apical impulse. Dependent edema, neck vein distention, and prolonged capillary refill time also may occur. In right ventricular failure, peripheral cyanosis occurs with fatigue, peripheral edema, ascites, jugular vein distention, and hepatomegaly.

Epiglottitis. In this life-threatening disorder, cyanosis is a late sign of hypoxemia resulting from airway obstruction by the swollen epiglottis. Earlier signs may include a high fever, muffled voice, sore throat, dysphagia, inspiratory stridor, use of accessory muscles of respiration, decreased breath sounds, tachycardia, anxiety, and drooling. The patient's history may reveal exposure to *Haemophilus influenzae*.

Laryngotracheobronchitis. In the acute stage of this life-threatening disorder, cyanosis can occur during a coughing episode. This harsh, barking cough typically is accompanied by accessory muscle use, restlessness, anxiety, stridor, and tachycardia. Auscultation reveals diminished breath sounds, crackles, and rhonchi. The patient may have a history of rhinitis, fever, malaise, and anorexia for 2 to 3 days before symptoms begin.

Peripheral arterial occlusion (acute). In this life-threatening disorder, central cyanosis of one arm or leg or, occasionally, of both legs occurs when the ischemic leg is placed in a dependent position. When elevated, the leg blanches. The cyanosis or pallor is accompanied by sharp or aching pain that worsens when the patient moves. Related findings in the affected limb include paresthesia, weakness, paralysis, and pale, cool skin. You may detect decreased or absent peripheral pulses, prolonged capillary refill time (greater than 2 seconds), and bruits over stenotic lesions.

Pneumonia. In this life-threatening disorder, central cyanosis typically is preceded by fever, shaking chills, and pleuritic chest pain that's exacerbated by deep inspiration. The patient may have a dry or productive cough, depending on the stage

and type of pneumonia. Sputum may be discolored and foul-smelling. Associated signs and symptoms can include decreased breath sounds, crackles, wheezing, dullness on percussion, whispered pectoriloquy, tachycardia, tachypnea, myalgia, fatigue, headache, dyspnea, abdominal pain, anorexia, and diaphoresis. Palpation may reveal increased fremitus.

Pneumothorax. A cardinal sign of life-threatening pneumothorax, central cyanosis is accompanied by dyspnea and sudden, sharp, severe chest pain. Often unilateral, this chest pain is rarely localized, and it increases with chest movement. When centrally located and radiating to the neck, the pain may mimic that of MI. Breath sounds are decreased or absent on the affected side with hyperresonance or tympany, subcutaneous crepitation, and decreased vocal fremitus. Asymmetrical chest expansion, accessory muscle use, nonproductive cough, tachypnea, tachycardia, anxiety, and restlessness also occur.

Pulmonary embolism. In this life-threatening disorder, central cyanosis occurs when a large embolus obstructs the pulmonary circulation. The cyanosis will be accompanied by the sudden dyspnea that's the hallmark of this disorder and by intense angina-like or pleuritic pain that's aggravated by deep breathing and thoracic movement. Other findings may include anxiety, tachycardia, tachypnea, nonproductive cough or one that produces blood-tinged sputum, low-grade fever, restlessness, diaphoresis, pleural friction rubs, crackles, diffuse wheezing, and dull percussion notes. The patient also may exhibit signs of circulatory collapse (a weak, rapid pulse and hypotension), signs of cerebral ischemia (transient unconsciousness, coma, and seizures), signs of hypoxia (restlessness), and—particularly in elderly patients—hemiplegia and other focal neurologic deficits.

Shock. With cardiogenic, hypovolemic, or septic shock, peripheral cyanosis or pallor develops in the hands and feet, which may also be cold and clammy. Related findings in these life-threatening disorders include lethargy, confusion, prolonged capillary refill time (greater than 2 seconds), and a rapid, weak pulse. You may also note tachypnea, hyperpnea, and hypotension.

Other causes. Cyanosis also results from bronchiectasis, Buerger's disease, chronic arteriosclerotic occlusive disease, chronic obstructive pulmonary disease, congenital heart defects that cause right-to-left intracardiac shunting, cystic fibrosis, deep vein thrombosis, lung cancer, methemoglobinemia, and Raynaud's disease.

_____ ❖

Dyspnea

Patients typically describe dyspnea as shortness of breath, but this symptom also refers to difficult or uncomfortable breathing. Its severity varies greatly and is often unrelated to the seriousness of the underlying cause. Dyspnea may arise suddenly or slowly and may subside rapidly or persist for years.

History
Explore your patient's problem by asking appropriate questions.
• When did the dyspnea first occur? Did it begin suddenly or gradually? Is it constant or intermittent? Does it occur during activity or while he's resting? Does anything seem to trigger, exacerbate, or relieve it? Has he ever had dyspnea before?
• Has the patient also had a productive or nonproductive cough or chest pain?
• Has the patient recently had an upper respiratory tract infection or experienced trauma? Does he smoke? If so, how much and for how long? Has he been exposed to any allergens or environmental pollutants? Does he have any known allergies?
• Which medications is he taking?

Physical examination
Observe the patient's respirations, noting their rate and depth, and any breathing difficulties or abnormal respiratory patterns. Check too for flaring nostrils, grunting respirations, inspiratory stridor, intercostal retractions during inspiration, and pursed-lip expirations.

Examine the patient for barrel chest, diaphoresis, neck vein distention, finger clubbing, and peripheral edema. Note the color, consistency, and odor of any sputum.

Palpate his chest for asymmetrical expansion, decreased diaphragmatic excursion, tactile

What causes ARDS?

Dyspnea is a characteristic sign in various conditions that may lead to adult respiratory distress syndrome (ARDS). The following list includes the most common underlying causes:
• aspiration of gastric contents
• drug ingestion and overdose
• hydrocarbon ingestion
• trauma and hemorrhagic shock
• near-drowning
• disseminated intravascular coagulation

• smoke or gas inhalation
• septic shock
• fat and air embolism
• severe pneumonitis (viral and other)
• oxygen toxicity
• cardiopulmonary bypass
• anaphylaxis
• uremia
• hemorrhagic pancreatitis
• head injury
• homologous blood transfusion
• pulmonary contusion.

fremitus, and subcutaneous crepitation. Also check the rate, rhythm, and intensity of his peripheral pulses.

As you percuss the lung fields, note dull, hyperresonant, or tympanic percussion sounds. Auscultate the lungs for bronchophony, crackles, decreased or absent unilateral breath sounds, egophony, pleural friction rubs, rhonchi, whispered pectoriloquy, and wheezing. Then auscultate the heart for abnormal sounds or rhythms, such as ventricular or atrial gallop, and for pericardial friction rubs and tachycardia. Be sure to monitor the patient's blood pressure and pulse pressure.

Causes
Your assessment may lead you to suspect one of these causes, all of which are potentially life-threatening.

ARDS. In life-threatening adult respiratory distress syndrome (ARDS), acute dyspnea is followed by accessory muscle use, crackles, grunting respirations, progressive respiratory distress, rhonchi, and wheezes. In the late stages, anxiety, cyanosis, decreased mental acuity, and tachycardia occur. Severe ARDS can produce signs of shock, such as cool, clammy skin and hypotension. The typical patient has no history of underlying cardiac or pulmonary disease but has sustained a recent pulmonary or systemic insult. (See *What causes ARDS?*)

Airway obstruction (partial). Inspiratory stridor and acute dyspnea occur as the patient tries to overcome the obstruction. Related findings in this potentially life-threatening disorder include accessory muscle use, anxiety, asymmetrical chest expansion, cyanosis, decreased or absent breath sounds, diaphoresis, hypotension, and tachypnea. The patient may have aspirated vomitus or a foreign body or been exposed to an allergen.

Asthma. In this life-threatening disorder, acute dyspneic attacks occur along with accessory muscle use, apprehension, dry cough, flushing or cyanosis, intercostal retractions, tachypnea, and tachycardia. On palpation, you'll detect decreased tactile fremitus. Hyperresonance occurs on chest percussion. On auscultation, you'll note wheezing and rhonchi or, during a severe episode, decreased breath sounds.

Congestive heart failure. Dyspnea usually develops gradually or occurs as chronic paroxysmal nocturnal dyspnea in this life-threatening disorder. In ventricular failure, dyspnea occurs with cough, basilar crackles, dependent peripheral edema, distended neck veins, fatigue, orthopnea, tachycardia, ventricular or atrial gallop, and weight gain. The patient may have a history of cardiovascular disease or may be taking drugs that can precipitate congestive heart failure (CHF), such as amiodarone, certain beta blockers, calcium channel blockers, or corticosteroids.

MI. Sudden dyspnea occurs with crushing substernal chest pain that may radiate to the back, neck, jaw, and arms in this life-threatening disorder. The patient's history may include heart disease, hypertension, hypercholesterolemia, or use of drugs that can precipitate myocardial infarction (MI), such as cocaine, dextrothyroxine sodium, estramustine phosphate sodium, or recombinant interleukin-2.

Pneumonia. Dyspnea occurs suddenly in this life-threatening disorder, usually accompanied by fever, pleuritic chest pain that worsens with deep inspiration, and shaking chills. The patient also has a dry or productive cough, depending on the stage and type of pneumonia. Sputum may be discolored and foul-smelling. Crackles, decreased breath sounds, dullness on percussion, and rhonchi may also be present. The history may include exposure to a contagious organism, hazardous fumes, or air pollution.

Pulmonary edema. In this life-threatening disorder, severe dyspnea is often preceded by signs of CHF, such as crackles in both lung fields, cyanosis, tachycardia, tachypnea, and marked anxiety. The patient may have a dry cough or one that produces copious amounts of pink, frothy sputum. The history may reveal cardiovascular disease – particularly mitral insufficiency, cardiomyopathy, or atrial fibrillation – cyanosis, fatigue, and pallor.

Pulmonary embolism. Severe dyspnea occurs with intense angina-like or pleuritic pain aggravated by deep breathing and thoracic movement in this life-threatening disorder. Other findings include crackles, cyanosis, diffuse wheezing, dull percussion sounds, low-grade fever, nonproductive cough, pleural friction rubs, restlessness, tachypnea, and tachycardia. The patient's history may include acute MI, CHF, hip or leg fractures, oral contraceptive use, pregnancy, prolonged bed rest, thrombophlebitis, or varicose veins.

Other disorders. Dyspnea may also result from anemia, anxiety, arrhythmias, cor pulmonale, inhalation injury, lung cancer, pleural effusion, and sepsis. ❖

Hemoptysis

The expectoration of blood or bloody sputum from the lungs or tracheobronchial tree is known as hemoptysis. Usually resulting from a tracheobronchial tree abnormality, hemoptysis is associated with inflammatory conditions or lesions that cause erosion and necrosis of bronchial tissues and blood vessels.

Sometimes, hemoptysis is confused with hematemesis: bleeding from the mouth, throat, nasopharynx, or GI tract. (See *Hemoptysis or hematemesis?*) Severe hemoptysis requires emergency endotracheal intubation and suctioning.

History

Explore your patient's problem by asking appropriate questions.
• When did the hemoptysis begin? How much blood or sputum is the patient expectorating? How often?
• Did the patient recently have a flulike syndrome? Has he had any recent invasive pulmonary procedures or chest trauma?
• Ask the patient if he smokes, or if he ever smoked. If so, how

RULE OF THUMB

Hemoptysis or hematemesis?

If your patient begins bleeding from his mouth, you'll need to determine if he's experiencing *hemoptysis* (coughing blood from the lungs) or *hematemesis* (vomiting blood from the stomach). Here's the rule of thumb for distinguishing the two conditions.
      It's hemoptysis if:
• it's bright red or pink, and frothy
• it's mixed with sputum
• it produces a negative litmus paper test (paper remains blue).
      It's hematemesis if:
• it's dark red, or has a coffee-ground appearance
• it's mixed with food
• it produces a positive litmus paper test (paper turns pink).

much? Does he have a history of cardiac, respiratory, or bleeding disorders?
• Which medications is the patient taking? Is he taking anticoagulants?
• Does he have a pulmonary artery catheter in place? If so, hemoptysis may indicate pulmonary artery rupture or infarction.

Physical examination

After assessing the patient's level of consciousness, examine his nose, mouth, and pharynx for sources of bleeding. Observe the rate and depth of his respirations, noting any breathing difficulty or abnormal breathing patterns. Also, as he breathes, look for abnormal chest movement, accessory muscle use, and retractions. Inspect the skin for central and peripheral cyanosis, diaphoresis, lesions, and pallor.

Palpate the rate, rhythm, and intensity of the peripheral pulses. Then feel the chest, noting abnormal pulsations, diaphragmatic tenderness, and fremitus. Check the level of the patient's diaphragm and assess respiratory excursion. If the patient has a history of trauma, carefully check the position of the trachea and note any edema.

As you percuss over the lung fields, note any dullness, flatness, hyperresonance, or tympany. Then auscultate the lungs for crackles, rhonchi, and wheezes, and the heart for bruits, gallops, murmurs, and pleural friction rubs. Be sure to monitor the patient's blood pressure and pulse pressure.

Causes

Your assessment may lead you to suspect one of the causes that follow.

Bronchitis (chronic). With this disorder, the patient usually has a productive cough that lasts at least 3 months and leads to expectoration of blood-streaked sputum. Other respiratory signs include dyspnea, prolonged expiration, scattered rhonchi, and wheezing.

Lung abscess. A patient with a life-threatening lung abscess expectorates copious amounts of bloody, purulent, foul-smelling sputum, especially if the abscess has penetrated the pulmonary vasculature. He also has anorexia, chills, diaphoresis, fever, headache, and pleuritic or dull chest pain. Lung auscultation may reveal tubular breath sounds or crackles. Percussion reveals dullness on the affected side. The patient may have a history of a recent pulmonary infection or evidence of poor oral hygiene with dental or gingival disease and is especially at risk if he's elderly or debilitated.

Lung cancer. In this life-threatening disorder, ulceration of the bronchus commonly causes recurring hemoptysis (an early sign), which can vary from blood-streaked sputum to blood. Related findings include anorexia, chest pain, dyspnea, fever, a productive cough, weight loss, and wheezing.

Pulmonary edema. A patient with life-threatening pulmonary edema may expectorate copious amounts of frothy, blood-tinged, pink sputum. He may also complain of dyspnea and orthopnea. On examination, you may detect diffuse crackles in both lung fields and a ventricular gallop.

Other disorders. Hemoptysis may also result from tracheal trauma, bronchiectasis, coagulation disorders, cystic fibrosis, primary pulmonary hypertension, and lung or airway injuries from diagnostic procedures, such as biopsy or pulmonary artery catheterization.

❖

Gastrointestinal signs and symptoms

Although abnormal bowel sounds may stem from a variety of causes, from benign to serious, abdominal pain often has a life-threatening cause that requires prompt action. A careful history-taking and physical examination can help determine the diagnosis.

Abdominal pain

Abdominal pain may originate in the abdominopelvic viscera, the parietal peritoneum, or the capsules of the liver, kidneys, or spleen. The pain may be acute or chronic, and diffuse or localized.

Visceral pain develops slowly into a dull ache that's poorly localized in the epigastric, periumbilical, or lower midabdominal region. By contrast, somatic pain develops quickly after an insult and is sharp and well localized. Moving or coughing aggravates it. Abdominal pain may also be referred from another site with the same or a similar nerve supply. (See *Recognizing types of abdominal pain*, pages 76 and 77.)

History

Explore your patient's problem by asking appropriate questions.
• When did the pain begin? What does it feel like? How long does it last? Where exactly is it? Does it radiate to other areas, such as the chest or back? Does it get better or worse when the patient changes position, moves, exerts himself, coughs, eats, or has a bowel movement?
• Find out if the patient had a fever during episodes of pain. Does he have appetite changes, constipation, diarrhea, nausea, pain with urination, pink or cloudy urine, vomiting, or urinary frequency or urgency?
• Does the patient have a history of adrenal disease, heart disease, recent infection, or recent blunt trauma to the abdomen, flank, or chest? Has he had any condition that could predispose him to emboli or that could narrow an arterial lumen? Has he recently undergone a urinary tract procedure or surgery? Has he traveled to a foreign country recently?
• Is the patient a woman of childbearing age? If so, what was the date of her last menses? Has her menstrual pattern changed? Could she be pregnant?
• Does the patient have a history of I.V. drug or alcohol abuse? Which prescription and over-the-counter drugs is he taking?

Physical examination

After assessing the patient's level of consciousness, observe his skin for diaphoresis, jaundice, and turgor. Then check for coolness, discoloration, and edema of the arms and legs. Inspect the abdomen and chest for signs of trauma: A bluish discoloration around the umbilicus (Cullen's sign) and around the flank area (Turner's sign) and ecchymosis of the scrotum or labia (Coopernail sign) can indicate blunt trauma. Obtain and record a baseline measurement of abdominal girth at the umbilicus.

Recognizing types of abdominal pain

AFFECTED ORGAN	VISCERAL PAIN
Stomach	Midepigastrium
Small intestine	Periumbilical area
Appendix	Periumbilical area
Proximal colon	Periumbilical area and right flank for ascending colon
Distal colon	Hypogastrium and left flank for descending colon
Gallbladder	Midepigastrium
Ureters	Costovertebral angle
Pancreas	Midepigastrium and left upper quadrant
Ovaries, fallopian tubes, and uterus	Hypogastrium and groin

After inspecting for neck vein distention, observe the rate and depth of respirations, noting any abnormal patterns. Observe the color and odor of the patient's urine.

Assess each abdominal quadrant with auscultation, percussion, and palpation. Auscultate first, because percussion and palpation can affect the frequency and intensity of bowel sounds. Listen for bowel sounds in each quadrant, noting whether the sounds are high pitched and tinkling, hyperactive, or absent. (See *Locating acute abdominal pain*, page 78.)

Then listen to the patient's heart and breath sounds for abnormalities. Be sure to monitor his blood pressure and pulse pressure. Also check peripheral pulses for rate, rhythm, and intensity.

Percuss each abdominal quadrant, noting tenderness, increased pain, and percussion sounds. The presence of dull percussion sounds indicates free fluid; hollow sounds, air.

As you systematically palpate the abdominal, pelvic, flank, and epigastric areas, note any enlarged organs, masses, rigidity, tenderness, rebound tenderness, or tenderness with guarding.

Causes
Your assessment may lead you to suspect one of these causes, some of which are life-threatening.

Abdominal aortic aneurysm (dissecting). In this life-threatening

PARIETAL PAIN	REFERRED PAIN
Midepigastrium and left upper quadrant	Shoulders
Over affected site	Midback (rare)
Right lower quadrant	Right lower quadrant
Over affected site	Right lower quadrant and back (rare)
Over affected site	Left lower quadrant and back (rare)
Right upper quadrant	Right subscapular area
Over affected site	Groin; scrotum in men, labia in women (rare)
Midepigastrium and left upper quadrant	Back and left shoulder
Over affected site	Inner thighs

disorder, constant, dull upper abdominal pain radiating to the lower back typically accompanies rapid aneurysmal enlargement and may herald a rupture. Palpation may reveal an epigastric mass that pulsates before rupture. On auscultation, you may detect a systolic bruit over the aneurysm. You may also note abdominal rigidity, increasing abdominal girth, and signs of hypovolemic shock.

Abdominal trauma. The patient may have generalized or localized abdominal pain along with abdominal ecchymosis, labial or scrotal ecchymosis (Coopernail sign), abdominal tenderness, or vomiting in this potentially life-threatening disorder. If he is hemorrhaging into the perito-

neal cavity, you may note abdominal rigidity, dullness on percussion, and increasing abdominal girth. The patient may have signs and symptoms of hypovolemic shock, if a large abdominal blood vessel has ruptured, or of septic shock, if intestinal contents have entered the peritoneum. You may hear hollow bowel sounds if an abdominal organ has been perforated, or bowel sounds may be absent. Bowel sounds heard in the chest cavity usually signal a diaphragmatic tear.

Appendicitis. The patient with this potentially life-threatening disorder may have sudden pain in the epigastric or umbilical region that increases over a few hours or days, along with flulike

Locating acute abdominal pain

These common causes of acute abdominal pain are grouped according to the abdominal quadrant where the pain may be felt.

Right upper quadrant
Acute cholecystitis
Biliary colic
Pancreatitis
Perforated duodenal ulcer
Hepatitis
Retrocecal appendicitis
Subphrenic abscess
Right-sided nephrolithiasis
Herpes zoster
Myocardial ischemia
Right-sided lower lobe
   pneumonia

Left upper quadrant
Gastritis
Gastric ulcers
Pancreatitis
Splenic rupture
Diverticulitis
Left-sided nephrolithiasis
Herpes zoster
Myocardial ischemia
Left-sided lower lobe
   pneumonia
Pulmonary embolism
Pericarditis

Right lower quadrant
Appendicitis
Cecal perforation
Regional enteritis
Intestinal obstruction
Crohn's disease
Diverticulosis
Ectopic pregnancy
Ovarian cyst
Salpingitis
Strangulated hernia
Kidney or ureteral stone

Left lower quadrant
Sigmoid perforation
Sigmoid diverticulitis
Early appendicitis
Ulcerative colitis
Colon perforation
Salpingitis
Ovarian cyst
Ectopic pregnancy
Strangulated hernia
Kidney or ureteral stone

symptoms. Anorexia, constipation or diarrhea, nausea, and vomiting precede the pain, which may be dull or severe. Pain localizes at McBurney's point in the right lower quadrant. Abdominal rigidity and rebound tenderness may also occur.

Ectopic pregnancy. Lower abdominal pain may be sharp, dull, or cramping, and either constant or intermittent. The pain may be accompanied by breast tenderness, nausea, vaginal bleeding, vomiting, and urinary frequency. The patient typically has a 1- to 2-month history of amenorrhea after sexual intercourse. Rupture of the fallopian tube produces sharp lower abdominal pain, which may radiate to the shoulders and neck and become extreme on cervical or adnexal palpation.

Hepatitis. Liver enlargement from any type of hepatitis causes discomfort or dull pain and tenderness in the right upper quadrant. Associated signs and symptoms of this potentially life-threatening disorder include anorexia, clay-colored stools, dark urine, jaundice, low-grade fever, pruritus, nausea, and vomiting.

Intestinal obstruction. With this life-threatening disorder, short episodes of intense, colicky, cramping pain alternate with pain-free periods. Accompanying signs and symptoms include constipation, pain-induced agitation, tympany, visible peristaltic waves, and abdominal distention, tenderness, and guarding. You may note high-pitched, tinkling, or hyperactive bowel sounds proximal to the obstruction and lower-pitched, hypoactive, or absent bowel sounds distal to the obstruction.

Pancreatitis. The characteristic symptom of pancreatitis is fulminating, continuous upper abdominal pain that may radiate to both flanks and to the back. Abdominal tenderness, fever, nausea, pallor, tachycardia, and vomiting may also occur. Some patients with this potentially life-threatening disorder have abdominal distention and rigidity, hypoactive bowel sounds, and rebound tenderness. The patient's history may include a family history of pancreatitis, alcohol abuse, gallbladder disease, trauma, a scorpion bite, or ingestion of a drug that can cause pancreatitis—such as a thiazide

diuretic. Pancreatitis often occurs after endoscopic procedures and cardiopulmonary bypass.

Other causes. Abdominal pain may result from adrenal crisis, cholecystitis, congestive heart failure, diabetic ketoacidosis, diverticulitis, hepatic abscess, mesenteric artery ischemia, myocardial infarction, an ovarian cyst, a perforated ulcer, peritonitis, pneumonia, pneumothorax, pyelonephritis, renal calculi, renal infarction, and splenic infarction. Also, salicylates and nonsteroidal anti-inflammatory drugs can produce abdominal pain.

❖

Abnormal bowel sounds

Abnormal bowel sounds are any sounds other than the soft bubbling of air and fluid moving through the bowel. Auscultating the abdomen to identify these sounds provides information on bowel motility and the underlying vessels and organs.

History

Explore your patient's problem by asking appropriate questions.
• Is the patient in pain? If so, when did the pain begin? Has it gotten worse? Where exactly is the pain? Is it localized or generalized? Does it radiate to another area?
• Ask if the patient has been vomiting. If so, find out when it started, how often it occurs, and whether the vomitus looks bloody.

Auscultating the abdomen

Warm the stethoscope and your hands before you begin auscultating a patient's abdomen. Muscular contraction in response to cold could alter your findings. You'll auscultate for bowel sounds throughout all four quadrants, using the diaphragm of the stethoscope. Then, using the bell of the stethoscope, listen for vascular sounds in the sites shown.

Auscultation sites for vascular sounds

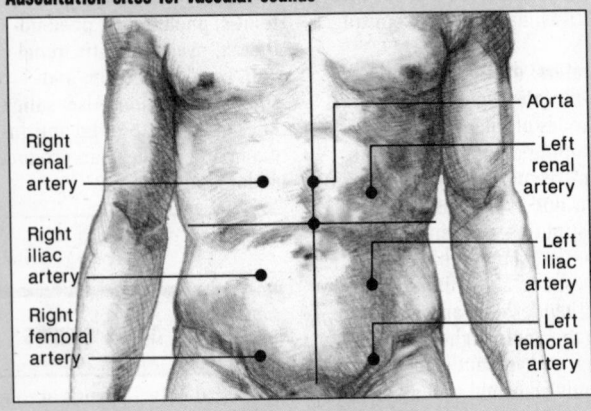

• Have the patient's bowel habits changed recently? Note if he's been constipated. Ask when he last had a bowel movement or expelled flatus. Has he had diarrhea or passed pencil-thin stools?
• Did the patient have an accident that could have caused vascular clots?
• Has the patient ever had a condition that could cause an obstruction—an abdominal tumor or hernia, for example? What about abdominal or pelvic surgery or radiation therapy that may cause obstruction or adhesions? Has the patient had a condition that could cause paralytic ileus, such as pancreatitis;

a bowel inflammation or a gynecologic infection, which may produce peritonitis; a toxic condition such as uremia; or a spinal cord injury?
• Is the patient taking any drugs that decrease peristalsis, such as opiates, anticholinergics, phenothiazines, tricyclic antidepressants, or vinca alkaloids?

Physical examination

After inspecting the patient's abdomen, use the diaphragm of the stethoscope to auscultate all four quadrants for bowel and vascular sounds. Be sure to auscultate for at least 2 to 5 minutes. (See *Auscultating the abdomen.*)

The normal sounds of peristalsis will have no regular pattern and are often interspersed with soft clicks and gurgles every 5 to 15 seconds. A hungry patient may have a familiar "stomach growl," a condition of hyperperistalsis called borborygmi. Rapid, high-pitched, loud, and gurgling, these *hyperactive* bowel sounds may occur normally. Sounds occurring at a rate of one every minute or longer are *hypoactive* and normally occur after bowel surgery or when the colon is filled with feces. Note any hyperactive or hypoactive sounds you don't think are related to digestion. Note any hepatic sounds such as friction rubs. (See *Identifying abnormal abdominal sounds,* page 82.)

Before reporting absent bowel sounds, be sure the patient has an empty bladder; a full bladder may obscure sounds. Gently pressing on the abdominal surface may initiate peristalsis and audible bowel sounds, as will having the patient eat or drink something.

Finally, use the bell of the stethoscope to auscultate for vascular sounds such as systolic bruits or a venous hum. (See *Detecting vascular sounds,* page 83.)

Causes

Your assessment may lead you to suspect one of these conditions or causes, some of which are life-threatening.

Mechanical intestinal obstruction. In this potentially life-threatening disorder, hypoactive bowel sounds follow a period of hyperactive bowel sounds. The patient may also have acute, colicky abdominal pain in the quadrant of obstruction, possibly radiating to the flank or lumbar regions.

Associated signs and symptoms include abdominal distention and bloating, constipation, nausea, and vomiting. The higher the blockage, the earlier and more severe the vomiting. You may palpate an abdominal mass. In the late stages, the patient may have a fever, rebound tenderness, and abdominal rigidity. Tachycardia, tachypnea, hypotension, and cool, clammy skin indicate shock associated with dehydration and hypovolemia.

Mesenteric artery infarction. After a brief period of hyperactivity, bowel sounds become hypoactive and then quickly stop in this life-threatening disorder. The patient feels sudden, colicky, severe midepigastric or periumbilical pain, which becomes more severe and generalized as the infarction progresses.

Other possible signs and symptoms include abdominal distention, copious vomiting, bloody diarrhea, constipation, fever, and bruits. Fever above 102° F (39° C), abdominal rigidity, and other signs of peritonitis signify necrosis.

Paralytic (adynamic) ileus. The cardinal sign of this life-threatening disorder is hypoactive bowel sounds that may stop. Associated signs and symptoms include abdominal distention, generalized discomfort, tympany, and constipation or flatus with small, liquid stools. If the disorder follows an acute abdominal infection, the patient may also have a fever and abdominal pain.

Identifying abnormal abdominal sounds

During abdominal auscultation you may hear several abnormal sounds, including abnormal bowel sounds, systolic bruits, venous hum, and friction rub. This chart lists the best places to listen for each sound and explains what they may mean.

SOUND AND DESCRIPTION	LOCATION	POSSIBLE CAUSE
Bowel sounds Sounds created by air and fluid movement through the bowel	• All four quadrants	• Hyperactive sounds unrelated to hunger: diarrhea or early intestinal obstruction • Hypoactive, then absent, sounds: paralytic ileus or peritonitis • High-pitched "tinkling" sounds: intestinal fluid and air under tension in a dilated bowel • High-pitched "rushing" sounds coinciding with an abdominal cramp: intestinal obstruction
Systolic bruits Vascular "blowing" sounds resembling cardiac murmurs	• Abdominal aorta • Renal artery • Iliac artery	• Partial arterial obstruction or turbulent blood flow, as in dissecting abdominal aneurysm • Renal artery stenosis • Hepatomegaly
Venous hum Continuous, medium-pitched tone created by blood flow in a large, engorged vascular organ such as the liver	• Epigastric region and umbilicus	• Increased collateral circulation between portal and systemic venous systems, as in hepatic cirrhosis
Friction rub Harsh, grating sound resembling two pieces of sandpaper rubbing together	• Hepatic	• Inflammation of the peritoneal surface of an organ, as from a liver tumor

His history may include recent abdominal surgery or any peritoneal insult. Paralytic ileus may also develop with a spinal, pelvic, or rib fracture; trauma; retroperitoneal hemorrhage; pyelonephritis; ureteral calculi; pneumonia; myocardial infarction; sepsis; or metabolic abnormalities.

Pancreatitis. In this potentially life-threatening disorder, hypoactive bowel sounds often accompany the cardinal signs of acute pancreatitis – abdominal rigidity and fulminating, continuous upper abdominal pain that may radiate to the flanks and back. To relieve the pain, the patient may bend forward, draw his knees to his chest, or move about restlessly. Other signs and symptoms include abdominal distention, abdominal tenderness, rebound tenderness, nausea, vomiting, fever, pallor, and tachycardia. Turner's or Cullen's sign may indicate hemorrhagic pancreatitis. The patient may have a history of alcohol abuse or use of drugs that may cause pancreatitis. His history may also include gallbladder disease, a scorpion bite, diabetes mellitus, or trauma.

Drugs. Certain drugs reduce intestinal motility, causing hypoactive bowel sounds. These include opiates such as codeine, anticholinergics such as propantheline bromide, phenothiazines such as chlorpromazine, tricyclic antidepressants such as amitriptyline, vinca alkaloids such as vincristine, and calcium channel blockers such as nifedipine. General or spinal anesthetics produce transient hypoactive sounds.

RULE OF THUMB

Detecting vascular sounds

Normally, on auscultation of the abdomen, you should detect no vascular sounds.

Detecting sounds over vascular areas signals a disorder that may be life-threatening. Bruits, for example, signify a narrowed or enlarged blood vessel that alters blood flow, causing turbulence.

Neurologic symptoms

Dizziness, headache, and paresthesia are common neurologic symptoms that may – or may not – accompany a serious disorder. A careful history that reveals details of onset, severity, and associated signs and symptoms will guide your physical assessment.

Dizziness

A common symptom, dizziness is a sensation of imbalance or faintness sometimes associated with blurred or double vision, confusion, and weakness. Dizziness may be mild or severe, and may start abruptly or gradually. It may be aggravated by standing up quickly and alleviated by lying down. Episodes are usually brief.

Dizziness typically results from inadequate blood flow and oxygen supply to the cerebrum and spinal cord. It may occur with anxiety, respiratory and cardiovascular disorders, and postconcussion syndrome. Dizziness is also a key symptom of certain serious disorders, including hypertension and vertebrobasilar artery insufficiency.

History
Explore the patient's problem by asking appropriate questions.
• When did the dizziness start? How severe is it? How often does it occur, and how long does each episode last? Does the dizziness abate spontaneously? Is it triggered by standing up suddenly or bending over?
• Does the patient have blurred vision, chest pain, a chronic cough, diaphoresis, a headache, or shortness of breath?
• Does the patient have a history of hypertension or another cardiovascular disorder? Also ask about diabetes mellitus, anemia, respiratory or anxiety disorders, and head injury.
• Which medications is the patient taking?

Physical examination
Assess the patient's level of consciousness, respirations, and body temperature. As you observe his breathing, look for accessory muscle use or barrel chest. Look also for finger clubbing, cyanosis, dry mucous membranes, and poor skin turgor. Then evaluate the patient's

motor and sensory functions and reflexes.

Palpate the extremities for peripheral edema and capillary refill. Then auscultate the patient's heart rate and rhythm and his breath sounds. Take his blood pressure while he's lying down, sitting, and standing. If the diastolic pressure exceeds 100 mm Hg, notify the doctor immediately and have the patient lie down.

Causes
Your assessment may lead you to suspect one of the causes that follow.

Cardiac arrhythmias. Dizziness lasts for several minutes or longer and may precede fainting in this potentially life-threatening disorder. Other signs and symptoms include blurred vision, confusion, hypotension, palpitations, paresthesia, weakness, and an irregular, rapid, or thready pulse.

Hypertension. Dizziness may precede fainting but may be relieved by rest in this potentially life-threatening disorder. Other findings include blurred vision; elevated blood pressure; headache; and retinal changes, such as hemorrhage, exudate discharge, and papilledema.

Transient ischemic attack. Dizziness of varying severity occurs in this potentially life-threatening disorder. Lasting from a few seconds to 24 hours, an attack may be triggered by turning the head to the side and typically signals an impending cerebrovascular accident. During an attack, blindness or visual field deficits, diplopia, hearing loss, numbness, paresis, ptosis, and tinnitus may also occur.

Other causes. Dizziness may result from anemia, generalized anxiety disorder, orthostatic hypotension, panic disorder, and postconcussion syndrome. Also, dizziness may be an adverse reaction to certain drugs, including antianxiety agents, central nervous system depressants, narcotic analgesics, decongestants, antihistamines, antihypertensives, and vasodilators.

Headache

The most common neurologic symptom, a headache may be mild to severe, localized or generalized, constant or intermittent. About 90% of all headaches are benign and can be described as vascular, muscle-contraction, or a combination of both.

Headaches can occasionally indicate a severe neurologic disorder. A generalized, pathologic headache may result from disorders associated with intracranial inflammation, increased intracranial pressure (ICP), meningeal irritation, or a vascular disturbance. A headache may also result from eye and sinus disorders and from the effects of drugs, tests, and treatments.

History

Explore your patient's problem by asking appropriate questions.
• When did the headache first occur? Is the pain mild, moderate, or severe? Is it localized or generalized? If it's localized, where does it occur? Is it constant or intermittent? If it's intermittent, how long does it last? Have the patient describe the pain: Is it stabbing, dull, throbbing, or viselike? Does anything trigger it or make it better or worse?
• Has the patient also experienced confusion, dizziness, drowsiness, eye pain, fever, muscle twitching, nausea, photophobia, seizures, speaking or walking difficulties, neck stiffness, visual disturbances, vomiting, or weakness?
• Has the patient been under unusual stress at home or at work? Has his family noticed any changes in his behavior or personality?
• Does he have a history of blood dyscrasia, cardiovascular disease, glaucoma, hemorrhagic disorders, hypertension, poor vision, seizures, or smoking? Has he had any recent traumatic injuries; dental work; or sinus, ear, or systemic infections?
• Which medications is the patient taking?

Physical examination

Check the rate and depth of the patient's respirations, and note any breathing difficulty or abnormal patterns. Then inspect his head for bruising, swelling, and sinus bleeding. Check also for Battle's sign, neck stiffness, otorrhea, and rhinorrhea.

Assess the patient's level of consciousness (LOC): Is he drowsy, lethargic, or comatose? Examine his eyes, noting pupil size, equality, and response to light. With the patient both at rest and active, note any tremors.

Gently palpate the skull and sinuses for tenderness. Unless head trauma has occurred, slowly move the neck to check for nuchal rigidity or pain. Then assess the patient's motor strength. Palpate his peripheral pulses, noting their rate, rhythm, and intensity.

Check for a positive Babinski's reflex. As you percuss for other reflexes, note any hyperreflexia. Then auscultate over the temporal artery, listening for bruits. Be sure to monitor the patient's blood pressure and pulse pressure.

Causes

After assessing the patient, you may suspect one of the causes that follow.

Brain abscess. A headache stemming from a brain abscess typically intensifies over a few days, localizes to a particular spot, and is aggravated by straining. The headache may be accompanied by a decreased LOC (drowsiness to deep stupor), focal or generalized seizures, nausea, and vomiting. Depending on the abscess site in this life-threatening disorder, the patient may also have aphasia, ataxia, impaired visual acuity, hemiparesis, personality changes, or tremors. Signs of an infection may or may not appear. The patient's history may include systemic, chronic middle ear, mastoid, or sinus infection; osteomyelitis of the skull or a compound fracture; or a penetrating head wound.

Brain tumor. In this life-threatening disorder, the headache initially develops near the tumor site and becomes generalized as the tumor grows. Pain is usually intermittent, deep-seated, dull, and most intense in the morning. It's aggravated by coughing, stooping, Valsalva's maneuver, and changes in head position.

Cerebral aneurysm (ruptured). The headache in this life-threatening disorder is sudden and excruciating. It may be unilateral and usually peaks within minutes of the rupture. The headache may be accompanied by nausea, vomiting, and signs of meningeal irritation. The patient may lose consciousness and experience seizures. His history may include hypertension or other cardiovascular disorders, a stressful lifestyle, or smoking.

Encephalitis. The patient with this life-threatening disorder has a severe, generalized headache accompanied by a deteriorating LOC over a 48-hour period. Fever, focal neurologic deficits, irritability, nausea, nuchal rigidity, photophobia, seizures, and vomiting may also develop. His history may reveal exposure to the viruses that commonly cause encephalitis, such as mumps or herpes simplex.

Epidural hemorrhage (acute). A progressively severe headache immediately follows a brief loss of consciousness in this life-threatening disorder. Then the patient's LOC rapidly and steadily declines. Accompanying signs and symptoms include increasing ICP, ipsilateral pupil dilation, nausea, and vomiting. The patient's history usually reveals head trauma within the past 24 hours.

Hypertension. Patients with potentially life-threatening hypertension may have a slightly throbbing occipital headache on awakening. During the day, the severity may decrease. But if the patient's diastolic blood pressure exceeds 120 mm Hg, the headache remains constant.

Meningitis. The patient with this life-threatening disorder experiences a severe, constant, generalized headache that starts suddenly and worsens with movement. He may also have chills, fever, hyperreflexia, nuchal rigidity, and positive Kernig's and Brudzinski's signs. His history may include recent systemic or sinus infection, dental work, trauma, ICP monitoring, or exposure to bacteria or viruses that commonly cause meningitis, such as *Haemophilus influenzae*, *Streptococcus pneumoniae*, enteroviruses, and mumps.

Migraine. A severe, throbbing headache, migraine may follow a 5- to 15-minute prodrome of dizziness; tingling of the face, lips, or hands; unsteady gait; and visual disturbances. Other signs and symptoms include anorexia, nausea, photophobia, and vomiting.

Subarachnoid hemorrhage. This life-threatening disorder causes a sudden, violent headache along with dizziness, hypertension, ipsilateral pupil dilation, nausea, nuchal rigidity, seizures, vomiting, and an altered LOC that may rapidly progress to coma. The patient's history may include congenital vascular defects, arteriovenous malformation, cardio-vascular disease, smoking, or excessive stress.

Subdural hematoma. In this life-threatening disorder, severe, localized headache usually follows head trauma that causes an immediate loss of consciousness, a latent period of drowsiness, confusion or personality changes, and agitation. Later, signs of increased ICP may develop. If the head trauma occurred within 3 days of the onset of signs and symptoms, the hematoma is acute; within 3 weeks, subacute; after more than 3 weeks, chronic. About 50% of patients with this disorder have no history of head trauma.

Other disorders. Cervical traction, acute angle-closure glaucoma, lumbar puncture, myelography, acute sinusitis, use of vasodilators, and withdrawal from vasopressors or sympathomimetic drugs can also cause headache. Indomethacin, digoxin, aspirin, and anticoagulants such as warfarin sodium can do the same.

Paresthesia

Paresthesia is an abnormal sensation commonly described as a numbness, prickling, or tingling, that's felt along peripheral nerve pathways. It may develop suddenly or gradually and be transient or permanent. A common symptom of many neurologic disorders, paresthesia may also occur in certain systemic disorders and with the use of certain drugs.

History

Explore your patients' problem by asking appropriate questions.
• When did the paresthesia begin? What does it feel like? Where does it occur? Is it transient or constant?
• Has the patient had recent trauma, surgery, or an invasive procedure that may have injured peripheral nerves? Has he been exposed to industrial solvents or heavy metals? Ask if he's had long-term radiation therapy. What about neurologic, cardiovascular, metabolic, renal, or chronic inflammatory disorders, such as arthritis or systemic lupus erythematosus?
• Which medications is the patient taking?

Physical examination

Focus on the patient's neurologic status, assessing his level of consciousness and cranial nerve function. Also note his skin color and temperature.

Test muscle strength and deep tendon reflexes in the extremities affected by paresthesia. Systematically evaluate light touch, pain, temperature, vibration, and position sensation. Then palpate his pulses.

Causes

Your assessment may lead you to suspect one of the causes that follow.

Arterial occlusion (acute). In this life-threatening disorder, the patient with a saddle embolism may complain of sudden paresthesia and coldness in one or both legs. Aching pain at rest,

intermittent claudication, and paresis are also characteristic. The leg becomes mottled, and a line of temperature and color demarcation develops at the level of the occlusion. Pulses are absent below the occlusion and capillary refill is diminished.

Brain tumor. Tumors that affect the parietal lobe are life-threatening and may cause progressive contralateral paresthesia accompanied by agnosia, agraphia, apraxia, homonymous hemianopia, loss of proprioception, and seizures.

Herniated disk. Herniation of a lumbar or cervical disk may cause acute or gradual paresthesia along the distribution pathways of the affected spinal nerves. Other neuromuscular effects include muscle spasms, severe pain, and weakness.

Herpes zoster. Paresthesia, an early symptom of herpes zoster, occurs in the dermatome supplied by the affected spinal nerve. Within several days, this dermatome is marked by a pruritic, erythematous, vesicular rash accompanied by sharp, shooting pain.

Spinal cord injury. Paresthesia may occur in a partial spinal cord transection after spinal shock resolves. The paresthesia may be unilateral or bilateral and occur at or below the level of the lesion in this potentially life-threatening disorder.

Other causes. Paresthesia may result from arthritis, a cerebrovascular accident, a migraine headache, multiple sclerosis, peripheral neuropathies, vitamin B_{12} deficiency, hypocalcemia, and heavy metal or solvent poisoning. Also, long-term radiation therapy, parenteral gold therapy, and certain drugs – such as phenytoin, chemotherapeutic agents, D-penicillamine, and isoniazid – may cause paresthesia.   ❖

Genitourinary sign

Among genitourinary signs and symptoms, hematuria is a cardinal sign of renal and urinary tract disorders. However, it can point to a range of upper and lower urinary tract disorders. Careful investigation into the onset and quality of the bleeding and associated complaints leads to a differential diagnosis.

Hematuria

The presence of blood in the urine, hematuria may be evident or confirmed by a urine test for occult blood. The bleeding may be continuous or intermittent, is often accompanied by pain, and may be aggravated by prolonged standing or walking. Dark or brownish blood indicates renal or upper urinary tract bleeding; bright red blood, lower urinary tract bleeding.

History
Explore your patient's problem by asking appropriate questions.
• When did the patient first notice the hematuria? Does it occur every time he urinates? Is he passing any clots? Has he ever had hematuria before?
• Does the patient have any pain? If so, does the pain occur only when he urinates, or is it continuous?
• Does the patient have bleeding hemorrhoids? Has he had any recent trauma or performed any strenuous exercise? Does he have a history of renal, urinary, prostatic, or coagulation disorders? Is the female patient menstruating?
• Which medications is the patient taking?

Physical examination
Check the urinary meatus for any bleeding or abnormalities. Palpate the abdomen and flanks, noting any pain or tenderness. Finally, percuss the abdomen and flanks, especially the costovertebral angle, to elicit any tenderness.

Causes
Your examination may lead you to suspect one of the following causes.

Bladder cancer. A primary cause of gross hematuria in men, bladder cancer may produce pain in the bladder, rectum, pelvis, flank, back, or leg. With this potentially life-threatening disorder, you may also note signs and symptoms of urinary tract infection.

Calculi. Both bladder and renal calculi produce hematuria, which may be accompanied by signs and symptoms of urinary tract infection. Both types of calculi are potentially life-threatening. Bladder calculi usually produce gross hematuria, pain referred to the penile or vulvar area and, in some patients, bladder distention. Renal calculi may produce either microscopic or gross hematuria.

Glomerulonephritis. Usually, acute glomerulonephritis begins with gross hematuria. This life-threatening disorder may also produce anuria or oliguria, flank and abdominal pain, and increased blood pressure. Chronic glomerulonephritis typically causes microscopic hematuria accompanied by generalized edema, increased blood pressure, and proteinuria.

Nephritis. Acute nephritis causes fever, a maculopapular rash, and microscopic hematuria. In chronic interstitial nephritis, the patient may have dilute, almost colorless urine along with polyuria. Both forms may be life-threatening.

Pyelonephritis (acute). A typical sign of life-threatening pyelonephritis is microscopic or macroscopic hematuria that progresses to grossly bloody hematuria. After the infection resolves, microscopic hematuria may persist for a few months. Other related findings include flank pain, high fever, and signs and symptoms of a urinary tract infection.

Renal infarction. Patients with renal infarction usually have gross hematuria. Other signs and symptoms of this life-threatening disorder include anorexia, costovertebral angle tenderness, and constant, severe flank and upper abdominal pain.

Other causes. Hematuria may result from benign prostatic hyperplasia, bladder trauma, obstructive nephropathy, polycystic kidney disease, renal trauma, and urethral trauma. Also, diagnostic tests — such as cystoscopy and renal biopsy — and drugs — such as anticoagulants, oxyphenbutazone, and thiabendazole — may cause hematuria.

3 Interpreting Puzzling Laboratory Findings

Coagulation tests

Cultures

Electrolyte tests

Fecal content tests

Hepatic enzyme tests

Immune function tests

Lipid and lipoprotein tests

Protein, protein metabolite, and pigment tests

Urinalysis

PUZZLING LAB
FINDINGS

Biopsies

With biopsies, laboratory findings may be compromised by poor collection technique. Tissue breaks down immediately after removal from the body, so a specimen must be placed immediately in fixing fluid and sent to the laboratory. If this isn't possible, refrigeration will preserve a specimen for up to 24 hours.

Bone marrow aspiration and biopsy

Bone marrow, the soft tissue contained in the medullary canals of long bone and in the interstices of cancellous bone, may be removed by aspiration or needle biopsy under local anesthetic.

Contraindicated in patients with severe bleeding disorders, these tests help diagnose thrombocytopenia; leukemia; granulomas; aplastic, hypoplastic, and pernicious anemia; and primary and metastatic tumors. Bone marrow biopsy can also determine the cause of infection, and aid in the staging of disease. Finally, it's used to evaluate the effectiveness of chemotherapy and to help monitor myelosuppression.

Normal findings

Both red and yellow marrow contain fat cells and connective tissue. Red marrow also contains hematopoietic cells.

Special stains that detect hematologic disorders produce these normal findings: The iron stain, which measures hemosiderin (storage iron), has a +2 level; the Sudan Black B (SBB) stain, which shows granulocytes, is negative; and the periodic acid-Schiff (PAS) stain, which detects glycogen reactions, is negative.

Problematic findings

Histologic examination of a bone marrow specimen can help detect myelofibrosis, granulomas, lymphoma, or cancer. Hematologic analysis, including the differential count and myeloid-erythroid ratio, can implicate a wide range of disorders.

In an iron stain, decreased hemosiderin levels may indicate a true iron deficiency. Elevated levels may accompany other types of anemia or blood disorders. A positive SBB stain can differentiate acute granulocytic leukemia from acute lymphocytic leukemia (SBB negative) or may indicate granulation in myeloblasts. A positive PAS stain may indicate acute or chronic lymphocytic leukemia, amyloidosis, thalassemia, lymphomas, infectious mononucleosis, iron-deficiency anemia, or sideroblastic anemia.

Interfering factors

Failure to obtain a representative specimen, to use a histologic fixative, or to send the specimen immediately to the laboratory may alter test results.

❖

Breast biopsy

Although mammography, thermography, and X-rays aid diagnosis of breast masses, only histologic examination of breast tis-

Precautions with lung biopsy

Needle biopsy shouldn't be used in patients with a lesion that's separated from the chest wall or that's accompanied by emphysematous bullae, cysts, or gross emphysema. It also shouldn't be used in patients with coagulopathy, hypoxia, pulmonary hypertension, or cardiac disease with cor pulmonale.

During the biopsy, observe your patient for signs of respiratory distress: shortness of breath, elevated pulse, and cyanosis (late sign). If any of these develop, report them immediately.

Because coughing or movement during the biopsy can cause the biopsy needle to tear the lung, the patient will be sedated before the biopsy to help him remain calm and still.

sue obtained by biopsy can confirm or rule out cancer.

Normal findings

Normally, breast tissue consists of cellular and noncellular connective tissue, fat lobules, and various lactiferous ducts. It's pink, more fatty than fibrous, and shows no abnormal development of cells or tissue elements.

Problematic findings

Abnormal breast tissue may exhibit varied benign or malignant pathology. Benign tumors include fibrocystic disease, adenofibroma, intraductal papilloma, mammary fat necrosis, and plasma cell mastitis (mammary duct ectasia). Malignant tumors include adenocarcinoma; cystosarcoma; intraductal, infiltrating, inflammatory, medullary or circumscribed, colloid, or lobular carcinoma; sarcoma; and Paget's disease.

The receptor assays evaluate tumors for estrogen and progesterone protein and assign a positive or negative value to the estrogen and progesterone receptors. This positive or negative value assists in the prognosis and treatment of breast cancer.

Interfering factors

Failure to obtain an adequate tissue specimen or to place the specimen in the proper solution container may interfere with test results.

❖

Lung biopsy

In a biopsy of the lung, a specimen of pulmonary tissue is excised by closed or open technique for histologic examination. The test confirms a diagnosis of diffuse parenchymal pulmonary disease and pulmonary lesions. (See *Precautions with lung biopsy*.)

PUZZLING LAB
FINDINGS

 Precautions with percutaneous liver biopsy

Percutaneous liver biopsy is contraindicated in a patient with a platelet count below 100,000/mm³; a prothrombin time longer than 15 seconds; empyema of the lungs, pleurae, peritoneum, biliary tract, or liver; a vascular tumor; hepatic angiomas; a hydatid cyst; or tense ascites. If extrahepatic obstruction is suspected, ultrasonography or subcutaneous transhepatic cholangiography should rule out this condition before the biopsy is considered.

During a biopsy, instruct the patient to hold his breath while the needle is in place.

Normal findings

Normal pulmonary tissue shows uniform texture of the alveolar ducts, alveolar walls, bronchioles, and small vessels.

Problematic findings

Histologic examination of a pulmonary tissue specimen can reveal squamous-cell or oat-cell carcinoma and adenocarcinoma. In confirming cancer or parenchymal pulmonary disease, histologic examination supplements the results of microbiological cultures, deep-cough sputum specimens, chest X-rays, computed tomography scans or magnetic resonance imaging, bronchoscopy, and the patient's physical history.

Interfering factors

Failure to obtain a representative tissue specimen or to store the specimens for histology and microbiology in the appropriate containers may interfere with test results.

❖

Percutaneous liver biopsy

Percutaneous biopsy of the liver is the needle aspiration of a core of tissue for histologic analysis. Performed under a local or general anesthetic, percutaneous liver biopsy can diagnose hepatic parenchymal disease, malignant tumors, and granulomatous infections. (See *Precautions with percutaneous liver biopsy*.)

Normal findings

A normal liver consists of sheets of hepatocytes supported by a reticulin framework. (See *Comparing normal and abnormal liver biopsies*.)

Problematic findings

Examination of the hepatic tissue may reveal diffuse hepatic disease, such as cirrhosis or hepatitis, or granulomatous infections such as tuberculosis. Primary malignant tumors include hepatocellular carcinoma, cholangiocellular carcinoma, and angiosarcoma, but hepatic metastases are more common.

Nonmalignant findings with a known focal lesion require further studies — laparotomy or laparoscopy with biopsy, for example.

❖

Percutaneous renal biopsy

In percutaneous renal biopsy, a core of kidney tissue is obtained by needle excision for histologic examination. Light, electron, and immunofluorescent microscopy is used. Percutaneous renal biopsy is used in the diagnosis of renal parenchymal disease. It also monitors the progress of renal disease and can help assess the effectiveness of treatment. (See *Precautions with percutaneous renal biopsy*, page 98.)

Normal findings

A section of normal kidney tissue shows Bowman's capsule (the area between two layers of flat epithelial cells), the glomerular tuft, and the capillary lumen. The tubule sections differ depending on the area of tubule involved. The proximal tubule is one layer of epithelial cells with microvilli that form a brush border. The descending Henle's loop has flat squamous epithelial cells, unlike the ascending, distal convoluted and collecting tubules, which are lined with cuboidal cells.

Problematic findings

Histologic examination of renal tissue can reveal malignancy or renal disease. Malignant tumors include Wilms' tumor, usually

Comparing normal and abnormal liver biopsies

The upper biopsy specimen shows normal liver tissue. The middle specimen confirms cancer of the liver, indicated by the small, dark malignant cells. The lower specimen confirms alcoholic cirrhosis, indicated by the fibrous septa that divide the liver into nodules.

Normal

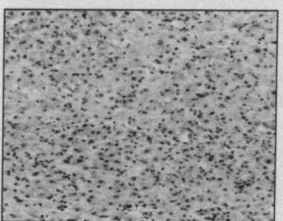

Liver cancer

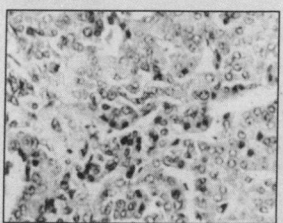

Alcoholic cirrhosis

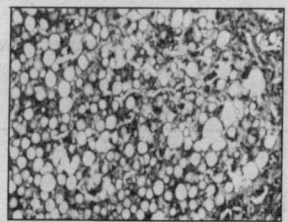

PUZZLING LAB FINDINGS

PUZZLING LAB FINDINGS

 Precautions with percutaneous renal biopsy

Percutaneous renal biopsy is contraindicated in patients with renal tumors, severe bleeding disorders, markedly reduced plasma or blood volume, severe hypertension, hydronephrosis, perinephric abscess, or advanced renal failure with uremia. It should also not be performed on a patient with only one kidney.

During a biopsy, instruct the patient to hold his breath and remain still whenever the needle or prongs are advanced into or retracted from the kidney.

Send the tissue specimen to the laboratory immediately to ensure accurate test results.

present in early childhood, and renal cell carcinoma, most prevalent in persons over age 40. Diseases indicated by characteristic histologic changes include systemic lupus erythematosus, amyloid infiltration, acute and chronic glomerulonephritis, renal vein thrombosis, and pyelonephritis.

Interfering factors

Failure to obtain an adequate tissue specimen, to store the specimen properly, or to send the specimen to the laboratory immediately may interfere with accurate determination of test results.

❖

Blood cell tests

Accurate results of these tests depend in part on proper handling of the blood sample. Hemoconcentration, hemodilution, hemolysis, and failure to use the proper anticoagulant or to adequately mix the sample and the anticoagulant can compromise results.

Complete blood count

This often-requested test gives a fairly complete picture of all the blood's formed elements. The following tests are usually included: hematocrit, platelet count, red blood cell (RBC) and white blood cell (WBC) counts, reticulocyte count, total hemoglobin, and WBC differential (see the following pages for test descriptions).

Complete blood count (CBC) data can detect types of anemia, determine their severity, and compare the status of specific blood elements. Thus, the CBC is especially useful for evaluating conditions in which hematocrit does not parallel the RBC count. Normally, as the RBC count rises, so does hematocrit. However, in patients with microcytic or macrocytic anemia, this natural correlation may not hold true. For example, a patient with iron deficiency anemia has undersized RBCs that cause his hematocrit to decrease, even though his RBC count may be reported as nearly normal. The reverse is true also: A patient with pernicious anemia has many oversized RBCs that cause his hematocrit to be higher than his RBC count.

❖

Erythrocyte sedimentation rate

This sensitive but nonspecific test is often the earliest indicator of disease when other chemical or physical signs are normal. The erythrocyte sedimentation rate (ESR) monitors inflammatory or malignant disease and aids in the detection and diagnosis of tuberculosis, tissue necrosis, or connective tissue disease.

Normal findings
Normal sedimentation rates range from 0 to 20 mm/hour; rates gradually increase with age.

Problematic findings
The ESR rises under the following conditions: pregnancy, acute or chronic inflammation, tuberculosis, paraproteinemia (especially multiple myeloma and Waldenström's macroglobulinemia), rheumatic fever, rheumatoid arthritis, and some malignancies. Anemia also tends to raise ESR; polycythemia, sickle cell anemia, hyperviscosity, or

low plasma fibrinogen or globulin levels tend to depress ESR.

Interfering factors
Failure to use the proper anticoagulant in the collection tube, to adequately mix the sample and the anticoagulant, and to send the sample to the laboratory immediately may alter test results. Hemolysis due to rough handling or excessive mixing of the sample may affect the sedimentation. Hemoconcentration due to prolonged tourniquet constriction also may alter test results.

❖

Hematocrit

This test aids diagnosis of abnormal states of hydration, polycythemia, and anemia. It's also used in calculating red cell indices.

Normal findings
Hematocrit (HCT) values vary, depending on the patient's sex and age, the type of sample, and the laboratory performing the test. (See *Age variations in normal hematocrit,* page 100.)

Problematic findings
Low HCT suggests anemia, hemodilution, or massive blood loss. A patient with high HCT may have polycythemia or hemoconcentration due to blood loss and dehydration.

Interfering factors
Failure to use the proper anticoagulant in the collection tube, to fill it appropriately, or to adequately mix the sample with the

Age variations in normal hematocrit

This chart shows normal hematocrit values for each age group.

Newborn
55% to 68%

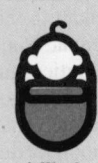
1 Week
47% to 65%

1 Month
37% to 49%

3 Months
30% to 36%

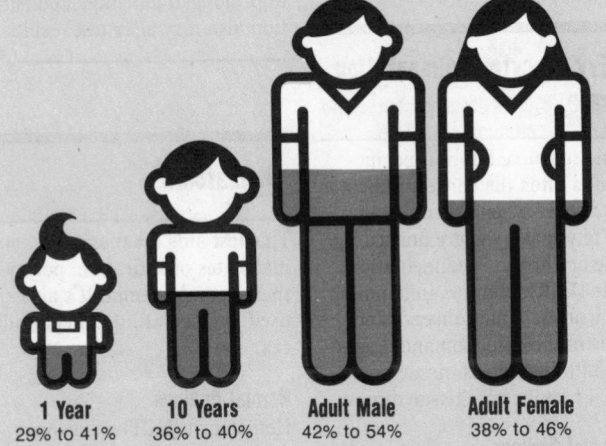
1 Year
29% to 41%

10 Years
36% to 40%

Adult Male
42% to 54%

Adult Female
38% to 46%

anticoagulant may alter test results. Hemolysis due to rough handling of the sample also may alter test results. Tourniquet constriction for longer than 1 minute causes hemoconcentration and typically raises HCT by 2.5% to 5%. Taking the blood sample from the same arm that's being used for I.V. infusion of fluids may cause hemodilution. If the sample must be drawn from the same arm, draw it from below the I.V. site.

——————————— ❖

Platelet count

Platelets, or thrombocytes, are the smallest formed elements in the blood. Vital to the formation of the hemostatic plug in vascular injury, they promote coagulation by supplying phospholipids to the intrinsic coagulation pathway. Platelet counts are used to evaluate platelet production and to assess the effects of chemotherapy or radiation therapy on platelet production. The test also aids in diagnosing thrombocytopenia and thrombocytosis. Finally, a platelet count confirms a visual estimate of platelet number and morphology from a stained blood film.

Normal findings

Normal platelet counts range from 130,000 to 370,000/mm³.

Problematic findings

A *decreased* platelet count (thrombocytopenia) can result from aplastic or hypoplastic bone marrow; infiltrative bone marrow disease, such as carcinoma, leukemia, or disseminated infection; megakaryocytic hypoplasia; ineffective thrombopoiesis due to folic acid or vitamin B_{12} deficiency; pooling of platelets in an enlarged spleen; increased platelet destruction due to drugs or immune disorders; disseminated intravascular coagulation; Bernard-Soulier syndrome; or mechanical injury to platelets.

An *increased* platelet count (thrombocytosis) can result from hemorrhage; infectious disorders; malignancies; iron deficiency anemia; recent surgery, pregnancy, or splenectomy; and inflammatory disorders, such as collagen vascular disease. In such cases, the platelet count returns to normal after the patient recovers from the primary disorder. However, the count remains elevated in primary thrombocythemia, myelofibrosis with myeloid metaplasia, polycythemia vera, and chronic myelogenous leukemia. When the platelet count is abnormal, diagnosis usually requires further studies, such as a complete blood count, bone marrow biopsy, a direct antiglobulin test (a direct Coombs' test), and serum protein electrophoresis.

Interfering factors

Failure to use the proper anticoagulant or to mix the sample and anticoagulant promptly and adequately may alter test results. Hemolysis due to rough handling of the sample or to excessive probing at the venipuncture site may also alter test results.

Certain medications may decrease platelet count, including acetazolamide, acetohexamide, antimony, antineoplastics, brompheniramine maleate, carbamazepine, chloramphenicol, ethacrynic acid, furosemide, gold salts, hydroxychloroquine, indomethacin, isoniazid, mephenytoin, mefenamic acid, methazolamide, methimazole, methyldopa, oral diazoxide, oxyphenbutazone, penicillamine, penicillin, phenylbutazone, phenytoin, pyrimethamine, quinidine sulfate, quinine, salicylates, streptomycin, sulfonamides, thiazide and thiazide-like diuretics, and tricyclic antidepressants. Heparin causes transient, reversible thrombocytopenia.

Platelet counts normally increase at high altitudes, in persistent cold temperature, and during strenuous exercise and excitement. They may decrease just before menstruation. ❖

Red blood cell count

A red blood cell (RBC) count supplies figures for computing the erythrocyte indices, which reveal RBC size and hemoglobin (Hb) content. It also supports other hematologic tests in the diagnosis of anemia and polycythemia.

Normal values

Normal RBC values vary, depending on age, sex, sample, and geographic location. In adult males, RBC counts range from 4.2 to 5.4 million/µl of venous blood; in adult females, 3.6 to 5.0 million/µl of venous blood; in children, 4.6 to 4.8 million/µl of venous blood. In full-term infants, values range from 4.4 to 5.8 million/µl of capillary blood at birth, fall to 3 to 3.8 million/µl at age 2 months, and increase slowly thereafter. Values are generally higher in persons living at high altitudes.

Problematic findings

An elevated RBC count may indicate absolute or relative polycythemia. A depressed count may indicate anemia, fluid overload, or hemorrhage beyond 24 hours. Further tests, such as stained cell examination, hematocrit, Hb, red cell indices, and white cell studies, are needed to confirm diagnosis.

Interfering factors

Failure to use the proper anticoagulant in the collection tube or to adequately mix the sample and anticoagulant may alter test results. Hemoconcentration due to prolonged tourniquet constriction and hemolysis due to rough handling of the sample also may alter test results. Taking the blood sample from the same arm that's being used for I.V. infusion of fluids may cause hemodilution. If the sample must be drawn from the same arm, it should be drawn below the I.V. site.

A high white blood cell count falsely elevates RBC count in semiautomated and automated counters.

Certain diseases that cause RBCs to agglutinate or form rouleaux falsely decrease RBC count.

❖

Red cell indices

Also referred to as erythrocyte indices, red cell indices use the results of the red blood cell (RBC) count, hematocrit, and total hemoglobin (Hb) tests. Used in the diagnosis and classification of anemia, they provide important information about the size, Hb concentration, and Hb weight of an average red cell. The indices include mean corpuscular volume (MCV), mean corpuscular hemoglobin (MCH), and mean corpuscular hemoglobin concentration (MCHC). They help distinguish normally colored (normochromic) red cells from paler (hypochromic) red cells.

Normal findings

The range of normal red cell indices is as follows:
• MCV: 84 to 99 fl
• MCH: 26 to 32 pg
• MCHC: 30 to 36 g/dl.

Problematic findings

The red cell indices aid in classification of anemia. Low MCV and MCHC indices indicate microcytic, hypochromic anemia caused by iron deficiency anemia, pyridoxine-responsive anemia, and thalassemia. A high MCV suggests macrocytic anemia caused by megaloblastic anemia, due to folic acid or vitamin B_{12} deficiency, inherited disorders of DNA synthesis, and reticulocytosis. Because the MCV index reflects the average volume of many cells, a value within the normal range can encompass RBCs of varying size, from microcytic to macrocytic.

Interfering factors

Failure to use the proper anticoagulant in the collection tube or to adequately mix the sample and anticoagulant may alter test results. Hemoconcentration due to prolonged tourniquet constriction and hemolysis due to rough handling of the sample also may alter test results.

A high white blood cell count falsely elevates the RBC count in semiautomated and automated counters and invalidates MCV and MCH results. Falsely elevated Hb values invalidate MCH and MCHC results. Certain diseases that cause RBCs to agglutinate or form rouleaux falsely decrease RBC count and invalidate test results.

Reticulocyte count

The purpose of this test is to aid in distinguishing between hypo- and hyperproliferative anemias. It also helps assess blood loss, bone marrow response to anemia, and therapy for anemia.

Normal findings

Reticulocytes compose 0.5% to 2% of the total red blood cell count. In infants, the percentage is normally higher, ranging from 2% to 6% at birth, but decreases to adult levels in 1 to 2 weeks.

Problematic findings

A low reticulocyte count indicates hypoproliferative bone marrow (hypoplastic anemia) or ineffective erythropoiesis (pernicious anemia). A high reticulocyte count indicates a bone marrow response to anemia caused by hemolysis or blood loss. The reticulocyte count may also rise after effective therapy for iron deficiency anemia or pernicious anemia.

Interfering factors

Falsely decreased test results can be caused by azathioprine, chloramphenicol, dactinomycin, and methotrexate. Falsely increased results can be caused by corticotropin, antimalarials, antipyretics, furazolidone (in infants), and levodopa. Sulfonamides can cause a false decrease or a false increase.

Failure to use the proper anticoagulant in the collection tube or to adequately mix the sample and anticoagulant may interfere with accurate determination of the reticulocyte count. Hemoconcentration due to prolonged tourniquet constriction, hemolysis due to rough handling of the sample, and recent transfusions may alter test results.

Age variations in normal hemoglobin levels

Except for infants, values for the age groups in the chart below are based on venous blood samples.

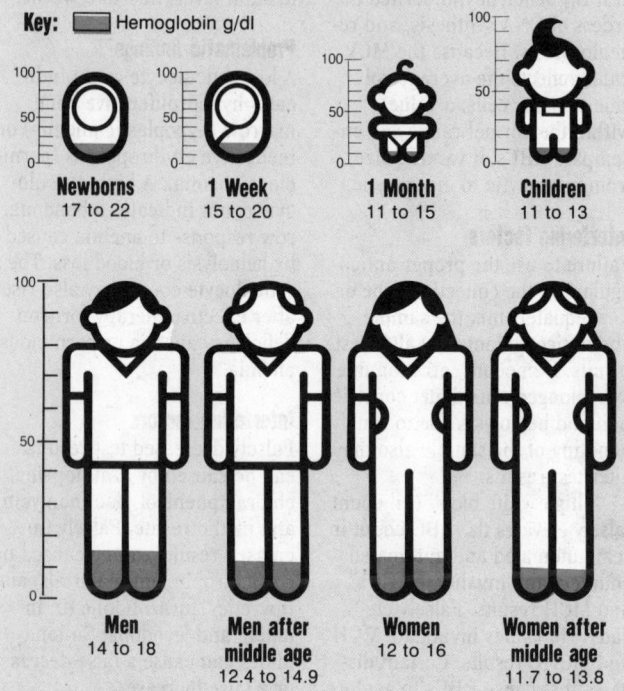

Key: ▨ Hemoglobin g/dl

Newborns
17 to 22

1 Week
15 to 20

1 Month
11 to 15

Children
11 to 13

Men
14 to 18

**Men after
middle age**
12.4 to 14.9

Women
12 to 16

**Women after
middle age**
11.7 to 13.8

Total hemoglobin concentration

This test measures the grams of hemoglobin (Hb) found in a deciliter (100 ml) of whole blood. This measurement determines the severity of anemia or polycythemia and helps monitor a patient's response to therapy. The test also supplies figures for calculating mean corpuscular hemoglobin concentration (the ratio of Hb to red blood cells).

Normal findings

Concentration of Hb varies, depending on the patient's age and sex, and on the type of blood sample drawn. (See *Age variations in normal hemoglobin levels*.)

Problematic findings

Low Hb concentration may indicate anemia, recent hemorrhage, or fluid retention, causing hemodilution. An elevated Hb concentration suggests hemoconcentration from polycythemia or dehydration.

Interfering factors

Failure to use the proper anticoagulant in the collection tube or to adequately mix the sample and anticoagulant may interfere with accurate test results. Hemoconcentration due to prolonged tourniquet constriction or hemolysis due to rough handling of the sample also may affect test results. Very high white cell counts, lipemia, or red cells that are resistant to lysis will falsely elevate Hb values.

White blood cell count

Part of the complete blood count, the white blood cell (WBC) or leukocyte count reports the number of WBCs found in a microliter (cubic millimeter) of whole blood. WBC count can determine infection or inflammation; help determine the need for further tests, such as the WBC differential or bone marrow biopsy; and help monitor a patient's response to chemotherapy or radiation therapy.

Normal findings

The WBC count ranges from 4,000 to 10,000/µl.

Problematic findings

An elevated WBC count (leukocytosis) often signals infection, such as an abscess, meningitis, appendicitis, or tonsillitis. A high count may also result from leukemia and tissue necrosis due to burns, myocardial infarction, or gangrene.

A low WBC count (leukopenia) indicates bone marrow depression that may result from viral infections or from toxic reactions, such as those following treatment with antineoplastics, ingestion of mercury or other heavy metals, or exposure to benzene or arsenicals. Leukopenia characteristically accompanies influenza, typhoid fever, measles, infectious hepatitis, mononucleosis, and rubella.

Interfering factors

Hemolysis due to rough handling of the sample may alter test results. Exercise, stress, or digestion raises the WBC count.

Some drugs, including most antineoplastic agents, anti-infectives (metronidazole and flucytosine), anticonvulsants such as phenytoin derivatives, thyroid hormone antagonists, and nonsteroidal anti-inflammatories such as indomethacin, lower the WBC count.

White blood cell differential

Although the white blood cell (WBC) count alone can suggest infection, a WBC differential adds a detailed evaluation of WBC distribution and morphology that can help confirm the

Interpreting the differential

To make an accurate diagnosis, the examiner must consider both relative and absolute values of the differential. Considered alone, relative results may point to one disease, while masking the true pathology that would be revealed by considering the results of the white blood cell (WBC) count. For example, consider a patient whose WBC count is 6,000/µl and whose differential shows 30% neutrophils and 70% lymphocytes. His relative lymphocyte count is high (lymphocytosis); but when this figure is multiplied by his WBC count—6,000 × 70% = 4,200 lymphocytes/µl—it is well within the normal range.

This patient's neutrophil count, however, is low (30%), and when this is multiplied by the WBC count—6,000 × 30% = 1,800 neutrophils/µl—the result is a low absolute number.

This low result indicates decreased neutrophil production, which may mean depressed bone marrow.

possibility of an infection, help determine the stage and severity of the infection, and suggest the type of organism (bacterial or viral). A differential may also indicate that the cause of the WBC count change is something other than infection, such as leukemia. It also detects allergic reactions and parasitic infections and assesses their severity (eosinophil count).

Normal findings

Normal values for the five types of WBCs that are classified in the differential—neutrophils, eosinophils, basophils, lymphocytes, and monocytes— vary according to age.

Problematic findings

For an accurate diagnosis, differential test results must always be interpreted in relation to the total WBC count. (See *Interpreting the differential.*) Evidence for a wide range of disease states and other conditions is revealed by abnormal differential patterns. (See *Influence of disease on white blood cell types.*)

Interfering factors

Failure to use the proper anticoagulant, to completely fill the collection tube, or to mix the sample and anticoagulant adequately may alter test results. Hemolysis caused by rough handling of the sample also may alter test results.

Influence of disease on white blood cell types

Counts of the following white blood cells are increased or decreased by certain disorders.

CELL TYPE	HOW AFFECTED
Neutrophils	*Increased by:* • Infections: osteomyelitis, otitis media, salpingitis, septicemia, gonorrhea, endocarditis, smallpox, chicken pox, herpes, Rocky Mountain spotted fever • Ischemic necrosis due to myocardial infarction, burns, carcinoma • Metabolic disorders: diabetic acidosis, eclampsia, uremia, thyrotoxicosis • Stress response due to acute hemorrhage, surgery, excessive exercise, emotional distress, third trimester of pregnancy, childbirth • Inflammatory disease: rheumatic fever, rheumatoid arthritis (RA), acute gout, vasculitis and myositis *Decreased by:* • Bone marrow depression due to radiation therapy or cytotoxic drugs • Infections: typhoid, tularemia, brucellosis, hepatitis, influenza, measles, mumps, rubella, infectious mononucleosis • Hypersplenism: hepatic disease and storage diseases • Collagen vascular disease such as systemic lupus erythematosus (SLE) • Deficiency of folic acid or vitamin B_{12}
Eosinophils	*Increased by:* • Allergic disorders: asthma, hay fever, food or drug sensitivity, serum sickness, angioedema • Parasitic infections: trichinosis, hookworm, roundworm, amebiasis • Skin diseases: eczema, pemphigus, psoriasis, dermatitis herpes • Neoplastic diseases: chronic myelocytic leukemia, Hodgkin's disease, metastases and necrosis of solid tumors • Miscellaneous: collagen vascular disease, adrenocortical hypofunction, ulcerative colitis, *(continued)*

Influence of disease on white blood cell types *(continued)*

CELL TYPE	HOW AFFECTED
Eosinophils *(continued)*	polyarteritis nodosa, postsplenectomy, pernicious anemia, scarlet fever, excessive exercise *Decreased by:* • Stress response due to trauma, shock, burns, surgery, mental distress • Cushing's syndrome
Basophils	*Increased by:* • Chronic myelocytic leukemia, polycythemia vera, some types of chronic hemolytic anemia, Hodgkin's disease, systemic mastocytosis, myxedema, ulcerative colitis, chronic hypersensitivity states, and nephrosis *Decreased by:* • Hyperthyroidism, ovulation, pregnancy, stress
Lymphocytes	*Increased by:* • Infections: pertussis, brucellosis, syphilis, tuberculosis, hepatitis, infectious mononucleosis, mumps, German measles, cytomegalovirus • Other: thyrotoxicosis, hypoadrenalism, ulcerative colitis, immune diseases, lymphocytic leukemia *Decreased by:* • Severe debilitating illness, such as congestive heart failure, renal failure, advanced tuberculosis • Defective lymphatic circulation, high levels of adrenal corticosteroids, immunodeficiency due to immunosuppressive drugs
Monocytes	*Increased by:* • Infections: subacute bacterial endocarditis, tuberculosis, hepatitis, malaria, Rocky Mountain spotted fever • Collagen vascular disease: SLE, RA, polyarteritis nodosa • Carcinomas, monocytic leukemia, lymphomas
Atypical lymphocytes	*Increased by:* • Infectious mononucleosis, hepatitis, viral pneumonia, systemic allergies

Blood gas tests

Certain drugs can alter the results of blood gas tests. With arterial blood gas analysis, exposing the blood sample to air and failing to transfer it immediately on ice to the laboratory are also prime factors that can affect test results.

Arterial blood gas analysis

Arterial blood gas (ABG) analysis evaluates gas exchange in the lungs by measuring the partial pressures of arterial oxygen (PaO_2) and arterial carbon dioxide ($PaCO_2$), and the pH of an arterial sample. PaO_2 indicates how much oxygen the lungs are delivering to the blood. $PaCO_2$ indicates how efficiently the lungs eliminate carbon dioxide. The pH indicates the acid-base level of the blood, or the hydrogen ion (H^+) concentration. Acidity indicates H^+ excess; alkalinity, H^+ deficit. Oxygen saturation (SaO_2) and bicarbonate (HCO_3^-) values also aid diagnosis. A blood sample for ABG analysis may be drawn by percutaneous arterial puncture or from an arterial line.

In addition to clarifying blood oxygen disorders, ABG levels can give considerable information about acid-base disorders. (See *Identifying acid-base disorders*, page 110.)

Normal findings

Normal ABG values fall within the following ranges:

PaO_2	75 to 100 mm Hg
$PaCO_2$	35 to 45 mm Hg
pH	7.35 to 7.42
SaO_2	94% to 100%
HCO_3^-	22 to 26 mEq/liter

Problematic findings

Low PaO_2 and SaO_2 levels with a high $PaCO_2$ value may be due to conditions that impair respiratory function, such as respiratory muscle weakness or paralysis (as in Guillain-Barré syndrome or myasthenia gravis), respiratory center inhibition (from head injury, brain tumor, or drug abuse, for example), and airway obstruction (possibly from mucus plugs or a tumor). Similarly, low readings may result from bronchiole obstruction caused by asthma or emphysema from an abnormal ventilation-perfusion ratio due to partially blocked alveoli or pulmonary capillaries or from alveoli that are damaged or filled with fluid because of disease, hemorrhage, or near-drowning.

When inspired air contains insufficient oxygen, PaO_2 and SaO_2 also decrease, but $PaCO_2$ may be normal. Such findings are common in pneumothorax, impaired diffusion between alveoli and blood (due to interstitial fibrosis, for example), or an arteriovenous shunt that permits blood to bypass the lungs.

Interfering factors

Exposing the sample to air affects PaO_2 and $PaCO_2$ levels. Venous blood in the sample may lower PaO_2 and elevate $PaCO_2$.

Failure to heparinize the syringe, place the sample correctly

PUZZLING LAB
FINDINGS

Identifying acid-base disorders

DISORDERS AND ARTERIAL BLOOD GAS FINDINGS	POSSIBLE CAUSES	SIGNS AND SYMPTOMS
Respiratory acidosis (excess CO_2 retention) pH <7.35 HCO_3^- >26 mEq/liter (if compensating) $PaCO_2$ >45 mm Hg	• Central nervous system depression from drugs, injury, or disease • Asphyxia • Hypoventilation due to pulmonary, cardiac, musculoskeletal, or neuromuscular disease	• Diaphoresis, headache, tachycardia, confusion, restlessness, apprehension
Respiratory alkalosis (excess CO_2 excretion) pH >7.42 HCO_3^- <22 mEq/liter (if compensating) $PaCO_2$ <35 mm Hg	• Hyperventilation due to anxiety, pain, or improper ventilator settings • Respiratory stimulation by drugs, disease, hypoxia, fever, or high room temperature • Gram-negative bacteremia	• Rapid deep respirations, paresthesia, light-headedness, twitching, anxiety, fear
Metabolic acidosis (HCO_3^- loss, acid retention) pH <7.35 HCO_3^- <22 mEq/liter $PaCO_2$ <35 mm Hg (if compensating)	• HCO_3^- depletion due to renal disease, diarrhea, or small bowel fistulas • Excessive production of organic acids due to hepatic disease, endocrine disorders, hypoxia, shock, or drug intoxication • Inadequate excretion of acids due to renal disease	• Rapid deep breathing, fruity breath, fatigue, headache, lethargy, drowsiness, nausea, vomiting, coma (if severe)
Metabolic alkalosis (HCO_3^- retention, acid loss) pH >7.42 HCO_3^- >26 mEq/liter $PaCO_2$ >45 mm Hg (if compensating)	• Loss of hydrochloric acid from prolonged vomiting, gastric suctioning • Loss of potassium due to increased renal excretion (as in diuretic therapy), corticosteroid overdose • Excessive alkali ingestion	• Slow shallow breathing, hypertonic muscles, restlessness, confusion, irritability, convulsions, coma

in an iced bag, or send the sample to the laboratory immediately alters test results.

Bicarbonate, ethacrynic acid, hydrocortisone, metolazone, prednisone, and thiazides may elevate $PaCO_2$ levels. Acetazolamide, methicillin, nitrofurantoin, and tetracycline may decrease $PaCO_2$ levels.

Special considerations
Wait at least 15 to 20 minutes before drawing arterial blood after making a change in oxygen therapy, starting or removing oxygen therapy, and suctioning.

Before sending the sample to the laboratory, include the following data on the laboratory slip:
• whether the patient was breathing room air or receiving oxygen therapy when the sample was drawn; if he was receiving oxygen therapy, give the flow rate
• the fraction of inspired oxygen and tidal volume, if the patient is on a ventilator
• the patient's rectal temperature and respiratory rate.

❖

Total carbon dioxide content

When the pressure of carbon dioxide (CO_2) in red blood cells exceeds 40 mm Hg, CO_2 spills out of the cells and dissolves in plasma. There it may combine with water (H_2O) to form carbonic acid (H_2CO_3), which, in turn, can dissociate into hydrogen ions (H^+) and bicarbonate ions (HCO_3^-). This test measures the total concentration of all such forms of CO_2 in serum, plasma, or whole blood samples.

For maximum clinical significance, test results must be considered with both pH and arterial blood gas values.

Normal findings
Total CO_2 levels normally range from 22 to 34 mEq/liter.

Problematic findings
High CO_2 levels may occur in metabolic alkalosis (due to excessive ingestion or retention of base bicarbonate), respiratory acidosis (from hypoventilation, for example, as in emphysema or pneumonia), primary aldosteronism, and Cushing's syndrome. CO_2 levels may also rise above normal after excessive loss of acids, as in severe vomiting and continuous gastric drainage.

Decreased CO_2 levels are common in metabolic acidosis (as in diabetic acidosis or renal tubular acidosis resulting from renal failure). Decreased total CO_2 levels in metabolic acidosis also result from loss of bicarbonate (as in severe diarrhea or intestinal drainage). Levels may fall below normal in respiratory alkalosis (from hyperventilation, for example, after trauma).

Interfering factors
CO_2 levels rise with administration of excessive corticotropin, cortisone, or thiazide diuretics, or with excessive ingestion of alkalis or licorice. The levels decrease with administration of salicylates, paraldehyde, methicillin, dimercaprol, ammonium chloride, acetazolamide, and accidental ingestion of ethylene glycol or methyl alcohol.

❖

Carbohydrate metabolism tests

Tests that measure the body's tolerance for carbohydrates rely on the patient's adherence to pretest dietary restrictions. They also depend on immediate specimen transfer to the laboratory or refrigeration to avoid glycolysis.

Fasting plasma glucose test

Commonly used to screen for diabetes mellitus, the fasting plasma glucose test measures plasma glucose levels following a 12- to 14-hour fast. The test also helps monitor drug or dietary therapy in diabetic patients.

Normal findings

The normal range for fasting plasma glucose varies according to the laboratory procedure used. Generally, normal values after a 12- to 14-hour fast are 70 to 100 mg of "true glucose" per 100 ml of blood when measured by the glucose oxidase and hexokinase methods.

Problematic findings

Fasting plasma glucose levels of 140 mg/100 ml or more obtained on two or more occasions confirm diabetes mellitus; however, borderline or transient elevated levels require the 2-hour postprandial plasma glucose test or the oral glucose tolerance test to confirm diagnosis. Although increased fasting plasma glucose levels most commonly occur

with diabetes, such levels can also result from pancreatitis, recent acute illness (such as myocardial infarction), Cushing's syndrome, acromegaly, and pheochromocytoma. Hyperglycemia may also stem from hyperlipoproteinemia (especially types III, IV, or V), chronic hepatic disease, nephrotic syndrome, brain tumor, sepsis, or gastrectomy with dumping syndrome, and is typical in eclampsia, anoxia, and convulsive disorders.

Depressed plasma glucose levels can result from hyperinsulinism, an insulinoma, von Gierke's disease, functional or reactive hypoglycemia, myxedema, adrenal insufficiency, congenital adrenal hyperplasia, hypopituitarism, malabsorption syndrome, and some cases of hepatic insufficiency.

Interfering factors

False-positive findings may be caused by acetaminophen when the glucose oxidase or hexokinase method is used. Other drugs known to elevate plasma glucose levels are chlorthalidone, thiazide diuretics, furosemide, triamterene, oral contraceptives (estrogen-progestin combination), benzodiazepines, phenytoin, phenothiazines, lithium, epinephrine, arginine, phenolphthalein, dextrothyroxine, diazoxide, large doses of nicotinic acid, corticosteroids, and recent I.V. glucose infusions. Ethacrynic acid may also cause hyperglycemia, but large doses can produce hypoglycemia in patients with uremia.

Decreased plasma glucose levels may be caused by beta blockers, ethanol, clofibrate, insulin, oral antidiabetic drugs, and monoamine oxidase inhibitors.

Failure to observe dietary restrictions may elevate plasma glucose levels. Recent illness, infection, or pregnancy can also elevate plasma glucose levels; strenuous exercise can depress them. Glycolysis due to failure to refrigerate the sample or to send it to the laboratory immediately can result in false-negative results.

Special considerations

Send the sample to the laboratory immediately because the blood glucose level decreases when the sample is left at room temperature. If transport is delayed, refrigerate the sample. On the laboratory slip indicate the time when the patient last ate, the sample collection time, and the time the last pretest insulin or oral antidiabetic drug dose was given (if applicable). ❖

Oral glucose tolerance test

The most sensitive method of confirming borderline cases of diabetes mellitus in selected patients, the oral glucose tolerance test measures carbohydrate metabolism after ingestion of a challenge dose of glucose. The test also aids diagnosis of hypoglycemia and malabsorption syndrome.

Normal findings

Normal plasma glucose levels peak at 160 to 180 mg/100 ml within 30 minutes to 1 hour after administration of an oral glucose test dose and return to fasting levels or lower within 2 to 3 hours. Urine glucose tests remain negative throughout.

Problematic findings

Depressed glucose tolerance, in which levels peak sharply before falling slowly to fasting levels, may confirm diabetes mellitus or may result from Cushing's disease, hemochromatosis, pheochromocytoma, or central nervous system lesions.

Increased glucose tolerance, in which levels may peak at less than normal, may indicate insulinoma, malabsorption syndrome, adrenocortical insufficiency (Addison's disease), hypothyroidism, or hypopituitarism. (See *Interpreting glucose tolerance curves*, page 114.)

Interfering factors

Elevated plasma glucose levels may result from chlorthalidone, thiazide diuretics, furosemide, triamterene, oral contraceptives (estrogen-progestin combination), benzodiazepines, phenytoin, phenothiazines, lithium, epinephrine, phenolphthalein, caffeine, arginine, dextrothyroxine, diazoxide, large doses of nicotinic acid, corticosteroids, and recent glucose I.V. infusions.

Depressed glucose levels may be caused by ingestion of beta blockers, amphetamines, ethanol, clofibrate, insulin, oral antidiabetic agents, and monoamine oxidase inhibitors.

Interpreting glucose tolerance curves

An oral glucose tolerance test measures both blood and urine glucose levels. As shown, various diseases other than diabetes mellitus produce abnormal glucose tolerance curves: (1) diabetes mellitus, myasthenia gravis, brain injury, Cushing's syndrome, acromegaly (early), and hemochromatosis; (2) alimentary glycosuria and glucose infusions; (3) normal; (4) insulin shock, spontaneous hypoglycemia, and hypoadrenalism (normal glucose tolerance until 2 hours after ingestion of the sugar load, then marked hypoglycemia); (5) pituitary deficiency and myxedema; (6) anorexia nervosa, panhypopituitarism, hyperinsulinism, and Addison's disease.

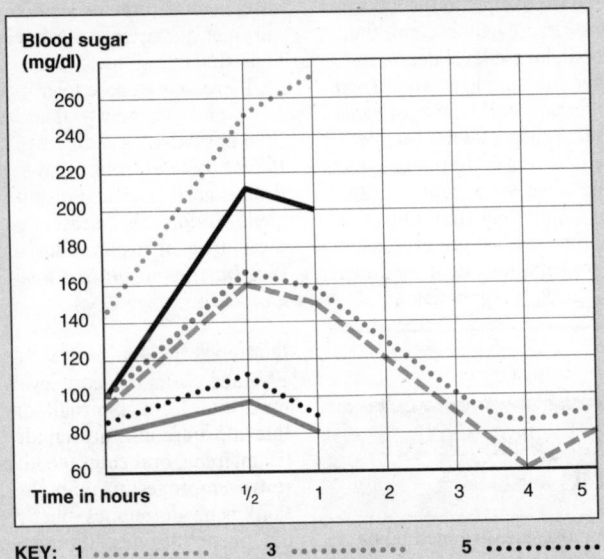

Adapted with permission from John D. Bauer, et al., *Clinical Laboratory Methods*, 8th ed. (St. Louis: Mosby-Year Book, Inc., 1974).

Failure to adhere to dietary and exercise restrictions may alter test results. Carbohydrate deprivation before the test can produce a diabetic response (abnormal increase in plasma glucose, with a delayed decrease) because the pancreas is unaccustomed to responding to high-carbohydrate load.

Recent infection, fever, pregnancy, or acute illness such as myocardial infarction may elevate glucose levels.

PREVENTIVE PRACTICE

 Precautions with oral glucose tolerance testing

If the patient develops severe hypoglycemia during an oral glucose tolerance test, notify the doctor. Draw a blood sample, record the time on the laboratory slip, and dis-continue the test. Have the patient drink a glass of orange juice to which sugar has been added, or administer glucose I.V. to reverse the reaction.

People over age 50 tend toward decreasing carbohydrate tolerance, which causes an increase in glucose tolerance, to upper limits of about 1 mg/100 ml for every year over age 50.

Special considerations

Send blood and urine samples to the laboratory immediately, or refrigerate them. Specify when the patient last ate, and the blood and urine sample collection times. As appropriate, record the time the patient received his last pretest insulin or oral antidiabetic drug dose. (See *Precautions with oral glucose tolerance testing.*)

❖

Two-hour postprandial plasma glucose test

Also referred to as the 2-hour postprandial blood sugar test, this test is a valuable screening tool for detecting diabetes mellitus. It's often performed when the patient demonstrates symptoms of diabetes (polydipsia and polyuria) or when results of the

fasting plasma glucose test suggest diabetes.

The 2-hour postprandial plasma glucose test is also used to monitor drug or diet therapy in patients with diabetes mellitus.

Normal findings

In a person without diabetes, postprandial glucose values are less than 145 mg/dl by the glucose oxidase or hexokinase method; levels are slightly elevated in persons over age 50. (See *Age variations in 2-hour postprandial plasma glucose levels*, page 116.)

Problematic findings

Two 2-hour postprandial blood glucose values of 200 mg/dl or higher indicate diabetes mellitus. High levels may also occur with pancreatitis, Cushing's syndrome, acromegaly, and pheochromocytoma. Hyperglycemia may also be caused by hyperlipoproteinemia (especially types III, IV, or V), chronic hepatic disease, nephrotic syndrome, brain tumor, sepsis, gastrectomy with dumping syndrome, eclampsia, anoxia, or convulsive disorders.

Depressed glucose levels occur in hyperinsulinism, an insulinoma, von Gierke's disease,

Age variations in 2-hour postprandial plasma glucose levels

The greatest difference in normal and diabetic insulin responses, and thus in plasma glucose concentration, occurs about 2 hours after a glucose challenge. Values of this test, however, can fluctuate according to the patient's age. After age 50, for example, normal levels rise markedly and steadily, sometimes reaching 160 mg/dl or higher. In younger patients, glucose concentration over 145 mg/dl suggests incipient diabetes and requires further evaluation.

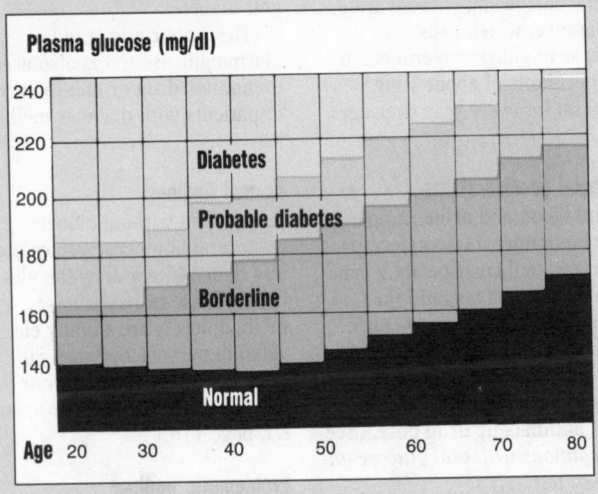

functional or reactive hypoglycemia, myxedema, adrenal insufficiency, congenital adrenal hyperplasia, hypopituitarism, malabsorption syndrome, and some cases of hepatic insufficiency.

Interfering factors

False-positive results may be caused by acetaminophen when the glucose oxidase or hexokinase method is used. Other drugs known to cause plasma glucose elevations are chlorthalidone, thiazide diuretics, furosemide, triamterene, oral contraceptives (estrogen-progestin combination), benzodiazepines, phenytoin, phenothiazines, lithium, epinephrine, arginine, phenolphthalein, dextrothyroxine, diazoxide, large doses of nicotinic acid, corticosteroids, and recent I.V. glucose infusions. Ethacrynic acid may also cause hyperglycemia, but large doses can cause hypoglycemia in patients with uremia.

Depressed glucose levels may result from the use of beta blockers, amphetamines, ethanol, clofibrate, insulin, oral antidiabetic agents, and monoamine oxidase inhibitors.

Recent illness, infection, or pregnancy may raise glucose levels; strenuous exercise or stress may depress them. Glycolysis caused by failure to refrigerate the sample or to send it to the laboratory immediately can depress glucose levels.

Special considerations
Send the sample to the laboratory immediately or refrigerate it. Specify on the laboratory slip the time when the patient last ate, the sample collection time, and the time the last pretest insulin or antidiabetic drug dose (if applicable) was given. If the sample is to be drawn by a technician, tell him the exact time the venipuncture must be performed.

Cardiac enzyme tests

With these tests, timing affects test results. Failure to draw blood samples on schedule may cause you to miss peak enzyme levels. With lactate dehydrogenase, it may cause you to miss the progressive elevation that spots myocardial infarction.

Creatine kinase

Creatine kinase (CK) is an enzyme that catalyzes the creatine-creatinine metabolic pathway in muscle cells and brain tissue. Because of its intimate role in energy production, CK reflects normal tissue catabolism; an increase above normal serum levels indicates trauma to cells with high CK content.

A CK test is used to detect and diagnose acute myocardial infarction (MI) and reinfarction (CK-MB—in cardiac muscle—is primarily used). It also helps evaluate possible causes of chest pain and monitors the severity of myocardial ischemia after cardiac surgery, cardiac catheterization, or cardioversion (CK-MB is primarily used). CK tests can detect skeletal muscle disorders that aren't neurogenic in origin such as Duchenne muscular dystrophy (total CK is primarily used) and early dermatomyositis.

Normal findings
Total CK values determined by ultraviolet or kinetic measurement range from 25 to 130 units/liter for men and from 10 to 150 units/liter for women. CK levels may be significantly higher in very muscular people. Infants up to age 1 have levels two to four times higher than adult levels, possibly reflecting birth trauma and striated muscle development. Normal ranges for isoenzyme levels are as follows: CK-BB—in the brain—undetectable; CK-MB, undetectable to 7

Serum enzyme and isoenzyme levels after myocardial infarction

Because they're released by damaged tissue, serum enzymes and isoenzymes—catalytic proteins that vary in concentration in specific organs—can help identify the compromised organ and assess the extent of damage. The following serum enzyme and isoenzyme determinations are most significant in myocardial infarction.

Isoenzymes
• Creatine kinase-MB (CK-MB): in the heart muscle, and a small amount in skeletal muscle
• Lactate dehydrogenase isoenzymes LD_1, LD_2: in the heart, brain, kidneys, liver, skeletal muscles, and red blood cells (RBCs).

Enzymes
• Hydroxybutyric dehydrogenase (HBD): an indirect measurement of LD_1 and LD_2
• Aspartate aminotransferase (AST): heart muscle and liver, and less extensively in skeletal muscles, kidneys, pancreas, and RBCs.

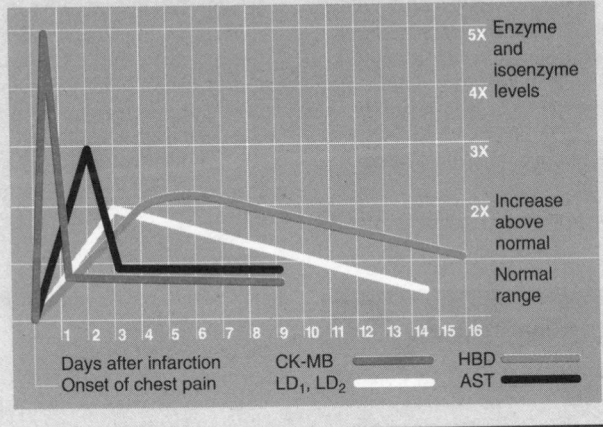

Days after infarction
Onset of chest pain

CK-MB   HBD
LD_1, LD_2 AST

units/liter; CK-MM—in skeletal muscle—5 to 70 units/liter.

Problematic findings
CK-MM constitutes over 99% of total CK normally present in serum. Detectable CK-BB isoenzyme levels may indicate brain tissue injury, certain widespread malignant tumors, severe shock, or renal failure. However, such elevations don't confirm a specific diagnosis.

CK-MB isoenzyme levels greater than 5% of total CK levels (or more than 10 units/liter) indicate MI, especially if the lactate dehydrogenase isoenzyme ratio (LD_1/LD_2) is greater than 1 (flipped LD). In acute MI and following cardiac surgery, CK-MB begins to rise in 2 to 4 hours, peaks in 12 to 24 hours, and usually returns to normal in 24 to 48 hours; persistent elevations or increasing levels indicate ongoing myocardial damage. Total CK levels follow roughly the same pattern but rise slightly later. (See *Serum enzyme and isoenzyme levels after myocardial infarction.*)

Serious skeletal muscle injury that occurs in certain muscular dystrophies, polymyositis, and severe myoglobinuria may produce mild CK-MB level elevation because a small amount of this isoenzyme is present in some skeletal muscles.

Rising CK-MM values follow skeletal muscle damage from trauma, such as surgery and I.M. injections, or from diseases, such as dermatomyositis and muscular dystrophy (values may be 50 to 100 times normal). A moderate rise in CK-MM levels develops in patients with hypothyroidism; sharp elevations occur with muscular activity caused by agitation, such as occurs in an acute psychotic episode.

Total CK levels may be elevated in patients with severe hypokalemia, carbon monoxide poisoning, malignant hyperthermia, postconvulsions, and alcoholic cardiomyopathy and, occasionally, in those who have suffered pulmonary or cerebral infarctions.

Interfering factors

Hemolysis may alter results. Failure to send the sample to the laboratory immediately or to refrigerate the serum if testing will be delayed for more than 2 hours may alter results. Failure to draw the samples at the scheduled time may cause missing of peak levels. Halothane and succinylcholine, alcohol, lithium, and large doses of aminocaproic acid as well as intramuscular injections, cardioversion, invasive diagnostic procedures, surgery, recent vigorous exercise or muscle massage and severe coughing and trauma raise total CK values.

Special considerations

Draw the sample before or within 1 hour of giving I.M. injections because muscle trauma raises total CK levels. Obtain the sample on schedule. On the laboratory slip, note the time the sample was drawn and the hours elapsed since chest pain started.

Be sure to handle the collection tube gently to prevent hemolysis. Send the sample to the laboratory immediately because CK activity diminishes significantly after 2 hours at room temperature.

Creatine kinase isoforms

An enzyme found in muscle tissue, creatine kinase (CK) has three isoenzymes: CK-MM, CK-MB, and CK-BB. CK-MM and CK-MB are found primarily in skeletal and heart muscle. Most prevalent in brain tissue, CK-BB is not usually seen in serum.

Isoforms, or subforms, of CK-MM and CK-MB isoenzymes are called $CK-MM_1$, $CK-MM_2$, $CK-MB_1$, and $CK-MB_2$. The CK-MB isoform can provide early confirmation of myocardial infarction (MI). It also helps evaluate reperfusion therapy.

Normal findings
$CK-MB_2$ concentrations are less than 1.0. The $CK-MB_2/CK-MB_1$ ratio is less than 1.5.

Problematic findings
Within 2 to 4 hours after MI, more than 50% of patients will have a $CK-MB_2/CK-MB_1$ ratio greater than 1.5. By 6 hours, more than 90% of patients will have a ratio of 1.5 or greater.

Giving thrombolytic drugs may restore coronary perfusion. The increased blood flow through the damaged area removes accumulated CK isoenzymes and causes the $CK-MB_2/CK-MB_1$ ratio to peak sooner.

Interfering factors
Hemolysis may alter results. Failure to draw the samples at the scheduled times may cause missing of peak levels. ❖

Lactate dehydrogenase

The purpose of this test is to aid differential diagnosis of myocardial infarction (MI), pulmonary infarction, anemia, and hepatic disease. It also can support creatine kinase (CK) isoenzyme test results in diagnosing MI or provide a diagnosis when CK-MB isoenzyme samples are drawn too late to display elevation. Lactate dehydrogenase (LD) can help monitor a patient's response to some forms of chemotherapy.

Normal findings
Total LD levels normally range from 45 to 90 units/liter. Normal distribution of LD isoenzymes is as follows:

LD_1	14% to 26% of total
LD_2	29% to 39% of total
LD_3	20% to 26% of total
LD_4	8% to 16% of total
LD_5	6% to 16% of total.

Problematic findings
Because many common diseases cause elevations in total LD levels, isoenzyme electrophoresis is usually necessary for diagnosis. In some disorders, total LD levels may be within normal limits, but abnormal proportions of each enzyme indicate specific organ tissue damage. For instance, in acute MI, the concentration of LD_1 is greater than LD_2 within 12 to 48 hours after onset of symptoms. (That is, the LD_1/LD_2 isoenzyme ratio is greater than 1.) This reversal of normal isoenzyme patterns is typical of myocardial damage and is referred to as flipped LD.

Interfering factors
Hemolysis due to rough handling of the sample may affect results. For diagnosis of acute MI, failure to draw the sample on schedule may interfere with test results. Failure to send the sample to the laboratory immediately may influence determination of LD isoenzyme patterns.

Recent surgery or pregnancy can cause elevated LD levels. Prosthetic heart valves may also increase LD levels because of chronic hemolysis.

Special considerations

Draw the samples on schedule to avoid missing peak levels, and mark the collection time on the laboratory slip. Handle the sample gently to prevent artifact blood sample hemolysis, because red blood cells contain LD_1. Send the sample to the laboratory immediately or, if transport is delayed, keep the sample at room temperature. Changes in temperature reportedly inactivate LD_5, thus altering isoenzyme patterns.

Coagulation tests

As with other tests that use a blood sample, these tests depend on proper procedure and proper handling of the sample to help ensure accurate results.

Activated partial thromboplastin time

The purpose of this test is to screen for deficiencies of the clotting factors in the intrinsic pathways and to monitor heparin therapy. The activated partial thromboplastin time (APTT) test evaluates all the clotting factors of the intrinsic pathway—except platelets—by measuring the time required for formation of a fibrin clot after the addition of calcium and phospholipid emulsion to a plasma sample. (See *Precautions with APTT testing.*)

PREVENTIVE PRACTICE

Precautions with APTT testing

When administering the activated partial thromboplastin time (APTT) test to a patient on anticoagulant therapy, you may need to apply additional pressure at the venipuncture site to control bleeding.

Normal findings

Normally, a fibrin clot forms 25 to 36 seconds after addition of reagents. For a patient on anticoagulant therapy, check with the attending doctor to find out the desirable values for the therapy being delivered.

Problematic findings

Prolonged times may indicate a deficiency of certain plasma clotting factors; the presence of heparin; or the presence of fibrin split products, fibrinolysins, or circulating anticoagulants that are antibodies to specific clotting factors.

Interfering factors

Failure to use the proper anticoagulant, fill the collection tube completely, mix the sample and the anticoagulant adequately, send the sample to the laboratory immediately, or place it on ice may alter test results. Hemolysis due to rough handling of the sample or excessive probing at the venipuncture site also may alter test results.

RULE OF THUMB

 When to stop the test

During administration of the bleeding time test, if the patient's bleeding doesn't diminish after 15 minutes, discontinue the test to avoid excessive blood loss.

Bleeding time

Bleeding time depends on the elasticity of the blood vessel wall and on the number and functional capacity of platelets. This test measures the duration of bleeding after a standardized skin incision. It's used to assess overall hemostatic function and to detect congenital and acquired platelet function disorders. Bleeding time may be measured by one of four methods: Duke, Ivy, template, or modified template. The template methods are the most frequently used and the most accurate.

Usually, the test isn't recommended for a patient whose platelet count is less than 75,000/mm³. (See *When to stop the test*.) However, some patients with altered platelet morphology may have normal bleeding times despite low platelet counts.

Normal findings
The normal range of bleeding time is from 2 to 8 minutes in the template method; from 2 to 10 minutes in the modified template method; from 1 to 7 minutes in the Ivy method; and from

1 to 3 minutes in the Duke method.

Problematic findings
Prolonged bleeding time may indicate the presence of many disorders associated with thrombocytopenia, such as Hodgkin's disease, acute leukemia, disseminated intravascular coagulation, hemolytic disease of the newborn, Schönlein-Henoch purpura, severe hepatic disease (cirrhosis, for example), or severe deficiency of factors I, II, V, VII, VIII, IX, and XI.

Prolonged bleeding time in a person with a normal platelet count suggests a platelet function disorder (thrombasthenia, thrombocytopathia) and requires further investigation with clot retraction, prothrombin consumption, and platelet aggregation tests.

Interfering factors
Sulfonamides, thiazides, antineoplastics, anticoagulants, nonsteroidal anti-inflammatory drugs, aspirin and aspirin compounds, and some nonnarcotic analgesics may prolong bleeding time. ❖

Plasma thrombin time

Also called the thrombin clotting time test, the plasma thrombin time test measures how quickly a clot forms when a standard amount of bovine thrombin is added to a platelet-poor plasma sample from the patient and to a normal plasma control sample. The test is used to detect fibrinogen deficiency or defect and to aid in the diagnosis of disseminated intravascular coagulation (DIC) and hepatic disease. It also monitors the effectiveness of treatment with heparin or thrombolytic agents.

Normal findings
Normal plasma thrombin time ranges from 10 to 15 seconds. Test results are usually reported with a normal control value.

Problematic findings
A prolonged plasma thrombin time may indicate heparin therapy, hepatic disease, DIC, hypofibrinogenemia, or afibrinogenemia.

Patients with a prolonged plasma thrombin time may require quantitation of fibrinogen levels; in suspected DIC, the test for fibrin split products is also necessary.

Interfering factors
Hemolysis caused by excessive probing during venipuncture or rough handling of the sample may alter test results. Failure to use the proper anticoagulant in the collection tube, mix the sample and the anticoagulant adequately, send the sample to the laboratory immediately, or place it on ice also may alter test results. Administration of heparin may prolong clotting time. ❖

Prothrombin time

The prothrombin time (PT), or *pro time*, test measures the time required for a fibrin clot to form in a citrated plasma sample after addition of calcium ions and tissue thromboplastin (factor III). It's used to evaluate the extrinsic coagulation system and to monitor a patient's response to oral anticoagulant therapy.

Normal findings
Normally, PT ranges from 10 to 14 seconds. However, times vary, depending on the source of tissue thromboplastin and the type of sensing devices used to measure clot formation. In a patient receiving oral anticoagulants, PT is usually maintained between 1½ and 2 times the normal control.

Problematic findings
Prolonged PT may indicate deficiencies in fibrinogen; prothrombin; or factors V, VII, or X (specific assays can pinpoint such deficiencies). It may also indicate vitamin K deficiency, hepatic disease, or ongoing oral anticoagulant therapy. Prolonged PT that exceeds 2½ times the control value is commonly associated with abnormal bleeding.

Prolonged PT can result from the use of corticotropin, overuse of alcohol, anabolic steroids, cholestyramine resin, I.V. heparin (within 5 hours of collection), indomethacin, mefenamic acid, para-aminosalicylic acid, methimazole, oxyphenbutazone, phenylbutazone, phenytoin, propylthiouracil, quinidine, quinine, thyroid hormones, and vitamin A.

Prolonged or shortened PT can follow ingestion of antibiotics, barbiturates, hydroxyzine, sulfonamides, salicylates (more than 1 g/day prolongs PT), mineral oil, or clofibrate.

Interfering factors

Hemolysis may alter test results. Failure to mix the sample and anticoagulant adequately or to send the sample to the laboratory promptly on ice may alter test results.

Fibrin or fibrin split products in the sample or plasma fibrinogen levels less than 100 mg/dl can prolong PT. Falsely prolonged results may occur if the collection tube is not filled to capacity with blood; then the amount of anticoagulant is excessive for the blood sample. Shortened PT can result from the use of antihistamines, chloral hydrate, corticosteroids, digitalis glycosides, diuretics, glutethimide, griseofulvin, estrogen-progestin combinations, pyrazinamide, vitamin K, and xanthines (caffeine, theophylline).

❖

Cultures

A proper collection technique that avoids introducing contaminants or destroying targeted pathogens is important to accurate culture results. Equally important is proper preservation of the specimen and quick transfer to the laboratory.

Blood culture

A blood culture is performed by inoculating a culture medium with a blood sample and incubating it for isolation and identification of the pathogens in bacteremia (bacterial invasion of the bloodstream) and septicemia (systemic spread of such infection). The test is used to confirm bacteremia and to identify the causative organism in bacteremia and septicemia.

Normal findings

Normally, blood cultures are sterile.

Problematic findings

Positive blood cultures don't necessarily confirm pathologic septicemia. Mild, transient bacteremia may occur during the course of many infectious diseases or may complicate other disorders. Persistent, continuous, or recurrent bacteremia reliably confirms the presence of serious infection. To detect most causative agents, blood cultures ideally are drawn on 2 consecutive days.

Isolation of most organisms takes about 72 hours; however, negative cultures are held for 1 week or more before being reported negative. For example, negative reports of cultures for suspected *Brucella* are held for about 4 weeks.

Common blood pathogens include *Neisseria meningitidis*, *Streptococcus pneumoniae*, other *Streptococcus* species, *Haemophilus influenzae*, *Staphylococcus aureus*, *Pseudomonas aeruginosa*, Bacteroidaceae, *Brucella*, and Enterobacteriaceae. Although 2% to 3% of the blood samples that are cultured are contaminated by skin bacteria, such as *Staphylococcus epidermidis*, diphtheroids, and *Propionibacterium*, these organisms may be clinically significant when isolated from multiple cultures or from immunocompromised patients.

Interfering factors

Improper collection technique may contaminate the sample. Previous or current antimicrobial therapy may give false-negative results; obtaining specimens before the start of antimicrobial therapy is preferable. Removal of culture bottle caps at the patient's bedside may prevent anaerobic growth; use of incorrect bottles and media may prevent aerobic growth.

❖

Nasopharyngeal culture

This test evaluates nasopharyngeal secretions for the presence and type of pathogenic organisms causing upper respiratory tract symptoms. It also identifies the proliferation of normal nasopharyngeal flora, which may prove pathogenic in debilitated and other immunocompromised patients. And it's used to detect asymptomatic carriers of infectious organisms such as *Neisseria meningitidis* and *Bordetella pertussis*.

Normal findings

Flora commonly found in the nasopharynx include nonhemolytic streptococci, alpha-hemolytic streptococci, *Neisseria* species (except *N. meningitidis* and *N. gonorrhoeae*), coagulase-negative staphylococci such as *Staphylococcus epidermidis* and, occasionally, the coagulase-positive *Staphylococcus aureus*.

Problematic findings

Pathogens include group A beta-hemolytic streptococci; occasionally groups B, C, and G beta-hemolytic streptococci; *B. pertussis; Corynebacterium diphtheriae; S. aureus;* and large amounts of *Haemophilus influenzae*, pneumococci, or *Candida albicans*.

Interfering factors

Recent antimicrobial therapy decreases bacterial growth. Improper collection technique may contaminate the specimen. Failure to place the specimen in a transport medium allows the specimen to dry out and the bacteria to deteriorate. Failure to send the specimen to the laboratory immediately after collection permits proliferation of organisms. Failure to keep a viral specimen cold allows the viruses to deteriorate.

Special considerations

Use gloves when performing the procedure and handling the specimen. Don't let the swab touch the sides of the patient's nostril or his tongue, to prevent specimen contamination.

On the laboratory slip, note recent antimicrobial therapy or chemotherapy. Also note if *C. diphtheriae* and *B. pertussis*, which need special growth media, are suspected.

Keep the container upright. Refrigerate a viral specimen, according to your laboratory's procedure.

❖

PREVENTIVE PRACTICE

 ## Precautions with sputum culture testing

Use gloves when performing the procedure and handling specimens. Because the patient may cough violently during suctioning, also wear a mask to avoid exposure to pathogens.

Tracheal suctioning is contraindicated in patients with esophageal varices or cardiac disease. In a patient with asthma or chronic bronchitis, watch for aggravated bronchospasms with use of more than 10% concentration of sodium chloride solution or acetylcysteine in an aerosol.

During tracheal suction-ing, suction for only 5 to 10 seconds at a time. *Never* suction longer than 15 seconds. If the patient becomes hypoxic or cyanotic, remove the catheter immediately, and administer oxygen.

Don't use more than 20% propylene glycol with water as an inducer for a specimen scheduled for tuberculosis culturing, since higher concentrations inhibit the growth of *Mycobacterium tuberculosis*. (If propylene glycol isn't available, use 10% to 20% acetylcysteine with water or sodium chloride solution.)

Sputum culture

Bacteriologic examination of sputum—material raised from the lungs and bronchi during deep coughing—is an important aid to the management of lung disease. A sputum culture can isolate and identify the cause of a pulmonary infection, thus aiding the diagnosis of respiratory diseases (most frequently bronchitis, tuberculosis, lung abscess, and pneumonia).

Certain precautions are advisable when administering a sputum culture. (See *Precautions with sputum culture testing.*)

Normal findings
Flora commonly found in the respiratory tract include alpha-hemolytic streptococci, *Neisseria* species, and diphtheroids. However, the presence of normal flora doesn't rule out infection.

Problematic findings
Since sputum is invariably contaminated with normal oropharyngeal flora, interpretation of a culture isolate must relate to the patient's overall clinical condition. Isolation of *Mycobacterium tuberculosis* is always a significant finding.

Interfering factors
Improper collection or handling of the specimen may alter test results. Failure to report current

or recent antimicrobial therapy prevents the laboratory from correctly interpreting decreased bacterial growth. Sputum collected over an extended period may allow pathogens to deteriorate or become overgrown by commensals and will not be accepted as a valid specimen by most laboratories.

❖

Stool culture

Bacteriologic examination of feces is valuable for identifying pathogens that cause overt GI disease — such as typhoid and dysentery — and carrier states.

Normal findings

Approximately 96% to 99% of normal fecal flora consist of anaerobes, including non-spore-forming bacilli, clostridia, and anaerobic streptococci. The remaining 1% to 4% consist of aerobes, including gram-negative bacilli (predominantly *Escherichia coli* and other Enterobacteriaceae, plus small amounts of *Pseudomonas*), gram-positive cocci (mostly enterococci), and a few yeasts.

Problematic findings

Isolation of some pathogens (such as *Salmonella*, *Shigella*, *Campylobacter*, *Yersinia*, and *Vibrio*) indicates bacterial infection in patients with acute diarrhea and may require antimicrobial sensitivity tests. Since normal fecal flora may include *Clostridium difficile*, *E. coli*, and other organisms, isolation of these may require further tests to demonstrate invasiveness or toxin production. Isolation of pathogens such as *Clostridium botulinum* indicates food poisoning; however, the pathogens must also be isolated from the contaminated food. In a patient undergoing long-term antimicrobial therapy, isolation of large numbers of *Staphylococcus aureus* or yeast, such as *Candida*, may indicate infection.

If a stool culture shows no unusual growth, detection of viruses by immunoassay or electron microscopy may diagnose nonbacterial gastroenteritis.

Interfering factors

Improper collection technique or the presence of urine may injure or destroy some enteric pathogens. Antimicrobial therapy may decrease bacterial growth in the specimen.

Failure to transport the specimen promptly or, if delivery is delayed, to use a transport medium that stabilizes pH (such as a buffered glycerol medium) may result in loss of some enteric pathogens or overgrowth of nonpathogenic organisms.

Special considerations

Use gloves when performing the procedure and handling the specimen. If the patient uses a bedpan or a diaper, avoid contaminating the stool specimen with urine.

Be sure to put the specimen container in a leakproof bag before sending it to the laboratory. Indicate the suspected cause of enteritis and current antimicrobial therapy on the laboratory slip.

Send the specimen to the laboratory immediately; be sure to

include mucoid and bloody portions. The specimen must always represent the first, middle, and last portion of the feces passed.

❖

Throat culture

A throat culture is used primarily to isolate and identify group A beta-hemolytic streptococci (*Streptococcus pyogenes*) — allowing early treatment of pharyngitis — and to prevent sequelae, such as rheumatic heart disease or glomerulonephritis. It also isolates and identifies pathogens, particularly group A beta-hemolytic streptococci, and screens asymptomatic carriers of pathogens, especially *Neisseria meningitidis*.

Normal findings

Normal throat flora includes nonhemolytic and alpha-hemolytic streptococci, *Neisseria* species, staphylococci, diphtheroids, some *Haemophilus* species, pneumococci, yeasts, and enteric gram-negative rods.

Problematic findings

Possible pathogens cultured include group A beta-hemolytic streptococci (*S. pyogenes*), which can cause scarlet fever or pharyngitis; *Candida albicans*, which can cause thrush; *Corynebacterium diphtheriae*, which can cause diphtheria; and *Bordetella pertussis*, which can cause whooping cough. The laboratory report should indicate the prevalent organisms and the quantity of pathogens cultured.

Interfering factors

Failure to report recent or current antimicrobial therapy on the laboratory slip may cause erroneous evaluation of bacterial growth.

Failure to use the proper transport media or delay of more than 15 minutes in sending the specimen to the laboratory may alter test results.

❖

Urine culture

Laboratory examination and culture of urine are necessary for evaluation of urinary tract infections, most commonly of bladder infections. Urine culture helps diagnose urinary tract infection and helps monitor microorganism colonization after urinary catheter insertion.

Normal findings

Culture results of sterile urine are normally reported as "no growth." Usually, this finding indicates the absence of urinary tract infection.

Problematic findings

Bacterial counts of 100,000 organisms/ml or higher of a single microbe species indicate probable urinary tract infection. Counts less than 100,000/ml may be significant, depending on the patient's age, sex, history, and other individual factors. However, counts less than 10,000/ml usually suggest that the organisms are contaminants, except in symptomatic patients, those with urologic disorders, or those whose urine specimens were collected by suprapubic aspiration. A special test for acid-fast bacteria isolates *Mycobacterium tuberculosis*, thus indicating tuberculosis of the urinary tract.

Isolation of more than two species of organisms, or of vaginal or skin organisms, usually suggests contamination and requires a repeat culture. Prolonged catheterization or urinary diversion may cause polymicrobial infection.

Interfering factors

Improper collection technique may contaminate the specimen. Fluid- or drug-induced diuresis and antimicrobial therapy may lower bacterial counts. Improper preservation or delays in sending the specimen to the laboratory may lead to inaccurate counts.

Special considerations

Use gloves when performing the procedure and handling specimens. Collect at least 3 ml of urine, but make sure you don't fill the specimen cup more than halfway. Seal the cup with a sterile lid, and send it to the laboratory immediately. If transport is delayed longer than 30 minutes, store the specimen at 39.2° F (4° C) or place it on ice, unless a urine transport tube containing preservative is used. ❖

Wound culture

A wound culture consists of microscopic analysis of a specimen from a lesion to confirm infection and to identify the infectious microbe.

Normal findings

Normally, no pathogenic organisms are present in a clean wound.

Problematic findings

The most common aerobic pathogens for wound infection include *Staphylococcus aureus*, group A beta-hemolytic streptococci, *Proteus*, *Escherichia coli* and other Enterobacteriaceae, and some *Pseudomonas* species; the most common anaerobic pathogens include some *Clostridium* and *Bacteroides* species.

Interfering factors

Poor collection technique (for example, exposing some specimens to oxygen) may contaminate or invalidate test results. Failure to report recent or current antimicrobial therapy on the laboratory slip may cause erroneous evaluation of bacterial growth. Failure to use the proper transport media may cause the specimen to dry up and the bacteria to die, altering test results.

Special considerations

Use gloves during the procedure and when handling the specimen, and take necessary isolation precautions when sending the specimen to the laboratory.

Cleanse the area around the wound thoroughly to limit contamination of the culture by normal skin flora, such as diphtheroids, *Staphylococcus epidermidis*, and alpha-hemolytic streptococci. However, *don't* cleanse the area around a perineal wound. Make sure no antiseptic enters the wound. Obtain exudate from the entire wound, using more than one swab.

Because some anaerobes die in the presence of even a small amount of oxygen, place the specimen in the culture tube quickly, take care that no air enters the tube, and check that double stoppers are secure. Keep the specimen container upright, and send it to the laboratory within 15 minutes to prevent growth or deterioration of microbes.

Electrolyte tests

For most of these tests, using a tourniquet for sample collection causes venous stasis, which can alter serum electrolyte levels. For all of them, rough handling of the sample can produce hemolysis, which also alters test results.

Serum calcium

This test measures serum levels of calcium, a predominantly extracellular cation that helps regulate and promote neuromuscular and enzyme activity, skeletal development, and blood coagulation. The test aids in diagnosing neuromuscular, skeletal, and endocrine disorders; arrhythmias; blood-clotting deficiencies; and acid-base imbalance.

Normal findings

Serum calcium levels range from 8.9 to 10.1 mg/dl (atomic absorption), or from 4.5 to 5.5 mEq/liter. In children, serum calcium levels are higher than in adults. Calcium levels can rise as high as 12 mg/dl or 6 mEq/liter during phases of rapid bone growth.

Problematic findings

Abnormally high serum calcium levels (hypercalcemia) may occur in hyperparathyroidism and parathyroid tumors (due to oversecretion of parathyroid hormone), Paget's disease of the bone, multiple myeloma, metastatic carcinoma, multiple fractures, or prolonged immobilization. Elevated serum calcium levels may also result from inadequate excretion of calcium, as in adrenal insufficiency and renal disease; from excessive calcium ingestion; or from overuse of antacids such as calcium carbonate.

Interfering factors

Using a tourniquet causes venous stasis and may alter test results. Excessive ingestion of vitamin D or its derivatives (dihydrotachysterol, calcitriol), and the use of androgens, calciferol-activated calcium salts, estrogen-progestin combinations, and thiazides can elevate serum calcium levels. Also, chronic laxative use, excessive transfusions of citrated blood, and administration of acetazolamide, corticosteroids, and mithramycin can alter results.

Serum chloride

This test quantifies serum levels of chloride, the major extracellular fluid anion. The test detects acid-base imbalance (acidosis and alkalosis) and helps evaluate fluid status and extracellular cation-anion balance.

Normal findings
Normally, serum chloride levels range from 95 to 105 mEq/liter.

Problematic findings
Chloride levels relate inversely to those of bicarbonate and thus reflect acid-base balance. Excessive loss of gastric juices or of other secretions containing chloride may cause hypochloremic metabolic alkalosis; excessive chloride retention or ingestion may lead to hyperchloremic metabolic acidosis.

Elevated serum chloride levels (hyperchloremia) may result from severe dehydration, complete renal shutdown, head injury (producing neurogenic hyperventilation), and primary aldosteronism.

Low chloride levels (hypochloremia) are usually associated with low sodium and potassium levels. Possible underlying causes include prolonged vomiting, gastric suctioning, intestinal fistula, chronic renal failure, and Addison's disease. Diabetic acidosis also reduces serum chloride levels by replacing chloride ions with ketone bodies. Congestive heart failure or edema resulting in excess extracellular fluid can cause dilutional hypochloremia.

Interfering factors
Elevated serum chloride levels may result from administration of ammonium chloride, cholestyramine, boric acid, oxyphenbutazone, phenylbutazone, or excessive I.V. infusion of sodium chloride. Serum chloride levels are decreased by thiazides, furosemide, ethacrynic acid, bicarbonates, or prolonged I.V. infusion of 5% dextrose in water. Hemolysis due to rough handling of the sample also may alter test results.

Serum magnesium

Vital to neuromuscular function, this often overlooked electrolyte helps regulate intracellular metabolism, activates many essential enzymes, and affects the metabolism of nucleic acids and proteins. Testing for serum magnesium helps evaluate electrolyte status and assess neuromuscular or renal function.

Normal findings
Serum magnesium levels normally range from 1.7 to 2.1 mg/dl (atomic absorption) or from 1.5 to 2.5 mEq/liter.

Problematic findings
Elevated serum magnesium levels (hypermagnesemia) most commonly occur in renal failure when the kidneys excrete inadequate amounts of magnesium. Adrenal insufficiency (Addison's disease) can also elevate serum magnesium.

Decreased serum magnesium levels (hypomagnesemia) most

commonly result from chronic alcoholism. Other causes include malabsorption syndrome, diarrhea, faulty absorption following bowel resection, prolonged bowel or gastric aspiration, acute pancreatitis, primary aldosteronism, severe burns, hypercalcemic conditions (including hyperparathyroidism), and certain diuretic therapy.

Interfering factors

Using a tourniquet causes venous stasis and may alter test results. Excessive use of antacids or cathartics, excessive infusion of magnesium sulfate, or hemolysis raises magnesium levels. Prolonged I.V. infusions without magnesium or excessive use of diuretics decreases magnesium levels. I.V. administration of calcium gluconate may falsely decrease serum magnesium levels.

Serum phosphate

This test measures serum levels of phosphate, the dominant cellular anion. Phosphate helps store and utilize body energy and helps regulate calcium levels, carbohydrate and lipid metabolism, and acid-base balance. This test aids in the diagnosis of renal disorders and acid-base imbalance. It also can detect endocrine, skeletal, and calcium disorders.

Normal findings

Serum phosphate levels normally range from 2.5 to 4.5 mg/dl (atomic absorption), or from 1.8 to 2.6 mEq/liter. Children have higher serum phosphate levels than adults. Phosphate levels can rise as high as 7 mg/dl or 4.1 mEq/liter during periods of increased bone growth.

Problematic findings

Since serum phosphate values alone are of limited use diagnostically (only a few rare conditions directly affect phosphate metabolism), they should be interpreted in light of serum calcium results.

Depressed phosphate levels (hypophosphatemia) may result from malnutrition, malabsorption syndromes, hyperparathyroidism, renal tubular acidosis, or treatment of diabetic acidosis. In children, hypophosphatemia can suppress normal growth.

Elevated levels (hyperphosphatemia) may result from skeletal disease, healing fractures, hypoparathyroidism, acromegaly, diabetic acidosis, high intestinal obstruction, and renal failure. Hyperphosphatemia is rarely clinically significant; however, if prolonged, it can alter bone metabolism by causing abnormal calcium phosphate deposits.

Interfering factors

Using a tourniquet causes venous stasis and may alter test results. Excessive vitamin D intake or therapy with anabolic steroids or androgens may elevate serum phosphate levels. Hemolysis of the sample falsely increases serum phosphate levels. Suppressed phosphate levels may result from excessive excretion due to prolonged vomiting and diarrhea, vitamin D deficiency, extended I.V. infusion of 5% dextrose in water, use of phosphate-binding antacids, and use of acetazolamide, insulin, and epinephrine.

❖

Serum potassium

This test quantifies serum levels of potassium, the major intracellular cation. Vital to homeostasis, potassium maintains cellular osmotic equilibrium and helps regulate muscle activity (it's essential in maintaining electrical conduction within the cardiac and skeletal muscles). Potassium also helps regulate enzyme activity and acid-base balance and influences kidney function.

This test evaluates clinical signs of potassium excess (hyperkalemia) or depletion (hypokalemia). It's also used to monitor renal function, acid-base balance, and glucose metabolism and to evaluate neuromuscular and endocrine disorders. Finally, serum potassium testing can detect the origin of arrhythmias.

Normal findings
Serum potassium levels normally range from 3.5 to 5 mEq/liter.

Problematic findings
Abnormally high serum potassium levels (hyperkalemia) are common in patients with burns, crushing injuries, diabetic ketoacidosis, and myocardial infarction—conditions in which excessive cellular potassium enters the blood. Hyperkalemia may also indicate reduced sodium excretion, possibly due to renal failure (preventing normal sodium/potassium exchange) or Addison's disease (due to the absence of aldosterone, with consequent potassium buildup and sodium depletion).

Interfering factors
Excessive or rapid potassium infusion, spironolactone or penicillin G potassium therapy, or renal toxicity from administration of amphotericin B, methicillin, or tetracycline elevates serum potassium levels. Insulin and glucose administration, diuretic therapy (especially with thiazides, but not with triamterine, amiloride, or spironolactone), or I.V. infusions without potassium suppress serum potassium levels. Excessive hemolysis of the sample or delay in drawing blood following the application of a tourniquet elevates potassium levels.

❖

Serum sodium

This test measures serum levels of sodium, the major extracellular cation. Sodium affects body water distribution, maintains osmotic pressure of extracellular fluid, and helps promote neuromuscular function; it also helps maintain acid-base balance and influences chloride and potassium levels. This test evaluates fluid-electrolyte and acid-base balance and related neuromuscular, renal, and adrenal functions.

Normal findings
Normally, serum sodium levels range from 135 to 145 mEq/liter.

Water imbalances

This chart shows the differences between hypervolemia and hypovolemia. In hypervolemia, fluid and electrolyte retention increases extracellular fluid volume. In hypovolemia, loss of fluid and electrolytes reduces extracellular fluid volume.

CAUSES	SIGNS AND SYMPTOMS	LABORATORY FINDINGS
Hypervolemia		
• Increased water intake • Reduced urine output due to renal disease • Congestive heart failure • Excessive ingestion or infusion of sodium chloride • Long-term administration of corticotropin • Excessive infusion of isotonic solutions	• Increased blood pressure, pulse rate, body weight, respiratory rate • Bounding peripheral pulses • Moist pulmonary crackles • Moist mucous membranes • Moist respiratory secretions • Edema • Weakness • Seizures and coma caused by cerebral edema	• Decreased red blood cell (RBC) count, hemoglobin (Hb) concentration, packed cell volume, serum sodium concentration (dilutional decrease), urine specific gravity
Hypovolemia		
• Decreased water intake • Fluid loss due to diarrhea, fever, vomiting • Systemic infection • Impaired renal concentrating ability • Fistulous drainage • Severe burns • Hidden fluid in body cavities	• Increased pulse rate, respiratory rate • Decreased blood pressure, body weight • Weak and thready peripheral pulses • Thick, slurred speech • Thirst • Oliguria • Anuria • Dry skin	• Increased RBC count, Hb concentration, packed cell volume, serum sodium concentration, urine specific gravity

Problematic findings

Sodium imbalance can result from a loss or gain of sodium or from a change in water volume. Remember, serum sodium results must be interpreted in light of the patient's state of hydration. (See *Water imbalances*.)

Elevated serum sodium levels (hypernatremia) may be due to inadequate water intake, water loss in excess of sodium loss (as in diabetes insipidus, impaired renal function, prolonged hyperventilation and, occasionally, severe vomiting or diarrhea), and sodium retention (as in aldosteronism). Hypernatremia can also result from excessive sodium intake.

Abnormally low serum sodium levels (hyponatremia) may result from inadequate sodium intake or excessive sodium loss due to profuse sweating, GI suctioning, diuretic therapy, diarrhea, vomiting, adrenal insufficiency, burns, or chronic renal insufficiency with acidosis. Urine sodium determinations are frequently more sensitive to early changes in sodium balance and should always be evaluated simultaneously with serum sodium findings.

Interfering factors

Most diuretics suppress serum sodium levels by promoting sodium excretion; lithium, chlorpropamide, and vasopressin suppress levels by inhibiting water excretion. Corticosteroids elevate serum sodium levels by promoting sodium retention. Antihypertensives, such as methyldopa, hydralazine, and reserpine, may cause sodium and water retention.

Hemolysis due to rough handling of the sample may alter test results.

❖

Fecal content tests

The patient's adherence to pretest drug and dietary restrictions is important to ensure accurate results in these fecal tests. Proper handling of the specimen is important as well, including immediate testing or transport of a sample for fecal occult blood testing.

Fecal lipids

Lipids excreted in feces include monoglycerides, diglycerides, triglycerides, phospholipids, glycolipids, soaps (fatty acids and fatty acid salts), sterols, and cholesterol esters. The fecal lipids test confirms steatorrhea.

Normal findings

Fecal lipids normally comprise less than 20% of excreted solids, with excretion of less than 7 g/ 24 hours.

Problematic findings

Both digestive and absorptive disorders cause steatorrhea. Digestive disorders may affect the production and release of pancreatic lipase or bile; absorptive disorders may affect the integrity of the intestine. In pancreatic insufficiency, impaired lipid digestion may result from insufficient production of lipase.

Pancreatic resection, cystic fibrosis, chronic pancreatitis, or ductal obstruction by stone or tumor may prevent the normal release or action of lipase. In impaired hepatic function, faulty lipid digestion may result from inadequate production of bile salts. Biliary obstruction, which may accompany gallbladder disease, may prevent the normal release of bile salts into the duodenum. Extensive small bowel resection or bypass may also interrupt normal enterohepatic circulation of bile salts.

Interfering factors
The following substances may alter test results by inhibiting absorption or affecting chemical digestion: azathioprine, bisacodyl, cholestyramine, kanamycin, neomycin, colchicine, aluminum hydroxide, calcium carbonate, alcohol, potassium chloride, and mineral oil.

Failure to observe pretest instructions pertaining to diet and ingestion of alcohol, use of a waxed collection container, contamination of the sample, and incomplete stool specimen collection (total weight less than 300 g) interfere with accurate testing.

Special considerations
Don't use a waxed collection container because the wax may become incorporated in the stool and alter test results. Tell the patient to avoid contaminating the stool specimen with toilet tissue or urine. Refrigerate the collection container between defecations, and keep it tightly covered. Wear gloves and handle the specimen carefully; it may be a source of infection.

Fecal occult blood

Fecal occult blood, invisible because of its minute quantity, can be detected by microscopic analysis or by chemical tests for hemoglobin, such as the guaiac or orthotoluidine test. Testing for fecal occult blood is done to detect GI bleeding and to aid the early diagnosis of colorectal cancer.

Normal findings
The test should reveal less than 2.5 ml/day of blood normally, resulting in a green reaction.

Problematic findings
A dark blue reaction that appears within 5 minutes indicates that the test is positive for occult blood; a strongly positive reaction within 3 to 4 minutes is always abnormal. A faint blue reaction is weakly positive and isn't necessarily abnormal. A positive test indicates GI bleeding, which may result from many disorders, such as varices, a peptic ulcer, carcinoma, ulcerative colitis, dysentery, or hemorrhagic disease. (See *Common sites and causes of GI blood loss.*)

Approximately 80% of people with colorectal cancer demonstrate positive test results.

Interfering factors
Failure of the patient to adhere to dietary restrictions before the test or failure to test the specimen immediately or to send it to the laboratory immediately may alter test results. If possible, the patient should not ingest meat or fish for 2 days before the test.

Common sites and causes of GI blood loss

Following are typical sites of GI blood loss and the possible causes.

Oral and pharyngeal
Hemangioma
Malignant tumor

Esophageal
Malignant and benign tumors
Eroding esophagus
Esophagitis
Varices
Peptic ulcer
Hiatal hernia

Hepatic
Liver cirrhosis (and other causes of portal hypertension)

Gastric
Varices
Diverticulum
Carcinoma
Benign tumor
Peptic ulcer
Gastritis
Erosions

Duodenal
Peptic ulcer
Duodenitis
Diverticulum
Ampullary tumor

Pancreatic
Pancreatitis
Eroding carcinoma

Jejunal and ileal
Peptic ulcer
Meckel's diverticulum
Mesenteric thrombosis
Intussusception
Benign tumor
Regional enteritis
Tuberculosis
Malignant tumor

Colonic and rectal
Polyps
Hemangioma
Malignant tumor
Diverticulitis or diverticulosis
Ulcerative colitis
Foreign body
Hemorrhoids
Fissure

Nonpathologic bleeding can result from the use of iron preparations, bromides, rauwolfia derivatives, indomethacin, colchicine, phenylbutazone, or corticosteroids. Ascorbic acid (vitamin C) can produce false-normal test results even in the presence of significant bleeding. Ingestion of 2 to 5 ml of blood, such as from bleeding gums, can cause abnormal results.

❖

Hepatic enzyme tests

Many drugs can falsely elevate or depress serum enzyme levels; if the drugs can't be temporarily withheld, their use must be noted on the laboratory slip. Hemolysis from rough handling of the sample can affect test results.

Alanine aminotransferase

Alanine aminotranferase (ALT) is one of two enzymes that catalyze a reversible amino group transfer reaction in the Krebs cycle (citric acid or tricarboxylic acid cycle) and are necessary for tissue energy production. Unlike aspartate aminotransferase (AST), the other aminotransferase, ALT primarily appears in hepatocellular cytoplasm, with lesser amounts in the kidneys, heart, and skeletal muscles, and is a relatively specific indicator of acute hepatocellular damage.

This serum test helps detect and evaluate treatment of acute hepatic disease—especially hepatitis, and cirrhosis without jaundice. It can help distinguish between myocardial and hepatic tissue damage (used with AST). It's also used to assess the hepatotoxicity of certain drugs.

Normal findings
Serum ALT levels range from 8 to 20 units/liter.

Problematic findings
Very high ALT levels (up to 50 times normal) suggest viral or severe drug-induced hepatitis or other hepatic disease with extensive necrosis. (AST levels are also elevated but usually to a lesser degree.) Moderate-to-high levels may indicate infectious mononucleosis, chronic hepatitis, intrahepatic cholestasis or cholecystitis, early or improving acute viral hepatitis, or severe hepatic congestion due to heart failure. Slight to moderate elevations of ALT (usually with higher increases in AST levels) may appear in any condition that produces acute hepatocellular injury—such as active cirrhosis, and drug-induced or alcoholic hepatitis. Marginal elevations occasionally occur in acute myocardial infarction, reflecting secondary hepatic congestion or the release of small amounts of ALT from myocardial tissue.

Interfering factors
Many medications produce hepatic injury by competitively interfering with cellular metabolism. Falsely elevated ALT levels can follow the use of barbiturates, griseofulvin, isoniazid, nitrofurantoin, methyldopa, phenothiazines, phenytoin, salicylates, tetracycline, chlorpromazine, para-aminosalicylic acid, and other drugs that affect the liver. Narcotic analgesics (morphine, codeine, meperidine) may also falsely elevate ALT levels by increasing intrabiliary pressure.

Ingestion of lead or exposure to carbon tetrachloride causes direct injury to hepatic cells and sharp elevations of ALT.

Hemolysis caused by rough handling of the sample also may alter test results.

❖

Alkaline phosphatase

Alkaline phosphatase (ALP) influences bone calcification and lipid and metabolite transport. Total serum levels reflect the combined activity of several ALP isoenzymes found in the liver, bones, kidneys, intestinal lining, and placenta.

Although both skeletal and hepatic diseases can raise ALP levels, this serum test is most useful for diagnosing metabolic bone disease. Additional liver function studies are usually required to identify hepatobiliary disorders. The test is also used to assess response to vitamin D in the treatment of deficiency-induced rickets.

Normal findings

Total ALP levels, when measured by chemical inhibition, range from 90 to 239 units/liter for males. For females under age 45, total ALP levels range from 76 to 196 units/liter; for women over age 45, the range widens to 87 to 250 units/liter.

Problematic findings

Although significant ALP elevations are possible with diseases that affect many organs, they are most likely to indicate skeletal disease or extrahepatic or intrahepatic biliary obstruction causing cholestasis. Many acute hepatic diseases cause ALP elevations before they result in any change in serum bilirubin levels. A moderate rise in ALP levels may reflect acute biliary obstruction from hepatocellular inflammation in active cirrhosis, infectious mononucleosis, and viral hepatitis. Moderate increases are also seen in osteomalacia and deficiency-induced rickets.

Sharp elevations of ALP levels may result from complete biliary obstruction by malignant tumors, infectious infiltrations, or fibrosis. Such markedly high levels are most common in Paget's disease and, occasionally, in biliary obstruction, extensive bone tumor metastases, or hyperparathyroidism. Metastatic bone tumors resulting from pancreatic cancer raise ALP levels without a concomitant rise in serum alanine aminotransferase levels.

Isoenzyme fractionation and additional enzyme tests – gamma glutamyl transferase, lactate dehydrogenase, 5'-nucleotidase, and leucine aminopeptidase – are sometimes performed when the cause of ALP elevations (skeletal or hepatic disease) is in doubt. Rarely, low levels of serum ALP are associated with hypophosphatasia and protein or magnesium deficiency.

Interfering factors

Recent ingestion of vitamin D may increase levels of ALP because of the effect of vitamin D on osteoblastic activity. Recent infusion of albumin prepared from placental venous blood causes extreme increases in serum ALP levels. Drugs that influence liver function or cause cholestasis, such as barbiturates, chlorpropamide, oral contraceptives, isoniazid, methyldopa, phenothiazines, phenytoin, and

FINDINGS

rifampin, can mildly elevate ALP levels; halothane sensitivity may increase levels drastically. Clofibrate decreases ALP levels.

Healing long bone fractures, age (infancy, childhood, adolescence, and ages 45 and older in women), and pregnancy (third trimester) can produce physiologic elevations of ALP levels.

Hemolysis due to rough handling of the sample or specimen analysis after 4 hours also may alter test results.   ❖

Aspartate aminotransferase

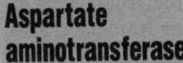

Aspartate aminotransferase (AST) is one of two enzymes that catalyze the conversion of the nitrogenous portion of an amino acid to an amino acid residue.

Although a high correlation exists between myocardial infarction (MI) and elevated AST, this serum test is sometimes considered superfluous for diagnosing MI because of its relatively low organ specificity; it doesn't enable differentiation between acute MI and the effects of hepatic congestion due to heart failure. Nevertheless, the test is used in the diagnosis of MI, particularly in correlation with creatine kinase and lactate dehydrogenase levels.

AST levels aid detection and differential diagnosis of acute hepatic disease. They're also used to monitor patient progress and prognosis in cardiac and hepatic diseases.

Normal findings

AST levels range from 8 to 20 units/liter. Normal values for infants are as high as four times those of adults.

Problematic findings

AST levels fluctuate in response to the extent of cellular necrosis and therefore may be transiently and minimally elevated early in the disease process and extremely elevated during the most acute phase. Depending on when during the course of the disease the initial sample was drawn, AST levels can rise—indicating increasing disease severity and tissue damage—or fall—indicating disease resolution and tissue repair. Thus, the relative change in AST values serves as a reliable monitoring mechanism.

Maximum elevations are associated with certain diseases and conditions. For example, very high elevations (more than 20 times normal) may indicate acute viral hepatitis, severe skeletal muscle trauma, extensive surgery, drug-induced hepatic injury, and severe passive liver congestion.

High levels (ranging from 10 to 20 times normal) may indicate severe MI, severe infectious mononucleosis, and alcoholic cirrhosis. High levels also occur during the prodromal or resolving stages of conditions that cause maximal elevations.

Moderate to high levels (ranging from 5 to 10 times normal) may indicate Duchenne muscular dystrophy, dermatomyositis, and chronic hepatitis. Moderate to high levels also occur during prodromal and resolving stages of diseases that cause high elevations.

Low to moderate levels (ranging from two to five times normal) may indicate hemolytic anemia, metastatic hepatic tumors, acute pancreatitis, pulmonary emboli, delirium tremens, and fatty liver. AST levels rise slightly after the first few days of biliary duct obstruction. Also, low to moderate elevations occur at some time during any of the preceding conditions or diseases.

Interfering factors
Chlorpropamide; opiates; methyldopa; erythromycin; sulfonamides; pyridoxine; dicumarol; antitubercular agents; large doses of acetaminophen, salicylates, and vitamin A; and many other drugs known to affect the liver cause elevated AST levels. Strenuous exercise and muscle trauma caused by intramuscular injections also raise AST levels.

Hemolysis due to rough handling of the sample may alter test results, as can missing peak AST levels by failing to draw the sample as scheduled.

Special considerations
To avoid missing peak AST levels, draw serum samples at the same time each day.

————————————————❖

Immune function tests

Careful handling of blood samples is paramount for most of these tests. Hemolysis and failure to send the sample immediately to the laboratory for testing can alter the results.

Antinuclear antibody test

In conditions such as systemic lupus erythematosus (SLE), scleroderma, and certain infections, the body's immune system may perceive portions of its own cell nuclei as foreign and may produce antinuclear antibodies (ANA). This test is used to screen for SLE and to monitor the effectiveness of immunosuppressive therapy for SLE.

Normal findings
Using Hep-2 cells, the test for ANA is negative at a titer of 1:40 or below. If mouse kidney substrate is being used, the test is negative at a titer less than 1:20.

Problematic findings
Although the test is a sensitive indicator of ANA, it is not specific for SLE. Low titers may occur in patients with viral diseases, chronic hepatic disease, collagen vascular disease, and autoimmune diseases and in some healthy adults; incidence increases with age. The higher the titer, the more specific the test is for SLE (titer often exceeds 1:256).

The pattern of nuclear fluorescence helps identify the type of immune disease present. A peripheral pattern is almost exclusively associated with SLE since it indicates the presence of antideoxyribonucleic acid (DNA) antibodies; anti-DNA antibodies are sometimes measured by radioimmunoassay if ANA titers are high or a peripheral pattern is observed. A homogeneous, or diffuse, pattern is also associated with SLE and with related connective tissue disorders; a nucleolar pattern, with scleroderma; and a speckled, irregular pattern, with infectious mononucleosis and mixed connective tissue disorders (for example, SLE and scleroderma).

A single serum sample, especially one collected from a patient with collagen vascular disease, may contain antibodies to several parts of the cell's nucleus. In addition, as serum dilution increases, the fluorescent pattern may change because different antibodies are reactive at different titers.

Interfering factors

Certain drugs—most commonly isoniazid, hydralazine, and procainamide—can produce a syndrome resembling SLE; other such drugs include para-aminosalicylic acid, chlorpromazine, clofibrate, phenytoin, griseofulvin, ethosuximide, gold salts, methyldopa, oral contraceptives, penicillin, propylthiouracil, phenylbutazone, methysergide, streptomycin, sulfonamides, tetracyclines, mephenytoin, quinidine, primidone, reserpine, and trimethadione. ❖

Complement assays

Complement is a collective term for a system of at least 20 serum proteins designed to destroy foreign cells and to help remove foreign materials. Complement can function as a defense by promoting removal of infectious agents, or as a threat by triggering destructive reactions in host tissues. Therefore, complement deficiency can increase an individual's susceptibility to infection and can predispose him to other diseases.

The complement assay is used to help detect immunomediated disease and genetic complement deficiency, as well as to monitor the effectiveness of therapy.

Normal findings

Complement values normally range as follows:
Total complement: 330 to 730 CH_{50} units
C1 esterase inhibitor: 7.8 to 23.4 mg/dl
C3: 57 to 125 mg/dl
C4: 10 to 54 mg/dl.

Problematic findings

Complement abnormalities may be genetic or acquired; acquired abnormalities are most common. Depressed total complement levels (which are clinically more significant than elevations) may result from excessive formation of antigen-antibody complexes, insufficient synthesis of complement, inhibitor formation, or increased complement catabolism, and are characteristic in conditions such as systemic lupus erythematosus (SLE), acute poststreptococcal glomerulonephritis, and acute serum sickness. Low levels may also occur in some patients with advanced cirrhosis of the liver, multiple myeloma, hypogammaglobulinemia, and rapidly rejecting allografts.

Elevated total complement levels may occur in obstructive jaundice, thyroiditis, acute rheumatic fever, rheumatoid arthritis, acute myocardial infarction, ulcerative colitis, and diabetes.

C1 esterase inhibitor deficiency is characteristic in hereditary angioedema, the most common genetic abnormality associated with complement; C3 deficiency is characteristic in recurrent pyogenic infection; C4 deficiency is characteristic in SLE.

Interfering factors
A history of recent heparin therapy, hemolysis due to rough handling of the sample, or failure to send the sample to the laboratory immediately may alter test results.

❖

Human immunodeficiency virus antibody test

This test detects antibodies to human immunodeficiency virus (HIV) in serum. It's used to screen for HIV in high-risk groups and to screen donated blood for HIV. (See *Precautions with HIV testing*.)

Test results should normally be nonreactive.

Problematic findings
The test detects previous exposure to the virus. However, it doesn't identify patients who have been exposed to the virus but who haven't yet made antibodies. Most patients with acquired immunodeficiency syndrome (AIDS) have antibodies to HIV. A positive test for the HIV antibody can't determine whether or not a patient harbors actively replicating virus or when the patient will present signs and symptoms of AIDS.

Precautions with HIV testing

When drawing a blood sample for human immunodeficiency virus (HIV) testing (or for any reason), always follow the universal precautions recommended by the Centers for Disease Control and Prevention. Use gloves, dispose of needles properly, and use blood-fluid precaution labels on tubes, as necessary.

Many apparently healthy people have been exposed to HIV and have circulating antibodies. *These are not false-positive results.* Furthermore, patients in the later stages of AIDS may exhibit no detectable antibody in their sera because they can no longer mount an antibody response.

Interfering factors
None.

❖

Human leukocyte antigen test

The human leukocyte antigen (HLA) test identifies a group of antigens present on the surfaces of all nucleated cells but most easily detected on lymphocytes. These antigens are essential to immunity and determine the degree of histocompatibility between transplant recipients and donors. The HLA test provides

PUZZLING LAB FINDINGS

histocompatibility typing of tissue recipients and donors. It's used in genetic counseling and in paternity testing.

Normal findings

In HLA-A, HLA-B, and HLA-C testing, lymphocytes that react with the test antiserum undergo lysis; they're detected by phase microscopy. In HLA-D testing, leukocyte incompatibility is marked by blast formation, deoxyribonucleic acid synthesis, and proliferation.

Problematic findings

Incompatible HLA-A, HLA-B, HLA-C, or HLA-D groups may cause unsuccessful tissue transplantation.

Many diseases have a strong association with certain types of HLAs. For example, HLA-DR5 is associated with Hashimoto's thyroiditis. B8 and Dw3 are associated with Graves' disease, whereas B8 alone is associated with chronic autoimmune hepatitis, celiac disease, and myasthenia gravis. Dw3 alone is associated with Addison's disease, Sjögren's syndrome, dermatitis herpetiformis, and systemic lupus erythematosus.

In paternity testing, a putative father who presents a phenotype (two haplotypes: one from the father and one from the mother) with no haplotype or antigen pair identical to one of the child's is ruled out as the father. A putative father with one haplotype identical to one of the child's *may* be the father; the probability varies with the incidence of the haplotype in the population.

Interfering factors

HLA from blood transfused within 72 hours before the collection of a sample or hemolysis due to rough handling of the sample may alter test results.

❖

Lymphocyte transformation tests

The transformation tests evaluate lymphocyte competency without requiring an injection of antigens into the patient's skin. This collection of in vitro tests eliminates the risk of adverse effects but can still accurately assess the ability of lymphocytes to proliferate and to recognize and respond to antigens.

The tests are used to assess and monitor genetic and acquired immunodeficiency states. They provide histocompatibility typing of both tissue transplant recipients and donors. They can also detect if a patient has been exposed to various pathogens, such as those that cause malaria, hepatitis, and mycoplasmal pneumonia.

Normal findings

Results depend on the mitogens used. Reference ranges accompany test results.

Problematic findings

In the mitogen and antigen assays, a low stimulation index or unresponsiveness indicates a depressed or defective immune system. Serial testing can be performed to monitor the effectiveness of therapy in a patient with an immunodeficiency disease.

In the mixed lymphocyte culture, the stimulation index is a measure of compatibility. A high index indicates poor compatibility. Conversely, a low stimulation index indicates good compatibility.

A high stimulation index, in response to the relevant pathogen, can also demonstrate exposure to malaria, hepatitis, mycoplasmal pneumonia, periodontal disease, and certain viral infections in patients who no longer have detectable serum antibodies.

Interfering factors
Pregnancy or the use of oral contraceptives depresses lymphocyte response to phytohemagglutinin and thus causes a low stimulation index. Chemotherapy may hinder accurate determination of test results unless pretherapy baseline values are available for comparison. A radioisotope scan performed within 1 week before the test and failure to send the sample to the laboratory immediately can affect accuracy of test results. ❖

Serum cytomegalovirus antibody screen

After primary infection, cytomegalovirus (CMV) remains latent in white blood cells (WBCs). In an immunocompromised patient, CMV can be reactivated to cause active infection. The presence of CMV antibodies indicates past infection with this virus.

This screen is used to detect past CMV infection in organ transplant donors and recipients. It's also used to detect past CMV infection in immunocompromised patients and especially in premature neonates who receive transfused blood products.

Normal findings
Patients who have never been infected with CMV have no detectable antibodies to the virus (less than 1:5). A serum specimen positive for antibody at this single dilution indicates that the patient has been infected with CMV and that the patient's WBCs contain latent virus capable of being reactivated in an immunocompromised host.

Problematic findings
Immunosuppressed patients who lack antibodies to CMV should receive blood products or organ transplants from donors who are also seronegative to avoid the morbidity and mortality associated with active infection with this virus. Patients with CMV antibodies can receive seropositive blood products.

Interfering factors
Hemolysis due to rough handling of the sample may alter test results. ❖

Serum herpes simplex antibody assays

Herpes simplex virus (HSV), a member of the herpesvirus group, causes various clinically severe manifestations, including genital lesions, keratitis or conjunctivitis, generalized dermal lesions, and pneumonia. Severe involvement is associated with intrauterine or neonatal infections and encephalitis; such infections are most severe in immunosuppressed patients. These tests can confirm systemic infections caused by HSV.

Normal findings
Sera from patients who have never been infected with HSV will have no detectable antibodies (less than 1:5). Patients who experience primary infections with HSV will develop both immunoglobulin M (IgM) and immunoglobulin G (IgG) class antibodies. Reportedly, over 50% of adults have IgG class antibodies to HSV because of prior infection. Reactivated infections caused by HSV can be recognized serologically only by an increase in IgG class antibodies between acute- and convalescent-phase sera.

Problematic findings
HSV infections can be ruled out in patients whose sera show no detectable antibodies to the virus. The presence of IgM or a fourfold or greater increase in IgG antibodies indicates active HSV infection.

Interfering factors
Hemolysis due to rough handling of the sample will alter test results.

─────────────────── ❖

Serum immune complex assays

When immune complexes are produced faster than they can be cleared by the lymphoreticular system, immune complex disease may occur: for example, postinfectious syndromes, serum sickness, drug sensitivity, rheumatoid arthritis (RA), and systemic lupus erythematosus (SLE). This test can demonstrate circulating immune complexes in serum, monitor patient response to therapy, and estimate the severity of disease.

Normal findings
Immune complexes are not normally detectable in serum.

Problematic findings
The presence of detectable immune complexes in serum has etiologic importance in many autoimmune diseases, such as SLE and RA. However, for definitive diagnosis, the presence of these complexes must be considered with the results of other studies. For example, in SLE, immune complexes are associated with high titers of antinuclear antibodies and circulating antinative deoxyribonucleic acid antibodies.

Because of their filtering function, renal glomeruli seem most vulnerable to immune complex deposition, although blood vessel walls and choroid plexuses (vascular folds in the ventricles of the brain) can be affected. Renal biopsy to detect immune complexes can provide conclusive evidence for immune complex glomerulonephritis, differentiating it from other types of glomerulonephritis.

Interfering factors
Failure to send the serum sample to the laboratory immediately can result in the deterioration of immune complexes and alter test results. The presence of cryoglobulins in the patient's serum and the inability to standardize rheumatoid factor inhibition tests and platelet aggregation assays can also alter test results. ❖

Serum thyroid-stimulating immunoglobulin test

Thyroid-stimulating immunoglobulin (TSI), formerly called long-acting thyroid stimulator, appears in the blood of most patients with Graves' disease. This autoantibody reacts with the cell-surface receptors that usually combine with thyroid-stimulating hormone. This test aids in the evaluation of suspected thyroid disease. It also helps diagnose suspected thyrotoxicosis (Graves' disease), especially in patients with exophthalmos, and helps monitor the treatment of thyrotoxicosis.

Normal findings
TSI doesn't normally appear in serum. However, it may be present in 5% of persons without hyperthyroidism or exophthalmos.

Problematic findings
Increased TSI levels are associated with exophthalmos, Graves' disease, and the recurrence of hyperthyroidism.

Interfering factors
Administration of radioactive iodine within 48 hours of the test or hemolysis due to rough handling of the sample may alter test results. ❖

T- and B-lymphocyte assays

Lymphocytes—key cells in the immune system—have the capacity to recognize antigens through special receptors found on their surfaces. The two main kinds of lymphocytes, T and B cells, originate in the bone marrow. The T cells mature under the influence of the thymus gland; B cells evolve without thymic influence. This test aids the diagnosis of primary and secondary immunodeficiency diseases, distinguishes between benign and malignant lymphocytic proliferative diseases, and monitors patient response to therapy. (See *Lymphocyte marker assays*, pages 148 and 149.)

Normal findings
Currently, T- and B-cell assays are being standardized, and values may differ from one laboratory to another, depending on test technique. Generally, T cells comprise 68% to 75% of total lymphocytes; B cells, 10% to 20%; and null cells, 5% to 20%. The total lymphocyte count

Lymphocyte marker assays

A normal immune response requires a balance between the regulatory activities of several interacting cell types—most notably, T-helper and T-suppressor cells. By using highly specific monoclonal antibodies, levels of lymphocyte differentiation can be defined, and both normal and malignant cell populations can be analyzed. Direct and indirect immunofluorescence, microcytotoxicity, and immunoperoxidase immunoassay techniques are used most frequently: These employ an anticoagulated blood sample combined with monoclonal antibodies that react with specific T- and B-cell markers. The chart below lists some commonly ordered lymphocyte marker assays and their indications.

LYMPHOCYTE MARKER ASSAY	PURPOSE
Pan T-cell marker	• To measure mature T cells in immune dysfunction
T-helper subset marker	• To identify and characterize the proportion of T-helper cells in autoimmune or immunoregulatory disorders • To detect immunodeficiency disorders, such as acquired immunodeficiency syndrome • To differentiate T-cell acute lymphoblastic leukemia from T-cell lymphomas and other lymphoproliferative disorders
T-suppressor subset marker	• To identify and characterize the proportion of T-suppressor cells in autoimmune and immunoregulatory disorders • To characterize lymphoproliferative disorders
T-cell/E-rosette receptor	• To differentiate lymphoproliferative disorders of T-cell origin, such as T-cell lymphocytic leukemia and lymphoblastic lymphoma, from those of non-T-cell origin
Pan-B (B1) marker	• To differentiate lymphoproliferative disorders of B-cell origin, such as B-cell chronic lymphocytic leukemia, from those of T-cell origin

Lymphocyte marker assays *(continued)*

LYMPHOCYTE MARKER ASSAY	PURPOSE
Pan-B (BA-1) marker	• To identify B-cell lymphoproliferative disorders, such as B-cell chronic lymphocytic leukemia
CALLA (common acute lymphoblastic leukemia antigen) marker	• To identify bone marrow regeneration • To identify non-T-cell acute lymphocytic leukemia
Lymphocyte subset panel (B, pan-T, T-helper, T-suppressor, and T-helper/T-suppressor ratio)	• To evaluate immunodeficiencies • To identify immunoregulation associated with autoimmune disorders • To characterize lymphoid malignancies
Lymphocytic leukemia marker panel (T-cell markers [E rosette receptor and Leu-9], B-cell markers [B-1 and BA-1], and CALLA)	• To characterize lymphocytic leukemias as T, B, non-T, or non-B, regardless of the stage of differentiation of the malignant cells

ranges from 1,500 to 3,000/mm³; the T-cell count varies from 1,400 to 2,700/mm³; and the B-cell count ranges from 270 to 640/mm³. These counts are higher in children.

Problematic findings

An abnormal T- or B-cell count suggests, but doesn't confirm, specific diseases. The B-cell count is elevated in chronic lymphocytic leukemia (thought to be a B-cell malignancy), multiple myeloma, Waldenström's macroglobulinemia, and DiGeorge's syndrome (a congenital T-cell deficiency). B cells decrease in acute lymphocytic leukemia and in certain congenital or acquired immunoglobulin deficiency diseases. In other immunoglobulin deficiency diseases, especially if only one immunoglobulin class is deficient, the B-cell count remains normal.

The T-cell count rises occasionally in infectious mononucleosis; it rises more often in multiple myeloma and acute lymphocytic leukemia. T cells decrease in congenital T-cell deficiency diseases, such as DiGeorge's, Nezlof's, and Wiskott-Aldrich syndromes, and in certain B-cell proliferative disorders, such as chronic lymphocytic leukemia, Waldenström's macroglobulinemia, and acquired immunodeficiency syndrome.

Normal T- and B-cell counts don't necessarily assure a competent immune system. In autoimmune diseases, such as systemic lupus erythematosus and rheumatoid arthritis, T and B cells, though present in normal numbers, may not be functionally competent.

Interfering factors

Failure to use the proper collection tube, to mix the sample and anticoagulant adequately, or to send the sample to the laboratory immediately can alter test results. T- and B-cell counts can change rapidly with changes in health status, from the effects of stress, or after surgery, chemotherapy, corticosteroid or immunosuppressive therapy, and X-rays. The presence of immunoglobulins, such as autologous antilymphocyte antibodies that sometimes occur in autoimmune disease, also can alter test results.

—————————————— ❖

Lipid and lipoprotein tests

Compliance with pretest dietary and alcohol restrictions and withholding or noting the use of certain compromising drugs can help ensure accurate results in these tests.

Lipoprotein-cholesterol fractionation

Cholesterol fractionation tests assess a patient's risk for coronary artery disease (CAD). They isolate and measure the cholesterol in serum – low-density lipoproteins (LDL) and high-density lipoproteins (HDL) – by ultracentrifugation or electrophoresis. The cholesterol in LDL and HDL fractions is significant: The Framingham Heart Study has shown that cholesterol in HDL is inversely related to the incidence of CAD. That is, the higher the HDL level, the lower the incidence of CAD; conversely, the higher the LDL level, the higher the incidence of CAD.

Normal findings

Since normal cholesterol values vary according to age, sex, geographic region, and ethnic group, check the laboratory for the normal values in your hospital. An alternate method (measuring cholesterol and triglyceride levels and separating out HDL by selective precipitation, and using these values to calculate LDL) provides normal HDL-cholesterol levels that range from 29 to 77 mg/100 ml and normal LDL-cholesterol levels that range from 62 to 185 mg/100 ml.

Problematic findings

High LDL levels increase the risk of CAD. Elevated HDL levels generally reflect a healthy state but can also indicate chronic hepatitis, early-stage primary biliary cirrhosis, or alcohol consumption. Rarely, a sharp rise (to as high as 100 mg/dl) in a second type of HDL (alpha$_2$-HDL) may signal CAD. Although cholesterol fractionation provides valuable information about the risk of heart disease, remember that sources of such risk besides cholesterol—diabetes mellitus, hypertension, cigarette smoking, and heredity—are at least as important.

Interfering factors

Values are increased by food intake, so the patient shouldn't eat or drink anything except water for 12 to 14 hours before the test.

Values are lowered by antilipemic medications, such as clofibrate, cholestyramine, colestipol, dextrothyroxine, niacin, probucol, and gemfibrozil. Oral contraceptives, disulfiram, alcohol, miconazole, and high doses of phenothiazines may increase values. Estrogens usually increase values, but they may also decrease them.

Failure to send the sample to the laboratory immediately may allow spontaneous redistribution of the lipoproteins and alter test results. Collecting the sample in a heparinized tube may produce false elevation of values through activation of the enzyme lipase, which, in turn, causes the release of fatty acids from triglycerides. The presence of bilirubin, hemoglobin, salicylates, iodine, vitamins A and D, and some other substances may alter test results. Some procedures (for example, Abell-Kendall) are less susceptible to interference than others. Concurrent illness, especially if accompanied by fever, recent surgery, or myocardial infarction, may alter test results. ❖

Phospholipids

This test aids in the evaluation of fat metabolism. Because a quantitative analysis of phospholipid levels adds minimal information to that provided by cholesterol levels, the test is not as useful as it once was. But it aids in diagnosing hypothyroidism, diabetes mellitus, nephrotic syndrome, chronic pancreatitis, obstructive jaundice, and hypolipoproteinemia.

Normal findings

Normal phospholipid levels range from 180 to 320 mg/dl. Although males usually have higher levels than females, values in pregnant females exceed those of males.

Problematic findings

Elevated levels may indicate hypothyroidism, diabetes mellitus, nephrotic syndrome, chronic pancreatitis, or obstructive jaundice. Decreased levels may indicate primary hypolipoproteinemia.

Interfering factors

Clofibrate and other antilipemics may lower phospholipid levels; estrogens, epinephrine, and some phenothiazines, such as chlorpromazine, increase levels. Failure of the patient to follow dietary restrictions may alter test results. ❖

Triglycerides

This test quantifies triglycerides – the main storage form of lipids – which constitute about 95% of fatty tissue. The test is used to screen for hyperlipemia, to help identify nephrotic syndrome, and to help determine a patient's risk of coronary artery disease (CAD).

Normal findings

Triglyceride values are age- and sex-related. Some controversy exists over the most appropriate normal ranges. Nonetheless, serum values of 40 to 160 mg/dl for adult men and 35 to 135 mg/dl for adult women are widely accepted.

Problematic findings

Increased or decreased serum triglyceride levels merely suggest a clinical abnormality, and additional tests are required for definitive diagnosis. For example, measurement of cholesterol may also be necessary, since cholesterol and triglycerides vary independently. High levels of triglycerides and cholesterol reflect an exaggerated risk of CAD.

Mild to moderate increases in serum triglyceride levels may indicate biliary obstruction, diabetes, nephrotic syndrome, endocrinopathies, or overconsumption of alcohol. Markedly increased levels without an identifiable cause reflect congenital hyperlipoproteinemia and necessitate lipoprotein phenotyping to confirm a diagnosis.

Decreased serum levels are rare, occurring mainly in malnutrition or abetalipoproteinemia.

In the latter, serum is virtually devoid of beta-lipoproteins and triglycerides because the body lacks the capacity to transport preformed triglycerides from the epithelial cells of the intestinal mucosa or from the liver. Decreased levels also appear with COPD.

Interfering factors

Failure of the patient to comply with dietary restrictions or use of glycol-lubricated collection tubes may alter test results.

Ingestion of alcohol within 24 hours of the test may cause elevated triglyceride levels. In fact, excessive consumption of alcohol is a common cause of excess concentration of triglycerides. Alcohol is heavily hydrogenated. As a result, this hydrogen has to be disposed of during alcohol metabolism; most of it ultimately ends up in triglycerides. Fatty liver is an early manifestation of this metabolic phenomenon.

Certain drugs lower cholesterol levels but raise or may have no effect on triglyceride levels. All antilipemics lower serum lipid concentration in the bloodstream, although their mechanism of action may differ. Cholestyramine lowers cholesterol; it raises or may have no effect on triglycerides. Colestipol lowers cholesterol; it raises or may have no effect on triglycerides. Long-term use of corticosteroids raises triglyceride levels, as does use of oral contraceptives, estrogen, furosemide, and miconazole. Clofibrate, dextrothyroxine, gemfibrozil, and niacin lower cholesterol and triglyceride levels.

Certain drugs have a variable effect. Probucol inhibits transport of cholesterol from the intestine and may also affect cholesterol synthesis. It lowers cholesterol but has a variable effect on triglycerides.

❖

Total cholesterol

The quantitative analysis of serum cholesterol, the total cholesterol test measures the circulating levels of free cholesterol and cholesterol esters. Of the total, 70% of cholesterol is esterified (combined with fatty acids) and 30% is in free form. The test is used to assess the risk of coronary artery disease (CAD), to evaluate fat metabolism, and to help diagnose nephrotic syndrome, pancreatitis, hepatic disease, and hypothyroidism and hyperthyroidism.

Normal findings

Total cholesterol concentrations vary with age and sex. The normal range is 170 to 200 mg/dl. Levels of 200 to 240 mg/dl are considered borderline or posing a high risk for CAD, depending on other concurrent risk factors. Levels above 240 mg/dl indicate higher risk of cardiovascular disease and require treatment.

Problematic findings

Elevated serum cholesterol (hypercholesterolemia) may indicate a risk of CAD, as well as incipient hepatitis, lipid disorders, bile duct blockage, nephrotic syndrome, obstructive jaundice, pancreatitis, and hypothyroidism. Hypercholesterolemia due to high dietary cholesterol intake

requires the modification of eating habits and, possibly, medication to retard absorption of cholesterol.

Low serum cholesterol (hypocholesterolemia) is commonly associated with malnutrition, cellular necrosis of the liver, and hyperthyroidism. Abnormal cholesterol levels frequently necessitate further testing to pinpoint the disorder, depending on the type of abnormality and the presence of overt signs. Abnormal levels associated with cardiovascular diseases, for example, may necessitate lipoprotein phenotyping.

Interfering factors

Cholesterol levels are lowered by cholestyramine, clofibrate, colestipol, dextrothyroxine, haloperidol, neomycin, niacin, and chlortetracycline. Levels are raised by epinephrine, chlorpromazine, trifluoperazine, oral contraceptives, and trimethadione. Androgens may have a variable effect on cholesterol levels.

Failure of the patient to follow dietary restrictions may interfere with test results. The patient should have nothing by mouth for 12 to 14 hours before the test.

❖

Protein, protein metabolite, and pigment tests

Checking the patient's medical history for certain drugs known to interfere with the results of these tests can help ensure accurate results. Also important is careful handling of the sample to avoid hemolysis.

the sample may also alter test results.

❖

Blood urea nitrogen fractionation

This test measures the nitrogen fraction of urea, the chief end product of protein metabolism. The blood urea nitrogen (BUN) level reflects protein intake and renal excretory capacity, but is a less reliable indicator of uremia than the serum creatinine level. Photometry is a commonly used test method. The BUN test is used to evaluate renal function and to aid the diagnosis of renal disease. It's also used to assess hydration.

Normal findings

BUN values normally range from 8 to 20 mg/dl, with slightly higher values in the elderly.

Problematic findings

Elevated BUN levels occur in renal disease, reduced renal blood flow (due to dehydration, for example), urinary tract obstruction, increased protein catabolism (as in burns), GI bleeding, and high protein diets. Depressed BUN levels occur in severe hepatic damage, malnutrition, and overhydration.

Interfering factors

Chloramphenicol can depress BUN levels, and nephrotoxic drugs—such as aminoglycosides, amphotericin B, and methicillin—can elevate BUN levels. Hemolysis due to rough handling of

Serum bilirubin

This test measures serum levels of bilirubin, the predominant pigment in bile. Bilirubin is the major product of hemoglobin catabolism. Serum bilirubin tests evaluate liver function; aid the differential diagnosis of jaundice and monitor the progression of this disorder; help diagnose biliary obstruction and hemolytic anemia; and determine whether a newborn requires an exchange transfusion or phototherapy because of dangerously high unconjugated bilirubin levels.

Normal findings

Normally, indirect serum bilirubin measures 1.1 mg/dl or less in an adult; direct serum bilirubin, less than 0.5 mg/dl. Total serum bilirubin in the newborn measures 1 to 12 mg/dl.

Problematic findings

Elevated indirect serum bilirubin levels often indicate hepatic damage in which the parenchymal cells can no longer conjugate bilirubin with glucuronide. Consequently, indirect bilirubin reenters the bloodstream. High levels of indirect bilirubin are also likely in severe hemolytic anemia, when excessive indirect bilirubin overwhelms the liver's conjugating mechanism. If hemolysis continues, both direct and indirect bilirubin levels may rise. Other causes of elevated indirect bilirubin levels include congenital enzyme deficiencies, such as Gilbert's disease and Crigler-Najjar syndrome; sickle cell anemia; congestive heart failure; and transfusion reactions.

Elevated direct serum bilirubin levels usually indicate biliary obstruction, in which direct bilirubin, blocked from its normal pathway from the liver into the biliary tree, overflows into the bloodstream. If the obstruction continues, both direct and indirect bilirubin levels eventually may be elevated due to hepatic damage. In severe chronic hepatic damage, direct bilirubin concentrations may return to normal or near-normal levels, but elevated indirect bilirubin levels persist.

In newborns, total bilirubin levels that reach 18 mg/dl indicate the need for exchange transfusion.

Interfering factors
Exposure of the sample to direct sunlight or ultraviolet light may depress bilirubin levels, confusing test results. Hemolysis due to rough handling of the sample may also alter test results.

Special considerations
Protect the sample from strong sunlight and ultraviolet light since bilirubin breaks down when exposed to light.

❖

nitrogen levels because renal impairment is virtually the only cause of creatinine elevation. The serum creatinine test is used to assess renal glomerular filtration and to screen for renal damage.

Normal findings
Creatinine concentrations in males normally range from 0.8 to 1.2 mg/dl; in females, from 0.6 to 0.9 mg/dl.

Problematic findings
Elevated serum creatinine levels generally indicate renal disease that has seriously damaged 50% or more of the nephrons. Elevated creatinine levels may also be associated with gigantism and acromegaly.

Interfering factors
Ascorbic acid, barbiturates, and diuretics may raise serum creatinine levels. Sulfobromophthalein or phenolsulfonphthalein given within the previous 24 hours can elevate creatinine levels if the test is based on the Jaffé reaction. Patients with exceptionally large muscle masses, such as athletes, may have above-average creatinine levels, even in the presence of normal renal function. Also, hemolysis due to rough handling of the sample may elevate results.

❖

Serum creatinine

A quantitative analysis of serum creatinine levels, this test provides a more sensitive measure of renal damage than blood urea

Serum uric acid

Used primarily to detect gout, this test measures serum levels of uric acid, the major end metabolite of purine. It's also used to identify kidney dysfunction.

Normal findings

Uric acid concentrations in men normally range from 4.3 to 8 mg/dl; in women, from 2.3 to 6 mg/dl.

Problematic findings

Increased serum uric acid levels may indicate gout or impaired renal function (levels don't correlate with severity of disease). Levels may also rise in congestive heart failure, glycogen storage disease (type I, von Gierke's disease), infections, hemolytic or sickle cell anemia, polycythemia, neoplasms, psoriasis, and leukemia. Depressed uric acid levels may indicate defective tubular absorption (as in Fanconi's syndrome and Wilson's disease) or acute hepatic atrophy.

Interfering factors

Loop diuretics, ethambutol, vincristine, pyrazinamide, thiazides, and low doses of aspirin may raise uric acid levels. With the colorimetric method, false elevations may be caused by acetaminophen, ascorbic acid, levodopa, and phenacetin. Aspirin in high doses may decrease uric acid levels. Starvation, a high-purine diet, stress, and abuse of alcohol may raise uric acid levels.

———————————————❖

Urinalysis

Proper collection procedure and immediate transfer for testing are important to the success of these urine tests to avoid introducing contaminants or destroying components. Noting the use of various interfering drugs also aids interpretation of results.

Routine urinalysis

Routine urinalysis is important in screening for renal or urinary tract disease or for metabolic or systemic pathologies unrelated to renal disorders.

Normal findings

Numerous macroscopic and microscopic elements exist in normal urine. (See *Normal findings in routine urinalysis.*)

Problematic findings

Nonpathologic variations in urine values may result from diet, nonpathologic conditions, specimen collection time, and other factors. For example, specific gravity influences urine color and odor: As specific gravity increases, urine becomes darker and its odor becomes stronger.

Urine pH, which is greatly affected by diet and medications, influences the appearance of urine and the composition of crystals. An alkaline pH (above 7) – characteristic of a vegetarian diet – causes turbidity, and formation of phosphate, carbonate, and amorphous crystals. An acid pH (below 7) – typical of a high-protein diet – produces turbidity, and formation of oxalate, cystine, leusine, tyrosine, amorphous urate, and uric acid crystals.

Normal findings in routine urinalysis

ELEMENT	FINDINGS
Macroscopic	
Color	Straw to dark yellow
Odor	Slightly aromatic
Appearance	Clear
Specific gravity	1.005 to 1.035
pH	4.5 to 8
Protein	None
Glucose	None
Ketones	None
Bilirubin	None
Urobilinogen	Normal
Hemoglobin	None
Erythrocytes (red blood cells [RBCs])	None
Nitrite (Bacteria)	None
Leukocytes (white blood cells [WBCs])	None
Microscopic	
RBCs	0 to 2/high-power field
WBCs	0 to 5/high-power field
Epithelial cells	0 to 5/high-power field
Casts	None, except 1 to 2 hyaline casts/low-power field
Crystals	Present
Bacteria	None
Yeast cells	None
Parasites	None
Nitrite (Bacteria)	None

Protein, normally absent from the urine, may be present in a benign condition known as orthostatic (postural) proteinuria. Most common in patients ages 10 to 20, this condition is intermittent, appears after prolonged standing, and disappears after recumbency.

Transient benign proteinuria can also occur with fever, exposure to cold, emotional stress, or strenuous exercise. Sugars, usually absent from the urine, may appear under normal conditions. The most common sugar in urine is glucose. Transient, nonpathologic glycosuria may result from emotional stress or pregnancy and may follow ingestion of a high-carbohydrate meal.

Centrifuged urine sediment contains cells, casts, crystals, bacteria, yeast and parasites. Red blood cells don't often appear in urine without pathologic significance, but hard exercise can cause hematuria.

The abnormal findings that follow generally suggest pathologic conditions.

• *Color:* Color change can result from diet, drugs, and many diseases.

• *Odor:* In diabetes mellitus, starvation, and dehydration, a fruity odor accompanies formation of ketone bodies. In urinary tract infections, a common fetid odor is associated with *Escherichia coli.* Maple syrup urine disease and phenylketonuria also cause distinctive odors.

• *Turbidity:* Turbid urine may contain red or white cells, bacteria, fat, or chyle, and may reflect renal infection.

• *Specific gravity:* Low specific gravity (< 1.005) is characteristic of diabetes insipidus, nephrogenic

diabetes insipidus, acute tubular necrosis, and pyelonephritis. Fixed specific gravity, in which values remain 1.010 regardless of fluid intake, occurs in chronic glomerulonephritis with severe renal damage. High specific gravity (> 1.035) occurs in nephrotic syndrome, dehydration, acute glomerulonephritis, congestive heart failure, liver failure, and shock.

• *pH:* Alkaline urine pH may result from Fanconi's syndrome, urinary tract infection, and metabolic or respiratory alkalosis. Acid urine pH is associated with renal tuberculosis, pyrexia, phenylketonuria, alkaptonuria, and acidosis.

• *Protein:* Proteinuria suggests renal failure or disease (including nephrosis, glomerulosclerosis, glomerulonephritis, nephrolithiasis, and polycystic kidney disease) or possibly multiple myeloma.

• *Sugars:* Glycosuria usually indicates diabetes mellitus but may result from pheochromocytoma, Cushing's syndrome, impaired tubular reabsorption, advanced renal disease, and increased intracranial pressure. Fructosuria, galactosuria, and pentosuria generally suggest rare hereditary metabolic disorders (except for lactosuria during pregnancy and lactation). However, an alimentary form of pentosuria and fructosuria may follow excessive ingestion of pentose or fructose. When the liver fails to metabolize these sugars, they spill into the urine since the renal tubules don't reabsorb them.

• *Ketones:* Ketonuria occurs in diabetes mellitus when cellular energy needs exceed available cellular glucose. In the absence of glucose, cells metabolize fat for energy. Ketone bodies – the end products of incomplete fat metabolism – accumulate in plasma and are excreted in the urine. Ketonuria may also occur in starvation states and following diarrhea or vomiting.

• *Bilirubin:* Bilirubin in urine may occur in liver disease resulting from obstructive jaundice or hepatotoxic drugs or toxins or from fibrosis of the biliary canaliculi (as in cirrhosis).

• *Urobilinogen:* Bilirubin is changed into urobilinogen in the duodenum by intestinal bacteria. The liver reprocesses the remainder into bile. Increased urobilinogen in the urine may indicate liver damage, hemolytic disease, or severe infection.

• *Cells:* Hematuria indicates bleeding within the genitourinary tract and may result from infection, obstruction, inflammation, trauma, tumors, glomerulonephritis, renal hypertension, lupus nephritis, renal tuberculosis, renal vein thrombosis, renal calculi, hydronephrosis, pyelonephritis, scurvy, malaria, parasitic infection of the bladder, subacute bacterial endocarditis, polyarteritis nodosa, and hemorrhagic disorders. Strenuous exercise or exposure to toxic chemicals may also cause hematuria. An excess of white cells in urine usually implies urinary tract inflammation, especially cystitis or pyelonephritis. White cells and white cell casts in urine suggest renal infection. Numerous epithelial cells suggest renal tubular degeneration.

• *Casts:* Plugs of gelled proteinaceous material or of high–molecular-weight mucoprotein, casts form in the renal tubules and collecting ducts by agglutination of protein cells or cellular debris and are flushed loose by urine flow. Excessive numbers of casts indicate renal disease.

• *Crystals:* Some crystals normally appear in urine, but numerous calcium oxalate crystals suggest hypercalcemia. Cystine crystals (cystinuria) reflect an inborn error of metabolism.

• *Other components:* Bacteria, yeast cells, and parasites in urinary sediment reflect genitourinary tract infection or contamination of external genitalia. Yeast cells, which may be mistaken for red blood cells, are identifiable by their ovoid shape, lack of color, variable size and, frequently, signs of budding. The most common parasite in sediment is *Trichomonas vaginalis*, which causes vaginitis, urethritis, and prostatovesiculitis.

Interfering factors

Failure to follow proper collection procedure, to send the specimen to the laboratory immediately, or to refrigerate the specimen may alter test results. Strenuous exercise before routine urinalysis may cause transient myoglobinuria, producing inaccurate results. Many drugs alter test results.

❖

Urinary calculi

Also called urinary stones, urinary calculi are insoluble substances – most commonly formed of the mineral salts calcium oxalate, calcium phosphate, magnesium ammonium phosphate, ur-

PUZZLING LAB FINDINGS

ate, or cystine—that may appear anywhere in the urinary tract.

Formation of calculi can result from reduced urinary volume, increased excretion of mineral salts, urinary stasis, pH changes, and decreased protective substances. Testing can detect and identify calculi in the urine.

Normal findings
Normally, calculi are not present in the urine.

Problematic findings
More than half of all calculi in urine are of mixed composition, containing two or more mineral salts; calcium oxalate is the most common component. Determination of the composition of calculi helps identify various metabolic disorders.

Interfering factors
None.

❖

Urine bilirubin

This screening test, based on a color reaction with a specific reagent, detects abnormally high urine concentrations of direct (conjugated) bilirubin. It's used to help identify the cause of jaundice.

Normal findings
Normally, bilirubin is not found in urine in a routine screening test.

Problematic findings
High concentrations of direct bilirubin in urine may be evident from the specimen's appearance (dark, with a yellow foam). To diagnose jaundice, however, the presence or absence of direct bilirubin in urine must be correlated with serum test results, and with urine and fecal urobilinogen levels.

Interfering factors
Dipstick testing, such as with Chemstrip or N-Multistix, is affected by large amounts of ascorbic acid and nitrite, which may lower bilirubin levels and cause false-negative test results. Phenazopyridine and phenothiazine derivatives, such as chlorpromazine and acetophenazine maleate, can cause false-positive results. Exposure of the specimen to room temperature or light can lower bilirubin levels, due to bilirubin degradation.

Special considerations
Use only a freshly voided specimen; bilirubin disintegrates after 30 minutes' exposure to room temperature or light. If the specimen is to be analyzed in the laboratory, send it immediately and record the time of collection on the patient's chart. If the specimen is tested at bedside, make sure 20 seconds elapse before interpreting the color change on the dipstick. Make sure lighting is adequate to make this color determination.

❖

Urine protein

This is a quantitative test for proteinuria. Normally, the glomerular membrane allows only proteins of low molecular weight to enter the filtrate. A damaged glomerular capillary membrane and impaired tubular reabsorption allow excretion of proteins in the urine. This test helps diagnose pathologic states characterized by proteinuria, primarily renal disease.

Normal findings
Normal values show up to 150 mg of protein excreted in 24 hours.

Problematic findings
Proteinuria is pathognomonic of renal disease. When proteinuria is present in a single specimen, 24-hour urine collection is subsequently required to identify specific renal abnormalities.

Proteinuria can result from glomerular leakage of plasma proteins (a major cause of protein excretion), from overflow of filtered proteins of low molecular weight (when these are present in excessive concentrations), from impaired tubular reabsorption of filtered proteins, and from the presence of renal proteins derived from the breakdown of kidney tissue.

Persistent proteinuria indicates renal disease resulting from increased glomerular permeability. *Minimal* proteinuria (less than 0.5 g/24 hours), however, is most often associated with renal diseases in which glomerular involvement is not a major factor, such as chronic pyelonephritis.

Moderate proteinuria (0.5 to 4 g/24 hours) occurs in several types of renal disease—acute or chronic glomerulonephritis, amyloidosis, toxic nephropathies—or in diseases in which renal failure often develops as a late complication (diabetes or heart failure, for example). *Heavy proteinuria* (more than 4 g/24 hours) is commonly associated with nephrotic syndrome.

When accompanied by an elevated white blood cell (WBC) count, proteinuria indicates urinary tract infection; with hematuria, proteinuria indicates local or diffuse urinary tract disorders. Other pathologic states (infections and lesions of the central nervous system, for example) can also result in detectable amounts of proteins in the urine.

Many drugs (such as amphotericin B, gold preparations, aminoglycosides, polymyxins, and trimethadione) inflict renal damage, causing true proteinuria. This makes the routine evaluation of urine proteins essential during such treatment.

Benign proteinuria can result from changes in body position. *Functional* proteinuria is associated with exercise, as well as emotional or physiologic stress, and is usually transient.

Interfering factors
Administration of tolbutamide, para-aminosalicylic acid, acetazolamide, sodium bicarbonate, penicillin, sulfonamides, iodine contrast media, and cephalosporins may cause false-positive results in acid precipitation tests. Contamination of the urine specimen with heavy mucus, vaginal

or prostatic secretions, or the presence of numerous WBCs can alter test results, regardless of the laboratory method used. Very dilute urine (which may result from forcing fluids) may depress protein values and cause false-negative results.

Special considerations
Tell the patient not to contaminate the urine with toilet tissue or stool. Refrigerate the specimen or place it on ice during the collection period.   ❖

4 Rapidly Caring for Acutely Ill Patients

Patients in cardiovascular crisis

Because a cardiovascular crisis can be quickly fatal, it demands immediate assessment and intervention. Each second counts, and your patient's life may well depend on your decisions. This section can help you understand five potentially fatal cardiovascular crises, including their causes and symptoms, and can give you the knowledge and confidence to act fast to avert brain damage or death.

Hypertensive crisis

This crisis is characterized by a rapid, sharp rise in blood pressure. Without prompt treatment, hypertensive crisis can lead to rapid death from brain damage or cerebrovascular accident (CVA) or to a more gradual death from renal impairment. The speed and severity of the increase in blood pressure can compromise your patient's cerebral, renal, and cardiovascular functions. In most patients, blood pressure is considered excessively elevated when mean systolic pressure exceeds 180 mm Hg and mean diastolic pressure exceeds 120 mm Hg. (See *Classifying blood pressure*.)

Causes

Hypertensive crisis can result from:
• untreated or inadequately treated essential hypertension

Classifying blood pressure

The Joint National Committee on the Detection, Evaluation, and Treatment of High Blood Pressure has revised its classification guidelines. The terms *mild*, *moderate*, and *severe* have been replaced with *normal* (systolic pressure below 130 mm Hg and diastolic pressure below 85 mm Hg), *high normal* (130 to 139 mm Hg systolic and 85 to 89 mm Hg diastolic), and four stages of hypertension, in order of increasing severity. They are:
• *Stage 1:* 140 to 159 mm Hg systolic and 90 to 99 mm Hg diastolic
• *Stage 2:* 160 to 179 mm Hg systolic and 100 to 109 mm Hg diastolic
• *Stage 3:* 180 to 209 mm Hg systolic and 110 to 119 mm Hg diastolic
• *Stage 4:* more than 209 mm Hg systolic and more than 119 mm Hg diastolic.

• renal disease, such as acute or chronic glomerulonephritis, pyelonephritis, and renal vascular disease
• eclampsia
• intracerebral hemorrhage
• acute left ventricular failure
• polycythemia
• pituitary tumors
• coarctation of the aorta
• adrenocortical hyperfunction
• monoamine oxidase inhibitor interactions.

Assessment

Your assessment should quickly explore any history of hypertension or its risk factors and should include a physical examination focused on hypertension's subtle neurologic and renal signs.

History

With your patient in crisis, you may not have time at first for a complete health history. Pose the following questions to the patient or his family; then proceed with a physical assessment.

Ask about a history of high blood pressure or of taking antihypertensive drugs. Has the patient had similar symptoms before? Did he consult a doctor? Has he had anginal pain and palpitations? Which prescription and nonprescription drugs is he taking? (Certain ones, such as cough medicines and analgesics, may raise blood pressure or make antihypertensive therapy less effective.)

When the patient's condition is stable, or as time permits, you can complete the history taking. If the patient has no history of hypertension, try to uncover possible causes of hypertensive crisis. Inquire about risk factors for hypertension, such as a history of heart or blood vessel disease, diabetes mellitus, hyperlipidemia, congenital heart defects, rheumatic fever, or syncope.

Ask about nosebleeds and about severe suboccipital or occipital headache, which may subside when he moves to an upright position. Listen for neurologic complaints of dizziness, weakness, numbness, or blurred vision. Expect reports of fatigue, bloody or cloudy urine, and nocturia, which may signal renal involvement. Ask if the patient uses alcohol, tobacco, caffeine, or recreational drugs.

Physical examination

Your examination should include careful funduscopic, cardiovascular, neurologic, and renal evaluations.

Funduscopic examination. Check for arteriolar narrowing, arteriovenous compression, hemorrhages, exudates, and papilledema. Determine the degree of hypertensive retinopathy by using the following scale, with Grade I representing the mildest form:
• Grade I – arterial narrowing or spasm
• Grade II – arteriovenous nicking
• Grade III – hemorrhages and exudates, indicating accelerated hypertension
• Grade IV – papilledema, representing malignant hypertension.

Cardiovascular examination. Note tachycardia, precordial heave, murmur of aortic insufficiency, a third or fourth heart sound, and arrhythmias. Also note dependent edema, lateral displacement of the point of maximal impulse (indicating cardiomegaly, which can trigger or result from hypertensive crisis), a bruit auscultated over the flanks or anteriorly over the renal vasculature, and weak peripheral pulses.

Neurologic examination. Assess the patient for confusion, somnolence, or stupor. Observe for visual and focal deficits, nystagmus, localized muscle weakness, and seizures.

Responding to hypertensive crisis

If your patient is in hypertensive crisis, your first priority is to maintain his airway and breathing while another nurse gets the doctor. Elevate the head of the patient's bed or stretcher and start oxygen at 2 liters/minute through a nasal cannula. Anticipating an order for I.V. medication, insert an I.V. line, according to hospital protocol. Have someone move the crash cart outside the room.

Reassure the patient that everything is under control. Then set up a cardiac monitor and automatic blood pressure cuff. Assess the patient's vital signs and level of consciousness.

When the doctor arrives, he'll order you to administer a vasodilator—such as I.V. nitroprusside, nitroglycerin, or enalapril—or an adrenergic blocker—such as methyldopa.

Most likely, you'll give I.V. diazoxide from the crash cart at 1 mg/kg/minute to a maximum of 150 mg. You may repeat the drug every 5 to 15 minutes until the patient's diastolic blood pressure drops below 100 mm Hg.

During this time, monitor the patient's blood pressure and electrocardiogram continuously, keep him supine, and elevate his legs to prevent injury from possible orthostatic hypotension.

Renal examination. Assess the patient for oliguria and azotemia.

Rapid intervention

If your patient is in hypertensive crisis, your first priority is to ask another nurse to call the doctor while you swiftly assess and maintain the patient's airway and breathing. (See *Responding to hypertensive crisis.*)

The doctor will order antihypertensive drugs to reduce the patient's blood pressure. When antihypertensive drug therapy begins, monitor the patient's blood pressure every 5 minutes for the first 15 minutes, every 15 minutes for the next hour, then every hour. These drugs have a rapid onset and may cause extreme vasodilation.

When administering drugs I.V., increase the infusion rate gradually until the patient's blood pressure begins to drop. When blood pressure stabilizes, the doctor will switch to oral drug administration. Throughout drug therapy, continue to assess the patient frequently for hypotension and signs and symptoms of heart failure, myocardial infarction, or CVA. Monitor his hemodynamic indicators—preferably with an arterial line or noninvasive blood pressure monitoring device—to evaluate the effectiveness of antihypertensive therapy.

Myocardial infarction

Myocardial infarction (MI) occurs when a portion of the myocardium is deprived of oxygenated coronary blood flow, resulting in cellular ischemia, tissue injury, necrosis (cell death), and loss of tissue function. Depending on the degree of imbalance between oxygen supply and demand, tissue changes may progress quickly from ischemia to acute injury. Interventions must begin at once to minimize cardiac damage and avert death.

Most infarctions are *transmural*, with tissue changes affecting the full myocardial thickness from epicardium to endocardium. *Subendocardial* infarctions involve the endocardium and some portion of the myocardium. A newer method of classifying MIs distinguishes those that cause Q-wave changes on an electrocardiogram from those that don't. (See *Coronary arteries and MI sites*, pages 168 and 169.)

Causes

MI results from significant occlusion of the coronary arteries, which disrupts the balance of oxygen supply and demand. The occlusion typically stems from a combination of factors, such as coronary artery disease, thrombosis, and coronary artery spasm.

Less common causes of MI include:
• arteritis from syphilitic or granulomatous lesions, polyarteritis nodosa, lupus erythematosus, rheumatoid arthritis, and ankylosing spondylitis
• coronary artery trauma from laceration or iatrogenic injury
• hematologic abnormalities, including polycythemia vera, thrombocytosis, disseminated intravascular coagulation, and thrombocytopenic purpura
• disproportional myocardial demand caused by aortic valvular disease, thyrotoxicosis, prolonged hypotension, carbon monoxide poisoning, use of amphetamines or cocaine, or pulmonary hypertension.

Assessment

Your assessment of an MI patient must include a complete health history of any significant chest discomfort and a thorough physical examination.

History

Find out if the patient has a history of cardiac or respiratory disease, cardiac surgery, chest trauma, or intestinal disease. Also determine if he drinks alcohol excessively, uses any illicit drugs, and which medications he is taking; all of these are risk factors.

Approximately 80% of patients with acute MI complain of chest discomfort. However, MI is just one of over 100 possible causes of chest discomfort. Suspect acute MI if your patient reports any of the following symptoms:
• dull, aching, gnawing, crushing, squeezing, or pressurelike pain (feelings of tightness, pressure, or a clenched-fist effect)
• pain in the midsternal area, pain that radiates to the left arm or left jaw, or even pain that diffuses across the entire chest
• pain brought on by exertion

Coronary arteries and MI sites

The permanent damage that myocardial infarction (MI) may cause depends on which coronary arteries are occluded and how well collateral circulation perfuses the affected area.

During recovery from acute MI, nearly 40% of patients develop collateral circulation in the area of main artery occlusion. In patients with a 75% or greater reduction in the coronary artery lumen, collateral circulation is especially well developed. Collateral circulation seems to reduce myocardial necrosis in patients with coronary artery occlusion. In those with extensive collateral vessel development, it can perfuse the area even if the artery is totally occluded—as long as no stress is placed on the heart.

The chart at right correlates the major regions and structures supplied by coronary arteries with the areas of infarction associated with obstruction of these arteries.

Anterior view

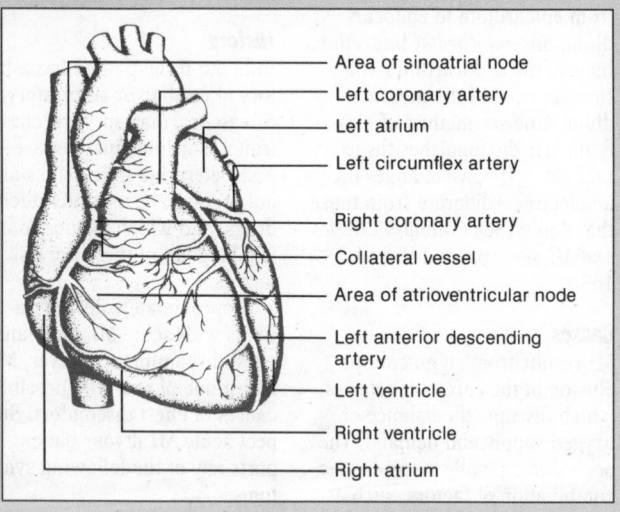

- Area of sinoatrial node
- Left coronary artery
- Left atrium
- Left circumflex artery
- Right coronary artery
- Collateral vessel
- Area of atrioventricular node
- Left anterior descending artery
- Left ventricle
- Right ventricle
- Right atrium

• pain that starts gradually, builds in intensity, and is constant rather than episodic
• shortness of breath, nausea, vomiting, and diaphoresis
• indigestion.

Keep in mind that roughly 20% of patients with acute MI experience no discomfort. Most of these patients are diabetic or elderly and have neuropathies that limit the sensation of discomfort.

CORONARY ARTERY	MAJOR AREAS AND STRUCTURES SUPPLIED	PRIMARY INFARCTION AREA
Right	• Sinoatrial (SA) node • Atrioventricular (AV) node • Bundle of His • Right atrium and right ventricle • Inferior and diaphragmatic surface of left ventricle • Posterior third of septum • Inferoposterior division of left bundle branch	• Inferior wall • Inferoposterior wall • Right ventricle
Left	• Massive left ventricular area	• Left ventricle
Left anterior descending	• Anterior wall of left ventricle • Anterior two-thirds of septum • Bundle of His • Right bundle branch • Anterosuperior division of left bundle branch • Inferoposterior division of left bundle branch	• Anterior wall • Septum • Anterolateral wall • Inferoapical wall • Apex
Left circumflex	• SA node • AV node • Inferior and diaphragmatic surface of left ventricle • Lateral wall of left ventricle • Left atrium • Posteroinferior division of left bundle branch	• Lateral wall • Inferolateral wall • Posterior wall • Inferoposterior wall

Physical examination

Your examination must be extremely thorough to assess the adequacy of the patient's cardiac output.

Palpation. Firmly palpate the area of discomfort; if the discomfort improves or worsens, you can suspect a musculoskeletal source and rule out MI and other cardiac causes.

Positional changes. Have the patient turn onto his right side, and then onto his left side. Then tell him to sit up. If a position change alters his discomfort, this may indicate a noncardiac source of pain. However, if he has pericarditis, the pain may be relieved by sitting up and leaning forward.

Respiration. Have the patient take a deep breath; if this action alters his discomfort, you can probably rule out MI. (However, if he has pericarditis as a complication of MI, a deep breath will exacerbate the discomfort.)

Cardiopulmonary status. Auscultate for S_4, a *lub-dub* sound that may occur late in diastole just before the first heart sound (S_1). You also may detect an acute systolic murmur if papillary muscle dysfunction has developed as a complication of MI. Pericarditis, another complication, produces an audible friction rub. If heart failure is complicating MI, you may auscultate S_3 and adventitious breath sounds (such as wheezes, crackles, or rhonchi). You may also detect jugular vein distention.

Vital signs. Expect a compensatory increase in heart rate and blood pressure in an attempt to boost perfusion and oxygenation. If compensation fails, you'll find decreased blood pressure, extreme tachypnea, and an extremely increased heart rate, possibly accompanied by arrhythmias. (See *Responding to lethal arrhythmias.*) Fever typically occurs 24 to 48 hours after MI as an inflammatory response to tissue injury.

Skin. You'll typically find pale, cool, moist skin in the patient with MI. Unless he's in shock, don't expect ashen or gray skin. Also assess his capillary refill; sluggish refill is one of the first signs of decreased perfusion.

Peripheral pulses. Assess the quality and amplitude of peripheral pulses. Quality may diminish slightly with MI. However, unless the patient is in shock, his pulses won't be thready or fleeting. Keep in mind that pulse amplitude reflects stroke volume (the volume ejected with each heartbeat).

Urine output. Urine output indirectly reflects cardiac output. An output below 400 ml/24 hours suggests decreased cardiac output.

Mentation changes. If cerebral perfusion is impaired, expect restlessness, agitation, and demanding behavior. Eventually, the patient becomes lethargic.

Rapid intervention

Immediate interventions focus on relieving pain, reducing myocardial oxygen consumption, restoring perfusion with thrombolytics, and maintaining cardiac output by manipulating preload and afterload.

Specific measures depend on the patient's signs and symptoms and any complications he has developed. However, all patients with acute MI need bed rest to reduce oxygen demand, supplemental oxygen, and I.V. line insertion to provide access for emergency medications. Infuse dextrose 5% in water at a keep-vein-open rate until drugs such

STAT CARE

 Responding to lethal arrhythmias

The American Heart Association (AHA) recommends the following advanced cardiac life support (ACLS) measures to treat life-threatening arrhythmias, such as ventricular fibrillation and pulseless ventricular tachycardia. The AHA identifies these arrhythmias by:
• a rapid, chaotic ventricular rhythm (indicating varying degrees of depolarization and repolarization) and unidentifiable QRS complexes
• a patient who is unconscious at onset
• absent pulses, heart sounds, and blood pressure
• dilated pupils
• the rapid development of cyanosis.

Even if you're not ACLS certified, the chart will help you know what to expect in such an emergency.

Establish responsiveness. Check pulse. If no pulse, then:

Perform CPR until a defibrillator is available.

Check rhythm. If ventricular fibrillation or tachycardia appears, then:

Defibrillate using 200 joules.

Defibrillate using 200 to 300 joules.

Defibrillate using 360 joules.

If ventricular fibrillation or tachycardia persists, then:

Continue CPR.

Intubate as soon as possible.

Establish I.V. access.

Administer epinephrine, 1:10,000, 1 mg I.V. push every 3 to 5 minutes.

Defibrillate using 360 joules, 30 to 60 seconds after epinephrine.

Administer lidocaine 1.5 mg/kg I.V. push.

Defibrillate using 360 joules.

Administer bretylium 5 mg/kg I.V. push. Defibrillate using 360 joules.

Administer bretylium 10 mg/kg I.V. push; consider sodium bicarbonate.

Defibrillate using 360 joules.

Repeat lidocaine or bretylium.

Defibrillate using 360 joules.

ACUTELY ILL
PATIENTS

as lidocaine (for arrhythmias), nitroglycerin and morphine (to relieve pain), and beta blockers (to prevent reinfarction) are administered. Thrombolytic therapy may also be ordered.

Pain relief

Your first priority is pain management because pain stimulates sympathetic nervous system (SNS) activity, leading to an even greater oxygen demand. I.V. nitroglycerin is the initial drug used, possibly in combination with morphine if the patient isn't hypotensive. I.V. nitroglycerin dilates coronary arteries and reduces preload by dilating peripheral arteries and veins. Titrate the dosage to achieve effective pain control, and monitor the patient's blood pressure carefully – nitroglycerin may cause hypotension.

Morphine depresses central nervous system activity, in turn reducing both anxiety and the heart's metabolic demands. The drug also dilates veins to decrease preload. Expect to administer morphine at prescribed intervals until the patient's chest pain subsides.

Don't administer nitroglycerin or morphine to a patient with a right ventricular MI because these drugs may depress an already low pulmonary artery wedge pressure (PAWP), causing a further drop in cardiac output. If PAWP is low, administer fluids, such as isotonic 0.9% sodium chloride solution, to boost diastolic filling in an attempt to improve cardiac output.

Oxygen consumption reduction

To reduce oxygen consumption and help manage pain, administer other prescribed drugs, such as nitrates, calcium channel blockers, beta-adrenergic blockers, or angiotensin-converting enzyme (ACE) inhibitors.

Calcium channel blockers, including nifedipine, diltiazem, and verapamil, block calcium influx into the cells, dilating coronary arteries and decreasing contractility. However, these drugs depress left ventricular function, so they're given only if left ventricular function is normal. Two new calcium channel blockers, felodipine and amlodipine, don't cause a decrease in left ventricular function. Stay alert for signs of congestive heart failure from reduced contractility.

Beta-adrenergic blockers, such as propranolol and metoprolol, block SNS stimulation, causing reductions in heart rate, contractility, and oxygen demand. Some beta blockers are $beta_1$-selective, acting primarily on the heart, whereas others are nonselective, acting on both the heart and peripheral blood vessels.

ACE inhibitors, such as captopril and enalapril, inhibit the enzyme that converts angiotensin I to angiotensin II, a potent vasoconstrictor. These drugs cause arterial dilation, which decreases afterload and oxygen demand. However, they can be used only if renal function is normal.

Thrombolytic therapy

Candidates for thrombolytic therapy include patients with acute ST-segment elevation and chest pain that has lasted no more than 6 hours. Timely use of thrombolytic agents can restore myocardial perfusion and prevent further damage from MI by lysing the clot in the occluded coronary artery. These drugs can also relieve chest pain, restore the ST segment to baseline, and induce reperfusion arrhythmias within 30 to 45 minutes. The most common thrombolytic drugs are alteplase, anistreplase, streptokinase, and urokinase.

Contraindications for thrombolytic therapy include surgery within the past 2 months, active bleeding, a history of cerebrovascular accident, intracranial neoplasm, arteriovenous malformation, aneurysm, uncontrolled hypertension, or prolonged cardiopulmonary resuscitation.

———————————————❖

Cardiogenic shock

A state of profoundly impaired tissue perfusion and reduced cardiac output, cardiogenic shock impairs the supply of blood, oxygen, nutrients, and electrolytes to body cells. As cardiac output reaches a perilous low, blood flow to the capillary bed—the site of gas exchange with cells—is bypassed. This leads to abnormal cellular metabolism, resulting in cellular injury.

Mortality from cardiogenic shock approaches 85%. Among survivors, the long-term prognosis is poor. Your immediate, expert intervention is the pa-tient's only hope for averting death.

Causes

Cardiogenic shock usually arises when at least 40% of the ventricle is dysfunctional. It can result from any condition that significantly reduces ventricular pumping, such as:

• ventricular impairment, typically stemming from coronary artery disease (CAD). By impairing myocardial perfusion, CAD causes tissue ischemia and, ultimately, myocardial infarction (MI) or necrosis. Myocardial necrosis reduces cardiac output by compromising contractility. The greater the extent of tissue damage from the MI, the greater the risk of cardiogenic shock.

• anterior-wall infarction, which is more likely to trigger cardiogenic shock than inferior-wall infarction because the anterior wall is the heart's main pumping muscle

• end-stage cardiomyopathy
• ruptured interventricular septum
• atrial thrombus that impedes intracardiac blood flow
• valvular heart disease (such as aortic stenosis and mitral insufficiency)
• cardiac tamponade
• massive pulmonary embolism
• arrhythmias
• papillary muscle dysfunction
• myocarditis.

Assessment

Your careful assessment of a patient in cardiogenic shock must include special attention to his health history and immediate recognition and treatment of shock.

Pinpointing the stage of cardiogenic shock

To recognize cardiogenic shock and prevent death, you must identify the compensatory mechanisms of its early phase. When these compensatory mechanisms are depleted, the patient displays the classic clinical profile of shock.

Early shock
Stimulation of the sympathetic nervous system causes various changes that may seem insignificant when considered alone but point to shock when correlated with each other and the patient's history. These changes include:
• *increased heart rate*. Typically, the heart rate rises about 20%.
• *arterial and venous constriction*. Look for signs of vasoconstriction—pallor, sluggish capillary refill, and reduced peripheral pulse quality. Pulse amplitude will increase from a normal +2 or +3 to +4. At this stage, the patient's pulses won't be weak or thready (+1).
• *coronary artery dilation*. This compensatory mechanism promotes myocardial

perfusion, making arrhythmias unlikely at this stage.
• *carotid artery dilation*. This compensatory mechanism increases oxygen flow to the brain and may cause a heightened awareness or a feeling of impending doom, fearfulness, restlessness, or anxiety. The patient may also exhibit demanding behavior at this time.
• *dilation of vessels supplying large muscles*. This response increases the patient's strength, perhaps necessitating safety precautions to avoid patient injury.
• *thirst stimulation*. Low cardiac output triggers stimulation of the thirst center in an attempt to enhance fluid volume, and thus boost perfusion, through increased fluid intake.

Late shock
Assessment findings reflect impaired perfusion to the capillary bed, cell damage, anaerobic metabolism, and acidosis. This phase is characterized by:
• *reduced cardiac output*. The heart rate typically measures

---

History
Determine if the patient has any risk factors, such as a history of MI, cardiomyopathy, CAD, embolism, valvular heart disease, or arrhythmias. Has he had more than one MI? Did the past MIs

present any additional problems?

Physical examination
Physical findings depend on the stage of shock. (See *Pinpointing the stage of cardiogenic shock*.)

less than 100 beats/minute. When auscultating heart sounds, you may hear an S_3, signifying ventricular gallop from increased ventricular filling pressure.

• *increased respiratory rate.* When you auscultate the lungs, you may hear crackles or wheezes from narrowed airways and increased fluid in the lungs.

• *reduced blood pressure.* Expect a mean arterial pressure less than 60 mm Hg and a systolic pressure less than 90 mm Hg (or at least 30 mm Hg lower than baseline). Pulse pressure narrows and peripheral pulses become weak and thready. You may detect arrhythmias on the electrocardiogram. The patient's skin is cold and clammy.

• *other changes.* Urine output may fall below 30 ml/hour. The patient may become less responsive and exhibit mentation changes. His skin will appear ashen, gray or even cyanotic, with mottled extremities. Expect slow capillary refill. Look for weak or floppy muscles.

Rapid intervention

Preventing further damage to the patient's heart is your overall priority in cardiogenic shock. This means taking measures to increase his myocardial oxygen supply, boost his cardiac output, increase contractility, and reduce his left ventricular workload, usually with a combination of cardiovascular drugs and mechanical-assist techniques.

First, assess the patient's airway, breathing, and circulation. If these are adequate and the patient is in respiratory distress, elevate the head of the bed to reduce discomfort. Start an I.V. line at a keep-vein-open rate.

As appropriate, arrange for patient transfer to the intensive care unit for vasoactive drug therapy and possible use of a mechanical-assist device.

If the patient has chest discomfort, administer morphine as prescribed. Insert an indwelling urinary catheter to allow precise measurement of hourly urine output, an indirect indicator of cardiac output. Prepare for insertion of hemodynamic monitoring lines.

To help support the failing heart, initiate oxygen therapy, as ordered, based on the patient's arterial blood gas values. Some patients may require mechanical ventilation. However, be aware that positive-pressure ventilation may further decrease cardiac output.

To reduce the heart's workload and oxygen demand, the doctor may insert an intra-aortic balloon pump. Enforce bed rest and administer prescribed afterload-reducing agents, such as vasodilators. Withhold negative inotropic drugs, such as beta blockers or calcium channel blockers, because they may depress contractility and worsen the existing problem. Notify the doctor any time you withhold a medication.

To improve contractility, administer prescribed positive inotropic drugs, such as digitalis glycosides, dopamine, dobutamine, and amrinone.

To optimize the patient's volume status, verify that he's hypervolemic by assessing for adventitious breath sounds, skin turgor, excessive jugular vein distention, sacral edema, and a positive hepatojugular reflex. Administer diuretics as ordered. Also give vasodilators, such as nitrates and morphine, as ordered.

Assess for desired and adverse effects of all administered drugs. Monitor the patient's hemodynamic values.

❖

Cardiac tamponade

This cardiovascular crisis occurs when excess fluid accumulates within the pericardial space, leading to compression of the heart. Ultimately, both stroke volume and cardiac output decrease, which may swiftly progress to cardiac arrest, cardiogenic shock, and death unless excess pericardial fluid is removed.

Cardiac tamponade may be acute or chronic. If fluid accumulates rapidly, as little as 150 ml can create a crisis. With slower accumulation (as in pericardial effusion associated with cancer), symptoms may not arise until 1 to 2 liters collect because the fibrous pericardial wall can stretch to accommodate the gradual increase.

Causes

Common causes of acute cardiac tamponade include acute pericarditis from:
• bacterial infections
• tuberculosis
• uremia
• connective tissue disorders, including rheumatoid arthritis, systemic lupus erythematosus, rheumatic fever, vasculitis, and scleroderma
• hemopericardium (bleeding into the pericardial cavity), stemming from ventricular rupture, a vascular pericardial tumor, penetrating or nonpenetrating chest wall trauma, or thoracic surgery.

Common causes of chronic cardiac tamponade include:
• infection, such as tuberculosis or a parasitic infection
• uremia
• neoplasm
• myxedema
• high cholesterol levels
• radiation therapy
• Dressler's syndrome
• postpericardiotomy syndrome.

Assessment

Your careful assessment of a patient with cardiac tamponade must include investigation of a history of any precipitating disorder and a physical examination centered on tamponade's cardinal signs.

History

Cardiac tamponade usually has an insidious onset. However, once signs and symptoms appear, the patient may progress rapidly to circulatory collapse. Stay alert for characteristic complaints of acute tamponade, such as sudden onset of dyspnea and chest pain. The patient may also report retrosternal pain or a feeling of fullness in the head. In chronic tamponade, expect vague complaints, such as malaise, chest discomfort, anorexia, and dyspnea.

Physical examination

Assess your patient's general appearance and demeanor, including his position. With acute tamponade, he may have to sit upright and lean forward to breathe. He may be orthopneic, diaphoretic, pale, and extremely anxious.

Look for the cardinal signs of cardiac tamponade: jugular vein distention (which indicates rising venous pressure and is present in 95% of patients with cardiac tamponade), decreasing systolic blood pressure with narrowing pulse pressure, muffled heart sounds, extreme tachycardia, and weak peripheral pulses.

When inspecting the patient's neck for jugular vein distention, remember that this sign won't appear if the patient is hypovolemic.

When measuring your patient's blood pressure, correlate the reading with the inspiratory phase of respiration. Cardiac tamponade typically causes pulsus paradoxus—an abnormal decrease in systolic pressure (more than 10 mm Hg) during inspiration. This sign results from impaired peripheral perfusion, a consequence of cardiac decompensation. As the patient inhales, venous return, ventricular filling, and pulmonary blood flow increase, as does the capacity of the pulmonary vascular space. As a result, pulmonary venous return to the left side of the

heart declines, reducing left ventricular filling and stroke volume. Expect an increased heart rate as the body desperately tries to improve stroke volume.

You may have trouble auscultating your patient's heart sounds because fluid sequestration in the pericardial sac increases the distance between the heart and the chest wall.

Rapid intervention

Your main responsibility is to maintain the patient's cardiac output until intrapericardial pressure is relieved. (See *Responding to cardiac tamponade*, page 178.)

Administer oxygen to enhance tissue perfusion and set a flow rate as ordered.

The doctor will probably insert a pulmonary artery catheter to monitor hemodynamic pressures. Check these pressures and assess the patient's blood pressure, pulse, and respirations every 5 to 10 minutes to help gauge cardiac output.

Assist the doctor during pericardiocentesis (needle aspiration of pericardial fluid). This procedure is usually done in acute tamponade if the patient's systolic pressure drops more than 30 mm Hg from baseline. Aspirating as little as 25 ml of pericardial fluid dramatically improves arterial pressure and cardiac output.

The doctor may order intravascular volume expanders and vasoactive drugs to maintain hemodynamic support. He usually orders colloids to maximize left ventricular filling and stroke volume, although initially he may order 0.9% sodium chloride so-

Responding to cardiac tamponade

If surgery causes cardiac tamponade, be prepared to assist with emergency thoracotomy. In extreme cases, thoracotomy is done at the patient's bedside in the intensive care unit.

Preparation

Gather a prepared thoracotomy tray and an emergency resuscitation cart with internal defibrillator paddles. Make sure that all equipment is turned on and operational.

Monitor the patient's blood pressure and hemodynamic indicators. As ordered, maintain volume infusion, vasopressor administration, or both, to support failing cardiac output.

Care during and after the procedure

During thoracotomy, assist the doctor while monitoring the patient's response.

After thoracotomy, monitor the patient's vital signs; they should improve immediately. Also monitor hemodynamic indices and arterial blood gas values, and auscultate for heart and breath sounds. Give analgesics as needed. Maintain the chest drainage system and monitor for complications, such as hemorrhage and arrhythmias.

lution or lactated Ringer's solution. As ordered, give the first 500 ml of colloid or I.V. solution over a 10-minute period; then infuse at a rate of 100 to 500 ml/hour, depending on the patient's hemodynamic response.

Administer other drugs as ordered. Isoproterenol is useful because it increases contractility. Arterial vasodilators, such as hydralazine and nitroprusside, reduce afterload and systemic vascular resistance and may be used to augment cardiac output. Depending on the cause of tamponade, the doctor also may order vitamin K, antibiotics, or protamine to promote clotting.

If the patient has chronic tamponade, ensure hemodynamic stabilization and prepare

him for diagnostic studies as ordered. Assess him regularly for warning signs of a drop in cardiac output.

❖

Cardiac arrest

The complete cessation of heart contraction, cardiac arrest severely impairs cardiac output and causes hypoperfusion of the capillary bed. Because brain damage and death occur within minutes, only immediate intervention can save your patient's life. Overall, men are four times more likely to experience cardiac arrest than women.

Causes

Immediate precipitating causes of cardiac arrest include:
• ventricular fibrillation, resulting from acute inferior-wall myocardial infarction (MI) with damage to the sinoatrial node; toxic doses of sympathomimetic drugs; or antiarrhythmic drugs, which decrease the fibrillation threshold
• ventricular asystole stemming from hypertrophic cardiomyopathy, acute anterior-wall MI complicated by bundle-branch block, or toxic doses of parasympathomimetic drugs
• electromechanical dissociation
• cocaine abuse
• invasive procedures that irritate the myocardium, such as pulmonary artery catheter insertion, cardiac catheterization, and pacemaker insertion
• vagal stimulation (which can lead to bradycardia), hypovolemia, hypoxemia, or hypercapnia during surgery; general anesthetics (which can induce asystole)
• the lethal postsurgical triad of hypothermia, acidosis, and hypokalemia, which can induce ventricular fibrillation.

Assessment

Your careful assessment of a patient in cardiac arrest must include asking family members or witnesses about the patient's history and performing a physical examination focusing on heart rate, pulses, and respirations.

History

Find out if the patient has a history of coronary artery disease. Also find out if he has received sympathomimetics or parasympathomimetics or if he uses cocaine. These drugs increase the risk of cardiac arrest.

Physical examination

Check the patient's heart rate. The patient in cardiac arrest has an absent or a chaotic heart rhythm (ventricular fibrillation).

Expect the patient to be pulseless and unresponsive. If he's attached to an electrocardiogram (ECG) monitor, check for ventricular fibrillation, ventricular asystole, or electromechanical dissociation. However, keep in mind that pulselessness *always* indicates cardiac arrest, regardless of which rhythm appears on the ECG monitor.

Assess him for signs and symptoms of failing cardiac output, such as loss of consciousness; absence of breath sounds; absence of capillary refill; and cool, pale or cyanotic, moist skin.

Rapid intervention

Because cardiac arrest occurs suddenly, successful intervention consisting of cardiopulmonary resuscitation and advanced cardiac life support measures can mean the difference between life and death. (See *Responding to cardiac arrest*, pages 180 and 181, and *Guide to ACLS drugs*, pages 182 to 187.) ❖

(Text continues on page 188.)

Responding to cardiac arrest

To survive, a patient in cardiac arrest depends on your ability to quickly assess his condition and initiate lifesaving measures.

During a cardiac arrest, code team members usually assume preassigned roles. Basic rescuer 1 calls for another rescuer and starts one-person cardiopulmonary resuscitation (CPR). Basic rescuer 2 calls the code team and performs two-person CPR with basic rescuer 1. The team leader has overall responsibility for running the code, overseeing resuscitation efforts, and directing major lifesaving interventions. The nurse-anesthetist, anesthesiologist, or respiratory therapist maintains a patent airway, intubates the patient as necessary, administers oxygen as directed, and monitors respiratory status.

The medication nurse brings a code cart and prepares and administers all medications. (In some hospitals, a pharmacist assists with medication preparation.) The equipment nurse sets up adjunctive emergency equipment, takes the patient's vital signs, and helps with medications as needed. The go-between nurse stays flexible, helping when needed. The recorder nurse documents resuscitation efforts and writes postarrest progress notes.

Initiating CPR
• Check for a pulse before initiating chest compressions. Performing compressions on a patient with a pulse can cause further myocardial damage.
• To begin CPR, perform chest compressions at a rate of 60 per minute.
• If the patient isn't breathing, insert an oral airway into a hand-held resuscitation bag and connect the bag to 100% oxygen. Deliver manual respirations (approximately 12 per minute) until the code team arrives.
• If the patient is sharing the room, have his roommate removed if possible.

Establishing I.V. access
• Bring an emergency equipment cart to the bed. Have a colleague insert a peripheral I.V. line and instill dextrose 5% in water at a keep-vein-open rate. Establishing early I.V. access for emergency medications is crucial. As circulatory collapse progresses, inserting an I.V. line becomes increasingly difficult. If I.V. access is unavailable, the endotracheal tube offers an alternative route for epinephrine,

atropine, and lidocaine delivery.

• Remove the headboard of the bed for easy access during intubation.

• Stay with the patient to provide pertinent information to the code team, including the patient's condition when you found him, his medical history, any allergies, and the attending doctor's name. As appropriate, carry out your duties as a member of the code team.

Initiating ACLS

• When the code team arrives, advanced cardiac life support (ACLS) begins. ACLS aims to provide adequate ventilation, initiate and maintain a hemodynamically effective heart rhythm, and maintain and support restored circulation. Specific therapies include CPR, drugs, electrocardiogram monitoring, I.V. access and management, intubation and management, defibrillation or cardioversion, and postarrest stabilization.

• The team may defibrillate (deliver an unsynchronized electrical current to the heart), causing massive simultaneous depolarization of myocardial cells. The cells then repolarize uniformly, allowing the sinoatrial node, the heart's normal pacemaker, to resume control of heart rhythm and rate. Defibrillation is less effective if the patient has acidosis, hypothermia, hypokalemia, or digitalis toxicity.

• If the patient has tachycardia associated with hypotension, the team may then deliver synchronized cardioversion. This technique synchronizes delivery of current with the R wave of the patient's QRS complex, depolarizing the myocardium to resume pacing control of the heart. Because it avoids the vulnerable period of the ventricle (the peak of the T wave), it reduces the risk of inducing a lethal arrhythmia such as ventricular fibrillation.

• The patient must continue to receive supplemental oxygen. Remember that ventilating with room air is inadequate and may lead to anaerobic metabolism, interfering with drug therapy, defibrillation, or cardioversion.

• The nurse-anesthetist, anesthesiologist, or respiratory therapist will intubate the patient with an oropharyngeal, nasopharyngeal, or esophageal obturator or an esophageal gastric tube airway. The fraction of inspired oxygen is determined by arterial blood gas values.

Guide to ACLS drugs

During cardiac arrest or other cardiovascular crises, you may be called on to administer these advanced cardiac life support (ACLS) drugs.

DRUG USES AND DOSAGES	SPECIAL CONSIDERATIONS
Adenosine • *For paroxysmal supraventricular tachycardia (PSVT):* initial dose of 6 mg by rapid I.V. push over 1 to 3 seconds, followed by 20-ml saline flush; if no response within 1 to 2 minutes, administer 12-mg dose by rapid I.V. push	• Remember, this drug depresses atrioventricular (AV) node and sinus node activity. It's used for PSVT because this arrhythmia usually involves a reentry pathway. If the arrhythmia isn't from reentry involving the AV node or sinus node, adenosine won't stop the arrhythmia but may clarify the diagnosis. • Watch for transient sinus bradycardia and ventricular ectopy (common after termination of supraventricular tachycardia with adenosine). • Be aware that PSVT may recur after drug delivery because of adenosine's short half-life (under 5 seconds). Consider giving additional doses of adenosine or a calcium channel blocker to treat recurrences. • Recognize that this drug produces few, if any, hemodynamic effects because of its short half-life, but facial flushing is common.
Atropine • *For sinus bradycardia with hemodynamic compromise or frequent ventricular ectopic beats:* 0.5 to 1 mg by I.V. push, repeated every 3 to 5 minutes to a maximum dose of 0.04 mg/kg • *For ventricular asystole:* 1 mg; can be repeated in 3 to 5 minutes; a total dose of 3 mg (0.04 mg/kg) results in full vagal blockade	• Don't use a full vagal blocking dose (except for asystole) because this can trigger tachyarrhythmias and increase myocardial oxygen demand. • Give the drug endotracheally if quick peripheral I.V. access is unavailable. Increase dose to 2 to 2½ times the I.V. dose, diluted in 10 ml of 0.9% sodium chloride solution or distilled water. Administer using a syringe with a catheter tip that protrudes beyond the end of the endotracheal (ET) tube; administer quickly and follow with several insufflations to ensure adequate drug dispersal.

Guide to ACLS drugs (continued)

DRUG USES AND DOSAGES	SPECIAL CONSIDERATIONS
Bretylium • *For resistant ventricular fibrillation:* 5 mg/kg by I.V. push followed by defibrillation; if fibrillation persists, increase to 10 mg/kg and repeat at 5-minute intervals (maximum: 30 mg/kg) • *For resistant ventricular tachycardia:* 5 to 10 mg/kg diluted to 50 ml with dextrose 5% in water (D_5W) and injected I.V. over 8 to 10 minutes; infuse continuously at 2 mg/minute if tachycardia persists	• Because bretylium isn't a first-line drug, use it only as follows: if ventricular fibrillation doesn't respond to drug therapy and defibrillation, if ventricular fibrillation recurs despite epinephrine and lidocaine therapy, if lidocaine and procainamide fail to control ventricular tachycardia associated with palpable pulse, or if lidocaine and adenosine fail to control wide-complex tachycardias.
Calcium salts • *For hypocalcemia, hyperkalemia, or calcium channel blocker toxicity:* calcium chloride 10%—1.4 to 2.8 ml I.V.; calcium gluceptate 22%—5 to 7 ml I.V.; calcium gluconate 10%—5 to 8 ml I.V.	• Avoid routine use of calcium salts in resuscitation efforts; they may be detrimental.
Dobutamine • *For low cardiac output, hypotension, or pulmonary congestion:* 2 to 20 mcg/kg/minute by I.V. infusion; use smallest effective dose, as indicated by hemodynamic parameters	• Be aware that this drug may induce reflex peripheral vasodilation. • Monitor the heart rate closely; a rise of 10% or more may increase myocardial ischemia.

ACUTELY ILL
PATIENTS

(continued)

Guide to ACLS drugs *(continued)*

DRUG USES AND DOSAGES	SPECIAL CONSIDERATIONS
Dopamine • *For hypotension with bradycardia:* initial dose of 2.5 to 5 mcg/kg/minute by I.V. infusion, titrated until desired response occurs	• Expect drug effects to vary with dosage. At 1 to 2 mcg/kg/minute, the drug dilates renal and mesenteric vessels without increasing heart rate or blood pressure. At 2 to 10 mcg/kg/minute, the drug increases cardiac output without peripheral vasoconstriction; at over 10 mcg/kg/minute, the drug causes peripheral vasoconstriction and a marked increase in pulmonary artery wedge pressure.
Epinephrine • *For cardiac arrest:* 1 mg I.V. (10 ml of 1:10,000 solution); repeat every 3 to 5 minutes during resuscitation if necessary	• Expect some clinicians to use a 1-mg dose initially, then raise subsequent doses to 5 mg. • Give the drug endotracheally if quick peripheral I.V. access is unavailable. Increase dose to 2 to 2½ times the I.V. dose, and dilute in 10 ml of 0.9% sodium chloride solution or distilled water. Administer using a syringe with a catheter tip that protrudes beyond the end of the ET tube; administer quickly and follow with several insufflations to ensure adequate drug dispersal. • Give the drug by intracardiac injection only if venous and endotracheal routes are unavailable.
Isoproterenol hydrochloride • *For torsades de pointes or temporary control of bradycardia:* 2 mcg/ml I.V. (obtained by diluting 1 mg [5 ml] in 500 ml of D$_5$W and infusing 2 to 10 mcg/minute), titrated according to heart rate and rhythm	• Use for immediate temporary control of hemodynamically significant bradycardia in heart transplant recipients, but not for cardiac arrest. • Be aware that this drug increases the cardiac workload and worsens ischemia and arrhythmias in patients with ischemic heart disease. • Use only until pacemaker therapy begins.

Guide to ACLS drugs *(continued)*

DRUG USES AND DOSAGES	SPECIAL CONSIDERATIONS
Lidocaine • *For ventricular tachycardia, ventricular fibrillation, premature ventricular contractions (PVCs), or cardiac arrest:* loading dose of 1 to 1.5 mg/kg by I.V. bolus, followed by 0.5 to 1.5 mg/kg by I.V. bolus every 5 to 10 minutes to a maximum of 3 mg/kg (300 mg over 1 hour) • *For persistent ventricular fibrillation if defibrillation and epinephrine fail:* 1.5 mg/kg by I.V. bolus initially, followed by a continuous infusion at 2 to 4 mg/minute (dilute 1 g of lidocaine in 250 ml of D₅W for a 0.4% solution, or 4 mg/ml)	• Avoid giving the drug prophylactically to prevent ventricular ectopy when myocardial infarction is suspected but unconfirmed, unless the ECG shows PVCs. • Keep in mind that this drug improves response to defibrillation if patient has ventricular fibrillations. • Give the drug endotracheally if quick peripheral I.V. access is unavailable. Increase dose to 2 to 2½ times the I.V. dose, and dilute in 10 ml of 0.9% sodium chloride solution or distilled water. Administer using a syringe with a catheter tip that protrudes beyond the end of the ET tube; administer quickly and follow with several insufflations to ensure adequate drug dispersal.
Magnesium sulfate • *For ventricular fibrillation or ventricular tachycardia:* 1 to 2 g in 100 ml of D₅W administered over 1 to 2 minutes • *For magnesium deficiency:* loading dose of 1 to 2 g mixed in 50 to 100 ml of D₅W over 5 to 60 minutes	• Use for torsades de pointes and to decrease the incidence of postinfarction arrhythmias. • Monitor the patient closely for significant hypotension and asystole.

ACUTELY ILL
PATIENTS

(continued)

Guide to ACLS drugs *(continued)*

DRUG USES AND DOSAGES	SPECIAL CONSIDERATIONS
Nitroglycerin • *For congestive heart failure or unstable angina:* continuous I.V. infusion (50 or 100 mg in 250 ml of D_5W or 0.9% sodium chloride solution) at 10 to 20 mcg/minute, increased by 5 to 10 mcg/minute every 5 to 10 minutes until desired hemodynamic or clinical response occurs	• Monitor for hypotension, which could worsen myocardial ischemia. • Provide a mean dosage range of 50 to 500 mcg/minute. Most patients respond to 200 mcg/minute or less. • Be aware that nonpolyvinylchloride plastic I.V. administration sets may elicit an increased drug effect. With regular I.V. administration tubing, expect a decreased drug effect resulting from the drug's increased binding to tubing. • Keep in mind that prolonged continuous administration (longer than 12 hours) may produce tolerance.
Nitroprusside • *For heart failure or hypertensive crisis:* 50 to 100 mg in 250 ml of D_5W or 0.9% sodium chloride solution; dosage range is 0.1 to 0.5 mcg/kg/minute up to 10 mcg/kg/minute	• Wrap the drug container in opaque material to prevent drug deterioration. • Monitor blood pressure with an intra-arterial line.
Norepinephrine • *For severe hypotension with low total peripheral resistance:* 4 mg norepinephrine or 8 mg norepinephrine bitartrate in 250 ml of D_5W with or without 0.9% sodium chloride solution to yield a concentration of 16 mcg/ml of norepinephrine or 32 mcg/ml of norepinephrine bitartrate; initial dosage is 0.5 to 1 mcg/minute titrated to effect; refractory shock may require 8 to 30 mcg/minute	• Avoid giving this drug if the patient has hypovolemia. • Monitor blood pressure with an intra-arterial line; a false-low blood pressure reading may occur with a standard cuff. • Be aware that cardiac output may increase or decrease, depending on vascular resistance, left ventricular function, and reflex response. • Avoid prolonged use, which may cause ischemia of vital organs. • Don't administer in the same I.V. line as alkaline solutions, which may inactivate the drug.

ACUTELY ILL
PATIENTS

Guide to ACLS drugs   (continued)

DRUG USES AND DOSAGES	SPECIAL CONSIDERATIONS
Procainamide • *For ventricular arrhythmias:* 20 mg/minute by I.V. infusion until arrhythmia is suppressed, hypotension ensues, QRS complex widens by 50% of original width, or a total of 17 mg/kg infuses; maintenance infusion rate is 1 to 4 mg/minute	• Use for ventricular arrhythmias, such as PVCs or tachycardia, when lidocaine is contraindicated or ineffective. • Lower the maintenance dosage for patients with renal failure. • Too-rapid infusion causes acute hypotension. • Monitor the ECG carefully; if the QRS complex widens more than 50% or if the PR interval appears prolonged, notify the doctor and discontinue the infusion as ordered. • Don't administer to patients with a preexisting prolonged QT interval or torsades de pointes.
Sodium bicarbonate • *For metabolic acidosis:* 1 mEq/kg initially, followed by half of the dose every 10 minutes thereafter	• If arterial blood gas analysis is available, guide therapy by the calculated base deficit or bicarbonate concentration. • Avoid giving this drug for initial resuscitation unless the patient clearly has preexisting acidosis (hyperventilation should be the primary therapy to control acid-base balance).
Verapamil • *For atrial arrhythmias:* initial dose of 2.5 to 5 mg I.V. over 2 minutes; if no therapeutic response, repeat doses of 5 to 10 mg may be administered every 15 to 30 minutes to a maximum dose of 20 mg	• Use for atrial arrhythmias, especially PSVT with AV node conduction. • Don't use to treat atrial arrhythmias in patients with Wolff-Parkinson-White syndrome. • Use cautiously and in lower doses for patients receiving beta blockers. • Monitor the patient for hypotension, severe bradycardia, and congestive heart failure.

ACUTELY ILL
PATIENTS

Patients in respiratory crisis

Because gas exchange is vital to the body's tissues, respiratory crises can swiftly involve other body systems, particularly the cardiovascular system. Your duties as a nurse may go beyond assessing and medicating the patient to include urgent life-support measures. This section covers all aspects of managing respiratory crises and safeguarding the patient.

Pulmonary embolism

A pulmonary embolism occurs when a mass partially or completely obstructs a branch of the pulmonary artery. When the embolus lodges in a narrower vessel, tissue infarction occurs distal to the occlusion. (See *Understanding embolism*, pages 190 and 191.)

This infarction may be so mild that it's asymptomatic, but a massive embolism (obstructing more than 50% of pulmonary arterial circulation) and infarction can cause rapid death.

Causes

A pulmonary embolus may be caused by:
• a substance produced by the body: a thrombus, fat, amniotic fluid, or tumor cells. (See *Other types of embolism*, pages 192 and 193.) About 90% of all pulmonary embolisms result from a dislodged thrombus originating in the deep veins of the leg; less

common sources of thrombi include the pelvic, renal, and hepatic veins, the right side of the heart, and the upper extremities.
• certain genetic tendencies, such as an antithrombin III deficiency and specific protein deficiencies, that predispose to venous thromboembolism by causing a hypercoagulability state and pulmonary embolism formation.
• a substance outside the body: air, clumps of bacteria, or foreign materials such as catheter fragments.

Assessment

You'll need to act quickly when you suspect pulmonary embolism, but don't skip history taking; it may provide a clue. Remember the three risk factors for pulmonary embolism: hypercoagulability of the blood, vascular wall abnormalities, and venous stasis, known as Virchow's triad.

History

Determine if the patient has a history of clotting disorders, polycythemia vera, sickle cell anemia, fever, or dehydration. Ask a female patient if she's pregnant or taking oral contraceptives. Keep in mind that local trauma, atherosclerosis, and varicose veins more readily cause thrombus formation in patients with vascular wall abnormalities. And extended bed rest, obesity, congestive heart failure, and advanced pulmonary disease promote venous stasis and thrombus formation.

Be alert for recent pelvic or long-bone fracture that may have led to fat emboli.

Also ask the patient about preexisting lung disease, hypercapnia, and hypoxemia. These cause polycythemia (elevation of the red blood cell count), thickening the blood and slowing the flow.

Physical examination
The most significant sign of pulmonary embolism is the sudden onset of dyspnea. The extent of lung damage, along with the size, number, and location of the emboli, determines the severity of symptoms. A large embolus may cause cyanosis, syncope, and distended neck veins. Total occlusion of the pulmonary artery results in severe dyspnea and cardiac arrest.

If the patient complains of chest pain, bear in mind that chest pain caused by pulmonary embolism mimics that caused by myocardial infarction. You may also note shortness of breath, tachycardia, tachypnea, and low-grade fever. If circulatory collapse has occurred, the patient will have a weak, rapid pulse rate and hypotension.

Other signs and symptoms include chest splinting, cough, leg edema, headache, hemoptysis, and nonradiating pleuritic pain on inspiration. Mental status changes include restlessness, irritability, confusion, and feelings of impending doom. Palpation may reveal a warm, tender area in the extremities, a possible area of thrombosis. Auscultation of the lungs may reveal crackles and a pleural friction rub.

When auscultating the heart, listen for a loud pulmonic closure (P_2), which may indicate pulmonary hypertension secondary to pulmonary embolism. Remember, the second heart sound (S_2) consists of the sound made by the aortic valve closing (A_2 followed by P_2). Normally, A_2 is louder than P_2. You may also note an S_3 and an S_4 gallop, with increased intensity of the pulmonic component of S_2.

Check for diaphoresis, pale cool skin, petechiae, flulike symptoms, and symptoms of phlebitis. And don't overlook dehydration—particularly common in older people—as a risk factor for the development of pulmonary emboli.

Rapid intervention
Your first goal in treating pulmonary embolism is to maintain cardiac and pulmonary function until the obstruction resolves. (See *Responding to pulmonary embolism,* page 194.)

Your second goal is to prevent a recurrence of the embolism by administering heparin by continuous infusion as ordered. Target the partial thromboplastin time to about 2 to 2½ times the control level; to achieve this, infuse approximately 25,000 units of heparin per 24 hours.

If your patient has a massive pulmonary embolism and is in shock, he may need fibrinolytic therapy with streptokinase, urokinase, or alteplase to lyse the existing clots. These thrombolytic agents initially dissolve clots within 12 to 14 hours; within a week, however, they are no more effective than heparin. ❖

(Text continues on page 194.)

Understanding embolism

Embolism is characterized by the release or entry of a solid, liquid, or gas into the vascular system. Blood flow then carries the embolus to a smaller vessel or bifurcation, where it lodges and obstructs circulation.

Two types of embolism

There are two general types of embolism: venous and arterial. *Venous emboli* originate in the venous system. They're released into other veins, the lymphatic system (which reroutes them back into the venous system), or the heart's right chambers; usually, they wind up blocking a branch of the pulmonary artery.

Arterial emboli originate mainly in the arterial system. The most common sites are the heart's left chambers and the large arteries. Some liquid venous emboli (such as fat and amniotic fluid emboli) can penetrate the microcirculation and pass through the pulmonary capillary bed into the arterial circulation. And any venous embolus can become arterial if the patient has a cardiac septal defect.

How emboli form

Virtually any substance can become an embolus. Its nature is important because it can affect the embolic process. For example, a thrombus, the most common type of embolus, is absorbable, as are fat, air, and calcium emboli. Other types of emboli, however, such as bits of glass, wood, or metal or a tiny piece of a plastic catheter, can't be absorbed.

The size and number of emboli affect their severity in pulmonary embolism. A single, small pulmonary embolism may cause mild or moderate symptoms, but if the embolus grows, the patient's condition will worsen. Multiple (or recurrent) pulmonary emboli, if sufficient in number, cause symptoms disproportionate to the area occluded because of concurrent pulmonary hypertension.

Serotonin and thromboxane cause this hypertension. Both these substances, which are found in blood vessels, are potent vasoconstrictors; serotonin is a bronchoconstrictor as well. Their vasoconstrictive effects impair ventilation and perfusion, causing unoxygenated blood to be shunted into the arterial circulation, provoking hypoxemia. To compensate, the patient's respiratory rate and effort increase, but this merely increases his oxygen consumption without improving his oxygen levels.

At first, excessive carbon

dioxide leaks from the capillaries and is removed by hyperventilation, creating a temporary state of hypocapnia and respiratory alkalosis. Later, metabolic acidosis sets in as a result of anaerobic metabolism and the kidneys' failure to excrete enough hydrogen ions. Eventually, pulmonary hypertension increases venous pressure and right ventricular afterload, causing engorged neck veins, hepatomegaly, cerebral congestion, and myocardial dysfunction. It also reduces cardiac output. Together with the hypoxemia that's already occurring, this effect causes ischemia of every major organ system, culminating in hypovolemic shock.

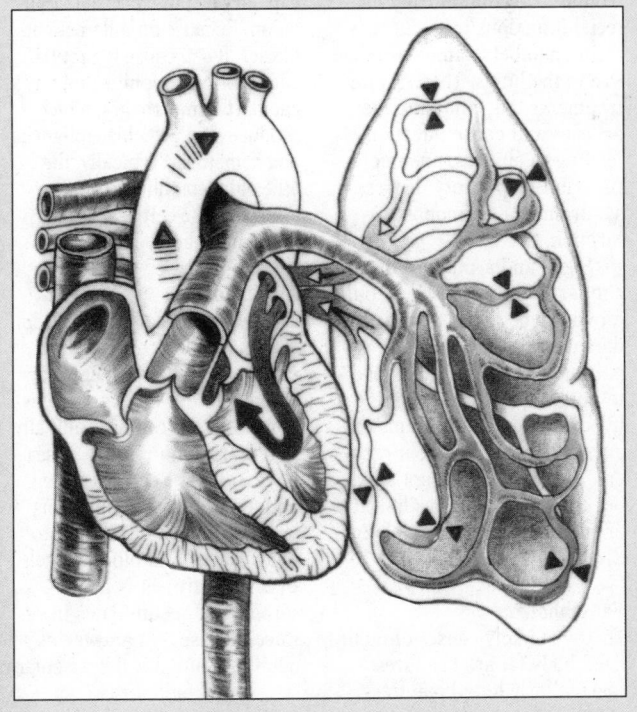

Other types of embolism

Besides thrombi, other types of embolism you should be familiar with are septic, fat, air, and amniotic fluid embolism. Usually venous in origin, they may all target the lungs.

Septic embolism

The most common causes of septic emboli in the lungs are septic deep vein thrombosis, septic abortion, abscesses, or wounds. Vegetation from bacterial infections in the heart's right chambers can also embolize to the lungs. These septic fragments lodge in pulmonary arteries and cause infection, leading to abscess, pneumonitis, adult respiratory distress syndrome, or pulmonary infarction.

Signs and symptoms are similar to those caused by pulmonary embolism. Besides the dangers of septicemia, impaired gas exchange can lead to potentially life-threatening hypoxia and acid-base imbalance. Even if the patient recovers, the prognosis is not good because healing leaves fibrotic areas that cause chronic lung disease.

Fat embolism

The most likely causes of mobilized body fat are fractures (particularly long-bone fractures such as of the femur), severe burns, and diabetic coma.

Fat flows in liquid form from bone marrow into body tissues; from there, it's pulled into the lymphatic system, then into the veins. In the blood, fat can combine with platelets to form a thrombotic mass that can occlude pulmonary artery blood flow.

Fat may also enter the pulmonary microcirculation in liquid form and pass through the capillary bed into arterial circulation. Because fat inflames capillaries, it can cause interstitial edema or pneumonitis and tiny capillary hemorrhages, which produce skin petechiae, oliguria, and hematuria. Typically, the 40% of fat emboli that become arterial cause cerebral, renal, and skin emboli.

Air embolism

The two main causes of air embolism are environmental and iatrogenic. Environmental air embolism follows exposure to atmospheric pressure radically different from pressure at sea level, such as deep-sea diving and high-altitude flying. This pressure forces nitrogen into body tissues and blood vessels. Because nitrogen is not absorbable, it accumulates in extracellular spaces and forms bubbles that enter the vascular system and embolize.

Iatrogenic air embolism may be caused by diagnostic or

therapeutic procedures—for example, cardiac catheterization, coronary arteriography, transcutaneous angioplasty, embolectomy, hemodialysis, central line insertion, open-heart surgery, and brain surgery performed with the patient in an upright position. The air embolus may then travel to vital organs through venous or arterial circulation. The most likely targets of air emboli are the heart's right chambers, pulmonary artery branches, and the cerebral venous sinuses. Arterial air emboli released during coronary arteriography or cardiac catheterization may invade coronary or cerebral arteries.

To prevent iatrogenic air embolism, check all catheter balloons, connections, and stopcocks carefully. Make sure that the taping on central lines is secure. Before a central line is inserted, place the patient in the Trendelenburg position, if he can tolerate it, to force direct air emboli toward the feet rather than toward the heart or brain. Also have him perform Valsalva's maneuver to increase intrathoracic pressure whenever the line is open (during connection changes, for example, or catheter insertion).

If you suspect a large amount of air has been pumped into a patient's vein, turn him on his left side and adjust the bed to the Trendelenburg position. This will trap the air embolus in the right side of the heart, where it can be absorbed.

Amniotic fluid embolism

Pregnant women are at risk for several types of embolism, including amniotic fluid embolism. During labor or abortion contractions, amniotic fluid leaks through torn fetal membranes and is pulled into uterine veins. Eventually, the fluid may pass through pulmonary capillary beds into arterial circulation, leaving fetal epithelial cells, lanugo, and meconium behind in pulmonary artery branches. The mother thus experiences massive pulmonary embolism and, possibly, arterial embolism.

As amniotic fluid travels to the lungs, it may combine with platelets to form a gel, risking disseminated intravascular coagulation and, possibly, uterine hemorrhage.

To detect amniotic fluid embolism, watch for sudden severe chest pain, dyspnea, and bronchospasm. Later signs include vaginal bleeding and shock. The mortality rate is about 80%.

Responding to pulmonary embolism

For the patient with pulmonary embolism, administer oxygen by nasal cannula at 4 liters/minute or by non-rebreather mask at concentrations up to 100%; the concentration depends on the degree of hypoxemia noted on arterial blood gas analysis. Keep the head of the patient's bed at a 90-degree angle to help him breathe; then apply a cardiac monitor.

Anticipate the doctor's order for anticoagulant or thrombolytic therapy. For anticoagulant therapy, you'll administer an initial I.V. bolus dose of 7,500 to 10,000 units of heparin.

For thrombolytic therapy, you'll administer heparin first, then 250,000 units of streptokinase, urokinase, or alteplase – also in an I.V. bolus dose – then another dose of heparin. (Thrombolytic therapy is contraindicated if the patient has had recent surgery or a cerebrovascular accident within the past 2 months, or currently has endocarditis or septic thrombophlebitis.)

Assess the patient's vital signs and cardiac output hourly, and continue to monitor him for arrhythmias. Check his respiratory rate, degree of dyspnea, and use of respiratory muscles.

Adult respiratory distress syndrome

A patient with adult respiratory distress syndrome (ARDS), a life-threatening condition, experiences painful hypoxemia and decreased lung compliance. Respiratory failure usually requires intubation and mechanical ventilation. Untreated, ARDS can quickly lead to acute respiratory failure and coma.

Causes

ARDS most often results from:
• direct or indirect injury to the lung (the most common cause of ARDS), possibly because fat emboli, sepsis, shock, pulmonary contusions, and multiple transfusions increase the likelihood of microemboli
• anaphylaxis
• aspiration of gastric contents
• diffuse viral pneumonia
• drug overdose or idiosyncratic drug reaction
• inhalation of noxious gases
• hemorrhage
• disseminated intravascular coagulation
• eclampsia
• near drowning
• oxygen toxicity
• shock
• multisystem organ failure.

Less often, ARDS results from complications of coronary artery bypass grafting, hemodialysis, leukemia, acute miliary tuberculosis, pancreatitis, thrombotic thrombocytopenic purpura, uremia, and venous air emboli.

Assessment

Assessing a patient with ARDS includes a health history, which may reveal lung trauma, and a physical examination, which should focus on the respiratory system.

History

First, find out if the patient has received a direct or an indirect injury to his lung in the past 48 to 72 hours. Has he aspirated gastric contents, recently received multiple blood transfusions, or inhaled noxious gases? Review other likely causes of ARDS.

Physical examination

In the first stage of ARDS, the patient may complain of dyspnea, especially on exertion. Respiratory and pulse rates will be normal to high. You may hear diminished breath sounds when you auscultate his lungs.

As respiratory distress becomes more apparent, the patient may have increased difficulty breathing. He'll begin using the accessory muscles of respiration. He may look pale and seem anxious and restless. He may have a dry cough or thick, frothy sputum and bloody, sticky secretions. His skin may feel cool and clammy. Tachycardia and tachypnea may accompany an elevated blood pressure. Auscultation may reveal basilar crackles.

As breathing difficulty increases, the patient may develop acute respiratory failure with severe hypoxia. He'll use his accessory muscles and will have a re-

spiratory rate above 30 breaths/ minute and tachycardia, often with premature ventricular contractions and a labile blood pressure. He'll probably need intubation and mechanical ventilation.

The patient may exhibit refractory hypoxemia or hypoxemia that doesn't respond to conventional treatments of oxygen therapy and positive end-expiratory pressure (PEEP). Spontaneous respirations usually aren't evident, and bradycardia with arrhythmias may accompany hypotension. Metabolic and respiratory acidosis develop, and mental status may deteriorate to coma. At this stage, the patient experiences a large intrapulmonary shunt because pulmonary blood is exposed to nonfunctioning alveoli and can't be oxygenated.

Rapid intervention

Administer oxygen with a tightly fitting mask to provide continuous positive airway pressure.

Monitor the patient's breathing. If his respiratory rate is greater than 35 breaths/minute and minute ventilation (respiratory rate multiplied by tidal volume) exceeds 10 liters/minute, he'll need to be intubated for mechanical ventilation.

Remember, the patient with ARDS usually requires oxygen therapy at greater than 50%. However, oxygen therapy at 50% for longer than 24 hours may cause oxygen toxicity, which can contribute to the development of ARDS. Use the lowest possible concentration of oxygen for the shortest possible period consistent with improving your patient's oxygenation.

Initially, the patient may require mechanical ventilation in the assist-control mode. Set the ventilator to deliver a tidal volume of 10 to 15 cc/kg, a respiratory rate of 12 to 16 breaths/minute, a fraction of inspired oxygen of 100%, and a PEEP of 3 to 5 cm H_2O.

Pressure-support ventilation may be used to provide positive airway pressure during the inspiratory cycle (the most difficult part of any breath). It improves the patient's oxygenation and reduces the airway resistance that occurs with traditional modes of mechanical ventilation.

Finally, pressure-controlled inverse ratio ventilation, which provides ventilation in direct opposition to normal breathing, may be used if the patient doesn't respond to oxygen and PEEP therapy.

Pneumothorax

An accumulation of air or gas between the parietal and visceral pleurae with lung collapse, pneumothorax is classified as tension, open (traumatic), or closed (spontaneous). It's also classified by size, with the amount of air or gas trapped in the pleural space determining the degree of lung collapse. A small pneumothorax occupies 15% or less of the pleural cavity; a moderate pneumothorax, 15% to 60%; and a large pneumothorax, more than 60%. In tension pneumothorax, air in the pleural space is under higher pressure than air in the adjacent lung and vascular structures. Without prompt treatment, a tension or large pneumothorax results in fatal pulmonary and circulatory impairment.

Causes

Causes of the three types of pneumothorax vary. Tension pneumothorax, in which air enters the pleural space but cannot escape, can be caused by:
• penetrating chest wound
• blunt trauma in which a tear in the pulmonary parenchymal tissue fails to seal
• chest tube occlusion or malfunction
• lung or airway puncture by a fractured rib associated with positive pressure ventilation
• mechanical ventilation (after chest injury) that forces air into the pleural space through damaged areas
• high-level positive end-expiratory pressure that causes alveolar blebs to rupture.

Open pneumothorax, in which air flows between the pleural space and the outside of the body, can be caused by:
• penetrating chest injury (such as a gunshot or knife wound)
• insertion of a central venous catheter
• chest surgery
• transbronchial biopsy
• thoracentesis
• closed pleural biopsy.

Closed pneumothorax, in which air reaches the pleural space directly from the lung, can be caused by:
• blunt chest trauma
• rupture of emphysematous blebs
• high intrathoracic pressures during mechanical ventilation

- tubercular or cancerous lesions that erode into the pleural space
- interstitial lung disease (such as eosinophilic granuloma)
- air leakage from ruptured, congenital blebs adjacent to the visceral pleural space
- leakage of blood into the pleural cavity (hemothorax), resulting from blunt or penetrating chest trauma, thoracic surgery, dissecting aortic aneurysm, or anticoagulation therapy.

Assessment
Your careful assessment of a patient with pneumothorax includes taking a causative patient history and performing a physical examination that focuses on palpation, percussion, and auscultation.

History
Review the patient's health history for possible causes of pneumothorax. Find out if normal chest movement, breathing, and coughing worsen chest pain. Ask the patient if he has been experiencing shortness of breath and, if so, for how long.

Physical examination
Inspect the patient for asymmetrical chest wall movement with overexpansion and rigidity on the affected side. Also assess for signs of cyanosis.

Palpation may reveal crackling beneath the skin, indicating subcutaneous emphysema and decreased vocal fremitus. Palpation may also reveal tympany on the affected side with unequal, diminished, or absent breath sounds.

Percussion may demonstrate hyperresonance on the affected side, and auscultation may disclose decreased or absent breath sounds over the collapsed lung.

Suspect tension pneumothorax if the patient reports sudden, sharp chest pain and shortness of breath. Tension pneumothorax is also likely if the patient on mechanical ventilation suddenly develops hypotension, high airway pressures, an increased respiratory rate, or increased anxiety. Other findings include a narrowed pulse pressure, dyspnea, rapid respirations, extreme anxiety, and a tracheal shift toward the unaffected side.

Rapid intervention
Tension pneumothorax must be treated immediately. It's confirmed by X-rays, so obtain an order for one immediately after the patient is stabilized.

If more than 30% of the lung collapses, chest tube drainage of air or blood is necessary. After the chest tube and drainage system are in place, encourage the patient to breathe deeply and exhale fully at least hourly to drain the pleural space and promote lung reexpansion. A flutter valve may be used in addition to or instead of a water seal to maintain one-way flow of drainage.

If less than 30% of the lung collapses, treatment is conservative, consisting of bed rest and careful monitoring of the patient's blood pressure, pulse rate, and respiratory rate. If symptoms are moderate, needle aspiration (thoracentesis) is performed.

Provide analgesics for pain. Monitor vital signs for indications of shock, respiratory distress, and mediastinal shift.

ACUTELY ILL PATIENTS

CLINICAL CLOSE-UP

 Understanding pulmonary edema

The pulmonary microcirculation consists of arterioles, capillaries, and venules. Normally, the thin capillary walls are permeable to fluid but not to blood cells and other large particles, such as proteins and glucose. Fluid constantly flows out through capillary walls into the interstitial space. An equal amount of fluid flows into the capillaries and the pulmonary lymphatic network.

Normal pulmonary fluid movement

This fluid movement ordinarily depends on the equal force of two opposing pressures, *pulmonary capillary hydrostatic pressure*, which forces fluid out of capillaries and into the interstitial space, and *plasma oncotic pressure*, which keeps fluid in the capillaries because of the force created by protein molecules.

Pulmonary capillary hydrostatic pressure is stronger in the arterioles, so fluid is pushed out of those vessels and into the interstitial space. In venules, however, plasma oncotic pressure is stronger, pulling fluid *into* the capillaries.

How pulmonary edema develops

Normally, the extensive pulmonary lymphatic network helps maintain a balance between these two pressures by absorbing any excess fluid. A small amount of fluid also evaporates in the alveoli and is exhaled.

Acute pulmonary edema develops when this delicate balance is upset. In cardiogenic pulmonary edema, abnormally high pulmonary capillary hy-

Pulmonary edema

A common complication of cardiac disease, pulmonary edema is an accumulation of fluid in the extravascular spaces of the lung. The disorder may be a chronic condition or may develop quickly and rapidly become fatal. Pulmonary edema may also progress to respiratory and metabolic acidosis with subsequent life-threatening cardiac or respiratory arrest. (See *Understanding pulmonary edema.*)

Causes

Pulmonary edema usually results from left ventricular failure caused by:
• ischemia from coronary atherosclerosis or occlusion
• cardiomyopathy
• hypertension
• valvular heart disease (most commonly mitral stenosis).

Cardiogenic pulmonary edema, the most common form of pulmonary edema, is marked by increased capillary hydrostatic pressure. It usually results from:
• myocardial infarction

drostatic pressure forces fluid out of the capillaries into the interstitial space. In most noncardiogenic types, however, the problem stems from increased capillary permeability, not high hydrostatic pressure. Leaky capillaries allow protein-rich fluid to escape. Because of its high oncotic pressure, this fluid tends to pull more fluid with it.

Normally, the right ventricle propels blood to the lungs, where gas exchange takes place. In cardiogenic pulmonary edema, left ventricular failure causes backward pressure, forcing fluid out of the vessels and impairing gas exchange. High hydrostatic pressure overcomes capillary oncotic pressure, forcing fluid out of the vessels and into the interstitial space and alveoli.

Normal

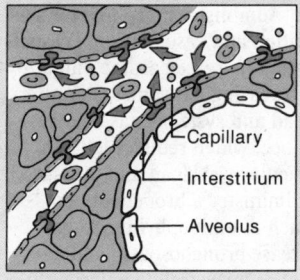

Capillary
Interstitium
Alveolus

Abnormal

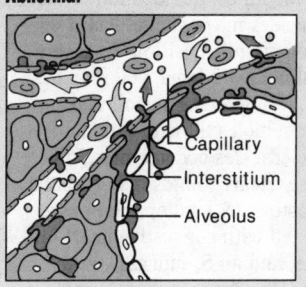

Capillary
Interstitium
Alveolus

• mitral stenosis
• decreased myocardial contractility
• left ventricular failure
• fluid overload.

Assessment
Your careful assessment of a patient with pulmonary edema should include a history of predisposing factors and a thorough physical examination.

History
Ask about a history of arteriosclerosis, cardiomyopathy, hypertension, or valvular heart disease. The patient will typically complain of a persistent, dry, hacking cough. He may report a cold, dyspnea on exertion, or orthopnea (increased dyspnea when lying flat). He may also describe paroxysmal nocturnal dyspnea (severe dyspnea and wheezing on awakening).

Physical examination
You may note restlessness, anxiety, and confusion. With severe pulmonary edema, the patient's breathing may be visibly labored and rapid. His cough may sound intense and produce frothy,

bloody sputum. In advanced stages, the patient's level of consciousness decreases, and respirations are shallow and rapid. You may observe Cheyne-Stokes respirations, indicating an underlying acid-base imbalance.

Inspect for neck vein distention. In acute pulmonary edema, the skin will feel sweaty, cold, and clammy. You may palpate fremitus over the chest. On percussion, you may detect dullness secondary to fluid accumulation in the dependent areas of the lung.

Auscultation may reveal crackles in the dependent areas of the lungs; the location of the crackles may change, based on the patient's position. In severe pulmonary edema, you may hear wheezing as the alveoli and bronchioles fill with fluid and the crackles become more diffuse. Heart sounds may reveal a diastolic (S_3) gallop, often associated with congestive heart failure, and an S_4 murmur. Additional findings include worsening tachycardia, falling blood pressure, thready pulse, and decreased cardiac output. In advanced pulmonary edema, breath sounds diminish.

Also assess for jugular vein distention, cyanotic extremities, prolonged peripheral capillary refill time, pulsus alternans, and a decreased urine output.

Rapid intervention

If you detect inspiratory crackles, a dry cough, or dyspnea, suspect pulmonary edema and notify the doctor immediately. Don't wait for chest X-ray results.

Treatment aims to reduce extravascular fluid, improve gas exchange and myocardial function, and correct the underlying disease (if possible).

High concentrations of oxygen to aid the patient's breathing can be administered by nasal cannula or mask, although many patients with pulmonary edema can't tolerate a mask. If the patient's arterial oxygen levels are still too low, assisted mechanical ventilation may improve oxygen delivery to the tissues and usually improves acid-base balance. Intubation and mechanical ventilation with positive end-expiratory pressure may be instituted to reduce intrapulmonary shunting.

Administer morphine for sedation and vasodilation. (Vasodilators increase cardiac output by decreasing left ventricular afterload and systemic vascular resistance, which reduces left ventricular workload and pressure.) Administer a bronchodilator such as aminophylline to decrease bronchospasm and enhance myocardial contractility.

Give diuretics, such as furosemide, ethacrynic acid, and bumetanide, to increase urine output, which helps to mobilize extravascular fluids.

Give inotropic medications, such as amrinone, dobutamine, or dopamine, to increase cardiac output by increasing myocardial contractility. Give antiarrhythmics such as lidocaine to treat cardiac arrhythmias caused by pulmonary edema. Cardiac glycosides may also be used to slow down the ventricular rate, especially when atrial fibrillation accompanies the rapid ventricular rate.

❖

Status asthmaticus

A complication of asthma, status asthmaticus is an asthma attack that may last for days to weeks and that fails to respond to conventional asthma therapy with bronchodilators. It may provoke respiratory alkalosis, respiratory acidosis, hypoxia, hypoxemia, and cyanosis. Ultimately, it can cause fatal respiratory failure even with optimal therapy. (See *Understanding status asthmaticus*.)

Causes

An asthma attack can be caused by a variety of stimuli or precipitating factors, including:
• dust, pollen, mold spores, and animal dander
• grains, food, and cooking odors
• perfume and cologne
• cleaning products
• cold, dry air and air pollutants
• exercise and emotional distress
• medications, such as aspirin, nonsteroidal anti-inflammatory drugs, and beta-adrenergic agents (including eyedrops)
• viral infections
• overuse of bronchodilators
• autonomic nervous system imbalance.

Assessment

Your assessment of the patient with status asthmaticus should include a history of precipitating factors, including failure to take medication, and a physical examination.

History

Ask the patient when the attack began and what he believes triggered it. Have the symptoms

---

CLINICAL CLOSE-UP

Understanding status asthmaticus

Status asthmaticus occurs when impaired gas exchange and heightened airway resistance increase the work of breathing. This flowchart shows the stages in its progression.

> Obstructed airways hamper gas exchange and increase airway resistance, leading to labored breathing.

> Initially, the patient hyperventilates, lowering the $PaCO_2$. Respiratory alkalosis and hypoxemia may develop quickly.

> The patient tires rapidly. His respiratory rate drops to normal.

> Later, $PaCO_2$ rises above the baseline level. (An asthmatic patient's $PaCO_2$ is usually low).

> The patient hypoventilates from exhaustion.

> Respiratory acidosis begins as the partial pressure of arterial oxygen drops and $PaCO_2$ continues to rise.

> Without treatment the patient experiences acute respiratory failure.

ACUTELY ILL PATIENTS

limited his walking, sleeping, and talking?

If his condition permits, review his medication history, especially since the attack began. Has he been taking his prescribed medications? How often does he use his metered-dose inhaler and what type of drug (such as the bronchodilators albuterol, metaproterenol, or theophylline) is he using? Also ask about any history of intubation or cardiac problems; patients requiring intubation or experiencing syncope during asthma attacks are at increased risk for a fatal attack.

Physical examination

Your examination will show a patient who is typically apprehensive, pale, breathless, and exhausted from fighting for air. Also, he is usually severely dyspneic and has great difficulty walking and talking. You may also detect signs of hypoxemia: anxiety, restlessness, and confusion. Also assess for tachypnea, tachycardia, and dehydration. Diaphoresis, cyanotic nail beds, and flaring nostrils may also be apparent.

You may hear wheezing without a stethoscope during inspiration and expiration. Often, the patient uses the accessory muscles of respiration. His expirations will be active and prolonged, with an inspiratory: expiratory ratio of 1:2 to 1:4. In a severe attack, you may not hear the patient's wheezing because he lacks sufficient air movement in his chest. Coughing may be almost impossible for him.

His heart sounds will be distant; his pulse, rapid and thready. You may also assess pulsus paradoxus, a drop of more than 12 mm Hg in systolic blood pressure during inspiration, indicating a severe airflow obstruction.

Chest percussion will reveal hyperresonance. Palpation may reveal vocal fremitus. Other assessment findings include increased pulse rate, respiratory rate, and blood pressure.

Rapid intervention

Your immediate priorities are reducing bronchoconstriction and treating hypoxemia.

Reduce bronchoconstriction by administering ordered bronchodilators. Provide emotional support and patient teaching to help reduce ineffective breathing as necessary. Regularly assess the patency of the I.V. line, or establish one if needed. Continually monitor vital signs and respiratory rate, pattern, and depth.

Treat hypoxemia with oxygen therapy to keep the partial pressure of arterial oxygen above 65 mm Hg or the arterial oxygen saturation (SaO_2) above 90%. Monitor oxygenation with periodic arterial blood gas samples and continuous pulse oximetry. Asthmatic patients don't tolerate a mask well, so use a nasal cannula at a fraction of inspired oxygen (FIO_2) of 2 to 4 liters/minute (30% to 35%).

Changes in patient position, intermittent airway plugging, and pulmonary vasodilation may result in decreasing SaO_2 levels. While monitoring the partial pressure of arterial carbon dioxide and the SaO_2, limit older patients with chronic airflow obstruction to an FIO_2 of 24% to 28%.

Rising carbon dioxide levels, a falling pH, and increasing respiratory fatigue are signs that the patient isn't responding to drug or oxygen therapy. Transfer him quickly to the intensive care unit for possible intubation and mechanical ventilation. ❖

Patients in neurologic crisis

Neurologic crises involve complex pathophysiologic and systemic interactions that may swiftly compromise other vital systems. Without early recognition and prompt treatment, your patient stands little chance of surviving a crisis or avoiding serious, perhaps irreversible, neurologic deficits. Because his condition may change rapidly, his chances may hinge on your ability to recognize when his condition is deteriorating.

Closed head injury

A head injury in which the skull remains intact or sustains only a linear fracture is a closed head injury (CHI). CHI can quickly cause extremely serious neurologic complications, including brain herniation, cerebral hemorrhage or hematoma, and systemic complications, such as pneumonia, seizures, and arrhythmias.

Types of CHI
Types of CHI include:
• concussion (jarring of the brain)
• contusion (bruising of the brain)
• coup injury (the head striking something and the brain striking the inside of the skull)
• contrecoup injury (the brain rebounding against the skull opposite the point of impact)
• acceleration injury (the head striking a moving object)
• deceleration injury (the head striking a stationary object)
• acceleration-deceleration injury, also called a coup-contrecoup injury (brain injury directly at and also opposite the point of impact)
• shearing injury (twisting of the brain on the brain stem)
• diffuse axonal injury (impact is spread throughout the entire brain, causing axons to stretch or become disrupted, altering their ability to conduct impulses).

CHI may further be classified as primary, resulting from direct impact, or secondary, resulting from a primary injury.

Causes
CHI results from head trauma that doesn't expose skull contents to air.

Assessment
If initial reports suggest CHI, assume that the patient has a spinal cord injury. Make sure that the patient has a cervical collar in place to immobilize the spine. Then proceed with your history and physical examination.

History

A patient with an altered level of consciousness (LOC) or memory loss may be unable to supply information about the injury or his medical history. You'll need to ask rescue workers or family members for a brief history. Focus on when and how the injury occurred; the mode of injury (a moving or stationary object); and the force, velocity, and point of impact. If the patient was in a motor vehicle accident, ask if he was wearing a seatbelt. Did his head strike the windshield or roof? Was he trapped in the vehicle? Did he lose consciousness and, if so, for how long?

Inquire if the patient's condition has deteriorated since the injury. Further ask about headache, neck pain, and vomiting.

Physical examination

Obtain vital signs and perform a brief examination to establish a baseline. Always assume that the patient has a spinal cord injury and take appropriate measures to immobilize the spine – or verify that rescue workers have done so. Evaluate the patient's neurologic status, and use the Glasgow Coma Scale score to gauge his LOC. Assess his pupils for equality, reaction to light, accommodation, and the consensual light reflex.

Next, test the patient's oculomotor responses and evaluate his respirations for abnormal patterns. Evaluate his motor strength and assess primitive reflexes, such as Babinski's, glabellar, and sucking reflexes.

Examine the patient's scalp for abrasions and lacerations, palpate his skull for elevations or depressions, and inspect his face for petechial bruising. If you find periorbital ecchymoses (raccoon's eyes) or posterior auricular ecchymosis (Battle's sign), suspect a basilar skull fracture. Also inspect the ears and nose for drainage, which may indicate a basilar skull fracture with associated cerebrospinal fluid leakage.

Assess for early and late signs of increased intracranial pressure (ICP). Early signs include restlessness, disorientation, lethargy, headache, contralateral hemiparesis, ipsilaterally dilated pupils with sluggish reaction, visual blurring, decreased visual acuity, and diplopia. The patient's vital signs are relatively stable and his temperature is normal. Late signs include increasing headache, coma, decorticate and decerebrate posturing and flaccid muscles (end stage), Cushing's triad (increased systolic blood pressure, widening pulse pressure, bradycardia), irregular respirations, fever, bilaterally dilated and fixed pupils, and possibly papilledema.

Rapid intervention

Maintain the patient's cervical collar until the doctor rules out cervical spine injury. Then assess and ensure an open airway, breathing, and circulation.

Next, perform a brief neurologic assessment. If the patient has a Glasgow Coma Scale score below 10, prepare him for intubation to maintain airway patency. Initiate hyperventilation therapy, as ordered, to constrict blood vessels and control cerebral blood flow and intracranial hypertension. Aim for a partial pressure of carbon dioxide in arterial blood of 33 to 35 mm Hg.

As ordered, arrange for an immediate computed tomography scan of the head. Insert a large-bore I.V. needle and draw blood for arterial blood gas (ABG) analysis, blood chemistry studies, a complete blood count, and blood typing and crossmatching. If appropriate, prepare the patient for insertion of an arterial line to permit frequent ABG evaluation.

If the patient has dilated pupils and an altered LOC, administer 50 to 100 g of mannitol I.V., as ordered, to reduce cerebral edema. Titrate the dose to the patient's weight. Elevate the head of the bed 30 to 45 degrees. Maintain mean arterial pressure (MAP) above 80 mm Hg and systolic blood pressure above 100 mm Hg. Monitor cardiac output, and notify the doctor if it falls below 5 liters/minute.

As ordered, administer 0.9% sodium chloride solution to expand volume. Insert an indwelling urinary catheter to permit accurate intake and output measurements. If the patient's Glasgow Coma Scale score registers 8 or below, prepare him for emergency surgery or placement of an ICP monitoring device as appropriate.

Managing ICP
After stabilizing the patient somewhat, focus on managing ICP and cerebral edema as ordered.

Obtain and document ICP readings every hour. Obtain MAP readings, and then calculate and document continuous positive pressure (CPP) hourly by subtracting ICP values from MAP values. To ensure normal CPP and maintain vascular volumes, maintain the patient at roughly two-thirds the normal volume restoration rate. Usually, this means ensuring a total I.V. fluid intake of approximately 100 ml/hour.

Keep the head of the bed elevated 30 to 45 degrees to help reduce ICP, and ensure proper head and neck alignment to promote venous drainage. Limit suctioning to 10 seconds to reduce stimulation and help reduce ICP.

Administer prescribed sedatives and analgesics judiciously, keeping in mind the patient's neurologic status and ICP.

Intersperse care with frequent rest periods to prevent overstimulating the patient, which could raise ICP. Dim the lights and minimize noise. Instruct the patient's family to speak in soft tones and use gentle touch.

Ruptured cerebral aneurysm

A cerebral aneurysm is a dilated cerebral vessel, usually an artery, that can produce neurologic symptoms by exerting pressure on cranial nerves and other surrounding structures. If an aneurysm ruptures, crippling subarachnoid hemorrhage (SAH) or death may follow. The patient requires close monitoring and expert care.

Aneurysms are classified according to size, shape, or underlying cause, as follows:

• Saccular (or berry) aneurysms are berry shaped and account for about 90% of cerebral aneurysms. They arise as a congenital defect in the medial layer of the vessel wall and usually occur at arterial bifurcations.
• Fusiform aneurysms are 3 cm or more in diameter and account for roughly 7% of cerebral aneurysms. They reflect a loss of elasticity in the vessel wall and involve the basilar, internal carotid, and vertebral arteries. Rarely rupturing, they compress surrounding structures instead.
• Microscopic aneurysms are associated with hypertension and commonly occur in the basal ganglia and brain stem.
• Mycotic aneurysms account for less than 1% of cerebral aneurysms and are usually multiple occurrences. They typically involve the middle cerebral artery, either in the sylvian fissure or distal artery, and may progress to acute inflammation of the vessel wall.
• Dissecting aneurysms also account for less than 1% of all cerebral aneurysms. Those associated with facial and skull fractures usually involve the carotid system. Others, stemming from atherosclerosis, force blood between layers of the vessel wall as the intima pulls away.

Causes

Aneurysms arise from:
• a congenital defect in the middle layer of the vessel wall (most common)
• atherosclerosis
• a head injury that damages the vessel wall
• septic emboli, resulting from bacterial endocarditis, that lodge in distal branches, leading to acute inflammation of the vessel wall
• hypertension
• syphilis.

Assessment

Your assessment of the patient with cerebral aneurysm must include a thorough history of any subtle neurologic signs, and a physical examination of a patient who may be comatose.

History

Most cerebral aneurysms produce no symptoms unless they rupture. Yet, before rupture, roughly half the patients experience certain warning signs and symptoms (prodrome) that suggest aneurysm expansion: localized head pain, diplopia, blurred vision, or palsy of the third, fourth, or sixth cranial nerve.

Find out if the patient has a history of head injury, hypertension, or infection.

If your patient has regained consciousness after an aneurysm rupture, he may report an intense headache, the worst he has ever had. Ask what triggered the headache, when it started, where it hurts, and what the pain feels like. He may report hearing a snapping or popping sound. Also note any complaints of a stiff neck, photophobia, and low-grade fever – signs of meningeal irritation from blood in the subarachnoid space.

With SAH, the patient may report a severe, migrainelike headache of sudden onset, which may be generalized or localized. A patient with a minor intracerebral hemorrhage may report nonfocal symptoms, such as malaise, generalized headache, nau-

PREVENTIVE PRACTICE

 Preventing cerebral rebleeding, vasospasm, and seizures

Prevent rebleeding by taking these precautions:
• enforcing bed rest
• keeping the head of the bed elevated (to promote venous drainage, decrease intracranial pressure, and prevent sudden blood pressure changes)
• darkening the room if the patient is photophobic
• restricting visitors
• maintaining sedation (usually with phenobarbital)
• giving analgesics for headache
• providing a soft-food, high-fiber diet

• having the patient avoid Valsalva's maneuver (for example, by giving stool softeners).

Prevent vasospasm by taking the following measures:
• administering intravascular volume expanders and antihypertensive agents (to improve perfusion and limit ischemia)
• administering calcium channel blockers.

Prevent seizures by taking the following measures:
• administering oxygen to prevent hypoxemia
• administering prophylactic anticonvulsants.

ACUTELY ILL
PATIENTS

sea and vomiting, and neck and back pain.

Development of nausea and vomiting after aneurysm rupture suggests increased intracranial pressure (ICP) from cerebral edema and hydrocephalus. These findings may be accompanied by papilledema, third and sixth cranial nerve palsy, and an altered level of consciousness (LOC) ranging from lethargy to coma.

Physical examination
Depending on the aneurysm's severity, physical findings may range from slight nuchal rigidity to deep coma. In the patient with SAH, expect transient to permanent loss of consciousness and temperature elevation. The patient with hydrocephalus usually has a decreasing LOC, pupil dilation

with reduced pupillary reflexes, and deviation of the eyes.

You may also detect lateralizing signs and symptoms after an aneurysm rupture. The result of cerebral vasospasms that impair blood flow to certain brain areas, these findings may be absent if bleeding is confined to the subarachnoid space.

Note any seizures or signs of pituitary dysfunction.

Rapid intervention
Guard against SAH by preventing or limiting the patient's ability to cough, sneeze, or strain; by banning all external stimuli, including TV, radio, and reading material; and by not giving enemas. (See *Preventing cerebral rebleeding, vasospasm, and seizures.*)

Arrange for an immediate computed tomography scan and, possibly, for a cerebral angiogram. Based on the results, the doctor may insert an intraventricular catheter to remove intraventricular blood, drain cerebrospinal fluid, or monitor ICP.

Check the patient's neurologic status every 30 minutes.

Limit the patient's fluid intake to 1,800 ml/day.

As ordered, give anticonvulsants to help prevent seizures, which increase the brain's oxygen needs and trigger increased ICP.

Arrange for laboratory tests and an electrocardiogram to establish a baseline for treatment. Depending on the clinical grade of the aneurysm, the patient may require intubation to maintain a patent airway and ensure adequate oxygenation.

———————————❖

Status epilepticus

In this disorder, the patient suffers a series of rapidly repeated seizures without recovering neurologic function between attacks. Although status epilepticus may involve any type of seizure, generalized tonic-clonic seizures are the most common type; they're also the most dangerous because they increase the risk of anoxia, arrhythmias, and systemic lactic acidosis. If seizures aren't arrested, irreversible brain damage may occur.

Most patients in neurologic critical care settings are at risk for posttraumatic seizures and metabolic disturbances stemming from their overwhelming injuries. Consider your patient's well-being, and know how to intervene in this medical emergency. (See *Responding to status epilepticus*.)

Causes
In most patients, the cause of status epilepticus remains unknown. However, factors that may precipitate it include:
• abrupt withdrawal of anticonvulsants or alcohol
• hypoglycemia
• brain tumor
• head injury
• high fever
• central nervous system infection
• poisoning.

Assessment
Your assessment of the patient with status epilepticus must include a history of any seizures and drug consumption and a rapid physical examination to help identify the type of seizure the patient is experiencing.

History
Obtain a brief history by asking family members if the patient has had a seizure before and when the most recent one occurred. Obtain a history of events occurring at the onset of the present attack. Also inquire about any prescription drugs the patient may be taking, and when he took his last dose. Ask about the use of recreational drugs and alcohol. Finally, inquire about any recent injury, especially head trauma, and about any recent illnesses.

STAT CARE

 Responding to status epilepticus

For the patient with status epilepticus, ensure a patent airway, but don't attempt to insert an artificial airway until the patient's muscles have relaxed. Otherwise, his tongue may occlude the airway or his teeth may break, creating a partial occlusion.

Keep emergency intubation equipment at hand in case the patient requires ventilatory support.

To reduce the risk of aspiration during a seizure, plan to perform pulmonary hygiene measures every 2 to 4 hours and mobilize secretions. Until the threat of aspiration passes, withhold all oral intake unless ordered otherwise. The doctor may insert a Salem sump tube to avert gastric distention and vomiting, which may cause aspiration.

Establish I.V. access
Establish an I.V. route to administer anticonvulsants and to allow blood withdrawal for analysis of arterial blood gases, electrolytes, and glucose.

Halt seizures
Expect to administer 5 to 10 mg of diazepam I.V. slowly. Repeat the dose every 15 minutes to a maximum of 30 mg. However, be aware that diazepam induces respiratory depression.

Alternatively, the doctor may order 4 to 8 mg of lorazepam I.V., repeated in 10 minutes, or 20 mg/kg phenytoin I.V. at a rate of 50 mg/minute. Because phenytoin may cause hypotension and slowed heart rate, monitor the patient's electrocardiogram. If bradyarrhythmia or heart block occurs, withhold the drug as ordered.

Take extended measures
If these drugs don't halt the seizure, the doctor may induce pharmacologic paralysis to ease intubation and ensure respiratory support. However, stopping visible seizure activity with a paralytic drug doesn't necessarily abolish the seizure. Seizure activity may continue and brain cells may die despite adequate oxygenation and blood pressure. To avoid clinical confusion about halting the seizure versus masking the motor responses, some hospitals use a short-acting, nondepolarizing muscle relaxant, such as vecuronium, in this circumstance for rapid clearance to prevent masking of the seizure activity and to eliminate fasciculations on clearance of the paralytic agent.

As long as the seizure continues, measures should be taken to determine the underlying cause, such as analyzing blood glucose levels for hypoglycemia and performing an echoencephalogram to detect cerebral hematoma.

Physical examination

You must first determine if the patient's seizures are partial (such as focal or psychomotor seizures) or potentially deadly generalized seizures (for example, tonic-clonic, myoclonic, or atonic seizures). Signs and symptoms of tonic-clonic seizures include nystagmus, bowel or bladder incontinence, diaphoresis, labored breathing, dyspnea, apnea, cyanosis, and mucus or saliva filling the mouth.

Rapid intervention

Ensuring a patent airway is your first priority. Typically, your patient may then be given such drugs such as diazepam to halt seizures and anticonvulsants or barbiturates to prevent seizure recurrence.

————————————◆

Cerebrovascular accident

The third most common cause of death in North America, cerebrovascular accident (CVA, or stroke) is the sudden nonconvulsant onset of neurologic deficits related to reduced blood supply to brain tissues. The sooner circulation is restored, the better the chances for recovery.

CVA accounts for roughly 200,000 deaths annually. An even greater number of patients are permanently disabled by cerebrovascular disease each year.

Causes

Possible causes of a CVA include:
• thrombus (most common), related to atherosclerosis
• embolism, usually related to heart disease
• hemorrhage, related to hypertension
• heart disease.

Assessment

Your assessment of the patient with CVA must include a thorough history of the timing of developing signs and symptoms and a physical examination that may yield different symptoms, depending on the CVA site.

History

Inquire about any factors that might increase the risk of CVA, such as a history of heart disease, atherosclerosis, or smoking. Ask the patient what signs and symptoms accompanied his CVA. He may report transient ischemic events, such as temporary loss of vision, numbness or weakness of extremities, or aphasia; or migraine headaches.

Ask the patient to describe the progression of the CVA, if possible. A *thrombotic stroke* occurs over time and produces progressive neurologic deficits; as arteries narrow, the blood supply to the brain decreases. In *evolving stroke syndrome*, signs and symptoms occur in a stepwise progression over several hours or days, usually leading to permanent neurologic deficits; the stroke is considered complete when deficits stabilize and symptoms no longer progress. An *embolic stroke* occurs without warning when a thrombus from the heart breaks loose and travels to the brain; symptoms develop rapidly and neurologic deficits are complete within a few minutes. In a *hemorrhagic stroke*, caused by cerebral artery rupture, symptoms occur within minutes or hours and persist for weeks to months until the clot is absorbed.

Ask the patient if he experienced any loss of consciousness.

Physical examination

Check the patient's circulation, neurologic status, and level of consciousness (LOC). Assessment findings vary with the location of the CVA (usually the middle cerebral artery), the extent of tissue damage, and the efficiency of the collateral circulation.

If the CVA occurred in the middle cerebral artery, your assessment may reveal contralateral hemiplegia, aphasia, hemianopia, alterations in LOC ranging from confusion to coma, and inability to recognize the paralyzed side.

If the CVA occurred in the anterior cerebral artery, your assessment may reveal contralateral foot and leg paralysis, impaired gait, paresis of the contralateral arm, abulia, flat affect, and amnesia.

If the CVA occurred in the posterior cerebral artery, you may detect hemianopia, memory deficits, and visual field deficits. If the penetrating branches were affected, you may detect signs of brain stem and thalamic impairment.

Rapid intervention

During the acute phase of a CVA, focus on helping the patient maintain vital functions and survive.

Maintain a patent airway, and closely monitor the patient's vital and neurologic signs until his condition stabilizes.

Then take appropriate steps to prevent complications. Continue monitoring vital and neurologic signs. Provide skin care to prevent skin breakdown, and perform passive range-of-motion exercises to prevent joint deformity. Maintain good pulmonary hygiene, and assess for adequate swallow and gag reflexes to prevent aspiration and ensure the patient's ability to eat properly. Institute measures to prevent deep vein thrombosis, and watch for signs of pulmonary embolism.

Medical interventions vary with the type of CVA. *A thrombotic* or *embolic stroke* relies on anticoagulants (heparin followed by warfarin) and, if indicated, an antiplatelet (aspirin or dipyridamole) to enhance circulation and to prevent further emboli. Anticoagulant dosage is calculated according to the patient's prothrombin time or his coagulation time. Drug therapy doesn't affect neurologic deficits.

In a *hemorrhagic stroke*, surgery may be performed to remove the blood clot or to treat an aneurysm. Other surgical interventions, which aim to correct predisposing conditions, are controversial. These include carotid endarterectomy and intracranial-extracranial bypass. The best surgical candidates include those without major neurologic deficits or underlying, uncontrolled systemic disease.

Meningitis

An inflammation of the meninges surrounding the brain and spinal cord, meningitis may affect the three meningeal membranes—the dura mater, the arachnoid membrane, and the pia mater. The prognosis is usually good for adults, especially if the disease is recognized early and the infecting organism is isolated and responds to the prescribed antibiotics. The prognosis is poorer for infants, children, and older adults. Without prompt treatment, the associated rise in intracranial pressure (ICP) can cause optical damage, deafness, permanent personality changes, coma, and paralysis, and 70% to 100% of patients in these age-groups die.

Causes

Meningeal infections can be caused by:
• bacteria (most common), such as *Neisseria meningitidis* (meningococcal meningitis), *Haemophilus influenzae*, *Streptococcus pneumoniae* (pneumococcal meningitis), *Escherichia coli*, or *Mycobacterium tuberculosis*
• viruses, such as enteroviruses, arboviruses, herpes simplex virus, mumps virus, or lymphocytic choriomeningitis virus
• protozoa
• fungi, such as *Cryptococcus;* cryptococcal meningitis is the most common fungal infection of the central nervous system.

Assessment

Your assessment and all subsequent treatment of meningitis hinge on a rapid, thorough patient history and physical examination identifying the probable cause and type of organism.

History

Ask the patient and his family to describe his symptoms. Family members typically report changes in mental status, behavior, and personality. Fully explore any history of recent infection (such as respiratory tract or ear) or other predisposing conditions (such as traumatic injury, surgery, or immunosuppression).

Physical examination

Assess for typical findings: fever, severe headache, photophobia, nuchal rigidity of the neck and back and, in some patients, opisthotonic posturing, vomiting, and seizures. Half of all patients with meningococcal meningitis present with a petechial, purpuric, or ecchymotic rash, usually over the lower body.

A neurologic examination shows further signs of meningeal irritation, such as a positive Brudzinski's or Kernig's sign.

Look for signs of increased ICP: decreased level of consciousness (ranging from memory impairment to stupor, unresponsiveness, and coma), pupil changes, widened pulse pressure, bradycardia, and irregular respiratory patterns. Left untreated, increased ICP can progress to brain herniation and death.

Before meningitis is evident or diagnosed, the patient may show signs of Waterhouse-Friderichsen syndrome: septicemia; abrupt onset of high fever; petechial hemorrhage on the face, arms, and legs; adrenal insufficiency; shock; and disseminated intravascular coagulation.

Rapid intervention

Promptly initiate appropriate antibiotic therapy, as ordered, usually with penicillin, ampicillin, or chloramphenicol, depending on the causative organism. You'll maintain the patient on large doses of parenteral antibiotics for 2 weeks, followed by a course of oral antibiotics. For some patients, the doctor may elect intrathecal administration. Other commonly ordered drugs may include mannitol and steroids for cerebral edema, anticonvulsants for seizures, sedatives for restlessness, and acetaminophen for headache and fever. Treatment also includes appropriate therapy for any coexisting conditions, such as pneumonia or endocarditis.

Institute vigorous supportive care, including bed rest, maintenance of normothermia, fluid and electrolyte replacement to prevent dehydration, and management of cerebral edema, seizures, and ICP.

Unless the patient has viral meningitis, maintain respiratory isolation for 24 hours after the start of antibiotic therapy. Follow strict aseptic and hand-washing techniques, and maintain infectious precautions for nasal and oral discharges and all used items.

Continually assess the patient for pupillary changes, signs of meningeal irritation, and alterations in mental status. Test for cranial nerve involvement, watching for such signs as pto-sis, strabismus, diplopia, and facial paresthesias.

Monitor vital signs, watch for signs of increased ICP, and frequently check the patient's temperature. Use tepid baths, ice packs, antipyretics, or a cooling blanket as needed. Routinely perform vascular assessments to detect early signs of circulatory compromise from septic emboli.

Monitor the patient's respiratory effort to ensure adequate oxygenation and ventilation. ❖

Malignant hyperthermia

A painful, life-threatening condition, malignant hyperthermia can develop, particularly after surgery, in patients with an inherited defect in muscle cells. It's characterized by constant, uncontrollable muscle contractions caused by an excess of intracellular calcium. The muscles' greatly increased demand for oxygen increases aerobic and anaerobic metabolism, leading to hypoxia and metabolic and respiratory acidosis. Without vigilant monitoring and proper treatment, a patient can develop arrhythmias, shock, renal failure, disseminated intravascular coagulation, cardiac failure, and pulmonary edema.

Causes

Malignant hyperthermia may be triggered by:
• certain anesthetics, such as halothane
• muscle relaxants, such as succinylcholine

- amide-type local anesthetics, such as lidocaine
- infections
- hypothermia
- pain
- trauma
- excessive physical activity
- stress.

Assessment

Your assessment of the patient with malignant hyperthermia includes history questions focusing on medication and other possible causes and a thorough physical examination.

History

Ask the patient or his family about any recent surgery and the types of drugs used, especially anesthetics and muscle relaxants. Also ask about any recent episodes of stress, such as illness, accidents, or unusually strenuous exercise.

Physical examination

Your assessment may reveal slight tachycardia and tachypnea, mottled and dusky skin, irregular pulse, and slight muscle rigidity—all early signs of malignant hyperthermia. Fever, however, is a late sign. Other late signs include hypotension, diaphoresis, nausea and vomiting, decreased urine output, pulmonary edema, cardiac arrhythmias, changes in serum electrolyte levels (such as hyperkalemia), and generalized skeletal muscle rigidity.

Rapid intervention

Start administering oxygen at 4 liters/minute through a nasal cannula and set up a cardiac monitor. Remove the patient's blankets and lower the room temperature, if possible, but don't let the room get too cold; shivering could cause temperature elevation. Call for a hypothermia blanket and ice packs to help lower the patient's temperature if it begins to rise. If severe hyperthermia develops, you may have to administer chilled 0.9% sodium chloride solution I.V. and iced solutions through a nasogastric tube to help lower his core body temperature.

Draw blood for an electrolyte profile. As ordered, administer I.V. dantrolene, the drug of choice for treating malignant hyperthermia, to decrease intracellular calcium levels. The doctor will most likely order an initial I.V. bolus dose of 2.5 mg/kg, repeated every 5 to 10 minutes until vital signs return to baseline and other signs and symptoms resolve, or until you've given a total dose of 10 mg/kg. (Because large amounts of chilled I.V. solutions may also be ordered, you may have to insert an indwelling urinary catheter.) Watch for dantrolene's adverse effects, such as muscle weakness and decreased gag reflex.

Have another nurse monitor the patient's vital signs every 5 minutes; his temperature could increase as rapidly as 1.8° F (1° C) every 5 minutes, and it could reach 111° F (43.9° C) or more. Have the nurse also monitor the patient for arrhythmias and signs of shock.

If the patient develops hyperkalemia, the doctor may order regular insulin (0.25 to 0.5 units/kg) and glucose (0.25 to 0.5 g/kg). He may also order mannitol (12.5 g I.V.) prophylactically to maintain renal function.

Patients in GI crisis

Any serious disruption of the GI system can have far-reaching metabolic effects and may lead to a life-threatening GI crisis. This type of crisis can occur as a primary disorder, as a consequence of chronic disorders or injuries, or as a complication of medications or diagnostic tests. This section details how to recognize and care for patients in a variety of GI crises, all potentially fatal.

Ruptured esophageal varices

When veins in the submucosa of the lower esophagus become varicosed (dilated and tortuous) and rupture, they may cause massive, life-threatening hematemesis (vomiting of blood). The patient with ruptured esophageal varices needs emergency treatment to control hemorrhage and prevent the progression to shock.

Causes

Esophageal varices nearly always result from portal hypertension – increased pressure in the portal vein caused by obstruction in the portal circulation. Usually, the underlying cause of portal hypertension is:
• a disorder of the liver or biliary system, such as alcoholic cirrhosis, hepatitis, biliary infection, liver or biliary tumors, cholelithiasis, congenital hepatic fibrosis, or schistosomiasis

• trauma or surgery involving the portal vein.

Assessment

Your assessment of the patient with ruptured esophageal varices must include a brief health history of any GI disease or alcoholism and a physical examination that centers on evaluating hematemesis.

History

Take a quick history from your patient or his family to determine the presence of underlying chronic liver disease or chronic alcohol abuse. Expect a complaint of bloody vomitus and of blood welling up in the back of the throat. Ask about the frequency of vomiting and the amount of vomitus. Also ask if the patient has noticed melena (black, tarry stools containing blood).

Inquire about pain – ruptured esophageal varices usually are painless.

Determine if the patient had a previous disorder or surgery of the biliary tract (such as gallstones, gallbladder surgery, abdominal trauma, or infection) or has a family history of GI tract disorders. Take a medication history, staying alert for drugs that may contribute to bleeding, such as aspirin, nonsteroidal anti-inflammatory drugs, and anticoagulants.

Determine if the patient recently traveled to a tropical climate where water or food may have been contaminated.

Physical examination

Sudden, profuse, painless vomiting of bright red blood is the hallmark of ruptured esophageal

RULE OF THUMB

 Determining blood loss from clinical findings

If your patient has ruptured esophageal varices, these rules of thumb will help you determine the severity of blood loss.

Loss of less than 500 ml
During initial bleeding, you may detect only weakness, restlessness, and diaphoresis. Body temperature may rise to between 101° and 102° F (38.3° and 39° C). Bowel sounds are hyperactive from bowel sensitivity to blood. Blood in the bowel acts as a cathartic, causing increased bowel sounds and diarrhea.

Loss of 500 to 1,000 ml
After moderate loss, a sympathetic nervous system response causes release of the catecholamines epinephrine and norepinephrine. This causes the heart rate to rise in an attempt to maintain blood pressure (more than 100 mm Hg systolic).

Loss of more than 1,000 ml
After heavy loss, expect classic signs and symptoms of shock. To boost blood flow to the brain and heart, catecholamine release now triggers vasoconstriction of the skin, lungs, intestines, liver, and kidneys. As blood flow to the skin diminishes, the patient's skin cools. With less blood flowing to his lungs, he hyperventilates to maintain adequate gas exchange. Expect blood pressure to drop—a sign of advanced shock indicating that the body's protective mechanisms have been overwhelmed. As intravascular volume diminishes, urine output decreases from renal reabsorption of water in response to the release of antidiuretic hormone.

varices. Assess vomitus for clots. Check stools for melena and occult blood. Observe for signs and symptoms of hypovolemic shock: restlessness, hypotension, tachycardia, diaphoresis, pallor, decreased urine output, and reduced central venous and pulmonary artery pressures. Other signs and symptoms depend partly on how much blood the patient has lost. (See *Determining blood loss from clinical findings*.)

Assess the patient for an altered level of consciousness or lethargy, jaundice, ascites, lower extremity edema, and muscle wasting. These signs reflect liver disease. You also may note dilated abdominal veins and abdominal distention.

Listen to bowel sounds to assess their quality and quantity. Blood in the GI tract typically causes hyperactive bowel sounds, so you should hear more than 20 sounds per minute instead of the normal 10 to 20.

Assess for abdominal tenderness or pain, and note the location of these symptoms. Palpate for masses and liver or spleen enlargement. Percuss the abdomen for shifting dullness, a sign of ascites.

Rapid intervention

The patient is at risk for shock and requires aggressive medical care and expert nursing care.

To stop the bleeding, the doctor will immediately insert a nasogastric (NG) tube and connect it to suction. He'll also use the NG tube for gastric lavage with 0.9% sodium chloride solution or water (iced or at room temperature). Accurately record the amount of fluid used for irrigation; then subtract it from the total amount of NG aspirate to assess the true amount of bleeding.

If gastric lavage doesn't control the bleeding, the doctor may insert a balloon tube (such as a Minnesota or Sengstaken-Blakemore tube) and apply pressure to the bleeding site. But recently, treatment with vasopressin has become increasingly popular. (See *Using vasopressin to treat ruptured esophageal varices*.)

Even if the patient doesn't have active bleeding, the doctor may insert an NG tube to prevent further hematemesis and allow accurate measurement of blood in vomitus.

Focus your nursing care first on ensuring and stabilizing the patient's airway, breathing, and circulation. As ordered, administer supplemental oxygen if the patient is hypoxic or in respiratory distress. If he can't breathe independently, he may need mechanical ventilation. If he experiences frequent bleeding, he may require endotracheal intubation to protect his airway.

Using vasopressin to treat ruptured esophageal varices

A posterior pituitary hormone, vasopressin is a potent vasoconstrictor that dramatically reduces mesenteric blood flow. It controls hemorrhaging by decreasing portal vein blood flow and pressure.

Vasopressin can be administered I.V. or intra-arterially; studies show that I.V. administration is equally effective, with fewer complications. Typically, I.V. vasopressin is initiated at 0.2 to 0.4 unit/minute and titrated according to patient response up to a maximum of 0.6 unit/minute.

Despite vasopressin's effectiveness, some studies show that it doesn't improve survival rates. Increasing dosages to improve survival would be risky; even in standard amounts, vasopressin can cause adverse hemodynamic reactions, including hypertension, bradycardia, electrocardiogram changes, and reduced cardiac output.

Some doctors combine vasopressin with nitroglycerin or nitroprusside to augment vasopressin's effect on portal pressure and counteract vasopressin's adverse effects, particularly reduced cardiac output. Combination therapy hasn't been extensively studied, but it seems to reduce complications and improve hemorrhage control.

Monitor the patient's blood pressure, heart rate, and respiratory rate. Initiate cardiac monitoring to check the heart rate and detect arrhythmias. Obtain noninvasive blood pressure equipment to allow blood pressure readings every 5 minutes.

Insert two or more large-bore I.V. lines to administer blood products and dextrose 5% in water or 0.9% sodium chloride solution, or both. Infuse at a rate of 250 to 500 ml/hour, as ordered, to replace volume lost through hematemesis or melena and to maintain normal vital signs.

Collect blood samples for type and crossmatch tests, complete blood count with differential, serum electrolyte levels, coagulation studies, liver function tests, and blood urea nitrogen levels. Draw an arterial sample to assess oxygenation.

❖

GI hemorrhage

Hemorrhage can occur at any place along the GI tract. Most cases involve upper GI tract bleeding. To avoid hypovolemic shock, organ failure, and brain death from massive fluid loss, the patient needs immediate treatment.

Causes
Hemorrhage of the lower GI tract may result from:
• ulcerative colitis
• diverticulosis
• fistulas
• cecal ulcers

• tumors
• angiodysplasia
• bowel infarction.
    Hemorrhage of the upper GI tract may result from:
• esophageal varices
• peptic ulcer
• prolapsed gastric mucosa
• Mallory-Weiss tear
• stress ulcer, typically in the esophagus, stomach, or duodenum, and stemming from central nervous system trauma or chronic ingestion of drugs that are toxic to the gastric mucosa (such as nonsteroidal anti-inflammatory drugs, alcohol, caffeine, nicotine, reserpine, corticosteroids, and phenylbutazone).

Assessment
Tailor your assessment to the patient's condition, postponing a detailed history until he's been stabilized. Because of the patient's pain, anxiety, or confusion, he may be unable to provide you with accurate information; but whatever his condition, assess carefully for the four stages of hemorrhage. Successful treatment hinges on your identification of the hemorrhage site (confirmed by X-ray).

History
If the patient reports nausea or vomiting, ask what seems to initiate or relieve it. Find out if he has noticed blood in his vomitus.
    Note any complaints of abdominal pressure, tenderness, or pain (which may be severe). Ask if the pain is localized and if it radiates. Have the patient describe its quality, duration, and intensity and the factors that aggravate or relieve it.
    Find out when the patient had his last meal. Has he re-

cently had any changes in taste, swallowing problems, pain after eating, weight loss, or change in bowel habits (such as frequency of bowel movements) or in the color or consistency of stools?

If the patient reports bright red or coffee-ground vomitus, suspect upper GI hemorrhage. Depending on the underlying cause, the patient may also have intense pain. Check for a history of previous bleeding or predisposing conditions, including surgery that might have contributed to GI hemorrhage.

If the patient reports lower abdominal pain and cramps or cramping pain with bowel movements, suspect lower GI hemorrhage.

Physical examination

Assess your patient for signs and symptoms of shock: weakness, pallor, tachycardia, hypotension, and an increased respiratory rate. Obtain vital signs, noting fever and rapid pulse rate.

Observe the patient's body position, and determine if position change or ambulation affects his symptoms, indicating the pain's source.

If he's vomiting, note the frequency and assess the vomitus for color, content, and odor. Inspect the patient's abdomen for guarded areas, distention, and rebound tenderness.

Physical findings vary with the underlying cause of hemorrhage and the amount of blood lost, classified in four stages:
• In *stage I* (up to 15% blood loss), compensatory mechanisms – essentially sympathetic nervous system (SNS) responses such as vasoconstriction – maintain homeostasis. The patient usually remains alert. Blood pressure remains normal, pulse rate is normal or slightly increased, and pulse quality remains strong. Respiratory rate and depth, skin color and temperature, urine output, and capillary refill time all remain normal.
• In *stage II* (up to 30% blood loss), baroreceptors detect decreased venous return and cardiac output, triggering stronger SNS response. Vasoconstriction continues to maintain adequate blood pressure, but with some difficulty. Blood shunts to vital organs, with decreased flow to intestines, kidneys, and skin.

The patient may become confused and restless. Skin turns pale, cool, and dry. Urine output decreases, possibly the first sign of hypovolemia because other signs and symptoms are still vague. Systolic pressure starts to fall; diastolic pressure may rise or fall, but it's more likely to rise (from vasoconstriction) or stay unchanged in an otherwise healthy patient with no underlying cardiovascular problem. However, orthostatic blood pressure changes may occur before systolic blood pressure changes because of hidden blood loss. Pulse pressure narrows, pulse quality weakens, respiratory rate increases, and the patient becomes tachycardic. Capillary refill time remains normal.
• In *stage III* (up to 40% blood loss), compensatory mechanisms become overtaxed. For example, vasoconstriction can no longer sustain diastolic pressure, which now begins to fall. Cardiac output and tissue perfusion continue to decrease, becoming potentially life-threatening.

Responding to GI hemorrhage

Emergency care for the patient with a GI hemorrhage focuses on preventing or halting shock and determining the source of the bleeding.
• To improve tissue perfusion and oxygenation, insert a large-bore peripheral venous catheter to replace lost fluids and infuse blood products.
• Prepare the patient for GI endoscopy or a GI X-ray to determine the source of the bleeding.
• Monitor arterial blood gas values, perform gastric lavage to arrest active bleeding, and administer drugs to inhibit gastric secretions as ordered.
• Because hemorrhage may induce arrhythmias, monitor the patient closely for hemorrhage-induced bradycardia, heart block, ventricular tachycardia, and ventricular fibrillation.
• As ordered, insert an indwelling urinary catheter to accurately measure urine output, which reflects fluid volume.
• Once the patient is stabilized and the bleeding site identified, you may need to prepare the patient for surgery, such as partial gastrectomy, bowel resection (for ruptured diverticulosis), pyloroplasty, or vagotomy.

The patient becomes more confused, restless, and anxious. Classic signs of hypovolemic shock appear: tachycardia; decreased blood pressure; tachypnea; and cool, clammy extremities. Capillary refill is delayed. Urine output continues to decrease. But even at this stage, the patient can still recover with prompt treatment.
• In *stage IV* (more than 40% blood loss), compensatory vasoconstriction becomes a complicating factor in itself, further impairing tissue perfusion and cellular oxygenation.

The patient becomes lethargic, drowsy, or stuporous. Signs of shock become more pronounced. Blood pressure continues to fall and pulse pressure narrows further (although if diastolic pressure "drops out," pulse pressure may widen). Arterial blood gas analysis reveals metabolic acidosis and respiratory alkalosis. Capillary refill is very delayed (more than 3 seconds). The patient becomes severely anuric (output below 20 ml/hour). Lack of blood flow to the brain and other vital organs ultimately leads to organ failure and death.

Rapid intervention
Immediate measures include identifying the source of hemorrhage and administering fluids and oxygen to maintain perfusion and oxygenation. (See *Responding to GI hemorrhage.*) ❖

Hepatic failure

An end stage of liver disease, hepatic failure may be acute and self-limiting or chronic and progressive. It's sometimes called hepatic coma because the patient's neurologic status gradually deteriorates. A life-threatening crisis may occur if the serum ammonia level rises, causing cerebral ammonia intoxication. In advanced stages of hepatic failure, the prognosis is poor despite vigorous treatment.

Causes

Hepatic failure can be idiopathic, but it usually arises as a complication of conditions that cause liver dysfunction, such as:
• cirrhosis
• hepatitis
• drug- or toxin-induced damage
• fatty liver
• portal hypertension or surgically created portal-systemic shunts that bypass the liver and allow toxins into the blood
• excessive protein intake (in patients with existing liver disease), which may cause cerebral ammonia intoxication by increasing serum ammonia level
• congestive heart failure or cardiomyopathy, which can decrease cardiac output, blood flow to the liver, and hepatic perfusion
• biliary obstruction.

Assessment

Your assessment of the patient with hepatic failure must include exploring underlying conditions and performing a physical examination that includes assessment for jaundice and the four stages of hepatic encephalopathy.

History

The patient may report fatigue and changes in mental status. If he's coherent at the time of admission, have him sign his name for a baseline handwriting sample. This will prove useful for later comparison because handwriting typically deteriorates as hepatic encephalopathy advances.

If the patient is incoherent, comatose, or otherwise neurologically impaired, question his family about causative conditions. Because hepatic failure is the terminal stage of liver disease, expect the history to reveal liver dysfunction. Also ask about exposure to hepatotoxic substances, and obtain a medication history.

Find out if the patient drinks alcohol; if so, determine the frequency and amount. Explore the family history for liver or biliary tract disease and for alcoholism. Obtain a dietary history and ask about recent appetite changes, indigestion, anorexia, and weight loss. Also inquire about recent changes in bowel habits, nausea, vomiting, or abdominal pain. If the patient has edema or ascites, find out when the problem first appeared.

Physical examination

Note the patient's general appearance. Liver disease usually causes jaundice, which produces icteric skin, sclerae, and oral mucosa. Also check for spider angiomas, peripheral edema, and ascites.

Obtain the patient's vital signs. Note rapid respirations,

which may result from pulmonary compression caused by liver enlargement or ascites. Hypotension and tachycardia may reflect decreased circulating blood volume from fluid shifts related to ascites.

Auscultate for abnormal bowel sounds associated with diarrhea or constipation, which commonly accompany liver disease. Palpate for right upper quadrant tenderness, hepatomegaly, and splenomegaly. Test for a fluid wave, and percuss the abdomen for shifting dullness; both are signs of ascites.

Hepatic encephalopathy. If hepatic failure has advanced to hepatic encephalopathy, assess it in four stages of progressively deteriorating levels of consciousness:
• In the prodromal stage, expect slight personality and mood changes, disorientation, forgetfulness, slurred speech, slight tremor, periods of lethargy and euphoria, inability to concentrate, and hyperactive reflexes. Sleep-wake patterns typically reverse, and handwriting ability starts to decline. Mild asterixis (flapping tremor) may appear. To elicit asterixis, ask the patient to extend his arms in front of him with hands flexed upward. Look for rapid irregular extensions and flexions of the wrists and fingers.
• In the impending stage, the patient grows more disoriented and drowsy. He may display inappropriate behavior, mood swings, agitation, and apraxia. Handwriting becomes illegible, and asterixis may become pronounced.

• In the stuporous stage, the patient becomes severely confused and may be combative, incoherent, and hard to arouse. He sleeps most of the time. You may detect hyperactive deep tendon reflexes and rigid extremities.
• In the comatose stage, the patient is comatose and doesn't react to stimuli. His pupils are dilated, and he lacks corneal and deep tendon reflexes. His extremities are flaccid, and he may assume decerebrate or decorticate posturing. The EEG is markedly abnormal.

Rapid intervention
Immediate treatment for a patient with hepatic encephalopathy focuses on reducing the serum ammonia level by hemodialysis and exchange transfusions. (These treatments offer only temporary improvement, however.)
• As ordered, administer antibiotics such as neomycin to sterilize the lower GI tract and suppress the bacterial flora that break down amino acids and produce ammonia. The doctor may also order sorbitol to induce catharsis and produce osmotic diarrhea. Administer lactulose rectally or through a nasogastric tube to reduce serum ammonia levels.
• Continually aspirate blood from the stomach, since blood, a protein, may serve as a source of amino acids contributing to the high serum ammonia level.
• Monitor the patient's vital signs every 15 minutes to 1 hour as indicated. Also monitor his electrocardiogram.
• Hemodialysis and exchange transfusions may also be used as

emergency treatments, but both have only a temporary effect. ❖

Patients in metabolic or endocrine crisis

Metabolic and endocrine crises can be difficult to identify and treat. Some are uncommon; others are so similar that telling them apart during an emergency is extremely difficult. In addition, patients may exhibit a decreased level of consciousness, signs of alcoholism, or bizarre behavioral disturbances, leading to misdiagnosis. Nevertheless, any delay in recognizing the condition may mean rapid death for your patient. This section presents the pertinent information you need to quickly identify and treat your patient.

Acute hypoglycemia

An abnormally low blood glucose level, acute hypoglycemia occurs when glucose burns up too rapidly, when the glucose release rate falls behind tissue demands, or when excessive insulin enters the bloodstream. If the blood glucose level isn't corrected immediately, the patient could experience seizures, permanent neurologic damage, or coma in addition to severe diabetic complications.

Causes

Acute hypoglycemia is caused by:
• excessive intake of insulin or oral antidiabetic medication or inadequate food intake (diabetic patients)
• delayed and excessive insulin production after carbohydrate ingestion (mildly diabetic patients)
• sharp increase in insulin output after a meal (nondiabetic patients)
• pancreatic islet cell tumor
• adrenal insufficiency.

Assessment

Your assessment of the patient with acute hypoglycemia must include a health history for previous hypoglycemic crises and a focused physical examination.

History

Find out when the patient's most recent meal or snack occurred, and how that corresponds to his intake of medication to control diabetes. The patient may report weakness, malaise, attention deficit, hunger, anxiety, headache, and visual disturbances such as blurred vision.

Physical examination

Assess for cool and clammy skin, greatly lowered blood pressure, and elevated pulse and respiratory rates. Neurologic changes may include nervousness and irritability. Also observe the patient for trembling and cold sweats.

Rapid intervention

Call for the blood glucose meter. Be sure that you have the crash cart available. You may have to ventilate your patient with a hand-held resuscitation bag if his respiratory effort diminishes.

Assess the patient's airway, and position him in the side-lying position to maintain a patent airway.

Perform a fingerstick to determine the patient's blood glucose level before giving any medications.

Normally, orange juice would be an excellent choice for hypoglycemia, but a weak patient with slow responses may aspirate it. Instead, the doctor will probably order I.V. glucose. As you're establishing I.V. access, draw blood for serum glucose and electrolyte levels and send it to the laboratory. Then begin an infusion of dextrose 5% in 0.45% sodium chloride solution, followed by 25 g of dextrose 50% by I.V. push as ordered. This solution is hypertonic, so it should be given slowly through a free-flowing I.V. line. Keep checking to ensure that the I.V. line is patent.

After 5 minutes, give another 25 g of dextrose 50% by I.V. push as ordered. If there has been a delay in starting the I.V. infusion, or if I.V. dextrose doesn't raise the patient's blood glucose level adequately, be prepared to give 0.5 to 1 mg of glucagon I.M. to stimulate the liver to convert its glycogen stores into glucose. Repeat the dose at 20-minute intervals, as ordered and needed, for two more doses.

Maintain the I.V. line, do a fingerstick each hour, and continue to monitor the patient until his blood glucose level is stable. ❖

Diabetic ketoacidosis

Also called diabetic coma, diabetic ketoacidosis (or DKA) is an acute complication of diabetes mellitus marked by pronounced hyperglycemia and ketonemia. Reflecting an insulin deficiency, it usually occurs in patients with Type I diabetes mellitus. For instance, it may arise if the patient has an illness that increases his insulin needs or if he omits or reduces his regular insulin dose. In some patients, DKA is the first manifestation of Type I diabetes mellitus.

DKA carries a mortality of 5% to 10%. Any delay in recognizing and treating the patient with DKA may lead to severe dehydration and metabolic acidosis, cerebral edema, or fatal arrhythmias (See *Responding to DKA*.)

Causes
DKA results from an absolute or relative deficiency of effective insulin. Causes of absolute insulin deficiency include:
• undiagnosed Type I diabetes mellitus
• failure to take prescribed insulin (patients with Type I diabetes mellitus).

Causes of relative insulin deficiency include:
• surgery
• stress resulting from infection
• urosepsis
• upper respiratory tract infection
• pneumonia
• trauma
• myocardial infarction
• perirectal abscess
• periodontal abscess

Responding to DKA

To combat dehydration in diabetic ketoacidosis (DKA), you'll administer fluids, electrolytes, and insulin as ordered.

Fluid replacement
Initial volume expansion lowers the patient's serum glucose level on its own, even without insulin administration. Usually, you'll give 0.9% sodium chloride solution or 0.45% sodium chloride solution at 1 liter/hour until the patient's blood pressure stabilizes and his urine output measures 60 ml/hour. Typically, this takes 1 to 2 hours.

Electrolyte replacement
Because osmotic diuresis in DKA causes total body potassium depletion, you'll administer potassium replacements simultaneously with fluids (except in patients with anuria or life-threatening hyperkalemia). (Note that insulin administration also reduces the serum potassium level by stimulating potassium uptake by adipose, muscle, and liver tissue.)

Bicarbonate administration is reserved for patients with severe acidosis (a pH below 7.1).

Insulin administration
Expect the doctor to order I.V. regular insulin to reverse hyperglycemia and acidosis. (Note that absorption of insulin by I.M. or S.C. routes can be erratic.) Typically, the doctor orders a continuous insulin infusion—usually 100 units of regular insulin I.V. in 500 ml of 0.9% sodium chloride solution, in a concentration of 0.2 unit/ml. Before initiating the infusion, allow 50 to 100 ml of the mixture to run through the tubing, and then discard this amount. This allows the tubing to absorb the insulin, limiting absorption during infusion.

Using an infusion pump, administer insulin at 0.1 unit/kg/hour initially. Keep in mind that the goal is to lower the serum glucose level by 80 to 100 mg/dl/hour. (When administered I.V., insulin quickly reaches a steady state in the bloodstream, eliminating the need for an initial bolus dose.)

Adjust the infusion rate according to your patient's hourly blood glucose levels, as determined by the laboratory or a portable blood glucose meter. If you're using a portable meter, check the manufacturer's guidelines to verify whether it can be used in patients with severe volume depletion, dehydration, hypovolemic shock, and extremes in hematocrit.

ACUTELY ILL PATIENTS

• Cushing's syndrome, thyrotoxicosis, acromegaly, or pheochromocytoma (less common).

Assessment

Your assessment of the patient with DKA must include a thorough health history and a multisystem physical examination seeking to gauge the degree of dehydration.

History

Because the patient's mental status may be impaired, you may need to obtain the health history from a family member. Ask how the patient was found and in what circumstances. Find out whether he has had similar symptoms before and, if so, what the outcome was. To help establish the severity of dehydration, ask about recent food or fluid intake.

Expect a history of increased fatigue, lethargy, dry mouth, and increased thirst and urination over the past few hours or days. The patient may also have had flulike symptoms, such as abdominal discomfort, nausea or vomiting, and generalized myalgia. As his condition worsened, he may have exhibited deep, rapid, sighing (Kussmaul's) respirations.

Find out if the patient had a recent illness or infection, such as a cold, upper respiratory tract infection, urinary tract infection, sore throat, or GI disturbance.

If he was previously diagnosed with diabetes mellitus, ask about his current insulin dosage and find out if he recently made changes in his regimen.

Physical examination

The patient with DKA will seem acutely ill and severely dehydrated. Assess for signs of dehydration: dry mucous membranes; warm, dry, flushed skin; and poor skin turgor.

Perform a complete neurologic assessment, evaluate reflexes, and check for muscle weakness and headache. Expect an altered level of consciousness ranging from confusion to coma.

Check for classic signs of DKA—acetone (fruity) breath odor and Kussmaul's respirations—to help rule out insulin shock.

Measure the patient's blood pressure, and suspect intravascular volume depletion if his systolic pressure drops 20 mm Hg when he moves from a supine to a sitting or standing position. Also assess neck vein filling, which will probably be reduced from dehydration.

Assess the patient's abdomen, listening closely for diminished or absent bowel sounds. Note abdominal tenderness, guarding, or rebound tenderness on palpation. These signs and symptoms probably stem from ketosis and usually resolve as the patient's biochemical status improves.

Rapid interventions

The patient with DKA has a life-threatening volume depletion—a fluid volume deficit of up to 10 liters. Be prepared to replace fluids and electrolytes rapidly. You'll also need to administer insulin.

❖

Adrenal crisis

Adrenal crisis (also called addisonian crisis or acute adrenal insufficiency) is the rapid and severe onset of adrenal hypofunction or insufficiency. The patient experiences metabolic and endocrine imbalances (hyponatremia, hypoglycemia, and hyperkalemia) and a precipitous drop in blood pressure and fluid volume.

Adrenal crisis is the most serious complication of adrenal insufficiency and is fatal if left untreated.

Causes

Adrenal crisis is typically caused by:
• unresponsiveness to hormone replacement therapy
• pronounced stress (such as from infection, trauma, or surgery) without sufficient glucocorticoid replacement
• abrupt withdrawal of glucocorticoid replacement in patients receiving high or chronic doses
• adrenal tumor
• burns
• hemorrhage associated with anticoagulant therapy
• hypermetabolic states
• bilateral adrenalectomy
• sudden cessation of antineoplastic therapy
• hypopituitarism
• hypothalamic suppression
• destruction of the adrenal cortex, as in Addison's disease.

Assessment

Your assessment of the patient in adrenal crisis must include a health history focusing on recent therapy and stress, and a physical examination that includes dehydration and hyperpigmentation.

History

Find out if the patient has a history of adrenal insufficiency, has been receiving steroid therapy, has undergone adrenal surgery, has recently had an infection, or has suffered pronounced physical or emotional stress. Obtain a medication history and ask if the patient has complied with his drug regimen.

Note any recent history of nausea, vomiting, diarrhea, abdominal pain, anxiety, irritability, fatigue, anorexia, muscle cramps, excessive thirst, headache, fever, or progressive muscle weakness. These symptoms reflect hyponatremia, hyperkalemia, and hypoglycemia from adrenal crisis. Also ask about reduced urine output, which reflects hypovolemia.

Physical examination

Measure the patient's vital signs, which may reveal an elevated temperature. Monitor for signs of shock, such as low blood pressure, weak and irregular pulse, and increased respiratory rate. Check for signs of dehydration (such as dry skin and mucous membranes), flaccid extremities, lethargy, confusion, restlessness, or a progressively diminishing level of consciousness.

If the patient has chronic adrenal insufficiency, inspect for a bronze coloration similar to a deep suntan on his elbows, knees, and knuckles and possibly on his lips, buccal mucosa, and scars. Vitiligo (depigmented skin patches) or abnormal hyperpigmentation may be evident, a result of excessive secretion of melanocyte-stimulating hormone and corticotropin (an effect of reduced cortisol secretion).

Rapid intervention

Emergency treatment for the patient in adrenal crisis focuses on reversing shock, replacing fluids, and replacing cortisol.

As soon as blood is drawn for laboratory studies, anticipate the doctor to order up to 3 liters dextrose 5% in 0.9% sodium chloride solution for rapid fluid replacement—usually given over the first few hours. He'll order diagnostic tests—cultures, abdominal magnetic resonance imaging scans, or skin tests—to investigate the underlying cause.

As ordered, replace cortisol by administering 100 mg of hydrocortisone I.V. As needed and ordered, administer plasma, oxygen, and short-term vasopressors. If the patient has an infection, give antibiotics as ordered.

Most of the metabolic and electrolyte abnormalities that accompany adrenal crisis resolve without further treatment. Because high-dose cortisol therapy has a mineralocorticoid effect, the patient probably won't need aldosterone replacement.

❖

Thyroid storm

Thyroid storm (thyrotoxic crisis) is an acute form of severe hyperthyroidism marked by sudden and excessive release of thyroid hormones into the bloodstream. Without immediate intervention, the patient may suffer heart failure, shock, hyperthermia, fatal arrhythmias, delirium, and coma. Mortality from thyroid storm is roughly 20%.

Causes

Thyroid storm is triggered by:
• stressful conditions (most common), such as trauma, surgery, infection, or emotional distress
• myocardial infarction
• pulmonary embolism
• abrupt withdrawal of antithyroid agents
• therapy with radioiodine (^{131}I) or an iodine-containing agent
• preeclampsia
• thyroid tumor
• subtotal thyroidectomy with excessive intake of synthetic thyroid hormone.

Assessment

Your expert assessment of the classic symptoms of hyperthyroidism could save the patient's life.

History

The patient's history may reveal an abrupt onset of symptoms after a typical precipitating event such as physical stress. Check for a family history of hyperthyroidism (Graves' disease), a common finding. The patient or an accompanying family member may report such classic symptoms as nervousness, heat intolerance, weight loss despite increased appetite, excessive sweating, diarrhea, tremors, and palpitations.

Physical examination

Measure the patient's vital signs and check for characteristic cardiovascular, GI, and sympathetic hypermetabolic activity, such as hyperpyrexia rising as high as 106° F (41.1° C). An obvious sign of hypermetabolism is tachyarrhythmia starting at 130 beats/minute and increasing to 300 beats/minute. Additional signs and symptoms that may bring on vascular collapse include angina, palpitations, respiratory distress, and atrial fibrillation.

Assess for hypermetabolic GI activity, such as nausea, vomiting, and diarrhea, possibly causing dehydration and hypovolemia. Hypermetabolic sympathetic activity may produce fine tremors, agitation, and restlessness progressing to manic or psychotic behavior.

Rapid intervention
Your treatment priorities are maintaining the patient's airway and ensuring tissue oxygenation, reversing hypovolemia, preventing further hypermetabolic decompensation, and decreasing thyroid hyperfunction.

Maintaining oxygenation
Administer oxygen via nasal cannula or mask, assess the patient's respiratory rate every 1 to 2 hours, and auscultate the lungs every 1 to 2 hours. Note tachypnea, dyspnea, pallor, or cyanosis. Provide chest physiotherapy, suctioning, and mechanical ventilation as needed.

Ensure that the patient is in a position that facilitates respiration, and turn him occasionally from side to side. Check his oxygenation status periodically by monitoring pulse oximetry or arterial blood gas values. (To prevent hypovolemia, the doctor will avoid sedatives or use them cautiously.)

Reversing hypovolemia
As ordered, give I.V. fluid replacement containing dextrose to reverse hypovolemia and prevent further glycogen depletion.

Reducing hypermetabolic decompensation
To lower the patient's body temperature, keep him cool with ice, fans, hypothermia blankets, and antipyretics. Give only non-aspirin-containing antipyretics, such as acetaminophen, to lower body temperature. (Aspirin further displaces thyroid hormones, worsening the hypermetabolic state.)

The doctor may order a beta-adrenergic blocker to reduce sympathetic nervous system activity and relieve arrhythmias; propranolol I.V. is preferred because it blocks further thyroid activity. The doctor may also place the patient on digoxin and diuretics to prevent or treat cardiac failure. If the patient is in shock or has adrenal insufficiency, the doctor may initiate hydrocortisone therapy.

Decreasing thyroid hyperfunction
Expect to give an antithyroid agent, as ordered, to halt the production of triiodothyronine and thyroxine. You'll probably give propylthiouracil or methimazole orally or by nasogastric tube, followed by an iodine preparation to prevent release of stored thyroid hormones. Give the iodine preparation 1 to 3 hours after the antithyroid agent to minimize hormone formation from the iodine. ❖

Syndrome of inappropriate antidiuretic hormone

The syndrome of inappropriate antidiuretic hormone, commonly known as SIADH, reflects excessive amounts of antidiuretic hormone (ADH). Secreted by the posterior pituitary gland, ADH acts as an antidiuretic and elevates blood pressure. Too much ADH seriously disrupts fluid and electrolyte balance and leads to increased water retention, greater extracellular fluid volume, hyponatremia, and cessation of urine output. SIADH calls for prompt treatment to avert seizures and death.

Causes

SIADH may result from:
• ectopic ADH release by a cancerous tumor, such as oat-cell lung carcinoma, thymomas, GI tumors, and lymphoid tumors
• autonomous ADH release by the lungs, such as in tuberculosis, viral pneumonia, chronic obstructive pulmonary disease, and lung abscess
• ADH release from the neurohypophysis secondary to neighboring inflammatory, neoplastic, or vascular lesions
• ADH release from the neurohypophysis secondary to drugs, such as acetaminophen, vincristine, clofibrate, tolbutamide, thiazide diuretics, cyclophosphamide, haloperidol, carbamazepine, nicotine, barbiturates, analgesics (such as morphine), antineoplastic drugs, anesthetics, or tricyclic antidepressants
• ADH release secondary to central nervous system disorders, such as brain tumor, head trauma, subdural hematoma, cardiovascular accident, pituitary adenoma, brain abscess, meningitis, encephalitis, cerebral atrophy, acute encephalopathy, acute psychosis, or Guillain-Barré syndrome
• other disorders, conditions, and procedures, such as lupus erythematosus, emotional stress, pain, and positive-pressure mechanical ventilation.

Assessment

Your assessment of the patient with SIADH must include a thorough causal health history and a physical examination of the potentially delirious patient.

History

A patient in the initial phase of SIADH may complain of headache, abdominal discomfort, nausea, and malaise. Sometimes nausea, vomiting, and weight gain (with or without edema) are the only initial signs and symptoms.

Try to determine if the patient has any risk factors for SIADH. If SIADH is severe, he may be unable to answer questions, so you'll need to interview family members. Check for any history of causative disorders or drugs.

Physical examiniation

Physical findings depend on the severity of water retention and hyponatremia. The patient with a serum sodium level of 125 mEq/liter or more usually is asymptomatic or complains only of mild GI discomfort. With acute hyponatremia (a serum sodium level below 125 mEq/liter), expect seizures and signs of diffuse cerebral edema, such as irritability, personality changes, and an altered level of consciousness ranging from disorientation and confusion to coma.

Measure the patient's heart rate and blood pressure, and check for signs of altered fluid and electrolyte status. However, be aware that edema is rare, despite weight gain, because the hypotonicity of extracellular fluid causes intracellular swelling.

Rapid intervention
Your priority is to restore normal serum osmolality without further expanding extracellular fluid volume. If the patient has severe hyponatremia, expect to infuse 200 to 300 ml I.V. hypertonic 0.9% sodium chloride solution over several hours until cerebral symptoms improve or the serum sodium level rises above 125 mEq/liter. However, use extreme caution when administering this solution because fluid overload may precipitate heart failure or circulatory collapse. If the patient has mild hyponatremia, fluid restriction may be the main treatment. I.V. furosemide will also usually be infused.

Other treatments focus on eliminating the underlying cause of SIADH: discontinuing a drug, eliminating an infection with antibiotics, treating adrenal insufficiency with corticosteroids, or cancer therapy. Carefully monitor the patient's blood urea nitrogen and creatinine levels, place the patient on seizure precautions, and perform frequent neurologic checks.

❖

Patients in systemic crisis

Systemic crisis is the progressive failure of several body systems in response to critical injury or illness. It can rapidly progress to irreversible damage and death, and you'll need to provide intensive nursing care to save the patient's life. (See *Nursing interventions for multisystem organ failure*, pages 232 to 235.)

Multisystem organ failure

Multisystem organ failure occurs when certain conditions cause injury that leads to stimulation of the sympathetic nervous system, damage to the endothelial lining of blood vessels, and an activation of the inflammatory response. These events trigger the release of tumor necrosis factor, interleukin-1, and other inflammatory mediators into the bloodstream and tissues. Normally, mediators help the body withstand and recover from an injury. But after massive injury, their responses may go unchecked, with potentially disastrous consequences.

The number of failing organs seems to correlate directly with the prognosis. Single-organ failure carries a mortality rate of 25% to 30%; two-organ failure, 50% to 60%; and three-organ failure, 75% to 85%. Failure of four or more organs is 100% fatal. In multisystem organ failure, prevention is paramount.

(Text continues on page 236.)

Nursing interventions for multisystem organ failure

Based on your assessment of the patient with multisystem organ failure, you'll develop specific nursing diagnoses and carry out appropriate nursing interventions.

Nursing diagnosis

Impaired gas exchange related to atelectasis, secretions, pulmonary edema, pulmonary microthrombi, and vasoconstriction

Assessment findings

- Pulmonary infiltrates on chest X-ray
- pH less than 7.35 or more than 7.45
- Partial pressure of arterial carbon dioxide less than 35 mm Hg or more than 45 mm Hg
- Partial pressure of arterial oxygen less than 10% of baseline
- Respiratory rate less than 12 breaths/minute or more than 20 breaths/minute
- Dyspnea; crackles; wheezes; thick, blood-tinged or color-tinged sputum

Nursing interventions

- Maintain a patent airway and keep the head of the bed at a 15- to 45-degree angle.
- Auscultate for breath sounds every 2 hours and as needed.
- Assess respiratory rate, depth, and rhythm every 2 hours and as needed.
- To help clear pulmonary secretions, turn the patient, encourage him to breathe deeply every 2 hours, and suction him as needed. (Placing the patient with an in-

jured or congested lung facing upward promotes ventilation-perfusion matching in the healthier lung.)

- After suctioning, document the amount, color, character, and odor of pulmonary secretions.
- Keep the patient well hydrated to enhance secretion removal.
- Administer supplemental oxygen as ordered.
- If the patient is on a mechanical ventilator, monitor ventilator settings: fraction of inspired oxygen, mode, tidal volume, and rate. Also monitor respiratory parameters: peak inspiratory pressure, compliance, and exhaled tidal volume.
- Administer antibiotics as ordered.
- Observe for adverse cardiopulmonary effects, such as respiratory distress, shallow respirations, decreased blood pressure, and tachycardia.

Nursing diagnosis

Decreased cardiac output related to decreased circulating volume, myocardial depression, and ventricular dysfunction

Assessment findings

- Cardiac output less than 4 liters/minute or inadequate to meet oxygen demands

Nursing interventions for multisystem organ failure (continued)

Assessment findings (continued)
• Cardiac index (CI) less than 2.5 liters/minute/m²
• Blood pressure 20 mm Hg or more below baseline
• Heart rate more than 100 beats/minute
• Capillary refill time more than 3 seconds
• Urine output less than 0.5 ml/kg/hour
• Decreased level of consciousness (LOC), weak pulses, cool skin
• Systemic vascular resistance (SVR) greater than 1,400 dynes/sec/cm⁻⁵ (usually) or less than 800 dynes/sec/cm⁻⁵ (when multisystem organ failure is associated with septic shock)
• Pulmonary artery wedge pressure (PAWP) more than 18 mm Hg

Nursing interventions
• Monitor heart rate and rhythm continuously.
• Take vital signs hourly.
• Obtain values for pulmonary artery pressure (PAP), PAWP, cardiac output, CI, SVR, and pulmonary vascular resistance every 2 to 4 hours.
• Administer I.V. fluids by infusion pump as ordered. Monitor for signs and symptoms of fluid overload: PAWP greater than 18 mm Hg, crackles, edema, weight gain, dyspnea, and pink frothy sputum.

• Administer vasoactive and inotropic drugs as ordered.
• Document fluid intake and output accurately.
• Administer sodium bicarbonate, as ordered, to treat acidosis, which can cause myocardial depression.
• Because "normal" cardiac output may still be inadequate to meet tissue oxygen demands, administer fluid and inotropic agents, as ordered, to drive cardiac output above usual normal values.

Nursing diagnosis
Altered tissue perfusion related to decreased circulating volume, microthrombi, reduced cardiac output, maldistribution of circulating volume, and altered cellular function.

Assessment findings
• Poor gas exchange (see assessment findings of *Impaired gas exchange*)
• Decreased bowel sounds, abdominal distention, diarrhea, upper and lower GI bleeding
• Urine output less than 0.5 ml/kg/hour
• Increased blood urea nitrogen, creatinine, potassium, and magnesium levels
• Decreased LOC, cardiac output, heart rate, and blood pressure
• Increased PAWP

(continued)

ACUTELY ILL
PATIENTS

Nursing interventions for multisystem organ failure (continued)

Assessment findings (continued)
• Increased liver enzyme levels
• Albumin level less than 4 g/dl
• pH less than 7.35

Nursing interventions
• To assess organ perfusion, monitor cardiac rhythm and blood pressure continuously; evaluate LOC hourly; obtain values for PAP, PAWP, and cardiac output every 4 hours and as needed; measure urine output hourly; auscultate for bowel sounds every 4 hours; test nasogastric aspirate every 4 hours; test all stools for blood; monitor pulses for regularity, amplitude, and rate; and check skin for temperature, color, dryness, and turgor.
• Enhance gas exchange and cardiac output by suctioning excess secretions as needed and providing hyperoxygenation before suctioning to minimize desaturation. Assess for respiratory failure and prepare for intubation, if appropriate. Have the patient cough and deep breathe every 4 hours and as needed.
• Administer antiarrhythmic drugs and monitor for any adverse effects.
• Provide support for individual organ systems — for example, with mechanical ventilation, hemodialysis, or vasoactive drugs.

• Administer sucralfate, antacids, and histamine₂ blockers, as ordered, to reduce the risk of stress ulcers.
• Continuously monitor mixed venous oxygen saturation to assess whether oxygen delivery matches tissue oxygen demands.

Nursing diagnosis
High risk for infection and superinfection related to invasive line and procedures, altered host defenses, and prolonged antibiotic therapy

Assessment findings
• White blood cell (WBC) count higher than 10,000/mm³
• Temperature higher than 98.6° F (37° C)
• Heart rate more than 100 beats/minute
• Glucose level higher than 110 mg/dl
• Cloudy urine
• Crackles; wheezes; thick, colored pulmonary secretions
• Purulent exudate from I.V. sites or wounds
• Oral or vaginal candidiasis

Nursing interventions
• Wash your hands frequently.
• Monitor temperature every 1 to 2 hours or continuously, using a rectal probe or a pulmonary artery catheter.
• Secure the artificial airway

Nursing interventions for multisystem organ failure (continued)

Nursing interventions
(continued)
to prevent aspiration and enhance oxygen delivery.
• Provide frequent oral care to reduce the patient's risk of aspirating contaminated oropharyngeal secretions.
• Use strict aseptic technique during placement and care of I.V. lines and urinary catheters.
• Assess all catheter insertion sites and wounds daily for edema, erythema, warmth, pain, and drainage.
• Monitor oral mucous membranes daily for candidiasis and other superinfections.
• Monitor results of WBC count, chest X-ray, and glucose testing daily.
• Observe urine, sputum, and wound drainage for changes in color and character.
• Remove all potential contaminants from the area—for example, cut flowers, soil, and standing water.

Nursing diagnosis
Altered nutrition (less than body requirements) related to lack of nutritional support, hypermetabolism, diarrhea, and altered GI function

Assessment findings
• Weight loss
• Muscle atrophy
• Total serum protein level less than 6 g/dl
• Negative nitrogen balance
• Absent bowel sounds
• Electrolyte imbalances

Nursing interventions
• Arrange for a nutritional support consultation within 24 hours of admission.
• Administer nutritional supplements enterally if possible. If total parenteral nutrition (TPN) is necessary, check solution, rate, and additives for accuracy.
• Provide meticulous tube, line, and I.V. site care. Both enteral and parenteral feeding increase infection risks.
• Assess bowel sounds and check for abdominal distention every 4 hours.
• Record the patient's weight at the same time each day.
• Monitor electrolyte levels, glucose level, and laboratory values indicating nutritional status (such as total lymphocyte count, albumin level, and transferrin level) every 4 to 8 hours or as ordered.
• Send a 24-hour urine specimen for urea nitrogen and nitrogen balance assessment once or twice a week.
• Monitor for complications of enteral feeding: aspiration, abdominal distention, tube dislodgment, diarrhea, and fluid and electrolyte imbalances.
• Monitor for complications of TPN: catheter sepsis, hyperglycemia, infiltration, and fluid and electrolyte imbalances.

ACUTELY ILL
PATIENTS

Causes

Multisystem organ failure may be triggered by:
• burns
• multiple trauma
• myocardial infarction
• cancer
• shock
• massive blood transfusion
• infection
• endotoxinemia.

Assessment

Your assessment of the patient at risk for multisystem organ failure must include a causative health history, and a thorough and ongoing physical examination.

History

Confirm any underlying medical problems and current medications, including allergies to medications. The patient may report a history of chronic pulmonary, cardiac, hematologic, or renal disease; recent onset of an infection, such as pneumonia or cholecystitis; or cancer.

Physical examination

The goal of your examination is to prevent multisystem organ failure from developing in the critically ill patient, especially in the patient with hypoperfusion and overwhelming inflammation, two factors which set the stage for multisystem organ failure. And your continuing assessment is vital to this goal. Monitor all body systems closely for signs and symptoms of cardiovascular instability, poor organ perfusion, and inflammatory or infectious complications.

However, be aware that any patient with multisystem organ failure can present a contradic-tory picture. The clinical manifestations of multisystem organ failure vary with the length of time that organ dysfunction continues. For example, in the early stages, respiratory rate, cardiac output, and temperature usually increase. As the process continues, they all may decrease. Also, the patient may be the victim of normal physiologic processes gone awry; responses designed to promote recovery could actually worsen his condition.

Rapid intervention

Your care of the patient with multisystem organ failure will vary with the assessment findings and nursing diagnosis.   ❖

Anaphylactic shock

An acute, systemic allergic reaction, anaphylactic shock (anaphylaxis) is characterized by immediate vascular and bronchial changes that cause profound hypovolemia and severe respiratory distress. To avert death, the patient needs immediate attention.

Causes

Anaphylactic shock results from an extreme hypersensitivity reaction to a foreign antigen, including:
• exposure to a substance to which the patient is highly sensitive
• antibiotics — most commonly, penicillin and its analogues, aminoglycosides, cephalosporins, sulfonamides, tetracycline, and vancomycin

• local anesthetics, including bupivacaine, lidocaine, procaine, and tetracaine
• chemotherapeutic drugs, including doxorubicin, bleomycin, cisplatin, cyclophosphamide, asparaginase, and melphalan
• other drugs, including corticotropin, aspirin, codeine, dextran, diuretics, histamine, meprobamate, and morphine
• diagnostic agents, such as sulfobromophthalein sodium dye, dehydrocholic acid, iodinated radiographic contrast media, and iopanoic acid
• mismatched blood products and antisera, such as cryoprecipitate, fresh frozen plasma, gamma globulin, packed red blood cells, and whole blood
• venom from bees, hornets, jellyfish, snakes, spiders, and wasps
• certain foods, including chocolate, eggs, grains, milk, nuts, seafood, shellfish, strawberries, and tomatoes
• immunotherapy.

Assessment
Your assessment of the patient in anaphylactic shock must include a rapid health history for substances ingested and exposure to venom, and a physical examination that includes assessing for wheals.

History
Quickly try to determine the cause of the anaphylactic reaction – but don't waste precious moments. Ask the patient, if possible, or his family what substances he's ingested or been exposed to recently. Find out if the patient previously reacted to the substance in question and, if so, to what degree.

At the onset of the reaction, the patient may report uneasiness, fear, or a feeling of impending doom. He may say he feels a lump in his throat, followed by hoarseness, coughing, sneezing, dyspnea, chest tightness, and stridor. He may complain of weakness, disorientation, flushing, diaphoresis, or feeling hot all over.

Physical examination
On inspection, you may note warm, flushed skin and detect circumscribed, discrete cutaneous wheals with erythematous, raised, serpiginous borders and blanched centers. The wheals may progress to diffuse erythema, then to generalized urticaria and angioedema, especially of the eyelids, lips, and tongue.

Inspect for a swollen uvula, vocal cords, and posterior pharynx. On auscultation, you may hear diffuse wheezes and prolonged expirations; these sounds, brought on by upper and lower airway obstruction from laryngeal edema, may signal respiratory failure.

Also assess for cardiovascular problems resulting from greatly decreased plasma volume caused by vasodilation and intravascular fluid leakage into the interstitial space. Expect hypotension and myocardial ischemia, possibly leading to myocardial depression, ventricular arrhythmias, and even myocardial infarction.

Note such neurologic signs and symptoms as dizziness, drowsiness, headache, restlessness, and seizures. Metabolic abnormalities may include signs and symptoms of lactic acidosis: lethargy, confusion, stupor, and other changes in level of consciousness; Kussmaul's respirations; cold, clammy skin that becomes warm and dry; arrhythmias; diminished muscle tone; and exaggerated deep-tendon reflexes.

Evaluate the patient for GI problems, although these are relatively rare in anaphylaxis.

Rapid intervention

First assess the patient's respiratory status. If he has a respiratory obstruction, administer oxygen as ordered until an endotracheal tube can be inserted. If laryngeal edema has closed off his airway, call for assistance, have someone notify the doctor, and be prepared to assist with an emergency tracheotomy.

If the patient was stung by an insect or just had an injection, wrap a tourniquet or blood pressure cuff above the affected site to obstruct venous return. If he's receiving blood or a medication I.V., stop the infusion immediately—it's the likely cause of the reaction.

In the early stages of anaphylaxis, you'll give epinephrine I.M. or S.C.; in severe reactions, when the patient is unconscious and hypotensive, give epinephrine I.V. Administer other drugs as ordered. Epinephrine is the drug of choice for acute anaphylaxis because it promptly reverses such life-threatening conditions as bronchoconstriction and hypotension. However, when administering this drug, stay alert for such adverse effects as tachycardia, hypertension, dyspnea, and electrocardiogram changes.

Expect to administer volume expanders, such as 0.9% sodium chloride solution or lactated Ringer's solution to restore fluid volume, increase blood pressure and cardiac output, and reverse lactic acidosis.

If cardiac arrest occurs, begin cardiopulmonary resuscitation. Watch for hypotension and shock.

❖

Septic shock

Septic shock refers to a state of impaired cellular function, decreased systemic vascular resistance, and increased cardiac output that occurs secondary to septicemia. Signifying failure of the body's defense mechanisms, it results in activated coagulation, cell injury, metabolic changes, and altered blood flow through the microcirculation.

Nearly 500,000 patients annually go into septic shock, and mortality is close to 25%. To ensure early detection and intervention, you must be familiar with its pathophysiology and clinical signs.

Causes

Septic shock usually occurs as a complication of another disorder or of an invasive procedure that allows entry of a pathogenic microorganism into the bloodstream. The microorganism produces septicemia in the already compromised patient. In about 66% of cases, the microorganism is a gram-negative bacteria, such as *Escherichia coli*, *Klebsiella*, *Serratia*, *Enterobacter*, or *Pseudomonas*. Under 3% of cases result from opportunistic fungi, mycobacteria, viruses, or protozoa.

Patients at high risk include neonates and elderly patients as well as patients with burns; traumatic wounds; recent surgery or invasive diagnostic or therapeutic procedures; invasive lines or indwelling urinary catheters; chronic cardiac, hepatic, or renal disorders; diabetes mellitus; immunosuppression; malnutrition; stress; and excessive use of antibiotics.

Assessment

Your assessment of the patient in septic shock must include a health history for causative procedures or conditions and a physical examination that includes differentiating between signs and symptoms of the two types of septic shock—hyperdynamic and hypodynamic.

History

Ask about any disorder or treatment capable of causing immunosuppression or sepsis, such as chemotherapy. Further inquire about recent invasive tests, treatments, surgery, or trauma.

At the onset of septic shock, the patient may report fever and chills; roughly 20% of patients are hypothermic.

Physical examination

Signs and symptoms vary with the hemodynamic pattern of septic shock. (See *Distinguishing between hyperdynamic and hypodynamic septic shock*, pages 240 to 242.) The *hyperdynamic* type of septic shock occurs most often in young, predominantly healthy individuals, such as one who develops sepsis after an appendectomy. It can progress to hypodynamic septic shock.

Hypodynamic septic shock occurs in individuals who have hypovolemia at the onset of septic shock. Its signs and symptoms are those of late shock. Your astute assessment can detect septic shock early and dramatically increase the patient's survival odds.

One of the earliest signs of sepsis is a change in the patient's level of consciousness. Other signs and symptoms depend on the type of shock. In hyperdynamic septic shock, expect signs and symptoms of increased cardiac output, peripheral vasodilation, decreased systemic vascular resistance, normal urine output, and warm, dry extremities.

In hypodynamic septic shock, expect signs and symptoms of decreased cardiac output, peripheral vasoconstriction, increased systemic vascular resistance, inadequate tissue perfusion, decreased urine output, and cold, cyanotic extremities.

Rapid intervention

Locating and eliminating the source of sepsis is essential. First, remove any I.V., intra-arterial, or urinary catheters and send them to the laboratory to help identify the sepsis-causing organism. Then you'll focus on maintaining the patient's oxygenation, increasing his intravascular volume by I.V. infusion, and initiating antimicrobial therapy.

Oxygen therapy

Initiate oxygen therapy, as ordered, to maintain arterial oxygen saturation above 95%. If respiratory failure occurs, the patient may need mechanical ven-

(Text continues on page 242.)

Distinguishing between hyperdynamic and hypodynamic septic shock

In hyperdynamic septic shock, vascular resistance decreases while cardiac output and stroke volume increase. Close assessment and prompt intervention can halt the progression of hypodynamic shock—even coma. Use this chart as an assessment guide.

BODY SYSTEM	FINDINGS IN HYPERDYNAMIC SHOCK	FINDINGS IN HYPODYNAMIC SHOCK
Cardiovascular		
• Assess and document pulse rate and blood pressure.	• Tachycardia, normal mean arterial blood pressure, widening pulse pressure	• Tachycardia, severe hypotension
• Assess peripheral pulses.	• Bounding	• Weak, thready
• Assess capillary refill time.	• Normal	• Prolonged
• Monitor cardiac output.	• Normal or increased above baseline	• Greatly decreased
GI		
• Check for ascites, abdominal masses, and occult blood in stools.	• Normal	• Abdominal pain
• Ask about recent changes in bowel habits.	• Constipation or diarrhea	• Constipation or diarrhea
• Auscultate for bowel sounds in all four quadrants.	• Bowel sounds present	• No bowel sounds

Distinguishing between hyperdynamic and hypodynamic septic shock *(continued)*

BODY SYSTEM	FINDINGS IN HYPERDYNAMIC SHOCK	FINDINGS IN HYPODYNAMIC SHOCK
Genitourinary		
• Assess for complaints of urinary burning or frequency or decreased urine output.	• Normal or below normal urine output	• Oliguria
• Check hourly intake and output.	• Normal or below normal urine output	• Below normal output (possibly below 25 ml/hour)
• Measure specific gravity once every shift.	• Normal specific gravity	• Increased specific gravity
• Weigh patient daily.	• Normal or increased weight	• Normal or increased weight
• Monitor blood urea nitrogen and serum creatinine levels.	• Increased levels	• Increased levels
• Check for glucose in urine.	• Glucose in urine	• Glucose in urine
Neurologic		
• Assess mental status and level of consciousness.	• Mild irritability, lethargy, slight restlessness, disorientation, inappropriate euphoria	• Extreme irritability, restlessness, confusion
• Take oral temperature.	• Normal, below normal, or elevated	• Below normal or elevated
Respiratory		
• Assess respiratory rate, rhythm, and effort.	• Tachypnea, hyperventilation	• Rapid, shallow breathing; respiratory distress
• Percuss and auscultate lungs, noting adventitious sounds.	• Crackles, decreased breath sounds	• Rhonchi, decreased breath sounds
• Obtain arterial blood gas values	• Respiratory alkalosis	• Respiratory alkalosis

(continued)

Distinguishing between hyperdynamic and hypodynamic septic shock (continued)

BODY SYSTEM	FINDINGS IN HYPERDYNAMIC SHOCK	FINDINGS IN HYPODYNAMIC SHOCK
Skin		
• Inspect and palpate skin; note its color, turgor, vascularity, moisture, temperature, texture, thickness, and mobility.	• Warm, dry, flushed skin; peripheral edema	• Cold and clammy skin • Peripheral mottling
• Observe for stomatitis or mucositis.	• Dry mouth	• Inflammation

tilation. Monitor the patient's blood pressure and pulse closely; any drop in blood pressure accompanied by a thready pulse may signal inadequate cardiac output.

I.V. infusion

Start an I.V. infusion with 0.9% sodium chloride solution or lactated Ringer's solution. Use a large-bore (14G to 18G) catheter to ease later administration of blood transfusions. Anticipate an order for colloid or crystalloid infusions to increase intravascular volume and raise blood pressure.

After sufficient fluid volume replacement, anticipate an order for a diuretic (such as furosemide) to maintain urine output above 25 ml/hour. If fluid replacement fails to increase the patient's blood pressure, give a vasopressor, such as dopamine, if ordered.

Antimicrobial therapy

As ordered, begin aggressive antimicrobial therapy for the causative organism, as determined by culture and sensitivity testing. In a patient with immunosuppression secondary to drug therapy, discontinue or reduce the dosage of the offending drug. The doctor may order granulocyte transfusions if the patient has severe neutropenia. ❖

5 Managing Medication Administration Problems

Subcutaneous medications

Intramuscular medications

Peripheral I.V. therapy

Blood transfusions

Central venous therapy

Parenteral nutrition

Patient-controlled analgesia

DRUG DIFFICULTIES

Safe drug administration

Regardless of your nursing specialty, you must be able to administer drugs safely and effectively. To do so, you need familiarity not only with drug names, indications, and dosages but also with drug interactions, alternate routes of administration, methods for avoiding injury during administration, and ways to overcome or prevent characteristic problems during therapy. This responsibility no doubt gives rise to numerous questions. You'll find many of them answered in this chapter.

How can I prevent drug interactions?

Most drug interactions can be prevented by checking and rechecking a medication before administration, and by understanding how reactions occur. The first step is to realize that a drug interaction may be either pharmacokinetic or pharmacodynamic.

Preventing pharmacokinetic drug interactions

Pharmacokinetic interactions are those in which the absorption, distribution, metabolism, or excretion of a drug is altered.

Altered absorption

Decreased or delayed absorption of a drug from the GI tract can reduce the drug's effectiveness. Here are some specific pharmacokinetic interactions that result in altered drug absorption.

Tetracyclines and metals. When tetracyclines combine with metal ions (calcium, magnesium, aluminum, and iron, for example) in the GI tract, they form complexes that are poorly absorbed, causing them to lose some of their effectiveness. That's why tetracycline shouldn't be taken with milk, which contains calcium. Nor should it be taken concurrently with certain other drugs, such as antacids (most of which contain metals) and iron preparations. To avoid tetracycline-antacid interactions, always administer the two drugs at least 1 hour apart.

Fluoroquinolones and metals. Metals also form complexes with the fluoroquinolone derivatives—ciprofloxacin, enoxacin, lomefloxacin, norfloxacin, and ofloxacin—and may markedly reduce fluoroquinolone absorption. Patients taking fluoroquinolones should avoid metal-containing products (such as antacids) or, if both drugs are necessary, should take them at least 2 hours apart. Antacids and sucralfate shouldn't be taken within 4 hours of certain fluoroquinolones such as lomefloxacin.

Cholestyramine or colestipol and other drugs. Cholestyramine and colestipol are resinous antilipemics that bind with bile acids and prevent their reabsorption. They can also bind with other drugs in the GI tract and reduce absorption. Therefore, the interval between administration of cholestyramine or colestipol and another drug should be as long as possible.

Food and antibiotics. Because food in the GI tract can affect absorption, you should give penicillins, tetracyclines, and fluoroquinolones, as well as several other antibiotics, at least 1 hour before or 2 hours after meals. Exceptions include penicillin V, amoxicillin, cephalosporins, doxycycline, lomefloxacin, minocycline, and certain formulations of erythromycin. Absorption of these drugs isn't appreciably affected by food.

Food may also greatly reduce the absorption of the antihistamine astemizole and the antiviral didanosine. Therefore, they must be administered on an empty stomach. (See *Which drugs to take—or not take—with food*, pages 248 and 249.)

Altered distribution

Another type of pharmacokinetic interaction can occur when the patient receives two drugs that bind to the same plasma protein. The drug with the greater affinity for the binding sites will displace the other, altering distribution of the second drug. Because only the unbound, or free, portion of a drug is pharmacologically active, the displacement of even a small fraction of a highly protein-bound drug may substantially alter the effects of the drug. Two examples follow.

Warfarin and phenylbutazone. If administered concurrently, phenylbutazone displaces much of the warfarin from the binding sites. This significantly increases the amount of active warfarin distributed through the body,

putting the patient at risk for hemorrhage.

Valproic acid and salicylates. Salicylates, such as aspirin, may displace valproic acid from plasma protein–binding sites and also alter its metabolism. The increased serum concentration of unbound valproic acid may be toxic. The anticonvulsant dosage may have to be reduced.

Altered metabolism

A number of drugs are metabolized in the liver. Many drug interactions result from one drug altering (either increasing or inhibiting) the metabolism of another.

For example, a drug may cause enzyme induction—that is, it increases the activity of liver enzymes. This causes a second drug that is metabolized by these enzymes to be metabolized and excreted faster than normal, thereby reducing its effects. Some examples follow.

Warfarin and phenobarbital. By causing enzyme induction, phenobarbital can accelerate warfarin metabolism. This reduces warfarin's effects, risking thrombus formation. To compensate, the warfarin dosage may be increased. Keep in mind that an equally hazardous situation could develop if the patient suddenly stopped taking phenobarbital and the warfarin dosage weren't reduced.

Cyclosporine and enzyme inducers. Enzyme inducers such as the barbiturates, phenytoin, and rifampin may increase the metabolism rate and reduce the

(Text continues on page 250.)

DRUG DIFFICULTIES

Which drugs to take—or not take—with food

To ensure optimal drug absorption, you need to know how a drug is affected by food. The following list should help. The key to the numbers listed after each drug is shown below.
1. Take with food or milk.
2. Take on empty stomach.
3. Don't take with milk or other dairy products.
4. Take before meals.
5. May take without regard to meals.

Drugs known equally well by generic and trade names are listed both ways. Trade names are capitalized.

A
acebutolol 5
Achromycin V.. 2, 3
allopurinol 1
Amcill 2
aminophylline .. 1
amiodarone 1
amoxicillin 5
amoxicillin/
  clavulanate
  potassium 5
Amoxil 5
ampicillin 2
aspirin 1
Augmentin 5
Azo Gantrisin ... 5
Azolid 1

B
Bactrim 5
bisacodyl 3
Butazolidin 1

C
Capoten 2
captopril 2
Carafate 2
Ceclor 5
cefaclor 5
Ceftin 1
cefuroxime
  axetil 1

cephalexin 5
chlorothiazide .. 1
cimetidine 1
Cipro 5
ciprofloxacin 5
Cleocin 5
clindamycin 5
cloxacillin
  sodium 2
Cloxapen 2
Colbenemid 1
Cordarone 1
co-trimoxazole .. 5
Cuprimine 2

D
Declomycin .. 2, 3
Deltasone 1
demeclocy-
  cline 2, 3
Depen 2
Desyrel 1
dicloxacillin 2
diflunisal 1
Diuril 1
Dolobid 1
Donnatal 4
Dopar 1
doxycycline
  hyclate 3, 5
Dulcolax 3
Dynapen 2

E
Ecotrin 3
E.E.S. 5
E-Mycin 5
enalapril 5
EYC 2
Ery-Tab 5
Erythrocin 2
erythromycin
  estolate 5
erythromycin
  ethylsuccinate .. 5
erythromycin
  stearate 2
etretinate 1

F
famotidine 5
Feldene 1
ferrous sulfate .. 3
Flagyl 1
flecainide 5
fluoxetine 5
Fulvicin 1
Furadantin 1

G
Gantrisin 5
glycopyrrolate .. 4
Grifulvin V 1
Grisactin 1
griseofulvin 1

DRUG DIFFICULTIES

effects of cyclosporine. The cyclosporine dosage may have to be significantly increased if the two are given concurrently.

Smoking and diazepam and other drugs. The polycyclic hydrocarbons in cigarette smoke may increase the activity of hepatic enzymes that metabolize certain drugs, such as diazepam, propoxyphene, theophylline, chlorpromazine, and amitriptyline. Therefore, the effects of these drugs may be diminished if the patient smokes cigarettes. Conversely, if the patient suddenly stops smoking, the effects of the drug could be dangerously increased.

Mercaptopurine and allopurinol or azathioprine and allopurinol. Allopurinol reduces uric acid production by inhibiting the enzyme xanthine oxidase. This enzyme helps metabolize such potentially toxic drugs as mercaptopurine and azathioprine. If xanthine oxidase is inhibited because of allopurinol therapy, the effects of mercaptopurine or azathioprine may be dangerously increased. When allopurinol is given in dosages of 300 to 600 mg/day concurrently with either drug, the mercaptopurine or azathioprine dosage should be one-fourth to one-third the usual dosage.

Benzodiazepines and cimetidine. Cimetidine inhibits the hepatic oxidative metabolic pathways through which most benzodiazepines (diazepam, for example) are normally metabolized. If cimetidine is administered with a benzodiazepine, the sedative effect of the benzodiazepine may be increased. However, cimetidine is not likely to affect the activity of lorazepam, oxazepam, and temazepam, which make them good alternative drugs for a patient receiving cimetidine.

Nonsedating antihistamines and macrolide antibiotics or ketaconazole. Certain anti-infectives, such as the macrolide antibiotics (erythromycin, for example) and the antifungal drug ketaconazole, block the metabolism of the nonsedating antihistamines (terfenadine and astemizole). Toxic serum levels result, and lethal arrhythmias can occur.

Altered excretion
A change in urinary pH will influence the activity of certain drugs, causing them to be reabsorbed or excreted to a greater extent than normal. For example, salicylates such as aspirin will be excreted faster, and therefore be less effective, when taken with an antacid that can increase urinary pH. Conversely, a more acidic urine will cause salicylates to diffuse more readily back into the blood, thereby enhancing their effects. Patients taking large doses of salicylates—for arthritis, for example—run the greatest risk of interaction.

A drug's effects may also be increased or prolonged because another drug inhibits its excretion by the kidneys. Two examples follow.

Penicillins and probenecid. By blocking renal tubular secretion of penicillins, probenecid can increase the serum concentrations of these drugs and prolong their activity.

Digoxin and quinidine. Serum digoxin levels rise significantly when digoxin is administered with quinidine, mainly because quinidine reduces renal clearance of digoxin. Quinidine also may reduce clearance of digoxin from tissue-binding sites.

Preventing pharmacodynamic drug interactions

Pharmacodynamic interactions result from concurrent administration of drugs having opposite or similar effects. They also occur when one drug alters the tissue sensitivity or responsiveness of another.

Drugs that produce opposite or similar effects

Interactions caused by drugs having opposite effects should be easy to detect, but sometimes they can be overlooked.

Thiazides and insulin. The thiazides and other diuretics are known to elevate blood glucose concentrations. If one of these diuretics is prescribed for a diabetic patient being treated with insulin or a sulfonylurea, such as glyburide, it may partially counteract the hypoglycemic action of the antidiabetic drug. As a result, the insulin or sulfonylurea dosage may need to be increased.

Beta-adrenergic agonists and beta-adrenergic blocking agents. Management of pulmonary disorders may be complicated by beta blockers (propranolol, for example); therefore, these drugs shouldn't be given to patients with conditions such as asthma. Concurrent use of a beta blocker and a beta-adrenergic agonist (for example, albuterol and metaproterenol sulfate) may reduce the effects of both drugs. The cardioselective beta blockers (for example, acebutolol, atenolol, and metoprolol tartrate) are less likely to cause complications of pulmonary disorders or to reduce the bronchodilating effect of the beta-adrenergic agonists.

Central nervous system depressants. One of the most common drug interactions results when the patient receives two or more drugs that depress the central nervous system (CNS). It's important to remember that many drugs can depress the CNS – for example, sedative-hypnotics, antipsychotics, tricyclic antidepressants, certain analgesics, most antihistamines, and some antihypertensive medications.

Alcohol and sedatives. The increased depressant effect caused by drinking alcoholic beverages while taking a sedative is a long-standing drug-related problem. The response of a patient will depend on many factors, including his tolerance for alcohol.

Antipsychotics, antiparkinsonian drugs, and antidepressants. Watch for an additive effect when two or more drugs that cause similar adverse reactions are administered to the same patient. For example, a patient being treated with an antipsychotic such as chlorpromazine may also receive an antiparkinsonian drug such as trihexyphenidyl to control extrapyramidal reactions. And because he is also depressed, a tricyclic antidepressant such as amitriptyline might be added to the therapy.

Each of these three drugs produces anticholinergic effects, which only increase when given in combination. Excessive anticholinergic effects can cause an atropine-like delirium, especially in elderly patients. In the case of the patient described above, this could be mistaken for an exacerbation of his psychiatric disorder, which might be treated by increasing the dosages of the drugs that are actually causing the problem.

Drugs with hypotensive effects.
Certain antihypertensive drugs, such as prazosin, as well as other drug classes (tricyclic antidepressants and calcium channel blockers, for example), can cause orthostatic hypotension resulting in dizziness, light-headedness, and even fainting. Older patients are more susceptible to this type of response and the associated risks, such as falls and injuries. Institute appropriate precautions with these drugs, whether giving them alone or in combination.

Drugs that alter electrolyte levels
Several important pharmacodynamic interactions may occur because a drug alters the concentrations of electrolytes, such as potassium and sodium. Some examples follow.

Digitalis glycosides and diuretics.
Most diuretics can cause excessive potassium loss within the first 2 weeks of therapy. This effect is common among the thiazide derivatives as well as bumetanide, chlorthalidone, ethacrynic acid, furosemide, inda-

pamide, metolazone, and quinethazone.

Hypokalemia can cause cardiovascular problems, so check serum potassium concentrations during diuretic therapy. Be especially alert if a digitalis glycoside, such as digoxin, is also ordered. If the patient loses too much potassium, his heart will become overly sensitive to the effects of the digitalis glycoside and he may develop arrhythmias.

To avoid potassium depletion, a potassium-sparing diuretic like amiloride, spironolactone, or triamterene can be given in combination with a potassium-depleting diuretic.

ACE inhibitors and potassium-sparing diuretics. The angiotensin-converting enzyme (ACE) inhibitors (for example, captopril and enalapril) may elevate the patient's serum potassium concentration. A potassium-sparing diuretic or a potassium supplement should be used concurrently only if hypokalemia is documented.

Lithium and diuretics. Sodium depletion, another effect of diuretics, reduces renal clearance of lithium. Even protracted sweating or diarrhea can cause enough sodium loss to reduce the patient's tolerance for lithium, thereby risking toxicity.

Drugs that cause interactions at receptor sites
Important pharmacodynamic interactions can occur at receptor sites. These include various interactions involving the use of the monoamine oxidase (MAO) inhibitors, such as isocarboxa-

zid, phenelzine, and tranylcypromine, and drugs with significant MAO-inhibiting effects, such as procarbazine and furazolidone. Several such interactions follow.

MAO inhibitors and sympathomimetics.
A primary function of the enzyme MAO is to break down catecholamines such as norepinephrine. If MAO is inhibited, the body will produce and store more norepinephrine than usual at receptor sites in adrenergic neurons. So a patient receiving an MAO inhibitor shouldn't be taking an indirect-acting sympathomimetic (such as amphetamines) that might release this norepinephrine. If he does, he may experience severe headache, hypertension, and cardiac arrhythmias from the release of excess norepinephrine.

MAO inhibitors and tyramine.
Serious reactions, including hypertensive crisis, have occurred in patients receiving MAO inhibitors after they have eaten foods high in tyramine, a pressor substance. These foods include certain cheeses (such as cheddar, Camembert, and Stilton), certain alcoholic beverages (Chianti, for example), pickled herring, and yeast extracts.

Why do these reactions occur? Because tyramine is metabolized by MAO in the intestinal wall and liver. The enzyme provides a built-in protection against the pressor actions of amines in foods. When MAO is inhibited, large amounts of unmetabolized tyramine can accumulate, resulting in the release of norepinephrine from adrenergic neurons.

MAO inhibitors and other antidepressants.
Severe atropine-like reactions, tremors, and hyperthermia may occur when an MAO inhibitor and a tricyclic antidepressant (amitriptyline and imipramine, for example) are used concurrently. Concomitant therapy with these drugs is contraindicated. In fact, an MAO inhibitor shouldn't be given until 7 to 14 days after therapy with the other antidepressant has been discontinued (and vice versa). However, combination therapy is effective in some patients who haven't responded to either drug alone or to other antidepressants. This concurrent therapy should be given only if the patient can be closely monitored and if the doctor is familiar with the risks involved.

Serious reactions and deaths have occurred in patients taking fluoxetine and an MAO inhibitor concurrently or in close proximity to each other, so the two should never be taken together. ❖

Which drugs can I combine in a syringe?

You can't combine drugs that are not compatible. (See *Compatibility of drugs combined in a syringe,* pages 254 and 255.) And you can't combine drugs when the combined doses exceed the amount of solution that can be absorbed from a single injection site. ❖

Compatibility of drugs combined in a syringe

The chart that follows illustrates how to combine selected drugs safely in a syringe.

KEY
Y = compatible for at least 30 minutes
P = provisionally compatible; administer within 15 minutes
P(5) = provisionally compatible; administer within 5 minutes
N = not compatible
* = conflicting data

(A blank space indicates no available data.)

	atropine sulfate	benzquinamide HCl	butorphanol tartrate	chlorpromazine HCl	cimetidine HCl	codeine phosphate	dimenhydrinate	diphenhydramine HCl	droperidol	fentanyl citrate	glycopyrrolate	heparin Na	hydromorphone HCl	hydroxyzine HCl	meperidine HCl	metoclopramide HCl
atropine sulfate		Y	Y	Y	Y		P	P	P	P	Y	P(5)	Y	Y	Y	P
benzquinamide HCl	Y										Y			Y	Y	
butorphanol tartrate	Y			Y	Y		N	Y	Y	Y				Y	P	
chlorpromazine HCl	Y		Y		N		N	P	P	P	Y	N	Y	P	P	P
cimetidine HCl	Y		Y	N				Y	Y	Y	Y	Y	Y	Y	Y	Y
codeine phosphate											Y			Y		
dimenhydrinate	P		N	N				P	P	P	N	P(5)		N	P	P
diphenhydramine HCl	P		Y	P	Y		P		P	P	Y		Y	P	P	Y
droperidol	P		Y	P	Y		P	P		P	Y	N		P	P	P
fentanyl citrate	P		Y	P	Y		P	P	P			P(5)	Y	Y	P	P
glycopyrrolate	Y	Y		Y	Y	Y	N	Y	Y				Y	Y	Y	
heparin Na	P(5)			N	Y		P(5)		N	P(5)					N	P(5)
hydromorphone HCl	Y			Y	Y			Y		Y	Y			Y		
hydroxyzine HCl	Y	Y	Y	P	Y	Y	N	P	P	Y	Y		Y		P	P
meperidine HCl	Y	Y	P	P	Y		P	P	P	P	Y	N		P		P
metoclopramide HCl	P			P			P	P	P	P		P(5)		P	P	
midazolam HCl	Y	Y	Y	Y	Y		N	Y	Y	Y	Y		Y	Y	Y	Y
morphine sulfate	P	Y	Y	P	Y		P	P	P	P	Y	N*		Y	N	P
nalbuphine HCl	Y				Y			Y			Y			Y		
pentazocine lactate	P	Y	Y	P	Y		P	P	P	P	N	N	Y	Y	P	P
pentobarbital Na	P	N	N	N	N		N	N	N	N	N		Y	N	N	
perphenazine	Y		Y	Y	Y		Y	Y	Y	Y					P	P
phenobarbital Na		N										P(5)				
prochlorperazine edisylate	P		Y	Y	Y		N	P	P	P	Y		N*	P	P	P
promazine HCl	P			P	Y		N	P	P	P	Y			P	P	P
promethazine HCl	P		Y	P	Y		N	P	P	P	Y	N	Y	P	Y	P
ranitidine HCl	Y			Y			Y	Y		Y	Y		Y	N	Y	Y
scopolamine HBr	P	Y	Y	P	Y		P	P	P	P	Y		Y	Y	P	P
secobarbital Na		N			N						N					
sodium bicarbonate											N					N
thiethylperazine maleate			Y										Y			
thiopental Na		N		N			N	N			N				N	

Drug	midazolam HCl	morphine sulfate	nalbuphine HCl	pentazocine lactate	pentobarbital Na	perphenazine	phenobarbital Na	prochlorperazine edisylate	promazine HCl	promethazine HCl	ranitidine HCl	scopolamine HBr	secobarbital Na	sodium bicarbonate	thiethylperazine maleate	thiopental Na
atropine sulfate	Y	P	Y	P	P	Y		P	P	P	Y	P				
benzquinamide HCl	Y	Y		Y	N		N					Y	N			N
butorphanol tartrate	Y	Y		Y	N.	Y		Y		Y		Y			Y	
chlorpromazine HCl	Y	P		P	N	Y		Y	P	P	Y	P				N
cimetidine HCl	Y	Y	Y	Y	N	Y		Y	Y	Y		Y.	N			
codeine phosphate																
dimenhydrinate	N	P		P	N	Y		N	N	N	Y	P				N
diphenhydramine HCl	Y	P		P	N	Y		P	P	P	Y	P				N
droperidol	Y	P	Y	P	N	Y		P	P	P		P				
fentanyl citrate	Y	P		P	N	Y		P	P	P	Y	P				
glycopyrrolate	Y	Y		N	N			Y	Y	Y	Y	Y	N	N		N
heparin Na		N*		N			P(5)		N							
hydromorphone HCl	Y			Y	Y			N*		Y	Y	Y			Y	
hydroxyzine HCl	Y	Y	Y	Y	N			P	P	P	N	Y				
meperidine HCl	Y	N		P	N	P		P	P	Y	Y	P				N
metoclopramide HCl	Y	P		P		P		P	P	P	Y	P		N		
midazolam HCl	■	Y	Y		N	N		N	Y	Y	N	Y			Y	
morphine sulfate	Y	■		P	N*	Y		P*	P	P*	Y	P				N
nalbuphine HCl	Y		■		N			Y		Y	Y	Y			Y	
pentazocine lactate		P		■	N	Y		P	Y	Y	Y	P				
pentobarbital Na	N	N*	N	N	■	N		N	N	N		Y		Y		Y
perphenazine	N	Y		Y	N	■		Y			Y					
phenobarbital Na							■				N					
prochlorperazine edisylate	N	P*	Y	P	N	Y		■	P	P	Y	P				N
promazine HCl	Y	P		Y	N			P	■	P	P					
promethazine HCl	Y	P*	Y	Y	N			P	P	■	Y	P				N
ranitidine HCl	N	Y	Y	Y		Y	N	Y	P	Y	■	Y		Y		
scopolamine HBr	Y	P	Y	P	Y			P		P	Y	■				Y
secobarbital Na													■			
sodium bicarbonate				Y										■		N
thiethylperazine maleate	Y		Y									Y			■	
thiopental Na		N			Y			N		N		Y		N		■

How can I avoid giving the wrong drug?

Medication errors can result in life-threatening complications for your patient. Hospital administration can help prevent errors by establishing and enforcing a policy that the hospital pharmacy be contacted before medication is obtained from any other source. You can safeguard against giving the wrong drug by following these guidelines.

Be alert

Pay attention at all times, even during routine procedures. Maintain good records and read them. Listen to the patient and record the information he gives you. Don't ignore a patient who says he's allergic to a certain medication. Before giving any drug, ask yourself if the drug corresponds with the patient's diagnosis.

Be informed

Read and follow drug labels. Never ignore a manufacturer's warning. Know the peculiarities – and particular dangers – for every drug you give. Before administering the first dose of a newly ordered medication, check the transcribed order against the doctor's order sheet. If you're unfamiliar with a drug, verify its dosage in a drug reference before giving it.

Be careful

Check and double-check the label before using a medication. Discard out-of-date drugs. Make sure your hospital storage procedure separates look-alike medications and separates medications from toxic chemicals.

Inject correctly

Aspirate before giving an injection I.M. Pull back on the syringe slightly. If a backflow of blood appears, you've punctured a blood vessel. Use accepted injection sites. Meperidine, for example, should be injected into the ventrogluteal, dorsogluteal, or vastus lateralis area. Use a needle of the right length. Standard needles will rarely deliver an I.M. injection in patients weighing more than 250 lb (112.5 kg). Many nurses use spinal needles for I.M. injections in obese patients. You could ask the prescribing doctor to specify in the order the size of needle to use and the injection site.

❖

How can I avoid needle-stick injuries?

Currently, I.V. system technology focuses on housings that either shield (recess) the needle or slide over it. (See *Avoiding needle sticks.*) The latest trend involves needleless systems, which eliminate the steel needle. These use a plastic "needle" or a special valve to connect a syringe or piggyback tubing to I.V. tubing or into an intermittent-infusion cap to infuse solutions. You can use needleless systems for every aspect of I.V. therapy except piercing the skin.

Because you use many more needles to give drugs and infusions than to access a vein directly, these devices greatly in-

Avoiding needle sticks

The latest I.V. products, some of which are shown here, make it easier than ever to avoid needle sticks.

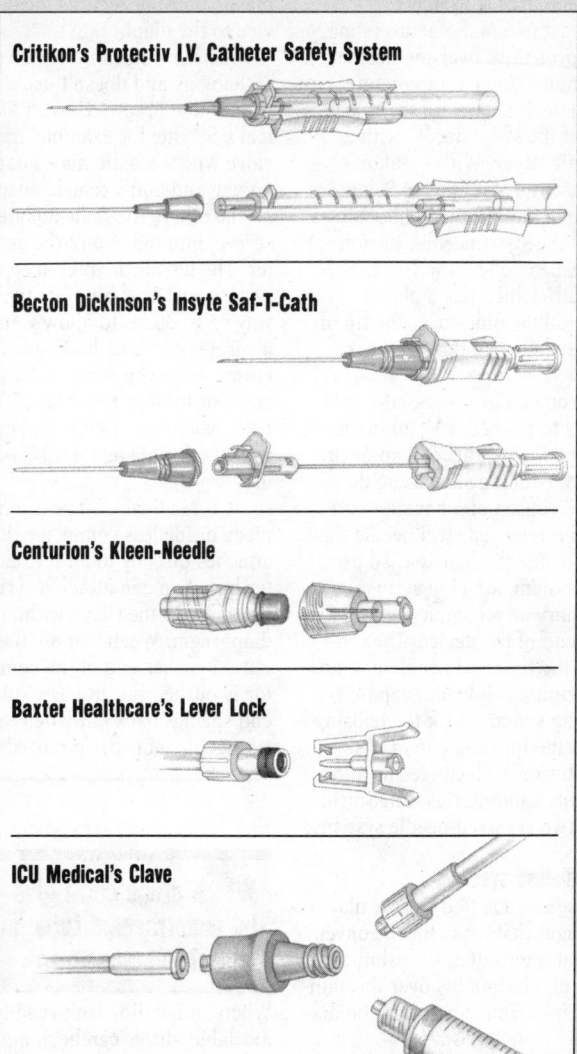

Critikon's Protectiv I.V. Catheter Safety System

Becton Dickinson's Insyte Saf-T-Cath

Centurion's Kleen-Needle

Baxter Healthcare's Lever Lock

ICU Medical's Clave

crease your safety. And they make connecting or disposing of I.V. components less risky. Following is a look at the latest products and how they work.

Needle-housing systems

At least two manufacturers market protective over-the-needle cannulas. After venipuncture, both devices enclose the sharp tip of the stylet needle with a plastic cover. With Critikon's Protectiv I.V. Catheter Safety System, a plastic chamber slides over the stylet needle. Becton Dickinson offers the Insyte Saf-T-Cath, which has a plastic shield that slides over the tip of the stylet when the stylet is retracted.

You can use recessed-needle units to connect I.V. tubing to an intermittent-infusion cap or primary Y-tubing site. These devices consist of a housing unit with a recessed steel needle that sits inside the housing. To use the system, attach a syringe or primary or secondary tubing to the end of the device. Then insert the recessed needle into an intermittent-infusion cap or Y-tubing site and lock the housing over the infusion cap or Y-site. Centurion's Kleen-Needle and Abbott Laboratories' LifeShield are two recessed-needle systems.

Needleless systems

These use a slitted rubber diaphragm that looks like a conventional intermittent-infusion cap. The diaphragm fits over the catheter hub. You can access the diaphragm in two ways. The first involves a plastic piercing needle enclosed in a plastic housing unit that resembles a clothespin, such as Baxter Healthcare's Le-

ver Lock. The second has a plastic needle covered with a drum-type plastic housing unit. With both, you penetrate the rubber split-septum of the diaphragm cap with the plastic needle. The plastic housing secures the device to the diaphragm.

Another system involves valve technology and doesn't use a rubber diaphragm. Burron Medical's Safsite, for example, has a valve with a plastic male adapter on one end and a female adapter on the other. The male adapter screws into the hub of the catheter. The female adapter accepts a syringe or I.V. tubing. Its two-way valve opens to allow you to aspirate or infuse fluid and closes when you remove the syringe or tubing. To maintain sterility, you place a dead-end cap over the female adapter between uses.

ICU Medical's Clave is a one-piece needleless connector that attaches directly to an I.V. catheter hub. You can attach a syringe or tubing to the Clave without a diaphragm. When you do, the recessed rubber end of the connector is pushed inward. The rubber end springs back out when the syringe or tubing is removed.

——————————————————— ❖

Which drugs can I give by endotracheal tube, and when?

When an I.V. line isn't readily available, drugs can be administered into the respiratory system through an endotracheal tube. Drugs commonly given by this route include naloxone, atropine,

Administering endotracheal drugs

Endotracheal administration of drugs in an emergency has become fairly common. To instill a drug correctly by this route, first calculate the drug dose. Advanced Cardiac Life Support guidelines for adults recommend that drugs be administered at 2 to 2½ times the recommended I.V. dose.

Next, use sodium chloride injection or sterile water for injection to dilute the drug to a volume of 10 to 25 ml. (This volume appears to provide the best absorption in the shortest amount of time.) Instill the solution into the tube, as shown below; then follow instillation with several insufflations of air using a hand-held resuscitation bag.

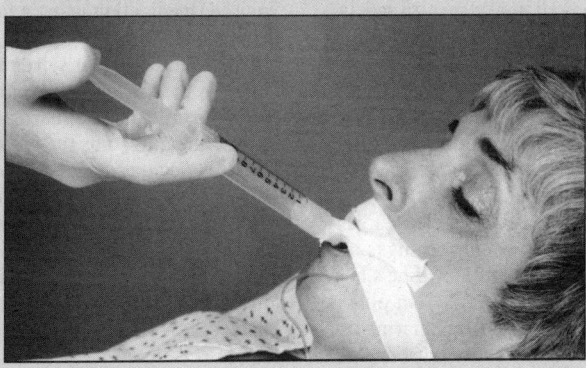

diazepam, epinephrine, and lidocaine. Endotracheal administration allows uninterrupted resuscitation efforts and avoids such complications as coronary artery laceration, cardiac tamponade, or pneumothorax, which can occur when emergency drugs are given intracardially.

When giving drugs by this route, remember that the duration of action is usually longer than if the drugs were given I.V. This is due to sustained absorption in the alveoli. You'll need to adjust repeat doses and continuous infusions to prevent adverse effects. (See *Administering endotracheal drugs*.)

❖

How can I ensure compliance?

To avoid having your patient refuse necessary medication, you must motivate him to participate in his own treatment and to see himself as the most important member of the health care team. Start by trying to anticipate any problems the patient might have in following instructions.

For example, if he has poor vision or poor muscle control, find a pharmacy that carries pre-loaded syringes or syringes with a spring release. Remember too, that a patient who has poor vision may not be able to read the label on his medication. Suggest that he use a magnifying glass or ask the pharmacist to use larger print. If the patient doesn't speak or understand English very well, make sure all labels and instructions are printed in his native language.

If your patient is annoyed about having to take too many pills, too many times a day, check with his doctor. The drug may be available in higher doses or in an extended-release form that would simplify things and ensure cooperation. If he's confused by all the different pills he has to take, ask the pharmacist to use color-coded caps on each pill bottle. If the patient has difficulty swallowing his pills, find out whether the drug also comes in liquid form.

Finally, if your patient is worried because the prescribed drug is too costly, discuss the problem with his doctor and pharmacist. A generic version may be available. If it is, make sure the doctor specifies on the prescription that a generic substitute can be used. If one isn't available, find out if a different, less expensive drug can be used instead.

❖

Can I use a fax machine to order medication?

Using a fax (facsimile) machine to order medication saves time and reduces errors. Although fax machines have their shortcomings (clarity, confidentiality issues, and the cost of machines and extra phone lines), they also offer many advantages, such as those that follow.

Less nursing and pharmacy time

To order medication using a fax machine, the unit secretary simply pulls off the doctor's order, puts it in the fax machine, and sends the order to the pharmacy. Neither the nurse nor the pharmacist is tied up unnecessarily. This process also gives the pharmacist a copy of the original order, which he needs for review and for his files. He doesn't have to rely on a courier who might inadvertently lose or misdirect the order.

Also, the time an order was sent and the health care facility it came from are automatically printed by the receiving fax machine. If a patient's identification information is missing or unclear, the pharmacist can immediately call the right nursing unit to get what he needs; he doesn't waste time tracking down the patient.

Less turnaround time

Orders can easily be filled on the same day, usually within 3 or 4 hours. In a hospital that doesn't use computers, orders can be faxed from the nursing unit to the pharmacy, which also shortens turnaround time. With a fax machine, a nurse no longer has to call for someone to come to the unit, pick up the order, and carry it to the pharmacy.

If an order can't be filled for some reason, the pharmacist can contact the doctor directly for a clarification or a new order. This reduces delays in filling orders—and the nurse doesn't waste time as a go-between.

Fewer errors

Before the pharmacist dispenses a drug, he and the nurse can interpret the doctor's order. As you're aware, a nurse and pharmacist may interpret an order differently. With the fax system, they can prevent errors by checking each other's work and talking with the doctor about unresolved problems. A fax also eliminates problems with sound-alike drug names and dosages that can be misunderstood over the phone. ❖

Topical medications

Applied directly to the skin, topical medications include creams, pastes, ointments, shampoos, lotions, sprays, powders, and assorted medicated dressings. The body absorbs topical medications through the epidermis and dermis. The variety of topical medications and the factors affecting absorption give rise to many questions.

Which topical drug form should I use?

Different topical drug forms have distinct properties, making some more suitable than others for certain disorders or for particular skin areas, such as the scalp and face. Ointments, for instance, have a fatty base, making them an ideal form for antimicrobial and antiseptic drugs. Common topical drug forms, their effects, and appropriate nursing considerations include those that follow.

Cream

An oil-in-water semisolid emulsion, cream acts as a barrier. To apply cream, thoroughly massage it into clean, dry skin. After application, observe the patient's skin for irritation.

Paste

A stiff mixture of powder and ointment, paste provides a uniform coating of medication, reducing and repelling moisture. Apply paste to clean, dry skin. Cover the medicated area to increase absorption and to protect the patient's clothing and bed linen.

Ointment

This semisolid suspension of oil and water retains body heat and provides prolonged contact with medication. To increase absorption, warm the patient's skin with heat packs or a warm bath before applying. As directed, apply a thin layer of ointment to clean, dry skin, and rub it in well. Use care when applying ointment to draining wounds.

DRUG DIFFICULTIES

Lotion

A suspension of insoluble powder in water or an emulsion without powder, lotion creates a sensation of dryness when applied to clean, dry skin. It leaves a uniform and powdery surface film that soothes, cools, and protects the skin. Before using, shake the container well. To increase absorption, warm the patient's skin with heat packs or a bath before applying. Thoroughly massage lotion into the skin. After application, observe the skin for irritation.

Powder

An inert chemical that may contain medication, powder promotes skin drying and reduces moisture, maceration, and friction. Apply powder to clean, dry skin. To keep the patient from inhaling powder, instruct him to turn his head to the side during application. If you're applying powder to the patient's face or neck, give him a cloth or a piece of gauze to mask his mouth. Direct him to exhale as you apply the powder.

❖

Which medicated dressing is right for my patient?

You may need to apply a permeable, a semipermeable, or an occlusive medicated dressing to treat skin problems—especially when the patient can't tolerate a bath, when the skin problem affects an area that can't be soaked, or when the skin needs long-term treatment and protection.

A permeable dressing allows air to reach the wound, whereas a semipermeable dressing allows oxygen to reach the wound. An occlusive dressing, which is impermeable to oxygen, reduces wound pain, speeds reepithelialization, and stimulates debridement and healing. No matter which dressing you use, be sure to apply it correctly. Incorrect application can macerate the skin and stain clothing and bed linen.

Open, wet dressing (permeable)

This type of dressing is used for acute inflammatory skin conditions, erosions, ulcers, and skin lesions with oozing exudate. It delivers medication and softens and heals the skin while absorbing pus and exudate. It also decreases blood flow to inflamed areas, helps promote drainage, and protects the site from contamination. You may use an open, wet dressing, for example, to apply a solution of water and aluminum sulfate.

When applying this medication-soaked dressing, leave the dressing uncovered. Remoisten the dressing when the water in the medication evaporates.

Closed, wet dressing (occlusive)

You'll use an occlusive dressing for such skin conditions as cellulitis, erysipelas, psoriasis, lichen simplex chronicus, and eczema. This type of dressing delivers medication, softens and heals the skin, and increases the effectiveness of medication. It also absorbs pus and exudate, increases blood flow to inflamed areas, and protects the site from contamination. You may use an occlusive dressing, for example, to apply desoximetasone and an insulative dressing to apply boric acid solution.

To use this medication-soaked dressing, apply it to the skin and cover with an occlusive or insulative bandage. Covering the dressing this way helps to prevent water evaporation and heat loss.

Wet-to-dry dressing (permeable)
Used for wound debridement, this type of dressing delivers medication and softens the skin. It also absorbs pus, exudate, debris, and eschar. As an example, you may use a wet-to-dry dressing to apply sodium hypochlorite.

Apply this dressing in the same way as you would the open, wet dressing. However, when the water evaporates, remove the dressing; don't remoisten it.

Dry dressing (semipermeable)
A dry dressing is used for neurodermatitis and stasis dermatitis to protect the skin from abrasion and the site from contamination. For example, you may use a dry dressing with a debriding agent such as collagenase. To use this ordinary gauze pad, simply apply it to the skin. ❖

How can I ensure proper absorption with transdermal drugs?

Transdermal drugs deliver constant, controlled medication directly into the bloodstream for prolonged systemic effect. Medi-cations currently available in transdermal form include nitroglycerin, used to control angina; nicotine, used to wean from smoking; scopolamine, used to treat motion sickness; estradiol for postmenopausal hormone replacement; clonidine, used to treat hypertension; and fentanyl, a narcotic analgesic used to control chronic pain. Ensuring proper absorption of these drugs depends on proper application along with appropriate patient teaching.

Application
To ensure effectiveness, don't apply transdermal drugs to broken or irritated skin, which would increase irritation, or to scarred or callused skin, which may impair absorption.

Reapply daily transdermal medications at the same time every day to ensure a continuous effect, but alternate the application sites to avoid skin irritation. Before reapplying nitroglycerin ointment, remove the plastic wrap, application strip, and any remaining ointment from the patient's skin at the previous site. Apply the new patch, wait 30 minutes, and then remove the old patch; this allows time for the new patch to begin working.

Avoid any area that may cause uneven absorption, such as skin folds, scars, and calluses, or any irritated or damaged skin areas. Also avoid applying the disk below the elbow or knee.

Patient teaching
With some precautions, a patient may avoid problems with his transdermal patch or disk. Use the following patient-teaching guidelines:

DRUG DIFFICULTIES

• Warn the patient not to get the disk wet. Tell him to discard the disk if it leaks or falls off, and then to clean the site and apply a new disk at a different site.

• Instruct the patient to apply the disk at the same time at the prescribed interval to ensure continuous drug delivery. Bedtime application is ideal because body movement is reduced during the night. Tell him to apply a new disk about 30 minutes before removing the old one.

• Advise him not to touch the gel because medication may rub off onto his fingers. Remind him to wash his hands after application to remove medication that may have rubbed off inadvertently. ❖

What's the best way to insert and remove an eye medication disk?

Small and flexible, the oval eye medication disk consists of three layers: two soft outer layers and a middle layer containing the medication. Floating between the eyelids and the sclera, the disk stays in the eye while the patient sleeps and even during swimming and athletic activities. The disk frees the patient from having to remember to instill his eyedrops. Once the disk is in place, ocular fluid moistens it, releasing the medication.

Inserting an eye medication disk

Arrange to insert the disk before the patient goes to bed. This minimizes the blurring that usually occurs immediately after disk insertion. Then perform the following steps:

• First, wash your hands and don gloves. Then press your fingertip against the oval disk so it lies lengthwise across your fingertip. It should stick to your finger. Lift the disk out of its packet.

• Gently pull the patient's lower eyelid away from the eye, and place the disk in the conjunctival sac, as shown below. It should lie horizontally, not vertically. The disk will adhere to the eye naturally.

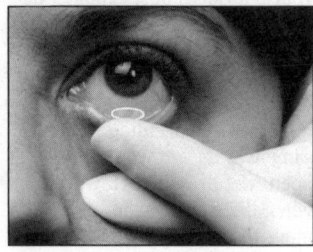

• Pull the lower eyelid out, up, and over the disk. Tell the patient to blink several times. If the disk is still visible, pull the lower lid out and over the disk again. Tell the patient that once the disk is in place, he can adjust its position by gently pressing his finger against his closed lid.

• If both of the patient's eyes are being treated with medication disks, replace both disks at the same time so that both eyes receive medication at the same rate.

• If the patient will continue therapy with an eye medication disk after discharge, teach him to insert and remove it himself. To check his mastery of these skills, have him demonstrate insertion and removal techniques for you.

Removing an eye medication disk

You can remove an eye medication disk with one or two fingers.

To use one finger, put on gloves and evert the lower eyelid to expose the disk. Then use the forefinger of your other hand to slide the disk onto the lid and out of the patient's eye.

To use two fingers, evert the lower lid with one hand to expose the disk. Then pinch the disk with the thumb and forefinger of your other hand and remove it from the eye.

❖

How can I help my patient use an inhaler?

Children or older patients with coordination problems often have trouble using metered-dose inhalers. They may inhale drug particles inefficiently, or larger particles may be deposited in the mouth or throat instead of in the respiratory tract.

For such patients, the addition of an extender, or spacer, may make the inhaler easier to use.

Newer models, such as the InspirEase extender, shown above, provide more dead-air space for medication mixing and have a reservoir bag that keeps the aerosolized drug suspended in the air for several seconds after activation of the inhaler. These modifications provide more effective inhalation and ensure that the larger particles are deposited in the respiratory tract, not in the mouth or throat.

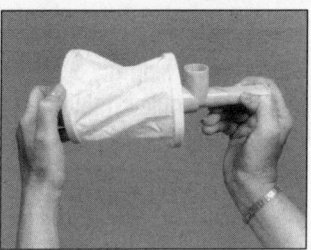

Because the extender mixes the drug dose with a larger volume of air than the metered-dose inhaler alone does, the patient may not be able to inhale all of it in one breath. He'll probably need to inhale twice to ensure that he receives the entire prescribed dose. Of course, each inhalation should be as slow and deep as possible, and the patient should hold his breath for 5 to 10 seconds afterward to allow the drug to reach the alveoli.

❖

Oral medications

You most likely administer oral medications to your patients on a routine basis and you administer them in many forms. Drugs for oral administration are available in tablets, enteric-coated tablets, capsules, syrups, elixirs, oils, liquids, suspensions, powders, and granules.

Many of these forms require special preparation. Some drugs shouldn't be combined with others. Many drugs mustn't be crushed or dissolved. And some may be difficult for certain patients to swallow.

Here are guidelines for handling these situations.

How can I help my patient swallow tablets or capsules?

If a patient can't swallow a whole tablet or capsule, ask the pharmacist if the drug is available in liquid form or if it can be administered by another route. If not, ask him if you can crush the tablet or open the capsule and mix it with food. Keep in mind, however, that many enteric-coated or timed-release medications and gelatin capsules should not be crushed. Remember to contact the doctor for an order to change the route of administration when necessary. ❖

How can I disguise a drug's unpleasant taste?

Some drugs, especially those in liquid or powder form, have an unpleasant taste. To promote patient compliance, consider these tips:
• Mix the drug with fruit juice or cola syrup if allowed. Have the patient sip the mixture through a straw.
• Use a syringe to instill the drug into the pocket between the patient's cheek and teeth.
• Suggest that the patient suck on ice chips just before taking the drug.
• Unless the patient is receiving a small amount of the drug, pour it over ice.
• Tell the patient to hold his nose as he swallows the drug.
• Chill oily medications.

• Offer a piece of hard candy or chewing gum after the patient swallows the drug, if allowed, or let him gargle or rinse his mouth. ❖

Which drugs mustn't be crushed or dissolved?

When you're preparing solid drugs for administration, be careful not to crush or dissolve a drug if doing so can impair its effectiveness or absorption. Many drug forms (such as slow-release, enteric-coated, encapsulated beads, wax matrix, sublingual, buccal, and effervescent tablet preparations) are formulated to release their active ingredient for a specified duration or at a predetermined time after administration. Disrupting these formulations by crushing can dramatically affect the drug absorption rate and increase the risk of adverse effects.

Other reasons not to crush a drug involve such considerations as taste, tissue irritation, and unusual formulation—for example, a capsule within a capsule, a liquid within a capsule, or a multiple, compressed tablet. ❖

Feeding tubes and buttons

If a patient can't ingest a medication orally, administration through a feeding tube or button is one alternative. However, to prevent adverse reactions, clogged tubes, and other potential complications, you need to consider the questions that follow.

Which drugs can I crush or dissolve for tube administration?

If a drug is available in both tablet and liquid form, administer the liquid whenever practical. Digoxin and acetaminophen, for example, are available as elixirs. But many oral drugs are available only as tablets or capsules. Some can be crushed (or, in the case of capsules, opened), mixed with water, and delivered by tube.

Crushing tablets
You can always crush simple compressed tablets, which are designed to dissolve immediately in the GI tract. Crushing the tablet allows it to enter the bloodstream slightly faster than it would if swallowed whole, but the difference is clinically insignificant.

This rule holds true even for tablets with sugar coatings, such as cimetidine and conjugated estrogen. The coating is intended to mask the bitter taste, not to delay tablet dissolution. (However, you should always confirm the type of coating with the pharmacy because sugar coatings resemble enteric coatings, and enteric-coated tablets shouldn't be crushed.)

Dissolving capsule contents
Although capsules shouldn't be crushed, you can open these types of capsules and mix the contents with water.

Hard gelatin capsules
Each capsule's gelatin envelope contains a powdered drug. Pull the capsule open (it's designed to separate in the middle) and mix the powder thoroughly in water. Ampicillin and doxycycline are two drugs available in this form.

Sustained-release capsules
Like sustained-release tablets, these capsules are designed to release the active drug slowly, over time. Feosol Spansules and Slo-bid Gyrocaps are common examples. The coated beads or pellets inside these capsules are designed to dissolve in the GI tract at different rates, prolonging the drug's duration of action. Obviously, crushing the capsules or their contents would destroy the timed-release trait.

If the doctor orders a sustained-release capsule, the best option is to ask him to order a liquid preparation of the drug instead. Theophylline, for example, is available in an elixir as well as a sustained-release capsule. Or the drug may be available as a simple compressed tablet that you could crush. (When changing to a formulation that isn't sustained-release, make sure the dosage frequency is increased appropriately.)

As an alternative, some capsules can be opened and their contents mixed with fluid or sprinkled on applesauce for ease in swallowing. As long as the protective coatings aren't disturbed, the medication will retain its sustained-release properties. Check with the pharmacist for advice.

Soft gelatin capsules
Drugs available in this form include chloral hydrate and various vitamin preparations. You can administer these drugs through a feeding tube by poking a pinhole in one end of the capsule and squeezing out the liquid contents or by drawing up the contents in a syringe. But don't use either of these methods if delivering an exact dose is important – no matter how careful you are, some of the drug is bound to remain inside the capsule.

If you want to make sure the patient gets the total dose, dissolve the capsule in warm water (15 to 30 ml for adults, 5 to 10 ml for children); then administer the drug-water mixture. Allow up to 1 hour for the capsule to dissolve.

❖

Which drugs can't be crushed?

Some types of tablets must not be crushed.
• Buccal or sublingual tablets, such as nitroglycerin and isosorbide, which are intended to be absorbed by veins under the tongue or in the cheek. The sublingual and buccal routes allow the drug to bypass the liver (avoiding the first-pass effect) and protect the drug from contact with other drugs, food, and GI secretions that could affect its potency or bioavailability. These

routes produce higher blood levels than the oral route, so dosages are smaller.
• Enteric-coated tablets, which are formulated to prevent release of the active drug until after the tablet has passed from the stomach into the intestine. Examples include bisacodyl and ferrous sulfate. Besides preventing premature drug release, the tablet's coating protects the stomach from irritation; crushing the tablet would destroy the coating.
• Uncoated gastric irritants, including aspirin. Although these drugs remain effective after crushing, they're more likely to cause adverse GI reactions, such as cramping or bleeding. Rather than crushing these tablets, ask the doctor for an alternative form or a different medication.
• Sustained-release tablets, which are designed to dissolve and release medication slowly. They actually contain two to three doses of the medication, so if you crushed them, the patient would get an overdose. Also, the intended beneficial effects wouldn't continue throughout the dosing interval.

❖

Can I give a medication with a tube feeding?

Whether or not you should give a medication with an enteral feeding depends on the specific drug, the feeding formula, and the patient's condition.

Schedule intermittent feedings to coincide with medication schedules, according to whether the medications should be taken

Can I mix drugs and enteral formulas in the feeding bag?

Avoid adding medications to enteral formulas in the feeding bag. Not only can this alter the drug's therapeutic effect, but it can also disrupt the integrity of the formula, causing it to resemble curdled milk. If the doctor orders the addition of a nonnutrient (such as sodium or potassium chloride) to the feeding bag, check with the pharmacist first to make sure the solutions are compatible. If so, shake the feeding bag thoroughly after adding the medication. Label the bag with the name and amount of the medication added and watch the formula for precipitation and other changes.

on a full or empty stomach. If the patient is receiving continuous feedings and needs drugs that should be taken on an empty stomach, discontinue the feeding 15 to 30 minutes before giving the medication to give the stomach time to empty. But if the tube is positioned beyond the pylorus, you can continue feeding the patient until just before you give the medication because there's no reservoir to hold the feeding solution.

Before giving the medication, check the residual volume to ensure that the patient is tolerating the feeding. If it's 20% greater than the volume to be given within 1 hour, wait a short period and check again. After giving the drug, flush the tube to prevent blockage and note the patient's response to assess whether he's getting the intended therapeutic benefit. If you have any questions, alert the doctor. (See *Can I mix drugs and enteral formulas in the feeding bag?*)

❖

Which drugs require special care when given by tube?

Here are some common examples of medications that must be handled carefully when given by tube.

Antacids
These liquids should be administered to the stomach only, so don't give them through a tube placed beyond the pylorus. Also, don't administer them in a tube that's smaller in diameter than a #10 French for adults (#6 to #8 French for children) or the tube may clog.

Ideally, you should give any other medications 15 minutes before an antacid dose to avoid potential interactions.

Antibiotics
Some antibiotics should be given with food, others on an empty stomach—check with the pharmacist or a drug reference for

DRUG DIFFICULTIES

guidelines applying to specific drugs. If the drug should be given on an empty stomach, stop continuous tube feedings for 15 to 30 minutes before giving the drug, and wait 15 to 30 minutes before resuming the feeding. Adjust the feeding schedule appropriately to meet the patient's nutritional needs over each 24-hour period.

Bulk-forming agents
Avoid giving psyllium (Metamucil) and other agents of this type by feeding tube whenever possible. Because they quickly congeal when mixed with water or juice, they can clog the tube. Check with the pharmacist for alternatives.

Phenytoin
Because the therapeutic range is so narrow for phenytoin, maintaining adequate blood levels is a problem when it's given by tube–the patient may need much higher doses than usual. Discontinue tube feedings for 1 to 2 hours before, and 1 to 2 hours after, giving phenytoin to enhance absorption. Because of these lengthy interruptions in the feeding routine, you'll need to adjust the patient's schedule to meet his nutritional needs over each 24-hour period.

Carefully monitor phenytoin levels and patient response, especially after any changes in the tube-feeding regimen–the dosage may need adjustment.

Theophylline
This drug may be poorly absorbed with continuous tube feedings. Monitor theophylline levels closely and alter the dosage as needed after tube feedings are discontinued.

Warfarin
Tube-feeding solutions contain vitamin K, and warfarin and vitamin K are pharmacologically antagonistic. Any change in the patient's feeding or medication regimen could cause adverse reactions such as bleeding. Monitor prothrombin times closely and adjust warfarin dosages as indicated.

❖

How can I avoid a clogged feeding tube?

Using the right-sized tube will help avoid clogs. For example, if the patient has both a nasogastric (NG) suction tube and a feeding tube, the NG tube is the preferred route for drugs. The reason: It's larger in diameter, so it's less likely to clog. Don't administer medications via a Miller-Abbott tube, which is intended to relieve intestinal obstructions. You don't want to risk clogging it.

Whenever possible, administer drugs in liquid form, rather than crushing the tablet form. (Digoxin and theophylline, for example, are available in both elixir and tablet forms.) Calculate equivalent liquid dosages carefully–many liquid medications are intended for pediatric use, so dosages may need adjusting for adults.

If you can't administer a preformulated liquid preparation, the next best alternatives are granule formulations, effervescent tablets or simple compressed tablets if available.

Dilute viscous liquids, such as clindamycin suspension, with 15 to 60 ml of water (depending on the tube's size and the liquid's viscosity). Also dilute hypertonic or irritating medications, such as potassium chloride elixir, with at least 15 ml of water; in some cases, you may need to use as much as 90 ml. Adjust water amounts appropriately for children and patients on fluid restrictions, and document the amount on the patient's intake and output record.

Flushing the tube after administering medication will also help prevent clogging. ❖

What should I do if a gastrostomy button pops out?

If your patient's gastrostomy button pops out (from coughing, for example), you or the patient will need to reinsert it. Perform the following steps:
• Gather gloves, the gastrostomy button, mild soap and water or povidone-iodine solution, an obturator, water-soluble lubricant and, if necessary, the ordered medication, a catheter adapter, and a catheter.
• Before reinsertion, wash your hands and put on gloves; then wash the button with soap and water and rinse it thoroughly.
• Check the depth of the stoma to make sure you have a button of

the correct size. Then clean around the stoma with soap and water or povidone-iodine solution and let it air-dry.
• Lubricate the obturator with a water-soluble lubricant and distend the button several times to ensure patency of the antireflux valve. Lubricate the mushroom dome and stoma. Gently push the button through the stoma into the stomach, as shown below.

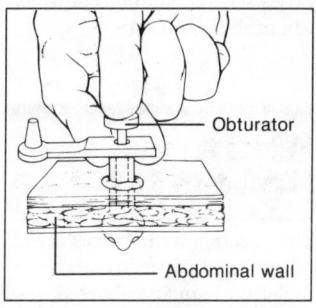

Obturator

Abdominal wall

• Remove the obturator by rotating it gently as you withdraw it to keep the antireflux valve from adhering. If the valve sticks, gently push the obturator back into the button until the valve closes.
• After removing the obturator, check the valve to make sure it's closed. Then close the flexible safety plug, which should be relatively flush with the skin surface.
• If you need to administer the drug right away, open the safety plug and attach the adapter and catheter. Deliver the drug as ordered. ❖

DRUG DIFFICULTIES

Subcutaneous medications

Injecting a medication into subcutaneous (S.C.) tissue allows the medication to move into the bloodstream more rapidly than if it's given by mouth. However, not all medications can be given by the S.C. route. Furthermore, this route of administration raises several questions of which you need to be aware.

What's the safest way to inject drugs S.C.?

The injection route makes use of adipose and connective tissue under the skin and above skeletal muscles to promote systemic drug action. The best sites yield a 1″ (2.5-cm) fat fold when pinched and have relatively few sensory nerve endings. Several factors determine how well the medication is absorbed from the site you've chosen: the patient's cardiovascular and fluid status, his physical build, the condition of his S.C. tissue, and your injection skills.

Preventing absorption problems
Absorption from an S.C. injection occurs by relatively slow diffusion into the capillaries—the rate is 1 to 2 ml/hour per injection site. So when a drug is given S.C. rather than by the I.M. route, initial blood concentrations of the drug will be lower but the drug's effects will last longer.

Be aware that the S.C. route's slow absorption rate, as well as the drug's effects, could markedly—and dangerously—increase if the patient exercises or warms or elevates the site after an injection. For example, an insulin-dependent diabetic patient could develop acute hypoglycemia from previously unabsorbed insulin if he goes for a 2-mile (3.2-km) jog.

Preventing tissue damage
To prevent S.C. tissue damage, irritating or concentrated drugs are usually given I.M. An irritating solution that's mistakenly given S.C. can cause tissue ischemia and necrosis. Also, concentrated drug solutions injected S.C. can cause sterile abscesses.

Sterile and nonsterile abscesses, cysts, granulomas, and nodules are common among drug abusers who inject suspensions made from capsules and tablets. These immune reactions can be caused by injecting irritating solutions, solutions containing invisible microcrystals (such as talc and cellulose found in oral dosage forms), or more than 1 ml of a drug per site. Overusing a site can also cause these problems. (See *Should I aspirate before giving an S.C. injection?*)

❖

Which drugs are safe to inject S.C.?

Although insulin is the drug most commonly injected S.C., the route is also appropriate for many other drugs that are wa-

DRUG DIFFICULTIES

RULE OF THUMB

 ## Should I aspirate before giving an S.C. injection?

Traditionally, you'd aspirate for blood before giving a drug S.C. to avoid inadvertently injecting some of it into a vein–which could cause serious adverse reactions if the patient were receiving certain drugs such as insulin or morphine. Heparin was the exception to this rule: If you traumatized the area during aspiration, heparin could allow a hematoma to form.

But for two reasons, some clinicians now believe that aspiration is unnecessary with any drug. First, some needles are made specifically for S.C. injections, and they're shorter than the needles you may have used in the past. If you have a needle of the correct length and the right site, hitting a vein would be anatomically impossible–the needle just wouldn't go in that far.

Second, today's needle tips have sharper edges and more sharply angled bevels, so they're less likely to lodge in a vein. Even if a vein were inadvertently pierced when the needle was inserted, this design would minimize the risk of the drug actually entering it.

Most of the time, you don't need to aspirate for blood before injecting insulin. But you should consider doing it for children, thin adults, or any patient who has many superficial blood vessels at the injection site or well-developed underlying muscle (as is common among diabetic athletes).

The best approach is to discuss this issue with your nurse-manager as a first step toward developing practice standards within the nursing department.

tery, noncytotoxic, nonirritating, and well-absorbed from adipose and connective tissue. Keep in mind that technique is important when injecting these drugs–the patient could have a dangerous response if you mistakenly inject certain drugs (such as insulin) I.M. instead of S.C.

Because of its high potency, epinephrine is usually effective when given S.C. for an acute allergic reaction. If it's accidentally injected I.M., it could cause life-threatening hypertension and arrhythmias.

❖

Which insulins are–and aren't–compatible?

Some insulins can be mixed together to fine-tune their onset, peak, and duration of action, thereby helping the patient to achieve better glucose control.

DRUG DIFFICULTIES

Most regular insulin can be combined in a syringe with all other types. Insulin zinc suspension (lente), prompt insulin zinc suspension (semilente), and extended insulin zinc suspension (ultralente) are compatible in any proportion. Regular insulin is compatible with protamine zinc suspension (PZI), but this mixture isn't usually recommended because its glycemic effects are unpredictable.

Before drawing up insulin suspension, gently roll and invert the bottle to ensure even drug particle distribution. Don't shake the bottle because this can cause foam or bubbles to develop in the syringe.

Don't mix human zinc suspension insulin (Velosulin Human) with insulin zinc suspension (lente) because their buffering systems aren't compatible. Furthermore, don't mix insulins of different purities or origins. Prompt insulin zinc suspension (semilente insulin) cannot be mixed with neutral protamine Hagedorn (NPH) insulin. Follow hospital policy regarding which insulin to draw up first. ❖

What caution is needed when injecting heparin?

When injecting heparin, your goal is to avoid local bleeding and irritation. Follow these guidelines:
• Locate the preferred site for heparin injection in the lower abdominal fat pad, 2″ (5 cm) beneath the umbilicus, between the right and the left iliac crests. In-

jecting heparin into this area, which isn't involved in muscular activity, reduces the risk of local capillary bleeding. Always rotate the sites from one side of the lower abdominal fat pad to the other.
• Don't administer any injections within 2″ of a scar, a bruise, or the umbilicus.
• Don't aspirate to check for blood return because this may cause bleeding into the tissues at the site.
• Don't rub or massage the site after the injection. Rubbing can cause localized minute hemorrhages or bruises.
• If the patient bruises easily, apply ice to the site for the first 5 minutes after the injection to minimize local hemorrhage, and then apply pressure. ❖

How can an infusion pump normalize blood glucose levels?

Changes in food consumption, problems with the insulin infusion pump, and other factors can contribute to abnormally high or low blood glucose levels. In some cases, you can correct these problems by adjusting the amount of insulin delivered by pump.

High blood glucose level
Consider the patient's blood glucose level to be high if it's more than 240 mg/dl on two consecutive readings. This problem can result from such causes as in-

creased food intake, illness, stress, menses, or decreased exercise. Intervene by reprogramming the insulin dosage as ordered. As well, high blood glucose levels may stem from a bolus dose of insulin delivered too soon (or not at all). If so, reprogram the insulin bolus dose.

High blood glucose levels may also result if the pump settings are incorrectly programmed, if the syringe is empty, or if the infusion set or syringe is leaking. Check all pump settings, including bolus doses, profiles, insulin concentration, and total insulin delivered; then reprogram settings as needed. Also check the syringe, and replace it if it's empty. Tighten the connection between the syringe and infusion set, or change the syringe and infusion set.

Air bubbles or obstruction in the infusion set or syringe, or irritation at the infusion site can also cause blood glucose levels to increase. Solve these problems by changing the infusion set and site.

Finally, if you can find no reasonable explanation for the patient's increased blood glucose level, test his urine for ketone bodies. If test results are positive, call the doctor; if they're negative, change the infusion set.

Low blood glucose levels

A low blood glucose level (below 60 mg/dl) may stem from reduced food intake or increased exercise or activity. To compensate, reprogram the insulin dosage as ordered. Decrease basal

or bolus doses before exercise if indicated.

Below normal blood glucose levels may also occur if pump settings are incorrectly programmed or if the infusion set is incorrectly disconnected from the syringe. Check pump settings, including bolus doses, profiles, insulin concentration, and total insulin delivered; then reprogram insulin settings as needed. Review correct disconnection procedures to prevent excessive insulin infusion.

A patient's blood glucose levels will decrease if he has consumed alcohol in the past 12 hours. Check with the doctor regarding the hypoglycemic effect of alcohol. Reprogram the insulin dosage as ordered.

If no reason can be found for the drop in blood glucose level, correct any hypoglycemia, reprogram the insulin dosage as ordered, and monitor pump program settings.

❖

Intramuscular medications

Intramuscular (I.M.) injections deposit medication deep into muscle tissue, which is well vascularized and can absorb it quickly. However, before giving an I.M. injection, you should consider which sites are appropriate for the injection, how to improve absorption, and how to make the injection less painful.

DRUG DIFFICULTIES

How do I choose the right I.M. injection site?

The I.M. injection site you choose will depend on the volume of the drug, how irritating the drug is, and the patient's age and muscle condition. Here's what you should know about these sites:

• The dorsogluteal site, shown below, may be the most dangerous – an injection given too low or too close to the buttocks crease could permanently damage the sciatic nerve or puncture the superior gluteal artery.

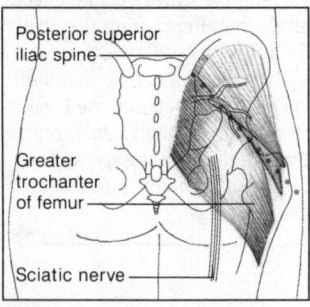

Posterior superior iliac spine

Greater trochanter of femur

Sciatic nerve

• The ventrogluteal site (gluteus medius and minimus), shown below, lacks major nerves or blood vessels and has dense muscles. It's a better choice for debilitated patients and a safe alternative to the dorsogluteal site.

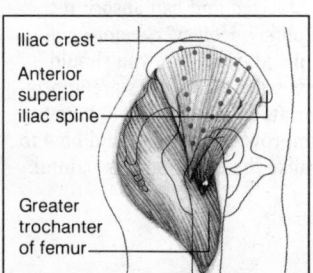

Iliac crest

Anterior superior iliac spine

Greater trochanter of femur

• The vastus lateralis site, shown below, which is also free from major nerves and blood vessels, is usually well developed in adults and walking children and is easily accessible. But, it does have a number of small nerve endings, so many patients complain of pain after the injection.

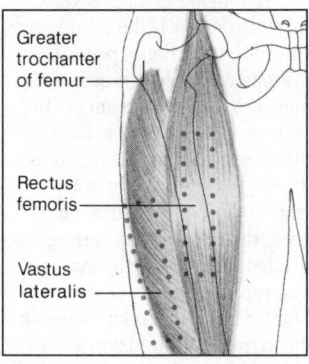

Greater trochanter of femur

Rectus femoris

Vastus lateralis

• The deltoid site, shown below, has a small muscle mass, so you can't give more than 2 ml of medication in a single injection. It's close to the radial nerve and the deep brachial artery. But it provides easy access for I.M. injections, such as tetanus toxoid boosters, that are often given in outpatient settings. Plus, medication is absorbed faster from this site.

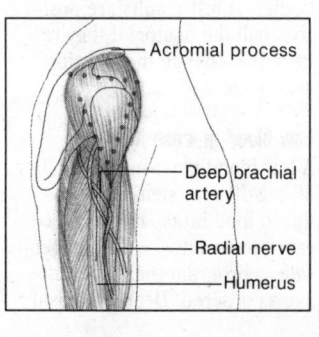

Acromial process

Deep brachial artery

Radial nerve

Humerus

How can I improve I.M. drug absorption?

Absorption rates from muscle tissue may vary from site to site. For example, absorption is faster from the arm than the thigh, and faster from the thigh than the buttock. In fact, studies have shown that blood flow in the deltoid muscle is 7% greater than that in the vastus lateralis and 17% greater than that in the gluteal muscles. So injections in the deltoid provide the fastest and highest peak serum concentrations of such drugs as haloperidol, lorazepam, and chlordiazepoxide hydrochloride.

Proper injection technique
But poor injection technique can impede absorption from any I.M. site. In a classic study, researchers measured serum levels of diazepam after one group of health professionals injected 10 mg of the drug into their patients' buttocks. Then they measured the levels of other patients after a second group injected the drug. The result: Serum levels were two-and-a-half times higher in the patients injected by the first group.

Technique seemed to account for the difference. The first group routinely used 1½″ (3.8-cm) needles; the second group used smaller 1¼″ (3.2-cm) needles, probably to save their patients from unnecessary pain.

As you know, needles are usually inserted to three-fourths of their length. So the second group who used the shorter needles probably injected the diazepam into S.C. tissue instead of muscle. No doubt the poor blood supply and high fat content of S.C. tissue limited the bioavailability of the diazepam, which tends to collect in fatty tissue anyway.

Proper drug choice
Compared with oral drugs, I.M. drugs are generally absorbed faster. But that doesn't always hold true. Chlordiazepoxide, diazepam, digoxin, and phenytoin are less dependable when given I.M. rather than orally. These I.M. solutions contain 10% alcohol (ethanol), 40% propylene glycol, and nearly 50% water. These drugs are rapidly diluted with tissue fluid, making them temporarily insoluble.

How can I make I.M. injections less painful?

You can reduce the pain of I.M. injections with expert patient preparation, injection technique, and aftercare.

Patient preparation
Encourage the patient to relax the muscle you'll be injecting. An injection into a tense muscle causes more bleeding and pain. The techniques that follow will relax the appropriate muscles.

For gluteal injections, the patient should lie facedown, stand with his toes pointed inward, or lie on his side with the upper leg drawn up in front of the lower one. For a vastus lateralis injection, the patient's toes should point in so the hip rotates internally. And for a deltoid injection, the patient should flex his elbow and support the lower arm.

Avoid especially sensitive areas. When you choose an injection site, roll the muscle mass with your fingers and watch for twitching, an indication that the area is too sensitive.

If the patient is very apprehensive, numb the site briefly by holding ice on it or by spraying an anesthetic coolant on it before you've applied an antiseptic. Then wait until the antiseptic is dry. Wet antiseptic could cling to the needle and cause pain when you insert it.

Injection technique
Follow these guidelines to help minimize pain:
• After you draw up the drug, change needles. A needle's point and bevel can be dulled when you puncture the drug vial's stopper, and dull needles hurt. By changing needles, you eliminate another source of pain: medication that clings to the outside of the needle when you draw medication out of the vial or ampule.
• Insert the needle smoothly and rapidly to minimize puncture pain. As you're doing so, try to distract the patient's attention.
• If the needle is properly placed, inject the drug slowly to avoid creating high pressure in the muscle.
• Withdraw the needle smoothly and rapidly.

Aftercare
Unless contraindicated by the medication (iron dextran, for example), gently massage the relaxed muscle to distribute the drug better and increase absorption. This helps reduce pain

caused by tissue stretching from a large-volume injection. (Lightly exercising the injected muscle does the same thing.) ❖

Peripheral I.V. therapy

Used to give drugs in large doses or drugs that can cause S.C. or I.M. damage, I.V. therapy presents several nursing challenges. For example, besides needing to know how to administer the medication properly, you'll also be charged with inserting the I.V. needle or catheter, initiating the therapy, caring for the site during therapy, and discontinuing therapy. The answers to the questions that follow will help you fulfill your duties properly.

How do I choose the right venipuncture device?

The venipuncture device you choose hinges on several factors, including your patient's age, weight, and condition. A rule of thumb is to select the device with the shortest length and the smallest diameter that allows for proper administration of the solution. Selection also depends on the type of solution to be used, the frequency and duration of the infusion, and the types of veins available.

You'll choose from among three types of venipuncture devices: an over-the-needle catheter, a through-the-needle catheter, and a winged infusion set. (See *Comparing peripheral venipuncture devices*, page 280.)

Over-the-needle catheters
The most commonly used device for peripheral I.V. therapy, the over-the-needle catheter, shown below, consists of a plastic outer catheter and an inner needle that extends just beyond the catheter. The needle pulls out after insertion, leaving the catheter in place. Available in lengths of 1″ (2.5 cm), 1¼″ (3 cm), and 2″ (5 cm) and gauges from 14G to 26G, over-the-needle catheters are used mainly for long-term therapy for the active or agitated patient.

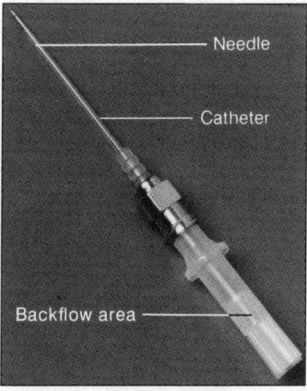

Through-the-needle catheters
This long, plastic, radiopaque catheter is used for placement in long arm veins, such as the antecubital. As shown at right, it consists of an 8″ to 12″ (20- to 30-cm), 14G to 19G catheter, whose tip lies inside the cannula of a 1½″ to 2″ (4- to 5-cm) introducer needle. A plastic sleeve protects the catheter from touch contamination as the catheter is gently pushed into the vein after

the needle is in place. When the catheter is in place, the needle is withdrawn and secured outside the skin with a plastic bevel cover. Because the catheter is radiopaque, placement can be confirmed by X-ray. You'll use a through-the-needle catheter when venous access is poor or when you administer caustic drugs or hypotonic solutions.

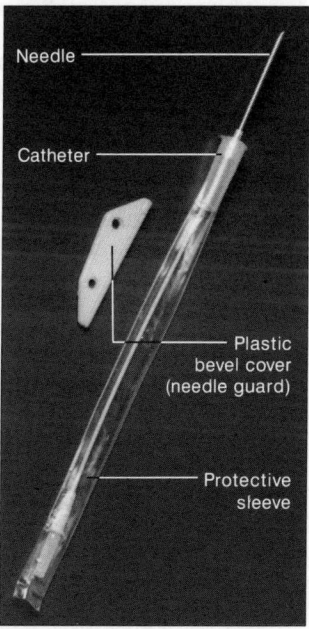

Winged infusion sets
Some venipuncture devices have flexible wings that you can grasp for easier insertion. The winged, over-the-needle catheter, shown on page 281, features short, small-bore tubing between the catheter and the hub. Available in a ¾″ (2-cm) length with narrow-gauge needles and a 1″ (2.5-cm) length with wider-gauge needles, the device is useful when you're using the patient's hand veins for infusion.

Comparing peripheral venipuncture devices

Most I.V. infusions are delivered through one of three basic types of venipuncture devices. The chart below details the advantages and disadvantages of each type to help you select the one that's right for your patient.

DEVICE	ADVANTAGES	DISADVANTAGES
Over-the-needle catheter	• Accidental puncture of the vein is less likely than with a needle. • The needle can be completely removed after insertion, greatly reducing the risk of catheter embolus. • The catheter is more comfortable for the patient once it's in place. • The device holds a radiopaque thread for easy location by X-ray. • Blood doesn't leak because the puncture made by the needle is the right size for the catheter.	• Insertion is more difficult than with other devices. • The apparatus is prone to touch contamination.
Through-the-needle catheter	• Accidental puncture of the vein is less likely than if you use a needle to deliver solution. • Once in place, this catheter is more comfortable for the patient than a needle. • The tubing holds a radiopaque thread for easy location by X-ray.	• Leakage may occur at the insertion site. • If a needle guard isn't used, the catheter may break. • Catheter embolus can occur if the catheter is withdrawn through the needle.
Winged infusion set	• This intravascular device is the easiest to insert. • The device is ideal for delivering medication by I.V. push. • The patient feels little discomfort on insertion. • The winged inserter reduces the risk of touch contamination.	• The patient is at higher risk for infiltration with a rigid-needle winged infusion device. • The set isn't suitable for delivery of highly viscous liquids or for long-term therapy.

Types of winged infusion sets include heparin locks, butterfly needles, and the Intima.

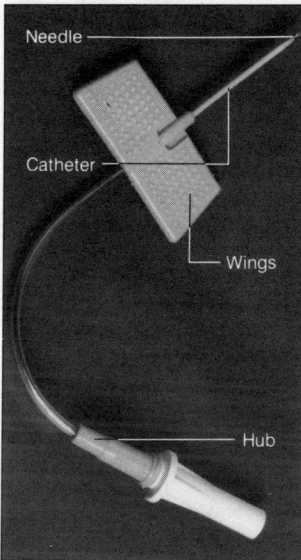

Needle

Catheter

Wings

Hub

Heparin lock
A variation of the winged, over-the-needle catheter is the intermittent infusion device—commonly called a heparin lock. On this device, which uses a steel needle, the tubing ends in a resealable, rubber injection port. When you use a heparin lock, the needle remains in the patient's vein. A plastic catheter isn't used.

Butterfly needle
Also called a winged, steel needle, a butterfly needle is thin-walled, has no hub, and lies flat on the skin. The needle is about ¾" (2 cm) long and its gauges range from 16G to 27G. Originally designed for children and elderly patients, this device can be used for any patient who is in stable condition, has adequate

veins, and requires short-term I.V. therapy.

Intima
Another variation of the winged, over-the-needle catheter is the device known as the Intima. A Y-shaped device with a latex cap, it comes in sizes 16G to 24G. The Intima allows continuous and intermittent therapy or simultaneous infusion of two compatible solutions.

❖

How do I select the best venipuncture site?

Successful I.V. therapy depends on selecting the best possible venipuncture site. You'll need to consider the vein's location and condition, the purpose of the infusion, and the duration of therapy. You'll also need to assess whether the patient can cooperate and determine which site he prefers. (See *Comparing venipuncture sites*, pages 282 and 283.)

Vein location and condition
If possible, choose a vein in the patient's nondominant arm or hand. The best sites are the cephalic and basilic veins in the lower arm, the branches extending from these veins, and the veins in the dorsum of the hand. Antecubital veins can be selected if no other veins are available, if you need to accommodate a large-bore needle, or if you must administer drugs requiring large volume dilution. If a patient will require long-term I.V. therapy, get maximum use from his arm

(Text continues on page 284.)

Comparing venipuncture sites

SITE	ADVANTAGES	DISADVANTAGES
Basilic vein Runs along ulnar side of forearm and upper arm	• Straight, strong vein suitable for large-gauge venipuncture devices	• Uncomfortable position for patient during insertion • Penetration of dermal layer of skin, where nerve endings are located, causes pain • Vein tends to roll during insertion
Cephalic vein Runs along radial side of forearm and upper arm	• Large vein that readily accepts large-gauge needles • Doesn't impair mobility	• Proximity to elbow may decrease joint mobility • Vein tends to roll during insertion
Antecubital veins Located in antecubital fossa (median cephalic, located on radial side; median basilic, on ulnar side; median cubital, in front of elbow)	• Large veins that facilitate drawing blood • Often visible or palpable in children when other veins won't dilate • May be used in an emergency or as a last resort	• Difficult to splint elbow area with armboard • Median cephalic vein crosses in front of brachial artery • Veins may be small and scarred if blood has been drawn frequently from same site
Accessory cephalic vein Runs along radial bone as a continuation of metacarpal veins of the thumb	• Large vein that readily accepts large-gauge needles • Doesn't impair mobility • Doesn't require an armboard in an older child or an adult	• Sometimes difficult to position catheter flush with skin • Venipuncture device placed at bend of wrist, so movement causes discomfort

Comparing venipuncture sites *(continued)*

SITE	ADVANTAGES	DISADVANTAGES
Median ante-brachial vein Begins at the palm and runs along ulnar side of forearm	• Vein that holds winged needles well • A last resort when no other site is available	• Many nerve endings in area may cause painful venipuncture • Infiltration occurs easily in this area, which increases the risk of nerve damage
Metacarpal veins Located on dorsum of hand; formed by union of digital veins between knuckles	• Easily accessible veins that lie flat on back of hand • In adult or large child, bones of hand act as splint	• Wrist mobility decreased unless a short catheter is used • Insertion painful because of the large number of nerve endings in hands • Site becomes inflamed easily
Digital veins Run along lateral and dorsal portions of fingers	• May be used for brief therapy • May be used when other sites aren't available	• Fingers must be splinted with a tongue blade, impairing hand mobility • Uncomfortable for patient • Infiltration occurs easily • Can't be used if metacarpal veins have already been used
Great saphenous vein Located at internal malleolus	• Large vein that is excellent for venipuncture	• May impair circulation of lower leg • Walking difficult with device in place • Increased risk of deep vein thrombosis
Dorsal venous network Located on dorsal portion of foot	• Suitable for infants and toddlers	• Vein may be difficult to see if edema is present • Walking difficult with device in place • Heightened risk of deep vein thrombosis

DRUG DIFFICULTIES

veins by starting the therapy in a hand vein and then switching to sites farther up his arm as necessary.

The least favored venipuncture sites are leg and foot veins because of the increased risk of thrombophlebitis. Keep in mind that some conditions contraindicate insertion of a peripheral I.V. line altogether. These include a sclerotic vein, an edematous or impaired arm or hand, the arm on the affected side of a mastectomy patient, burns in the area, or an arteriovenous fistula.

When you're performing a venipuncture in an arm or leg previously used for I.V. therapy – or in a previously injured vein – take care to insert the line proximal to the former site.

————————————❖

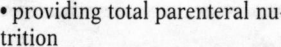

When should I use a filter?

Using an in-line filter helps reduce the risk of phlebitis by removing impurities from the I.V. solution. But because in-line filters are expensive and their installation cumbersome and time-consuming, they're not routinely used. Many health care facilities require a filter only for administering an admixture. If you're unsure of whether or not to use a filter, check the policy of your health care facility.

When to use a filter
You can expect to use an in-line I.V. filter when:
• administering solutions to an immunodeficient patient

• providing total parenteral nutrition
• using additives comprising many separate particles, such as antibiotics requiring reconstitution, or when administering several additives
• repeatedly using rubber injection sites or plastic diaphragms
• phlebitis is likely to occur.

Be sure to change the in-line filter according to the manufacturer's recommendations (typically every 24 to 96 hours). If you don't, bacteria trapped in the filter release an endotoxin, a pyrogen small enough to pass through the filter into the bloodstream.

When infusing lipid emulsions and albumin mixed with nutritional solutions, use an add-on filter with a larger pore size (1 to 2 microns).

When not to use a filter
Don't use an in-line filter when:
• administering solutions with large particles that will clog a filter – for example, blood and its components, suspensions, lipid emulsions, and high-molecular-volume plasma expanders
• administering 5 mg or less of a drug (because the filter may absorb the drug).

When to use a filter needle
You'll use a filter needle when removing drugs from a glass ampule and when mixing and drawing up drugs in powder form. If the top of an ampule breaks off, microscopic slivers of glass could fall into the drug solution. So before withdrawing the drug from an ampule, place the filter needle on the syringe. Remove and discard it before injecting the drug into the diluent.

When removing a reconstituted drug from a vial, use a filter needle to filter out any glass or undissolved particles. Injecting foreign particles into a patient's peripheral vein could cause an embolism.

_____ ❖

How can I locate "hard-to-find" veins?

Sometimes, palpation and visualization techniques aren't enough to help you find an appropriate peripheral vein for I.V. therapy. The Landry Vein Light Venoscope lets you perceive veins that otherwise are not easily seen or palpated. It illuminates the S.C. tissue while freeing your hands to perform venipuncture.

The Landry Vein Light Venoscope
A new device, the Landry Vein Light Venoscope has two fiber-optic probes that rest on the skin a few inches apart and shine intense beams into the patient's S.C. tissue. Veins absorb the light and appear as dark lines against the pinkish illumination of the skin, thus giving you easy targets to work with during the entire procedure.

The battery-operated Venoscope won't replace palpation and visualization techniques that, for many patients, may be more convenient to use than this device. And you should keep in mind that it needs to be used in a dimly lit or dark environment, presenting unique challenges. To use it, you'll have to become accustomed to working with shades drawn and lights turned down—a contrast to the bright illumination traditionally used during venipuncture.

Used properly, though, this device can help when peripheral veins aren't readily visible and are difficult to detect through palpation. It will become even more useful as the aging of the patient population leads to more I.V. therapy at home and in the hospital. Critically ill and elderly patients frequently require multiple attempts to get an I.V. line started.

The Venoscope not only makes veins easier to see, but also secures the vessels and prevents them from rolling. It reveals their size and course, the presence of bifurcations, and unusual angles. As you know, this information helps you choose appropriate veins and the right-sized cannula.

The Venoscope can be used on patients of any age or size and on virtually any part of the body. Here's a step-by-step guide on how to use it.

Getting started
First, attach disposable tips, or skids, to the fiber-optic arms. The skids should be replaced for each patient to prevent spreading infection.

Locating a vein
Turn off the lights or dim them to the lowest possible level. Draw the shades or pull the curtains to block out sunlight. Apply a tourniquet in the usual manner. Put the Venoscope on its

brightest setting and position the adjustable fiber-optic probes a finger's length apart, tilted toward each other. Run the probes across the skin. Veins will appear as dark lines.

Verifying a vein
Push the probes down on each side of the vein you intend to use. You'll know it's a vein if it collapses and disappears, then reappears when you relieve the pressure. Keep in mind that a vein that doesn't collapse and refill may be thrombosed from unsuccessful venipuncture attempts or long-term I.V. therapy. Try finding another one. Once you've verified a vein, use the twin beams to track it proximally to ensure a successful path for the I.V. cannula.

Securing the Venoscope
Use the Velcro strap to secure the Venoscope at the planned puncture site. Tighten it enough to slightly depress the skin – but not so much that the vein collapses.

Performing the venipuncture
In addition to the twin beams, the Venoscope has a tiny spotlight to help guide you in the darkness while you prepare the skin for venipuncture and assess the needle's bevel position before insertion. Pull the skin back away from the insertion site. Insert the cannula at a point just beyond the spot between the probes, angling the cannula down slightly as you begin insertion, as shown above.

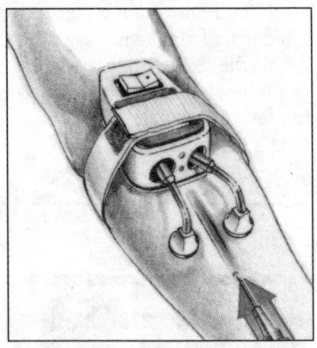

Threading the cannula
After you've penetrated the vein, use the spotlight to check for blood return. Reduce the angle of approach before advancing the cannula farther; then thread the cannula and complete the procedure as you normally would. Now you can turn the room lights back on or up. ❖

How can I keep veins from rolling?

Prevent the vein from rolling by maintaining it in a taut, distended, stable posititon. Because the wrist and hands are flexible, hand veins are generally easier to immobilize than arm veins. Hand veins may also be easier to cannulate because they're usually surrounded with less fatty tissue. And they enlarge with age as they lose elasticity, providing a bigger target. Use these techniques to immobilize hand and arm veins:
• To immobilize a hand vein, grasp the patient's hand with your nondominant hand. Place your fingers under his palm and

fingers, with your thumb on top of his fingers below the knuckles. Pull his hand downward to flex his wrist, creating an arch. To maintain the proper angle, make sure his elbow remains on the bed. Use your thumb to stretch the skin over the knuckles to stabilize the vein. Grip the patient's hand firmly throughout venipuncture.

• To stabilize the cephalic vein along the thumb side of the arm, ask the patient to clench his fist. Grasp his fist and pull it laterally downward. Although this maneuver may make the vein harder to see, it keeps it stable, which is crucial.

❖

What's the easiest way to cannulate a vein?

Although a deep arm vein is a challenge to cannulate, sometimes you have no choice because it's all that's available. However, cannulating an arm vein has the virtue of freeing the patient's hand so he can move around easily. An arm vein is also less likely to become phlebitic.

When you stretch a deep arm vein to immobilize it, it may seem to disappear because stretching may flatten it slightly. So you must be able to "see" it by palpating it with your fingers.

Cannulating a deep vein
To cannulate a vein that's palpable but hard to see, follow these steps:

• Ask the patient to clench his fist. Stretch the extremity and

vein while placing the fingers of your nondominant hand on top of the vein where the shaft of the cannula will lie. Using moderate pressure, retract the skin away from the insertion site to stabilize the vein.

• Grasp the cannula with your fingers touching only the hub, so you can easily see blood return. Aim the cannula tip at the vein you feel under your fingers, and insert it in one smooth, aggressive motion.

• Use your nondominant hand to maintain vein stretch. Lower the cannula angle and continue advancing it until you see blood return in the hub, indicating that the tip has entered the vein.

• Place a protective pad under the hub; then remove the stylet. As you remove the stylet, blood will flow into the backflow chamber. If the vein or cannula is large, the chamber can fill very rapidly.

• Remove the tourniquet and connect the I.V. tubing to the hub. Remove your gloves; apply a dressing, tape, and a label; and document the procedure.

❖

Which I.V. site dressing is better—transparent or gauze?

Select a dressing that you won't have to constantly manipulate to check the site—such handling can lead to contamination. Your choices include traditional gauze dressings and transparent dressings.

Several studies have shown that transparent dressings tend

to keep the I.V. device more stable and, in the long run, cost less to maintain than gauze dressings. Because you can see the insertion site through a transparent dressing, you'll save time checking it, too.

Although all dressings should be changed at least once every 24 hours, one study suggests that transparent dressings can be worn for a longer time than gauze dressings without increasing the risk of contamination. The study found that transparent dressings worn for up to 7 days were comparable to gauze dressings worn for an average of 2.4 days in terms of the incidence of infections and phlebitis.

❖

Which flushing solution is better – heparin or saline?

Recommended practices for maintaining patency of a heparin lock vary, depending on your health care facility's policy. According to results of a nationwide practice survey, 40% of the respondents use 100 units/ml of heparin to flush heparin locks, 37% use 10 units/ml of heparin, and 18% use 0.9% sodium chloride solution. The remaining 5% use other solutions or dilutions, but if the patient has a clotting disorder, use 1 to 2 ml of 0.9% sodium chloride solution instead of heparin flush solution.

If you're giving a bolus injection of a drug that's incompati-

ble with dextrose 5% in water, such as diazepam or phenytoin, flush the device with 0.9% sodium chloride solution.

❖

How can I ensure patient safety when giving I.V. bolus injections?

Commonly called an I.V. push, an I.V. bolus injection allows rapid drug delivery and a maximum, or peak, drug level in the patient's bloodstream immediately. Used in emergencies, the technique also allows administration of a drug that can't be diluted – for example, phenytoin, digoxin, furosemide, diazoxide, diazepam, many chemotherapeutic drugs, and diagnostic contrast media. Usually, you'll give a bolus injection directly into an existing peripheral primary I.V. line, an existing intermittent infusion device, or a vein.

I.V. bolus precautions

For certain drugs, the manufacturer supplies specific administration directions such as the appropriate injection rate. If you don't have such directions, keep the following precautions in mind:

• Don't give an I.V. bolus when you need to dilute a drug – an antibiotic or a vitamin, for example – in a large-volume parenteral solution before it enters the bloodstream.

• Avoid an I.V. bolus whenever the rapid administration of

a drug, such as potassium chloride, could be life-threatening.

• Finish each bolus injection by recording the type and amount of drug given and the administration times on the patient's medication record. Record all I.V. solutions used to dilute the drug and flush the line on the patient's intake and output record.

• Keep in mind that drug tolerance declines in patients with decreased cardiac output, diminished urine output, pulmonary congestion, or systemic edema. To compensate, you'll need to dilute the prescribed drug more than usual and administer it at a slower rate.

❖

How can I safely piggyback an incompatible drug?

If you're delivering a piggyback drug that's incompatible with the primary I.V. solution, consult the pharmacist and check with the drug manufacturer for directions. You should be able to flush the line with 2 to 3 ml of 0.9% sodium chloride solution, administer the drug, again flush the line, and then restart the flow of the primary I.V. solution.

If you can't do this, insert a venipuncture device to deliver the medication or use a T-connector.

❖

How can I prevent postinfusion complications?

Peripheral venous therapy can produce both local and systemic complications. Here are some of the most common complications as well as the possible causes, signs and symptoms, nursing interventions, and prevention techniques.

Local complications

Common local complications include phlebitis, extravasation and infiltration, occlusion, venous irritation, severed catheter, hematoma, venous spasm, and thrombosis.

Phlebitis

You'll identify phlebitis by a redness at the catheter tip that continues up the vein. The patient may complain of tenderness along the catheter and above it. Plus, the vein may feel hard, and the surrounding tissue may be edematous and warm.

Causes. Possible causes of phlebitis include a clot at the tip of the catheter, catheter movement within the vessel, and poor blood flow around the catheter. Phlebitis may also result when a catheter is left in the vessel too long or when the infused solution has a particularly high or low pH or a high osmolarity.

Treatment. Remove the catheter immediately and apply warm soaks to the affected area. If the patient develops a fever, notify his doctor.

DRUG DIFFICULTIES

Prevention. You can prevent phlebitis or its recurrence by using one of these measures:
• When inserting a new catheter, use either a larger vein or a smaller gauge catheter to ensure adequate blood flow around it.
• Employ a filter. This may prevent phlebitis by filtering out small particles that may cause irritation.
• Anchor the venipuncture device securely to avoid any irritating movement.
• Change the catheter site at routine intervals and at the first sign of vein tenderness or redness.

Extravasation and infiltration
Both common complications of I.V. therapy, extravasation is the leakage of a vesicant solution into the surrounding tissues and infiltration is the leakage of a nonvesicant solution into the surrounding tissues. When either occurs, you'll note swelling at and above the I.V. site, and decreased skin temperature and blanching around the site. The drip rate will slow considerably. If you're using a pump, the flow rate may continue despite an occlusion. The patient may complain of burning, tightness, and pain at the I.V. site.

Cause. Catheter dislodgment is the most common cause of extravasation and infiltration. Besides catheter dislodgment, you may suspect partial retraction from the vein or infiltration into the surrounding tissues.

Treatment. Extravasation of vesicants requires emergency treatment. Follow policy. Essential

steps should include the following:
• Stop the I.V. flow and remove the I.V. line, unless you need the needle to infiltrate the antidote.
• Estimate the amount of extravasated solution and notify the doctor.
• Instill the appropriate antidote according to hospital protocol. (See *Antidotes to vesicant extravasation*.) Usually, you'll give an antidote for vesicant extravasation in one of two ways—either you'll instill it through an existing I.V. line to infiltrate the area or you'll inject small amounts S.C. in a circle around the infiltrated area, using a 1-ml syringe. With the latter method, you should change needles before each injection.
• Elevate the arm and apply either ice packs or warm compresses to the affected area.
• If skin breakdown occurs, apply silver sulfadiazine cream and gauze dressings or wet-to-dry povidone-iodine dressings as ordered. If severe debridement occurs, the patient may need surgery and physical therapy.
• Record the location of the extravasation site, the patient's symptoms, the estimated amount of infiltrated solution, and the treatment. Also record the time you notified the doctor and the doctor's name. Continue documenting the site's appearance and associated symptoms.
   If partial retraction from the vein is the cause, make sure the I.V. line isn't tangled in the patient's clothes or bed linen. If the I.V. solution hasn't infiltrated the surrounding tissues, retape the I.V. without pushing the catheter back into the vein. If the solution has infiltrated, re-

Antidotes to vesicant extravasation

The following chart lists common antidotes you may administer. Some will be used in combination with others.

ANTIDOTE	DOSE	EXTRAVASATED DRUG
Ascorbic acid injection	50 mg	dactinomycin
Edetate calcium disodium (calcium EDTA)	150 mg	cadmium copper manganese zinc
Hyaluronidase 15 units/ml	Mix a 150-unit vial with 1 ml of 0.9% sodium chloride solution for injection; withdraw 0.1 ml and dilute with 0.9 ml of 0.9% sodium chloride solution to get 15 units/ml; give five 0.2 ml S.C. injections around site	aminophylline calcium solutions contrast media dextrose solutions (concentrations of 10% or more) nafcillin potassium solutions total parenteral nutrition solutions vinblastine vincristine vindesine
Hydrocortisone sodium succinate 100 mg/ml, then topical 1% hydrocortisone cream	50 to 200 mg (25 to 50 mg/ml of extravasate)	doxorubicin vincristine
Phentolamine mesylate	Dilute 5 to 10 mg with 10 ml of 0.9% sodium chloride solution for injection	dopamine epinephrine metaraminol norepinephrine
Sodium bicarbonate 8.4%	5 ml	carmustine daunorubicin doxorubicin vinblastine vincristine
Sodium thiosulfate 10%	Dilute 4 ml with 6 ml of sterile water for injection; administer 10 ml	dactinomycin mechlorethamine mitomycin plicamycin

DRUG DIFFICULTIES

move the I.V. line and insert a new one. Make sure the I.V. catheter and tubing are securely taped to the patient.

Prevention. To avoid infiltration, check the I.V. site often, especially if an infusion pump is being used. Don't apply tape or tight restraints above the site. And tell the patient to report any discomfort, pain, or swelling as soon as possible.

Keep in mind that seeing a blood return in an I.V. catheter doesn't confirm that the catheter is in the vein. Similarly, if you don't see a blood return, you can't assume that the catheter is not in the vein. If the patient has low venous pressure, or if the catheter and vein are too small, the I.V. catheter may not show a blood return even if it is in the vein. Conversely, sometimes the I.V. solution may have infiltrated and you'll still see a blood return because the tip of the catheter is partially out of the vein. (See *Preventing extravasation.*)

Occlusion
Look for two indications of occlusion: a backflow of blood into the I.V. tubing and a flow rate that doesn't increase when the bag is elevated.

Causes. Occlusion may result from an interruption of the I.V. flow rate during a piggyback infusion, from a heparin lock that's not flushed, or from a backflow of blood into the tubing when the patient moves around.

Treatment. To attempt to clear the line, use the following aspiration-irrigation procedure:

• Insert a 3- or 5-ml syringe with a 20G or 21G needle into the distal injection port on the I.V. tubing. After clamping the tubing between the catheter and the port, aspirate 3 to 5 ml of I.V. fluid into the syringe. Then unclamp the tubing. Note: If the I.V. fluid contains medication, use 0.9% sodium chloride solution instead of I.V. fluid.
• Clamp the tubing close above the port where the needle and syringe are inserted. Then, after straightening the catheter by stretching the skin area at the I.V. insertion site, forcefully aspirate fluid through the syringe.
• If blood appears, discard the syringe and then irrigate with a new saline-filled syringe. If no blood appears, inject the solution with slight to moderate pressure. *Important:* Don't force the injection if you feel strong resistance. Try aspirating, then irrigating again. If you still feel resistance, remove the catheter and restart the I.V. at a new site. (See *Is it OK to irrigate a peripheral I.V. line?* page 294.)

Prevention. To avoid occlusion, check the I.V. line frequently and maintain the I.V. flow rate. Also encourage the patient to walk with his arm across his chest to avoid a backflow of blood. (See *Preventing clotted I.V. lines,* page 295.)

Venous irritation
Your patient may feel irritation or pain during an I.V. infusion. The site may blanch during a venous spasm, or the skin over the vein may turn red.

Causes. Venous irritation may be a preliminary sign of phlebitis.

Preventing extravasation

Extravasation—the leakage of a vesicant drug or solution into the surrounding tissues—can result from a punctured vein or from leakage around an I.V. site. Because vesicant drugs or fluids cause blistering, severe local tissue damage often results.

Prevention
To prevent extravasation when giving vesicants, use proper administration techniques and follow these guidelines:
• Don't use an existing I.V. line unless its patency is ensured. Perform a new venipuncture to ensure correct needle placement and vein patency.
• Check the site carefully. Use a distal vein that allows successive proximal venipunctures. To avoid tendon and nerve damage from extravasation, avoid using the hand's dorsal surface. Also avoid the wrist and fingers (they're hard to immobilize) and areas previously damaged or with compromised circulation.
• Don't probe for a vein—you may cause trauma. Stop and begin again at another site.
• Start the infusion with dextrose 5% in water (D_5W) or 0.9% sodium chloride solution.
• Use a transparent semipermeable dressing to allow inspection of the site.

• Check for extravasation before starting the infusion. Apply a tourniquet above the needle to occlude the vein and see if the flow continues. If the flow stops, the solution isn't infiltrating. Another method is to lower the I.V. container and watch for blood backflow. This method is less reliable because the needle may have punctured the opposite vein wall yet still may rest partially in the vein. Flush the needle with 0.9% sodium chloride solution to ensure patency. If swelling occurs at the I.V. site, the solution is infiltrating.
• Give vesicants by slow I.V. push through a free-flowing I.V. line or by a small-volume (50- to 100-ml) infusion.
• During administration, observe the infusion site for erythema or extravasation. Tell the patient to report burning, stinging, pain, pruritus, or temperature changes.
• After drug administration, instill several milliliters of D_5W or 0.9% sodium chloride solution to flush the drug from the vein and to prevent drug leakage when the needle is removed.
• Administer vesicants last when multiple drugs are ordered. If possible, avoid using an infusion pump to administer vesicants because a pump will continue the infusion after extravasation occurs.

DRUG DIFFICULTIES

Is it OK to irrigate a peripheral I.V. line?

The possibility of pulmonary emboli and infection makes this a controversial issue. Pulmonary emboli can occur if irrigation pushes a clot into the pulmonary vasculature. Infection can occur if bacteria have colonized the occluding clot.

However, some clinicians argue that pulmonary emboli aren't likely to occur because clots typically originate in the leg's deep veins—not in veins normally used for I.V. insertion. What's more, the likelihood of infection is low be-

cause a clot in an I.V. catheter typically hasn't been established long enough to colonize bacteria. Those in favor of I.V. irrigation consider the risks slight when compared to the alternative of restarting the I.V.

All clinicians, however, agree that you should never risk forcing a blood clot into the bloodstream by using high irrigation pressure. So, if you observe an occlusion in your patient's I.V. line, the rule of thumb is to use the aspiration-irrigation procedure.

Certain I.V. solutions may also cause irritation, including potassium chloride, vancomycin, nafcillin, phenytoin, or any solution with a high or low pH or high osmolarity.

Treatment. To relieve the patient's discomfort, slow the infusion and use an infusion pump to maintain a steady flow. The I.V. medication may be diluted in 250 ml of solution rather than 100 ml. Check with the doctor and pharmacist to see if the solution can be buffered with sodium bicarbonate. If the irritating solution is to be given over a long period, the doctor may recommend using a central I.V. line. Ice or heat over the I.V. site may alleviate discomfort during the infusion.

Prevention. To avoid venous irritation, use strict aseptic tech-

nique when inserting the I.V. line and when performing tubing changes, dressing changes, and site care. Avoid inserting the I.V. line in or near joints if possible. Use the largest vein available to promote hemodilution. Tape the cannula hub securely to prevent movement; use an armboard if necessary. Dilute medications when possible. Rotate I.V. sites every 48 to 72 hours.

Severed catheter
If you notice solution leaking from the catheter, a severed catheter may be the cause.

Causes. A catheter may be severed when accidentally cut with scissors, or when the needle is reinserted into the catheter.

Treatment. If a catheter is severed, try to retrieve the broken part if it's visible. Otherwise, ap-

PREVENTIVE PRACTICE

 ## Preventing clotted I.V. lines

Here are some helpful hints to avoid clotted I.V. lines.

Insert the catheter correctly
When starting an I.V., insert the catheter with its tip away from the extremity's flexion and extension areas. This will help prevent catheter kinking and stasis of blood at its tip.

Use heparin locks
Use heparin locks instead of slow keep-vein-open I.V. lines as much as possible. If your patient must have a keep-vein-open I.V. line, open the clamp wide for a fast flush—3 to 4 seconds every few hours (providing the medication in the I.V. fluid would produce no ill effects).

Flush immediately
Flush I.V. lines or heparin locks with either heparin or saline immediately after infusion of any solution or drug, especially drugs which tend to precipitate—phenytoin sodium, diazepam, or antibiotics, for example.

Elevate the solution
To prevent blood from backing up and clotting in the catheter or tubing, keep the I.V. solution elevated at least 36″ (91 cm) above the catheter insertion site. If your patient is active, he's especially vulnerable to blood backup because activity increases peripheral venous pressure. Also, movement may cause the catheter tip to lodge against the vein wall, preventing I.V. flow.

Retract the catheter
If the I.V. rate is sluggish despite efforts to improve it, try this: Remove the tape and dressing from the catheter insertion site; then pull the catheter out about ¼″. This helps if the catheter is lodged against a vein wall or located in a valve or narrow section of the vein. *Note:* Never attempt to push the catheter farther into the vein because that would introduce bacteria into the bloodstream.

---

ply a tourniquet above the I.V. site.

Prevention. To avoid this problem, don't use scissors while inserting a catheter and don't reinsert the needle into it. If you're unable to insert the catheter, remove the catheter and needle together.

Hematoma
If the patient has a hematoma, you'll notice that you're unable to advance the catheter beyond a certain point. You may also notice a bruise around the insertion site, and the patient may complain of tenderness at the site.

DRUG DIFFICULTIES

Causes. A hematoma may result if the opposite vein wall is punctured during insertion or if infiltration causes blood leakage into the surrounding tissue.

Treatment. If you notice a hematoma, remove the catheter and reinsert it at a new site. Apply pressure to the area and recheck periodically for bleeding. Once the bleeding has stopped, apply warm soaks.

Prevention. To avoid hematoma, select a vein that can accommodate the size of the venipuncture device. As soon as insertion is successful, release the tourniquet.

Venous spasm

If the patient complains of pain along the vein, he may be experiencing venous spasm. You'll notice that the I.V. flow rate is sluggish even when the roller clamp is fully open.

Causes. Venous spasm may result from solutions that irritate the vein, from the administration of cold medications, and from a rapid infusion rate.

Treatment. Apply warm soaks for 10 to 15 minutes over the area and slow the infusion rate.

Prevention. You can prevent venous spasm by allowing solutions to reach room temperature before administration, by choosing a large vein for I.V. insertion, and by diluting medications when possible.

Thrombosis

With thrombosis, the vein will be painful, reddened, and swollen.

The I.V. flow rate will be sluggish or may have stopped completely.

Causes. Thrombosis results from injury to the endothelial cells of the vein wall, allowing platelets to adhere and a thrombus to form.

Treatment. In the case of thrombosis, remove the I.V. line immediately and reinsert it in another limb if possible. Apply warm soaks and monitor the site for infection.

Prevention. To avoid thrombosis, select the largest vein available for I.V. insertion and avoid using veins in the legs or over joints. Tape the cannula hub securely to prevent movement; use an armboard if necessary.

Systemic complications

Four systemic complications may result from I.V. therapy: circulatory overload, systemic infection, speed shock, and allergic reaction.

Circulatory overload

In circulatory overload, the patient may show signs of congestive heart failure (CHF), increased blood pressure, crackles, neck vein distention, and shortness of breath.

Causes. Typically caused by an increased flow rate over time, circulatory overload can be lifethreatening.

Treatment. Notify the doctor immediately. Raise the head of the patient's bed; then administer

DRUG DIFFICULTIES

oxygen and medications as ordered.

Prevention. To prevent circulatory overload, use a pump when administering I.V. therapy to patients who have problems eliminating fluids. Such patients include those with a history of CHF, decreased renal function, and decreased cardiac output. Check and monitor the flow rate frequently.

Systemic infection

With systemic infection, the patient has chills, fever, and malaise without an apparent cause.

Causes. This complication may result from not using aseptic technique. It may also result from severe phlebitis, prolonged use of a venipuncture device, and poor taping that allows the catheter to slide back and forth within the vein when the patient moves, thus introducing skin microorganisms into the vein.

Treatment. Notify the doctor, obtain a culture of the infected site, and give any ordered medications.

Prevention. To avoid systemic infection, always use aseptic technique when inserting a new catheter. Change sites, tubing, and solutions when appropriate, and make sure all connections are secure. (See *Preventing contamination of I.V. tubing*, page 298.)

Speed shock

A patient with speed shock will have a headache, syncope, a flushed face, tightness in his chest, an irregular pulse and, possibly, shock and cardiac arrest.

Causes. More common with bolus injections than with other methods, speed shock occurs when a medication is administered too quickly, causing plasma levels to reach toxicity.

Treatment. If you suspect speed shock, discontinue the infusion immediately and notify the patient's doctor. You may give dextrose 5% in water at a keep-vein-open rate. You can prevent speed shock by making sure you're familiar with the manufacturer's recommendations for administering a medication.

Prevention. To prevent speed shock, follow the administration guidelines recommended for the medication and know its expected actions and potential adverse effects. Use an I.V. pump if possible. Monitor the flow rate and the patient's response.

Allergic reaction

If your patient has an allergic reaction to a medication, you may note itching, bronchospasm, wheezing, urticaria, and edema at the I.V. site.

Treatment. If you detect these signs and symptoms, stop the infusion immediately and notify the patient's doctor. Help maintain the patient's cardiopulmonary status. If ordered, give corticosteroids, nonsteroidal anti-inflammatory drugs, and epinephrine.

DRUG DIFFICULTIES

Preventing contamination of I.V. tubing

Constant manipulation of the I.V. device may cause contamination as well as separation of the I.V. tubing from the cannula hub. Multiple medication pushes and tubing changes increase the risk of in-line contamination. You can reduce that risk by following these guidelines:
• Use strict aseptic technique when changing I.V. tubing — particularly when connecting (or disconnecting) the tubing to the solution container or cannula hub. Because the cannula can easily be shifted during this procedure, extravasation often occurs.
• Change the cannula and primary tubing simultaneously whenever possible.
• When piggybacking solutions into the injection port, rub the port with alcohol swabs before inserting the needle.
• When a piggyback solution is discontinued (and before starting a new infusion), take precautions in removing the I.V. needle and extension set, which may harbor contaminants. Dispose of them properly to protect other personnel and equipment from contact with solutions or contaminated blood.
• Change tubing every 72 hours, as recommended by the Centers for Disease Control and Prevention. This procedure is often neglected because of rotating staffing practices, use of agency nurses, random accountability for performing this task, and failure to label tubing.
• Never leave a contaminated needle or I.V. dressing attached to I.V. tubing not being used; doing so may cause upward contamination of the entire tubing and solution.
• Never let I.V. tubing touch the floor; contamination may occur through microscopic pores in the tubing.

Prevention. To avoid allergic reactions, you should know the patient's allergy history before administering any medications.

Keep in mind that a patient may experience a delayed repeat allergic reaction hours after an initial reaction.

Blood transfusions

Transfusing blood safely requires strict adherence to transfusion protocol and also careful patient monitoring. To ensure that your patient receives the utmost benefit from his transfusion, and that the transfusion is completed without complication, you need to know the answers to the questions that follow.

When must I discard blood?

You must discard blood if you cannot begin the transfusion within 30 minutes after receiving the unit. That's the amount of time it takes for the blood's temperature to exceed 50° F (10° C) once it's been removed from storage. The Food and Drug Administration requires blood to be stored at a temperature range of 33° to 42° F (1° to 6° C).

❖

When and how should I heat blood?

You'll need to heat blood for rapid transfusions, for exchange transfusions in neonates, or when a patient risks transfusion-induced hypothermia. Such a patient may be a trauma victim who requires massive transfusion, or a patient who has cold agglutinin disease – a condition in which an antibody in the patient's plasma reacts at cold temperatures against an antigen on his own red blood cells, causing their destruction.

To heat blood, use a blood-warming device – never a microwave oven or hot water immersion. A blood warming device passes blood through warm tubing or coils to maintain the blood at a temperature between 89.6° and 98.6° F (32° and 37° C).

❖

Do I infuse differently for acute blood loss?

You'll use a special infusion pump or pressure bag, similar to a blood pressure cuff, to replace blood rapidly following acute loss. Place the blood bag into the sleeve of the cuff and, using a pressure manometer, inflate the cuff. Monitor the gauge as the unit of blood empties, and reinflate as needed. If the peripheral I.V. catheter is less than 20G, be alert for signs of infiltration.

❖

What's the best way to infuse blood slowly?

A syringe pump or an electronic infusion pump delivers blood at a rate that's rigidly controlled or slower than you can obtain with the flow-control clamp on a blood-administration set. Follow your hospital's protocol and the manufacturer's instructions to prevent the pump from hemolyzing red blood cells.

❖

DRUG DIFFICULTIES

What should I do if the transfusion stops?

First, check the distance between the I.V. container and the insertion site. Make sure it's at least 3' (1 m) above the site. Next, check the flow clamp and make sure it's open. Also make sure the blood completely covers the filter. If it doesn't, squeeze the drip chamber until it does, as shown below.

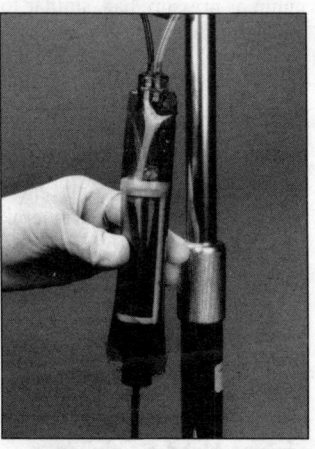

Now, rock the bag back and forth gently to agitate blood cells that may have settled to the bottom. Squeeze the tubing and flashbulb to get the fluid moving again.

Untape the dressing over the insertion site, and make sure the needle or catheter is still correctly placed in the vein. Reposition if necessary.

Finally, close the primary line's flow clamp. Lower the blood bag and open the 0.9% sodium chloride solution line. Dilute the blood with 50 to 100 ml of this solution to facilitate blood flow. ❖

What should I do if a hematoma develops at the needle site?

Stop the transfusion immediately. Remove the needle or catheter, and cap the tubing with a new needle and guard. Then notify the doctor. Expect an order to apply ice intermittently to the site for 24 hours and warm compresses after that. Promote reabsorption of the hematoma by gently exercising the involved limb. Finally, document your observations and actions. ❖

What's the best way to manage transfusion reactions?

Many transfusion-related complications, including transfusion reactions, are immediate, but others can be delayed up to 96 hours. Although a transfusion reaction typically results from incompatibility, contaminated blood, or too rapid an infusion, other complications stem from mechanical malfunction or other problems with the transfusion equipment.

Transfusion reactions can occur after single transfusions, or massive or multiple transfusions. Unlike a transfusion reaction, an infectious disease transmitted during a transfusion may go undetected until days, weeks, or even months later, when it produces signs and symptoms.

Hemolytic reaction

Caused by an ABO or Rh incompatibility or by improper storage of the blood unit, a hemolytic reaction may cause such signs and symptoms as shaking, chills, fever, nausea, vomiting, chest pain, dyspnea, hypotension, oliguria, hemoglobinuria, flank pain, and abnormal bleeding.

If you note any of these signs and symptoms, stop the transfusion immediately. Keep the vein open with a secondary line of 0.9% sodium chloride solution. Treat the patient's shock by giving oxygen, fluids, and epinephrine as ordered. Maintain his renal circulation by giving mannitol or furosemide, and collect blood and urine samples for the laboratory. In a hemolytic reaction, the blood will show hemolysis, and the urine will contain hemoglobin. Record fluid intake and output, and watch for signs of diuresis or oliguria.

Prevention

One way to prevent a hemolytic reaction is to make sure the blood you're administering is compatible with the patient's blood type. Always double-check the patient's identification before starting the transfusion, and begin the transfusion slowly. Stay with the patient for at least the first 15 minutes of the transfusion.

Febrile reaction

A common reaction, although not usually a serious one, a febrile reaction results from the presence of bacterial lipopolysaccharides. The patient's antihuman leukocyte antigen antibodies react with the transfused lymphocytes or platelet cell membranes. He may experience signs ranging from mild chills and fever to the more serious signs and symptoms of a hemolytic reaction.

For mild cases, administer antipyretics and antihistamines as ordered. Treat severe cases as you'd treat a hemolytic reaction.

Prevention

You can help prevent this reaction by keeping the patient covered and warm. Using a leukocyte-removal filter during the transfusion may prevent febrile reaction, as may administering saline-washed red blood cells (RBCs) or frozen saline-washed packed cells. You may administer antipyretics orally during blood administration. Never add antihistamines or any other substances to the blood bag.

Allergic reaction

Like a febrile reaction, an allergic reaction is common but shouldn't become serious. An allergic reaction results from an atopic substance in the blood. The patient may experience pruritus, urticaria, facial swelling, chills, fever, nausea, and vomiting. If you note any of these signs and symptoms, notify the doctor and give parenteral antihistamines. (See *How do I manage a severe reaction?* page 302.)

Prevention

To prevent an allergic reaction, find out if the patient has ever had such a reaction to a transfusion. If so, he has a two-in-three chance of having another one.

DRUG DIFFICULTIES

How do I manage a severe reaction?

Act promptly if the patient develops wheezing and bronchospasm—possible signs of an allergic reaction or anaphylaxis. If, after a few milliliters of blood are transfused, a patient becomes dyspneic and shows generalized flushing and chest pain (with or without vomiting and diarrhea), he could be having an anaphylactic reaction. Stop the blood and change the tubing. Start a slow infusion of 0.9% sodium chloride solution. Then ask another nurse to stay with the patient and administer oxygen while you call the doctor. Monitor the patient's vital signs, and keep the head of the bed elevated if the vital signs allow it. Make sure you tell the patient what's happening. Expect epinephrine and corticosteroid administration and intubation as emergency treatments.

Send the blood bag and its tubing to the blood bank, collect a urine specimen, and call the laboratory to request a repeat crossmatching if the patient shows signs worse than a rash or slight fever. Remember, only laboratory tests can determine whether a severe reaction is hemolytic, pyrogenic, severely allergic, or anaphylactic.

Blood contamination

Although blood contamination is rare, it's a serious complication. Caused by cold-growing, gram-negative bacteria, such as *Pseudomonas* or *Achromobacter*, blood contamination may cause chills, fever, vomiting, abdominal cramping, diarrhea, shock, and signs of renal failure. Notify the doctor at the first indication of blood contamination. He may order a broad-spectrum antibiotic and corticosteroids.

Prevention

To prevent blood contamination, examine the blood for gas, clots, or a dark purple color. Make sure that blood storage is strictly controlled, and use aseptic technique during administration. Change the blood tubing and filter every 4 hours, and transfuse each unit of blood over 2 to 4 hours.

Circulatory overload

Common and fairly easy to treat, circulatory overload occurs when too large a transfusion is given and the patient cannot handle the extra fluid over a short period. The patient may have engorged neck veins, constricting chest pain with breathing difficulties, moist crackles and, eventually, acute edema.

If these signs and symptoms occur, stop the transfusion and notify the doctor immediately. He may prescribe a diuretic. Once the transfusion is stopped, give dextrose 5% in water—not 0.9% sodium chloride solution—to keep the vein open.

Prevention

To prevent circulatory overload, the doctor may order packed RBCs rather than whole blood. He also may order a diuretic before or during the transfusion. You should keep the patient warm and in a sitting position. With high-risk patients, transfuse the blood at a reduced rate.

Hypothermia

The result of a rapid transfusion of large amounts of cold blood, hypothermia decreases myocardial temperature. The patient may experience shaking, chills, and hypotension. If his core temperature falls below 86° F (30° C), the patient may experience ventricular fibrillation and cardiac arrest.

To treat hypothermia, stop the transfusion and warm the patient with blankets. You should also obtain an electrocardiogram to assess for any heart irregularities.

Prevention

To prevent hypothermia in a patient receiving multiple transfusions, use a blood warmer to warm the blood to 95° to 98.6° F (35° to 37° C) before transfusing it.

❖

How can I protect my patient from transmissible diseases?

Even though blood and blood products undergo many tests that screen for transmissible diseases, you can never be sure the blood you're transfusing is dis-ease-free. These five diseases may be transmitted through a blood transfusion: acquired immunodeficiency syndrome (AIDS), hepatitis, malaria, syphilis, and a viral syndrome, such as those caused by cytomegalovirus or Epstein-Barr virus. The causes and incubation times vary for each, as do the methods of detection, treatment, and prevention.

AIDS

Caused by the presence of the human immunodeficiency virus (HIV) in the blood, AIDS has an incubation time of months to years. AIDS antibodies develop within 6 weeks to 6 months after infection. The presence of the antibodies in the blood confirms the presence of the virus. These antibodies can be detected by two tests, the enzyme-linked immunosorbent assay and the Western blot assay.

Prevention

Although antiviral drugs may reduce a carrier's ability to infect another, no drug cures HIV infection. To prevent transmission of the virus through blood transfusion, potential donors should be educated about the disease and the need for strict compliance with the Centers for Disease Control and Prevention's universal precautions.

Hepatitis

The greatest risk of hepatitis B and hepatitis C transmission is carried by pooled plasma, fibrinogen, and concentrates of factors VII and IX. Immune serum, globulin, plasma protein fraction, and normal serum albumin pose no risk. Hepatitis C (for-

DRUG DIFFICULTIES

merly called non-A, non-B hepatitis) accounts for 85% of blood-borne hepatitis cases. The incubation time for this disease is 2 weeks to 6 months.

If a patient does contract hepatitis, he may exhibit these signs and symptoms: anorexia, vomiting, abdominal discomfort, enlarged liver, diarrhea, headache, fever, and jaundice. Once diagnosed with hepatitis, a patient must be isolated to avoid infecting others. He should receive immune globulin therapy and nursing care that promotes his comfort.

Prevention

To avoid hepatitis transmission, make sure the blood is tested for the hepatitis B surface antigen and the anti-hepatitis C virus before you administer it. All donor blood products should receive a radioimmunoassay for hepatitis B. Only healthy, reliable donors should be accepted. If potential donors are suspected hepatitis carriers, arrange for epidemiologic follow-up tests. ❖

Central venous therapy

Inserted through a major vein—such as the subclavian or jugular—a central venous (CV) catheter allows for multiple infusions of fluid, blood, medications, or total parenteral nutrition. Caring

for a patient with such a line, however, requires special nursing skills. The answers to the following questions should help you gain the knowledge you need to care for a CV line safely.

Which drugs can—and can't—I give by CV line?

Many hospitals prohibit central venous (CV) administration of amphotericin B because it increases the likelihood of hypokalemia, which may cause cardiac arrhythmias. Some hospitals prohibit CV delivery of dopamine because this drug can also cause arrhythmias. Others, in contrast, specify that dopamine must be given only through a CV line because of the risk of extravasation with a peripheral line.

Despite the controversy about which drugs can and can't be administered safely through a CV line, experts generally agree on which ones should always be given this way. For instance, most hospitals require CV therapy for delivering highly osmolar fluids, such as hypertonic sodium chloride solution, dextrose 50% in water (often used in total parenteral nutrition), and certain chemotherapeutic agents.

Make sure that you consult your hospital's policy to find out which drugs can and can't be given through a CV line.

What's involved in maintaining a CV catheter?

While your patient has a central venous (CV) catheter in place, you'll care for the insertion site and maintain the setup to prevent complications. Routine care involves changing the dressing, changing the injection cap, and flushing the catheter at regular intervals.

CV catheter dressing changes

In general, hospital infection-control practices and the Intravenous Nurses Society (INS) standards of practice require you to change the catheter's dressing every 48 hours or whenever it becomes soiled, moist, or loose. When you do so, use sterile technique. And make sure that you find out which type of dressing your hospital recommends for catheter insertion sites. Recent studies show that transparent dressings may increase the risk of infection because they allow moisture to accumulate under the dressing. In light of these findings, some hospitals elect to use gauze and tape dressings.

Injection cap changes

Guidelines on changing the catheter's injection caps also vary among hospitals (although INS standards specify injection cap changes at least weekly). Generally, the more often you puncture an injection cap, the more

often it should be changed; repeated punctures increase the risk of infection. Besides, pieces of the rubber stopper may break off after repeated punctures, placing the patient at risk for an embolism.

Catheter flushing

As a general rule, flush all lumens of a multilumen CV catheter regularly. (Most experts recommend daily flushing.) However, flushing isn't necessary for a single-lumen CV catheter in use for a continuous infusion.

Hospital policies vary widely regarding flush solutions. Most hospitals use a heparin flush solution that's available in premixed 10-ml multidose vials. Recommended heparin concentrations range from as little as 10 units/ml to as much as 100 units/ml. However, some hospitals do not use heparin. They rely instead on 0.9% sodium chloride solutions because some studies show that heparin isn't always needed to keep the CV line open.

The recommended amount of flush solution can vary. (See *How much flush solution should I use?* page 306.) Keep in mind, too, that different catheters require different amounts of solution. A catheter that's been cut to fit the patient, for example, needs less flush solution. Whatever the flush solution volume, use a 10-ml catheter to reduce the risk of rupturing the catheter.

RULE OF THUMB

 How much flush solution should I use?

The amount and the strength of heparin to be infused varies with the patient's body size. Follow these guidelines:
• For patients weighing less than 11 lb (5 kg), infuse 1 ml of 10 units/ml every 12 hours.
• For pediatric patients weighing more than 11 lb, infuse 1 ml of 100 units/ml every 12 hours.
• For adult patients, infuse 1½ ml of 100 units/ml every 12 hours.

How soon after catheter placement can a VAP be used?

The vascular access port (VAP) can be used immediately after placement, although some edema and tenderness may persist for about 72 hours. This makes the device initially difficult to palpate and slightly uncomfortable for the patient. Place an ice pack over the area for several minutes to alleviate discomfort from the needle puncture.

How often should I change a Huber needle?

Commonly, the needle is left in place for several days for continuous infusions. For intermittent or cycled infusions, you can also leave the needle in the port and heparinize the injection cap, extension tubing, needle, and port between uses. For most infu-sions, the needle will be changed every 3 to 7 days.

Some home-care patients receiving cycled total parental nutition infusions prefer to insert a new needle every day. They'll remove the needle after the infusion so that they can participate in certain activities. The skin over the port may become irritated if the needle is left in place between infusions and the patient is very active. Using the muscles of the upper body may also cause the needle to move, resulting in an ulcerated or craterlike appearance around the needle. ❖

What if I can't flush or withdraw fluid from a VAP?

Inability to obtain blood could mean that the catheter leading from the vascular access port (VAP) is lodged against the vessel wall. Ask the patient to raise his arms, perform Valsalva's maneuver, or change position to free the catheter.

If this doesn't work, consider other possible causes. Check the I.V. tubing for kinks and the pump for malfunction. Also check the needle for proper placement. If the needle is placed incorrectly, reposition the needle and advance the tip to the bottom of the reservoir. Verify correct positioning by blood aspiration.

If none of these measures corrects the problem, a fibrin sleeve on the distal end of the catheter may be occluding the opening. Flush the catheter with 3 ml of sterile 0.9% sodium chloride solution and repeat if necessary. Increase the frequency of flushing to prevent sheath formation. If clots are occluding the port, use a declotting or fibrinolytic agent such as urokinase as ordered. If the problem stems from a kinked catheter or port rotation, contact the doctor.

How often should I change the dressing over a PICC line?

Determining when to change the dressing over a peripherally inserted central catheter (PICC) line really depends on your health care facility's policy. Every 3 to 7 days is the norm for transparent film dressings and every 24 to 48 hours is usual for dry sterile dressings. Make sure you use a sterile dressing and sterile technique. Write the type and length of line, the insertion date, the date of the dressing change, and the date of the next change on the dressing.

What shouldn't I do for a patient with a PICC line?

Don't take the patient's blood pressure or draw blood from the arm where the peripherally inserted central catheter (PICC) line was inserted – the blood pressure cuff could damage the catheter or the needle could puncture the catheter.

How do I remove a PICC line?

After taking off the dressing, gently tug on the peripherally inserted central catheter (PICC) line. It should come out easily. If you feel resistance, place tension on the line and tape it down; then try again in a few minutes. You shouldn't have trouble – in fact, PICC lines can fall out easily, which is why anchoring them securely is so important.

What should I do if my patient develops a PICC line problem?

When caring for a patient with a peripherally inserted central catheter (PICC) line, you can anticipate such problems as occlusion; a damaged, broken, or disconnected catheter; inability to infuse fluid; and inability to draw blood. Here's how to intervene appropriately.

DRUG DIFFICULTIES

Occlusion

This problem may indicate thrombus formation or improper flushing. If thrombus formation has occluded the line, try repositioning the patient; then check for flow. If the line hasn't been flushed properly, attempt to aspirate the clot, taking care not to force it. If these measures don't work, notify the doctor; he may wish to increase the flow rate.

Occlusion also may be caused by precipitate that forms when incompatible substances are infused through the line. Infusing thrombolytic agents, such as streptokinase or urokinase, may correct the problem.

Finally, occlusion may occur if the catheter is improperly positioned in the vein or if the catheter tip is against the vessel wall. A possible solution is to remove the catheter. (It may be repositioned in the vein with verification by X-ray.) Be sure to document your interventions.

Damaged or broken catheter

To detect pinholes, leaks, or tears in the catheter, examine for drainage after flushing. Follow the recommended clamping procedure and remove the catheter if ordered.

To prevent this problem, avoid using sharp objects near the catheter and avoid injection of needles larger than 1″ through the injection cap.

Inability to infuse fluid

First check the infusion system and clamps and make sure none of the clamps are closed. If this doesn't work, try changing the patient's position: The catheter may be displaced or kinked.

Finally, inability to infuse fluid may indicate thrombus formation. Have the patient cough, breathe deeply, or perform Valsalva's maneuver. Remove the dressing and examine the external portion of the catheter. If a kink isn't apparent, obtain an X-ray order. Try to withdraw blood. Also try a gentle flush with saline solution.

Inability to draw blood

Inability to draw blood may result from a closed clamp, a displaced or kinked catheter, a thrombus, or catheter movement against the vessel wall with negative pressure. To intervene, first check the infusion system and clamps. Then change the patient's position. Have the patient cough, breathe deeply, or perform Valsalva's maneuver. Remove the dressing and examine the external portion of the catheter. Finally, obtain an X-ray order.

Disconnected catheter

This problem can result from patient movement or from the catheter not being securely connected to the tubing. To intervene, apply a catheter clamp if one is available. Place a sterile syringe or a catheter plug in the catheter hub. Change the extension set. Don't reconnect contaminated tubing. Clean the catheter hub with alcohol or povidone-iodine. Don't soak the hub. Connect clean I.V. tubing or a heparin lock plug to the site. Then restart the infusion.

How can I spot complications of CV therapy?

Complications can occur at any time during central venous (CV) therapy. Generally, though, traumatic complications, such as a punctured subclavian artery, occur during CV catheter insertion; systemic complications such as infection occur later during infusion therapy. Here are some common complications, their signs and symptoms, and possible causes. (For interventions, see *Managing complications of CV therapy*, pages 310 and 311.)

Air embolism
Suspect air embolism if your patient develops low blood pressure; a weak, rapid pulse; and loss of consciousness. Air embolism may be caused by air introduced into the CV circulation during catheter insertion or tubing changes. To help prevent it, have the patient perform Valsalva's maneuver during catheter insertion and removal.

Catheter embolism
Caused by a piece of broken-off catheter, catheter embolism produces cardiac arrhythmias, chest pain, cyanosis, weak pulse, decreased blood pressure, and altered level of consciousness or loss of consciousness.

Clotted catheter
Your patient's catheter may be clotted if you meet resistance when attempting to flush the catheter, or if you're unable to infuse I.V. solutions or medica-

tions. This complication results from blood coagulating in the lumen.

Hydrothorax
Suspect hydrothorax if your patient develops sudden, sharp, needlelike chest pain; a wet cough; and shortness of breath. Auscultation may reveal decreased breath sounds on the affected side. This problem may result if the catheter punctures the lung during insertion or exchange over a guide wire. It may also result from a punctured lymph node and leaking lymphatic fluid or from I.V. solution infiltrating the chest from the catheter.

Infection
You'll recognize infection by its classic signs and symptoms—fever, chills, and malaise—along with nausea and vomiting. Inspection may reveal tenderness, redness, warmth, or swelling at the insertion site. You may also detect drainage at the site and local rash or pustules. Infection may stem from failure to maintain aseptic technique during catheter insertion or maintenance, or failure to comply with dressing change protocol. It may also be caused by immunosuppression, a contaminated catheter or I.V. solution, frequent opening of the catheter, or longterm use of a single I.V. access site.

Pneumothorax
Suspect pneumothorax if your patient develops sudden, sharp, needlelike chest pain; cough; and shortness of breath. Auscultation may reveal decreased breath sounds on the affected

DRUG DIFFICULTIES

Managing complications of CV therapy

Complications that occur during central venous (CV) therapy demand prompt, assured intervention. To manage common problems effectively, follow these guidelines.

Air embolism
• Clamp the catheter immediately.
• Administer 100% oxygen through a nonrebreather face mask to improve oxygen concentration in the blood.
• Place the patient on his left side with his head down. This position displaces the air to the apex of the heart, where the air can be reabsorbed or aspirated.
• Ask another nurse to put the crash cart outside the room and have someone else call the doctor immediately.
• Place a pressure dressing over the original dressing to prevent more air from entering the circulation.

• Be sure to reassure the patient and explain what you're doing; he's probably frightened.

Catheter embolism
• Stop the procedure.
• Prepare the patient for fluoroscopy, as ordered, to locate and retrieve the foreign particle.
• Monitor the patient's electrocardiogram.
• Administer oxygen and turn the patient on his left side with his head down. This position displaces air traveling with the foreign body to the apex of the heart, where the air can be reabsorbed or aspirated.

Clotted catheter
• Clamp the catheter immediately.
• Have the patient change position, or attempt to reposition the catheter by having the patient raise his arms and cough.

side. Pneumothorax may occur if the lung is punctured by the catheter during catheter insertion or exchange over a guide wire.

Punctured subclavian artery
Resulting when the cannulation needle punctures the artery, this complication is heralded by bright-red blood pulsating from the insertion site. Later, hemorrhage, tracheal compression, and respiratory distress may develop.

Venous thrombosis
This complication produces unilateral edema on the side of catheter insertion, beginning at the fingers and progressing to the neck. It may also cause difficulty in maintaining the infusion flow rate and occlusion, signaled by the infusion pump's alarm. Venous thrombosis may stem from sluggish flow rate, preexisting limb edema, infusion of irritating solutions, or preexisting cardiovascular disease.

• Obtain a doctor's order to use urokinase to lyse the clot.

Hydrothorax
• Stop the insertion procedure.
• Apply ointment and a dressing over the insertion site.
• Obtain a chest X-ray (and, possibly, contrast studies).
• Set up equipment and assist with insertion of chest tubes.
• Administer oxygen as ordered.

Infection
• Frequently monitor vital signs, including temperature, to detect infection as soon as possible.
• Obtain blood for culture studies in accordance with hospital policy.
• Provide antibiotic therapy as ordered.

Pneumothorax
• Stop the insertion procedure.

• Apply ointment and a dressing over the insertion site.
• Obtain a chest X-ray.
• Set up equipment and assist with insertion of chest tubes.
• Administer oxygen as ordered.

Punctured subclavian artery
• Remove the cannulation needle.
• Apply digital pressure over the site for 10 minutes.

Venous thrombosis
• Prepare the patient for venography to verify thrombosis.
• Avoid using or removing the catheter.
• Use a peripheral line to begin a continuous heparin infusion as needed or ordered.
• Don't use the limb on the affected side for subsequent venipunctures.
• Apply warm, moist compresses locally.

DRUG DIFFICULTIES

Parenteral nutrition

Parenteral nutrition (PN) involves the infusion of a solution of dextrose, proteins, electrolytes, vitamins, and trace elements in amounts that exceed a patient's energy expenditure. Because the solution is extremely concentrated, it requires special care. When faced with caring for a patient receiving PN, you may find you have many questions.

Also, because many patients may now receive PN at home, you need to be prepared to answer their questions.

Should I use a peripheral or a central vein for PN?

Parenteral nutrition (PN) given through a peripheral vein is indicated for patients who have interrupted enteral intake, but can resume enteral feedings in 5 to 7 days. This route is also indicated for patients with mild to moderate malnutrition, normal or mildly elevated metabolic rate, and no fluid restrictions. You'll need to supplement enteral feedings as ordered.

Use a central venous (CV) line to administer the solution if the patient is unable to tolerate enteral intake for more than 7 days. Also use a CV line for patients with moderate to severe malnutrition that can't be corrected with enteral feedings, moderately or severely elevated metabolic rates, and restricted fluid intake. Finally, use this route if the patient has poor or inaccessible peripheral veins and a readily accessible central vein.

❖

How long is PN solution stable at home?

Some hospitals send patients home on a three-in-one parenteral nutrition (PN) mixture. The patient or pharmacy must then mix all three components (fat, carbohydrates, and amino acids) into one bag. This procedure significantly lowers the cost of home PN, and because the solution isn't premixed, the patient is aware of its exact composition.

If the three-in-one solution is mixed by the pharmacy, it should remain stable for 7 days. But if the patient is preparing the solution, he should mix only 1 day's supply each day. This helps limit the growth of bacteria in case the solution is inadvertently contaminated. It also helps cut down on medication errors.

❖

How often should the site dressing be changed at home?

A dressing made of semipermeable membrane can stay in place for 7 days, while one made of gauze and tape should be changed two to three times a week. Some home parenteral nutrition programs advocate using no dressing.

Change the dressing over the catheter according to the policy at your health care facility, usually every 24 to 72 hours or whenever the dressing becomes wet, soiled, or nonocclusive. Always use strict aseptic technique. When performing dressing changes, watch for signs of phlebitis or catheter retraction from the vein. Measure the catheter length from the insertion site to the hub for verification.

Change the tubing and filters every 24 to 72 hours or according to the policy at your health care facility.

Always document the times of the dressing, filter, and solution changes; the condition of the catheter insertion site; your observations of the patient's condition; and any complications and resulting treatments.

❖

Can I use the PN line for other functions?

Exercise caution when using the parenteral nutrition (PN) line for other purposes. If you're using a single-lumen central venous (CV) catheter, don't use the line to infuse blood or blood products, to give a bolus injection, to administer simultaneous I.V. solutions, to measure CV pressure, or to draw blood for laboratory tests. Never add medication to a PN solution container. Also, don't use a three-way stopcock, if possible, because add-on devices increase the risk of infection. In addition, don't administer PN solution through a pulmonary artery catheter because of the high risk of phlebitis. After infusion, flush the catheter with heparin or 0.9% sodium chloride solution according to the policy of your health care facility.

How can I handle complications of PN?

Catheter-related sepsis is the most serious complication of parenteral nutrition (PN). Although rare, a malpositioned subclavian or jugular vein catheter may lead to thrombosis or sepsis.

An air embolism, a potentially fatal complication, can occur during I.V. tubing changes if the tubing is inadvertently disconnected. An embolism may

also result from undetected hairline cracks in the tubing. Extravasation of PN solution can cause necrosis, with sequential sloughing of the epidermis and dermis. (See *Managing complications of parenteral nutrition*, pages 314 to 317.)

Patient-controlled analgesia

Patient-controlled analgesia allows a patient to control the amount and timing of I.V. analgesic he receives. When using this system, the patient simply presses a button on a delivery device to receive a dose of analgesic. Patients who control their own analgesia typically use less narcotic, experience less pain, and return to normal activities sooner. You'll need to know how, and under what circumstances, to use this system.

Is my patient a good candidate for PCA?

It is essential that patients receiving patient-controlled analgesia (PCA) therapy be mentally alert and able to understand and comply with instructions and procedures. Patients with limited respiratory reserve, a history of drug abuse, or a psychiatric disorder are ineligible for PCA.

(Text continues on page 317.)

DRUG DIFFICULTIES

Managing complications of parenteral nutrition

Patients receiving parenteral nutrition (PN) risk developing certain metabolic, mechanical, and other problems. Use this chart to review common problems associated with PN, their characteristics, and the appropriate interventions.

COMPLICATIONS	SIGNS AND SYMPTOMS	INTERVENTIONS
Metabolic problems		
Hepatic dysfunction	Elevated serum aspartate aminotransferase, alkaline phosphatase, and bilirubin levels	Reduce total caloric and dextrose intake, making up lost calories by administration of lipid emulsion. Change to cyclical infusion. Use specific hepatic formulations only if the patient has encephalopathy.
Hypercapnia	Heightened oxygen consumption, increased carbon dioxide production, measured respiratory quotient of 1 or greater	Reduce total caloric and dextrose intake, and balance dextrose and fat calories.
Hyperglycemia	Fatigue, restlessness, confusion, anxiety, weakness, polyuria, dehydration, elevated serum glucose levels and, in severe hyperglycemia, delirium or coma	Restrict dextrose intake by decreasing either the rate of infusion or the dextrose concentration. Compensate for calorie loss with administration of lipid emulsion. Begin insulin therapy.
Hyperosmolarity	Confusion, seizures, lethargy, hyperosmolar nonketotic syndrome, hyperglycemia, dehydration, and glycosuria	Discontinue dextrose infusion. Administer insulin and 0.45% sodium chloride solution with 10 to 20 mEq/liter of potassium to rehydrate the patient.

DRUG DIFFICULTIES

Managing complications of parenteral nutrition (continued)

COMPLICATIONS	SIGNS AND SYMPTOMS	INTERVENTIONS
Metabolic problems (continued)		
Hypocalcemia	Polyuria, dehydration, and elevated blood and urine glucose levels	Increase calcium supplements.
Hypoglycemia	Sweating, shaking, and irritability after the infusion has stopped	Increase dextrose intake or decrease exogenous insulin intake.
Hypokalemia	Muscle weakness, paralysis, paresthesia, and arrhythmias	Increase potassium supplements.
Hypomagnesemia	Tingling around the mouth, paresthesia in fingers, mental changes, and hyperreflexia	Increase magnesium supplementation.
Hypophosphatemia	Irritability, weakness, paresthesia, coma, and respiratory arrest	Increase phosphate supplements.
Metabolic acidosis	Elevated serum chloride level, reduced serum bicarbonate level	Increase acetate and decrease chloride in PN solution.
Metabolic alkalosis	Diminished serum chloride level, elevated serum bicarbonate level	Decrease acetate and increase chloride in PN solution.
Zinc deficiency	Dermatitis, alopecia, apathy, depression, taste changes, confusion, poor wound healing, and diarrhea	Increase zinc supplements.

DRUG DIFFICULTIES

(continued)

Managing complications of parenteral nutrition (continued)

COMPLICATIONS	SIGNS AND SYMPTOMS	INTERVENTIONS
Mechanical problems		
Clotted I.V. catheter	Interrupted flow rate, resistance to flushing and blood withdrawal	Attempt to aspirate the clot. If unsuccessful, instill urokinase to clear the catheter lumen as ordered.
Cracked or broken tubing	Fluid leaking from the tubing	Apply a padded hemostat above the break to prevent air from entering the line.
Dislodged catheter	Catheter out of the vein	Apply pressure to the site with a sterile gauze pad.
Too-rapid infusion	Nausea, headache, and lethargy	Adjust the infusion rate and, if applicable, check the infusion pump.
Other problems		
Air embolism	Apprehension, chest pain, tachycardia, hypotension, cyanosis, seizures, loss of consciousness, and cardiac arrest	Clamp the catheter. Place the patient in a steep, left lateral Trendelenburg position. Administer oxygen as ordered. If cardiac arrest occurs, begin cardiopulmonary resuscitation. When the catheter is removed, cover the insertion site with a dressing for 24 to 48 hours.
Extravasation	Swelling and pain around the insertion site	Stop the infusion. Assess the patient for cardiopulmonary abnormalities; a chest X-ray may be required.

Managing complications of parenteral nutrition *(continued)*

COMPLICATIONS	SIGNS AND SYMPTOMS	INTERVENTIONS
Other problems *(continued)*		
Phlebitis	Pain, tenderness, redness, and warmth	Apply moist heat at 105° F (40.5° C) to the area, and elevate the insertion site if possible.
Pneumothorax and hydrothorax	Dyspnea, chest pain, cyanosis, and decreased breath sounds	Assist with chest tube insertion and apply suction as ordered.
Septicemia	Red and swollen catheter site, chills, fever, and leukocytosis	Remove the catheter and culture the tip. Obtain a blood culture if the patient has a fever. Give appropriate antibiotics.
Thrombosis	Erythema and edema at the insertion site; ipsilateral swelling of the arm, neck, face, and upper chest; pain at the insertion site and along the vein; malaise; fever; tachycardia	Remove the catheter promptly. If not contraindicated, systemic thrombolytic therapy may be used. Apply warm compresses to the insertion site and elevate the affected extremity. Venous flow studies may be done.

DRUG DIFFICULTIES

How can I best determine bolus doses and lock-out intervals?

Follow these suggestions for determining bolus doses for bolus-only patient-controlled analgesia pumps and lock-out intervals in bolus-only or bolus plus continuous infusion devices.

Determining bolus doses

If the patient has only intermittent pain, simply estimate a dose and increase or decrease it until you determine the amount that relieves pain. Calculate the number of milligrams per dose and the total dose (or number of boluses) that he may receive per hour.

Determining lock-out intervals for bolus doses

For I.V. boluses (whether bolus only or bolus plus continuous infusion), set the lock-out interval for 6 minutes or more. Typically, pain relief following an I.V. narcotic bolus takes 6 to 10 minutes.

For S.C. boluses (whether bolus only or bolus plus continuous infusion), set the lock-out interval for 30 minutes or more. Typically, pain relief following an S.C. bolus takes 30 to 60 minutes.

For spinal boluses (whether bolus only or bolus plus continuous infusion), set the lock-out interval for 60 minutes or more. Typically, pain relief following a spinal bolus takes 30 to 60 minutes.

❖

What should I do if an epidural catheter disconnects from the PCA tubing?

A disconnected catheter from the patient-controlled analgesia (PCA) tubing is a potential conduit for microorganisms to migrate into the epidural space, so your main concerns are preventing an epidural infection and relieving the patient's pain.

Immediate interventions

Do not reconnect the catheter. While you explain to the patient what happened, cover the tip of the catheter with a heparin lock adapter or a sterile dressing and tape the catheter securely to his

back. Have another nurse notify the doctor and get an alternative analgesic for the patient. (Make sure the dosage is equianalgesic.)

Catheter repair or removal

Some hospitals permit only certified nurses to repair or remove epidural catheters. If repair is ordered and you're qualified, put on sterile gloves and, using sterile scissors, cut 1″ (2.5 cm) off the catheter's distal end. Place a new sterile connector tightly on the end. Flush the air out of the new PCA pump catheter tubing; then connect the tubing to the epidural catheter. Tape the catheter tubing to the patient's back.

If removal is ordered and you're qualified to do it, use nonsterile gloves. After carefully removing the butterfly bandages, grasp the catheter close to the insertion site and slowly pull it straight toward you.

If it doesn't come out easily and stretches instead, ask the patient to bend forward at the waist. (This increases the distance between the spinous processes and makes catheter removal easier.) If the catheter still doesn't come out, stop pulling and notify the anesthesiologist.

Aftercare

Once you've removed the catheter, check its proximal tip for a black dot or some similar marking. This indicates that you've gotten all of it. Send the tip for culture and sensitivity testing, and discard the catheter in the needle bin.

Assess the site for redness, swelling, and exudate. Apply antimicrobial ointment on the site and cover it with an adhesive bandage. Document the amount of drug remaining in the infusion device and discard the remaining drug according to hospital protocol.

❖

What should I teach my patient about PCA?

Your patient must understand how patient-controlled analgesia (PCA) works for therapy to succeed. Although some patients receive excellent preoperative teaching, not all patients who receive PCA go through planned surgery. Often you are in the best position to teach him and his family about PCA. And you may have to reinforce your teaching several times.

When your patient plans to receive PCA therapy at home, make sure that he and his family fully understand the method. Explain how the pump works and precisely how he can increase or decrease his dose. Also, make sure that he and his caregivers know when to contact the doctor.

Managing doses
A narcotic analgesic relieves pain best when taken before the pain becomes intense. Stress that the patient shouldn't increase the dose or the frequency of administration. If he misses a dose, he should take it as soon as he remembers. But, if it's almost time for the next dose, tell him to skip the missed dose. Advise the patient never to double-dose.

Using caution
Advise the patient to get up slowly from his bed or a chair because the drug may cause postural hypotension. Instruct him to eat a high-fiber diet, to drink plenty of fluids, and to take a stool softener if one has been prescribed. Caution him against drinking alcohol because this may enhance central nervous system depression.

Calling the doctor
Your patient should notify his doctor if the drug loses its effectiveness. His family should report signs of an overdose: slow or irregular breathing, pinpoint pupils, or loss of consciousness. Teach family members how to maintain respiration until help arrives.

❖

How can I manage complications of PCA?

The primary complication of patient-controlled analgesia (PCA) is respiratory depression. Other complications include anaphylaxis, nausea, vomiting, constipation, postural hypotension, and drug tolerance. Infiltration into the S.C. tissue and catheter occlusion may also occur, and these can cause the drug to back up into the primary I.V. tubing.

Respiratory depression
Watch for respiratory depression during administration. If the patient's respiratory rate declines to 10 or fewer breaths per minute, call his name and touch him. Tell him to breathe deeply.

If he can't be roused, or is confused or restless, notify the doctor and prepare to give oxygen. If ordered, give a narcotic antagonist such as naloxone. Respiratory depression during PCA isn't common. That's because if a patient receives too much narcotic, he'll fall asleep and be unable to press the bolus button. Make sure family or staff members don't give extra doses of the narcotic when a patient hasn't requested them.

Anaphylaxis
In case of anaphylaxis, treat the symptoms and give another drug for pain relief as ordered.

Nausea and vomiting
If a patient has persistent nausea and vomiting during therapy, the doctor may change the medication. If ordered, give the patient an antiemetic such as chlorpromazine.

Constipation
To prevent constipation, give the patient a stool softener and, if necessary, a senna-derivative laxative. Provide a high-fiber diet and encourage the patient to drink fluids. Regular exercise may also help. In case of urine retention, monitor the patient's intake and output.

Postural hypotension
Guard against accidents. Keep the side rails raised on the patient's bed. If the patient is mobile, help him out of bed and assist him in walking. Encourage him to practice coughing and deep breathing to promote ventilation and to prevent pooling of secretions, which could lead to respiratory difficulty.

Drug tolerance
Evaluate the effectiveness of the drug at regular intervals. Is the patient getting relief? Does the dosage need to be increased because of persistent or worse pain? Is the patient developing a tolerance to the drug? Although you should give the smallest effective dose over the shortest time period, narcotic analgesics shouldn't be withheld or given in ineffective doses. Psychological dependence on narcotic analgesics occurs in fewer than 1% of hospitalized patients.

❖

6 Mastering Problematic Procedures

Skin and wound procedures

Cardiopulmonary support

By providing emergency resuscitative support, these procedures restore spontaneous heart rate and respirations and prevent hypoxic damage to the brain and other vital organs.

Managing a code

Responding to a code swiftly and effectively is essential to saving a patient's life. Without such a response, the patient will stop breathing, his heart will stop beating, and his brain and other vital organs will suffer damage from hypoxia. Managing a code successfully requires a team of health care workers trained in advanced cardiac life support (ACLS), although training in basic life support (BLS) may qualify you as part of the team. In most hospitals, ACLS-trained nurses often perform the first resuscitative efforts, administering cardiac medications and performing defibrillation before the doctor arrives. Of course, the scope of your responsibilities in any situation depends on your hospital's policies and procedures and your state's nurse practice act.

Preparation
You, all other personnel, and all requisite equipment must be ready for a code at any time. (See *Organizing your crash cart*, page 324.) You should also be familiar with the cardiac drugs you may have to administer.

Key steps
If you're the first to arrive at a code site, follow these key steps:
• Assess the patient's airway, breathing, circulation, and level of consciousness, and then call for help immediately.
• Begin cardiopulmonary resuscitation (CPR). Use a pocket mask, if available, to ventilate the patient.
• When a second BLS provider arrives, have that person call a code and retrieve the emergency equipment.
• Once the emergency equipment arrives, have the second BLS provider place the cardiac arrest board under the patient and then assist with two-rescuer CPR. Meanwhile, have the nurse assigned to the patient quickly relate the patient's history and any precipitating events.
• A third person, either a nurse certified in BLS or a respiratory therapist, will then attach the hand-held resuscitation bag to the oxygen source and ventilate the patient with 100% oxygen.
• When the ACLS-trained nurse arrives, she'll expose the patient's chest and apply defibrillator pads. She'll then apply the paddles to the patient's chest to quickly check the patient's cardiac rhythm. If the patient is in ventricular fibrillation, ACLS protocol calls for immediate defibrillation with 200 joules. The ACLS-trained nurse will act as code leader until the doctor arrives.
• Apply electrocardiogram electrodes (if not already in place), and attach the patient to the defibrillator's cardiac monitor.

Organizing your crash cart

When responding to a code, you can't waste time searching the drawers of your crash cart for the equipment you need. One way to make sure you know the precise location of everything is to follow the ABCD plan; label the crash cart drawers with the letters A, B, C, and D and fill them as follows.

A: Airway control drawer
This drawer should contain all the equipment necessary for maintaining a patient's airway. It should include oral, nasal, and endotracheal airways; an intubation tray containing a laryngoscope and blades; an extra laryngoscope; lidocaine ointment; tape; a 10-ml syringe to inflate the endotracheal balloon; extra batteries and light bulbs; and suction devices.

B: Breathing drawer
This drawer should contain all of the equipment needed to support the patient's oxygenation and ventilation. Oxygenation is maintained with nasal cannulas, face masks, and Venturi masks. Ventilation is supported by maintaining gastric compression with nasogastric tubes.

C: Circulation drawer
In this drawer, place anything needed to start a central or peripheral I.V. line, such as catheters, tubing, start kits, pump tubing, and 250-ml or 500-ml bags of I.V. solutions (dextrose 5% in water and 0.9% sodium chloride solution).

D: Drug drawer
This drawer should contain all medications needed for advanced cardiac life support.

Avoid placing electrodes on bony prominences and hairy areas. Also avoid the defibrillator pads and areas where chest compressions will be given.
• As CPR continues, you or an ACLS-trained nurse will then start two peripheral I.V. lines with large-bore I.V. catheters. Use only a large vein, such as the antecubital vein, to allow for rapid fluid administration and to prevent drug extravasation.
• As soon as the I.V. catheter is in place, begin an infusion of 0.9% sodium chloride solution or lactated Ringer's solution to help prevent circulatory collapse. Recent ACLS guidelines encourage the use of 0.9% sodium chloride solution or lactated Ringer's solution—not dextrose 5% in water (D_5W)—because D_5W can provoke hyperglycemia during cardiac arrest.
• While one nurse starts the I.V. lines, the other nurse will set up portable or wall suction equipment and suction oral secretions to maintain an open airway.

• The ACLS-trained nurse will then prepare and administer emergency cardiac drugs as needed. Drugs administered through a central line reach the myocardium more quickly than those given through a peripheral line.

• If the patient doesn't have an accessible I.V. line, administer medications such as epinephrine, lidocaine, and atropine through an endotracheal (ET) tube. Dilute the drugs in 10 ml of 0.9% sodium chloride solution or sterile water and then instill them into the ET tube. Afterward, manually ventilate the patient to distribute the drug throughout the bronchial tree, to aid absorption.

• The ACLS-trained nurse will also prepare for, and assist with, ET intubation. Don't interrupt CPR for longer than 30 seconds during intubation.

• After the patient has been intubated, assess his breath sounds to ensure proper tube placement, and suction as needed. If the patient has diminished or absent breath sounds over the left lung field, the doctor will pull back the ET tube slightly and reassess. When the tube is correctly positioned, tape it securely. To serve as a reference, mark the point on the tube that's level with the patient's lips.

• Throughout the code, check the patient's carotid or femoral pulses before and after each defibrillation. Also check the pulses frequently during the code to evaluate the effectiveness of cardiac compressions.

Special considerations

During the code, you or another team member must document the events in as much detail as possible. Note whether the arrest was witnessed or unwitnessed, the time of the arrest, the time CPR was begun, the time the ACLS-trained nurse arrived, and the total resuscitation time. Also document the number of defibrillations, the times they were performed, the joule level, the patient's cardiac rhythm before and after the defibrillation, and whether or not the patient had a pulse.

Other duties include prompting participants about when to perform certain activities, such as checking the pulse and taking vital signs, overseeing the effectiveness of CPR, and keeping track of the time between therapies. Each team member should also know every other member's role to prevent duplicating efforts. Finally, someone from the team should make sure that the primary nurse's other patients are reassigned to another nurse.

Document all drug therapy, including dosages, routes of administration, and patient response. Record all procedures, such as peripheral and central line insertion, pacemaker insertion, and ET tube insertion, with the time performed and the patient's tolerance of the procedure. Also keep track of all arterial blood gas results.

Finally, document any complications and the measures taken to correct them. Once your documentation is complete, have the doctor and ACLS-trained nurse review and then sign the document.

❖

Opening an airway

The basic cardiopulmonary resuscitation procedure begins with ensuring that the patient's airway is open. Remember, if you suspect a head or neck injury, move the patient as little as possible to reduce the risk of paralysis.

Preparation

Place the patient in the supine position on a hard, flat surface. When moving him, roll his head and torso as a unit. Avoid twisting or pulling his neck, shoulders, or hips. Kneel near the patient's shoulders. This position will give you easy access to his head and chest.

Key steps

Remember that the back of the tongue and the epiglottis commonly obstruct the airway of an unconscious patient.

If the patient doesn't appear to have a neck injury, use the head-tilt, chin-lift maneuver to open his airway. Place one hand on the patient's forehead and tilt the patient's head back. Next, place the fingertips of your other hand under the bony part, never the soft tissue, of his lower jaw near the chin. Placing your fingertips on the soft tissue may inadvertently obstruct the airway you're trying to open. Now lift the patient's chin, keeping his mouth partially open, to open his airway.

If you suspect a neck injury, use the jaw-thrust maneuver instead of the head-tilt, chin-lift maneuver. (See *Two maneuvers to open a patient's airway.*)

Kneel at the patient's head with your elbows on the ground. Rest your thumbs on his lower jaw near the corners of his mouth, with your thumb pointing toward his feet. Then place your fingertips around the lower jaw. To open the airway, lift the lower jaw with your fingertips. Tilting the head back and moving the lower jaw (chin) forward lifts the tongue and the epiglottis from the back of the throat and usually opens the airway. ❖

Clearing an obstructed airway

A patient with an obstructed airway (due to a foreign body lodged in the throat or bronchus) will be unable to speak, cough, or breathe. Your interventions will depend on the degree of obstruction and the patient's age, weight, and level of consciousness.

Preparation

Determine a conscious patient's degree of obstruction by tapping his shoulder and asking, "Are you choking?" If he makes crowing noises, his airway is partially obstructed, and you should encourage him to cough. This will either clear the airway or make the obstruction complete. If he has complete airway obstruction, he won't be able to answer because the obstruction will block airflow to his vocal cords.

Two maneuvers to open a patient's airway

Depending on the circumstances, you may use one of two methods to open a patient's airway. When performing cardiopulmonary resuscitation, you'll typically use the head-tilt, chin-lift maneuver, illustrated below left. However, if you suspect a neck injury, use the jaw-thrust maneuver, as shown below right. This maneuver opens the patient's airway without moving his head.

Head-tilt, chin-lift maneuver

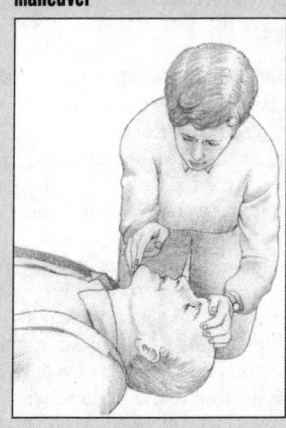

Jaw-thrust maneuver

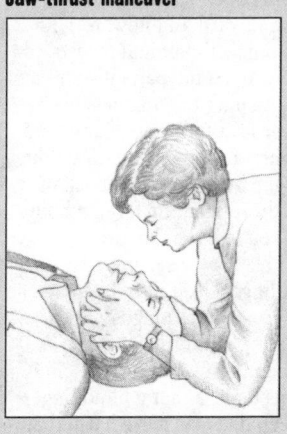

Key steps

If the patient is conscious, use the abdominal thrust maneuver to dislodge the obstruction. This maneuver creates enough diaphragmatic pressure in the static lung below the foreign body to expel the obstruction.

If the patient is unconscious, perform an abdominal thrust followed by a finger-sweep maneuver to manually remove the foreign body from the patient's mouth.

Conscious adult

• First, tell a conscious adult you're going to try to dislodge the foreign body.
• Then, standing behind the patient, wrap your arms around his waist. Make a fist with one hand and press your thumb against his abdomen, slightly above the umbilicus but well below the xiphoid process. Then grasp your fist with the other hand.
• Press the patient's abdomen with quick inward and upward thrusts. Each thrust must be separate, distinct, and forceful enough to create an artificial

cough to dislodge an obstruction. The thrusts should be repeated until the foreign body is expelled or the victim becomes unconscious.

Unconscious adult
• First, kneel astride the patient's thighs.
• Then, place the heel of one hand on top of the other. Place your hands between the patient's umbilicus and the tip of his xiphoid process at the midline. Push inward and upward with five quick abdominal thrusts.
• Now open the patient's airway by grasping the tongue and lower jaw with your thumb and fingers. Lift the jaw to draw the tongue away from the back of the throat and the foreign body.
• If you can see the foreign body, remove it by inserting your index finger deep into the throat at the base of the tongue with a hooking motion.
• Keep in mind that some clinicians believe that a blind finger-sweep does far more harm than good, because your finger acts as a second obstruction. They believe that if you cannot see the foreign body, the tongue-jaw lift should be enough to dislodge the obstruction.

Obese or pregnant adult
• If the patient is conscious, stand behind her and place your arms under her armpits and around her chest.
• Place the thumb side of your clenched fist against the middle of the sternum, avoiding the margins of the ribs and the xiphoid process. Grasp your fist with your other hand and perform chest thrusts with enough force to expel the foreign body.

• If you are unsuccessful and the patient loses consciousness, carefully lower her to the floor.
• Then kneel close to her side and place the heel of one hand just above the bottom of her sternum. The long axis of the heel of your hand should align with the long axis of the patient's sternum. Place the heel of your other hand on top of that, making sure your fingers don't touch the patient's chest. Deliver each thrust forcefully enough to remove the obstruction.

Conscious or unconscious child
• If the child is conscious and can stand, perform up to five quick, upward, abdominal thrusts using the same technique that you would with an adult, but with less force.
• If he's unconscious or lying down, kneel at his feet; if he's a large child, kneel astride his thighs. If he's lying on an examination table, stand by his side. Deliver up to five abdominal thrusts as you would for an adult patient, but with less force. Then attempt to ventilate the patient.

Conscious or unconscious infant
• Place a conscious or unconscious infant face down so he's straddling your arm with his head lower than his trunk. Rest your forearm on your thigh and strike the infant up to five times with the heel of your hand between his shoulder blades.
• If this maneuver doesn't remove the obstruction, place your free hand on the infant's back. Supporting his neck, jaw, and chest with your other hand, turn him over onto your thigh. Keep his head lower than his trunk.

• Draw an imaginary line between the infant's nipples and place the index finger of your free hand on his sternum, just below this line. Now place the middle and ring fingers of your free hand next to your index finger and lift your index finger off his chest. Deliver up to five chest thrusts as you would for a child, but more slowly.

• If the infant vomits while you are performing these abdominal thrusts, quickly wipe out his mouth with your fingers.

• Continue the sequence of performing back blows, chest thrusts, and mouth checks until the infant breathes. Even if your efforts to clear the airway don't seem to be effective, keep trying. As oxygen deprivation increases, smooth and skeletal muscles relax, making your maneuvers more likely to succeed.

Special considerations

Don't perform these maneuvers if the patient has an incomplete or a partial airway obstruction or if he can breathe well enough to dislodge the foreign body by coughing. Also, don't perform the abdominal thrust if the patient is pregnant, is markedly obese, or has recently undergone abdominal surgery. For such patients, use a chest-thrust maneuver, which forces air out of the lungs to create an artificial cough.

Positioning your hands for CPR chest compression

Positioning your hands is crucial to safe, effective cardiopulmonary resuscitation (CPR). Study the following illustrations for proper hand placement on an adult, a child, and an infant.

Adult

Slide your fingers along the lower rib margin to the notch where the ribs and sternum meet.

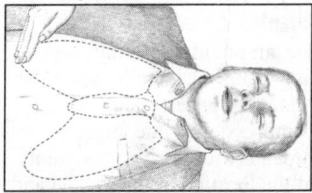

Place your middle finger on this spot.

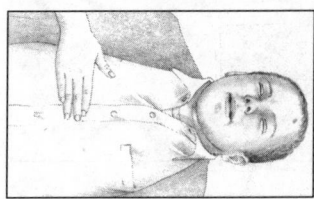

Then place the heel of your other hand on the sternum, one fingerbreadth above the middle finger.

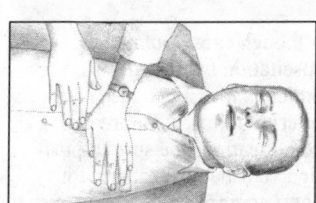

Child

Move your fingertips along the lower rib margin to the notch where the ribs and sternum meet. Place your middle finger on the notch and your index finger next to your middle finger. Then place the heel of the other hand next to the index finger.

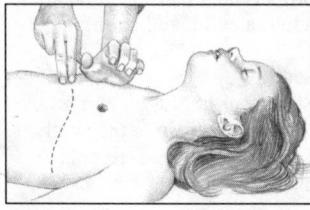

Infant

For an infant, place the index finger of your hand between the infant's nipples. The area of compression is one finger-breadth width below this point, at the location of the middle and ring fingers.

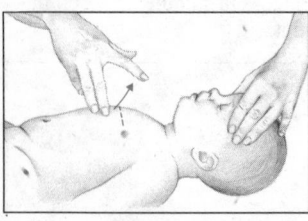

Avoiding CPR hazards

Although cardiopulmonary re-suscitation (CPR) can save your patient's life, it can also cause internal injuries. To prevent complications, be sure to position your hands properly for chest compressions. If you suspect any of the following compli-cations, notify the doctor – but don't stop CPR – and follow these immediate treatment guidelines.

Fractured rib

Once the patient's condition stabilizes, you can detect fractured ribs by palpating for bone displacement and crepitus (a crunching sound). The patient will need rest and analgesics for a fractured rib. If he has a serious fracture, his rib cage may need to be splinted.

Lacerated liver

Although rare, liver laceration from CPR can trigger hemorrhage, resulting in shock and abdominal distention. You may have trouble distinguishing it from shock caused by respiratory or cardiac arrest. If you suspect liver laceration, tell the doctor. After the patient's condition stabilizes, the doctor may order diagnostic studies such as peritoneal fluid analysis. Treatment includes fluid resuscitation and surgical repair.

Punctured lung

If a broken rib punctures the patient's lung, a tension pneumothorax may develop. In this complication, air enters – but can't escape – the pleural space. Positive pressure then builds in the thoracic cavity and collapses the lung.

Other signs of a tension pneumothorax include asymmetrical chest movement, no breath sounds on the side of the pneumothorax and, as the condition grows worse, a shift of the trachea away from the affected side. A chest X-ray confirms the diagnosis.

Treatment involves inserting a chest tube or a large-bore needle into the pleural space (at about the second intercostal space) to relieve the pressure caused by trapped air.

Distended stomach

A common and seemingly trivial complication of CPR, gastric distention results from delivering too much air during ventilation. Gastric distention can promote regurgitation, thereby increasing the risk of aspiration.

If you notice the patient's stomach becoming distended during CPR, immediately retilt his head, thus repositioning his airway. Then make sure that his chest, not his stomach, rises and falls during ventilation. If retilting isn't effective, turn the patient on his side and apply pressure over the epigastrium to induce regurgitation. (The need for a continued air supply overrides the risk of aspiration.) In the unconscious patient, sweep out the airway or suction it, and continue CPR.

❖

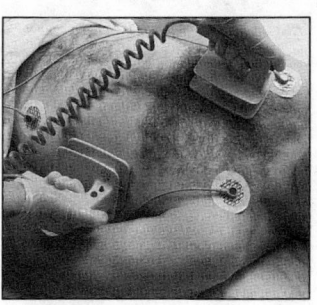

Key steps

Place the paddles as follows:
• Expose the patient's chest.
• Apply conductive pads at the paddle placement positions shown above.

❖

Placing defibrillator paddles correctly

When positioning defibrillator paddles, place one paddle to the right of the upper sternum, just below the right clavicle. Place the other paddle at the fifth or sixth intercostal space in the left anterior axillary line. This position is known as the standard or anterolateral position.

Conducting synchronized cardioversion

Used to treat tachyarrhythmias, cardioversion delivers an electrical charge to the myocardium at the peak of the R wave. This causes immediate depolarization, interrupting reentry circuits and allowing the sinoatrial node to resume control. Synchronizing the electrical charge with the R wave ensures that the current won't be delivered on the vulnerable T wave and disrupt repolarization.

Synchronized cardioversion is the treatment of choice for atrial tachycardia, atrial flutter, atrial fibrillation, or symptomatic ventricular tachycardia that doesn't respond to vagal massage or drug therapy. Cardioversion may be elective or urgent, depending on how well the patient tolerates the arrhythmia. Left untreated, persistently rapid heart rates or highly irregular rhythms may impair cardiac output.

Preparation

Check the patient's recent serum potassium and magnesium levels, digoxin levels, and arterial blood gas results. Patients taking digitalis glycosides tend to require lower energy levels to convert; if the patient is taking digoxin, withhold the dose the day of the procedure. Also withhold all food and fluids for 6 to 12 hours before the procedure.

Obtain a 12-lead electrocardiogram (ECG) to serve as a baseline, check whether or not the doctor has ordered administration of any cardiac drugs before the procedure, and verify that the I.V. line is patent in case drug administration becomes necessary. Connect the patient to a pulse oximeter and an automatic blood pressure cuff if available.

Now place the patient in the supine position, and assess his vital signs, level of consciousness, cardiac rhythm, and peripheral pulses. Remove any oxygen delivery equipment just before cardioversion to avoid combustion. Have epinephrine, lidocaine, and atropine available at the patient's bedside.

Key steps

If hospital protocol permits you to perform cardioversion, follow these key steps:
• Administer a sedative as ordered. Ensure that the patient can breathe adequately. Carefully monitor his blood pressure and respiratory rate until he recovers from the procedure.

• Press the POWER button to turn on the defibrillator. Next, push the SYNC button to synchronize the machine with the patient's QRS complexes; it should flash with each QRS complex.
• Turn the energy SELECT dial to the ordered amount of energy. Advanced cardiac life support protocols call for delivery of 50 to 360 joules for a patient with stable paroxysmal atrial tachycardia, 75 to 360 joules for a patient with unstable paroxysmal supraventricular tachycardia, 100 joules for a patient with atrial fibrillation, 50 joules for a patient with atrial flutter, 100 to 360 joules for a patient who has ventricular tachycardia with a pulse, and 200 to 360 joules for a patient with ventricular tachycardia with no pulse.
• Remove the paddles from the machine and prepare them as you would if you were defibrillating the patient. Place the conductive gel pads or paddles in the same positions as you would to defibrillate.
• Make sure everyone is clear of the bed; then push the discharge buttons. Hold the paddles in place and wait for the energy to be discharged – the machine has to synchronize the discharge with the QRS complex.
• Check the waveform on the monitor. If the arrhythmia fails to convert, repeat the procedure two to three more times at 3-minute intervals. Gradually increase the energy level with each additional countershock.

Special considerations

If the patient is attached to a bedside monitor or telemetry device, disconnect the unit before cardioversion. The electric current could damage the equipment.

Improper synchronization may result if the patient's ECG tracing contains artifact-like spikes, such as peaked T waves or bundle-branch blocks when the R' wave is taller than the R wave.

If the patient develops ventricular fibrillation or ventricular tachycardia and doesn't have a pulse, turn off the synchronizer switch on the cardioverter and defibrillate the patient. Have emergency medications available.

Hypokalemia, hypomagnesemia, acute myocardial ischemia, and digitalis or quinidine toxicity may increase the risk of ventricular fibrillation following cardioversion.

Although the electric shock of cardioversion won't usually damage an implanted pacemaker, avoid placing the paddles directly over the pacemaker. If the paddles have been recharged but you're not going to use them, clear the charge by turning the machine off, adjusting the energy selector dial, or placing the paddles in their protective housing and discharging them into the machine—never against each other or into the air.

Cardioversion is not recommended for patients with digitalis toxicity, but it may sometimes be necessary for severe arrhythmias. Administer a bolus dose of 50 to 100 mg of lidocaine immediately before cardioversion.

Cardiovascular procedures

Because cardiovascular problems are among the most likely to affect your patient, you'll perform cardiovascular procedures most often. Of the procedures that follow, vagal maneuvers aim to slow an accelerated heart rate, while autologous transfusion aims to reinfuse the patient's own blood safely.

Performing vagal maneuvers

Vagal maneuvers, including Valsalva's maneuver and carotid sinus massage, stimulate nerve endings, which in turn stimulate the autonomic nervous system to increase vagal tone and decrease the heart rate. They're usually performed at the patient's bedside, either by a specially trained nurse or a doctor. If you don't perform the maneuver, your job is to prepare the patient, gather the necessary equipment, assist the doctor, and monitor for complications.

Valsalva's maneuver and carotid sinus massage are contraindicated for patients with severe coronary artery disease, acute myocardial infarction, or hypovolemia. Carotid sinus massage is contraindicated for patients with digitalis toxicity or cerebrovascular disease and for patients who've had carotid surgery.

Complications

Possible complications of Valsalva's maneuver include bradycardia accompanied by a decrease in cardiac output, possibly leading to syncope. This maneuver can also mobilize venous thrombi and provoke bleeding.

Possible complications of carotid sinus massage include ventricular fibrillation, ventricular tachycardia, and ventricular standstill as well as worsening atrioventricular block leading to junctional or ventricular escape rhythms. Carotid sinus massage can also cause cerebral damage from inadequate tissue perfusion (especially in elderly patients) or cerebrovascular accident from decreased perfusion.

Key steps

To perform vagal maneuvers properly, follow these essential steps.

Valsalva's maneuver

Your role in this maneuver consists of instructing and monitoring the patient, as follows:
• Tell the patient to take a deep breath, hold it, and then bear down, as if trying to defecate. If he doesn't feel light-headed or dizzy, and if no new arrhythmias occur, have him hold that breath and bear down for 10 seconds.
• If he does feel dizzy or light-headed, or if you see a new arrhythmia on the monitor, asystole for more than 6 seconds, frequent premature ventricular contractions (PVCs), ventricular tachycardia, or ventricular fibrillation, tell the patient to stop the maneuver.
• After 10 seconds, ask the patient to exhale and breathe normally. If the maneuver was successful, the monitor will show his heart rate slowing before he exhales.

Carotid sinus massage

If you're trained to perform this procedure, your role includes massaging the patient's carotid sinus artery and monitoring his electrocardiogram (ECG), as follows:
• Obtain a rhythm strip, using the lead showing the strongest P waves.
• Auscultate both carotid sinuses. If you detect bruits, don't proceed.
• Before applying manual pressure to the patient's right carotid sinus, locate the bifurcation of the carotid artery on the right side of the neck.
• Turn the patient's head slightly to the left and hyperextend the neck. This brings the carotid artery closer to the skin and moves the sternocleidomastoid muscle away from the carotid artery.
• Now, using a circular motion, gently massage the right carotid sinus between your fingers and the transverse processes of the spine for 3 to 5 seconds. Don't massage for more than 5 seconds to avoid life-threatening complications.
• If the procedure has no effect within 5 seconds, stop massaging the right carotid sinus and start massaging the left. If this also fails. the doctor may administer a cardiotonic drug. Remember that a brief period of asystole – from 3 to 6 seconds – and several PVCs may precede conversion to normal sinus rhythm.

Special considerations

Monitor the patient's ECG throughout the procedure. If it indicates complete heart block or asystole, start basic life support at once, if you're trained to do so.

Proceed cautiously when performing carotid sinus massage on elderly patients, patients receiving digitalis glycosides, and those with heart block, hypertension, diabetes mellitus, or hyperkalemia. The procedure may cause arterial pressure to plummet in these patients (particularly elderly patients with heart disease), although it usually rises quickly afterward. Have the crash cart handy for emergency treatment if a dangerous arrhythmia occurs.

Monitor the patient's cardiac rhythm closely. Vagal maneuvers also occasionally cause bradycardia or complete heart block. Bradycardia will usually pass quickly; if it doesn't, or if it advances to complete heart block or asystole, begin basic life support and, if necessary, advanced cardiac life support.

————————————❖

Managing autologous transfusion

Also called autotransfusion, autologous transfusion is the collection, filtration, and reinfusion of the patient's own blood. The procedure is performed before, during, or after surgery and after traumatic injury. It is safer than blood bank transfusions, which can cause transfusion reactions and transmit diseases such as human immunodeficiency virus and hepatitis, although these occurrences are rare. However, autologous transfusion may still provoke citrate toxicity, coagulation, emboli, sepsis, and other hazards.

The three techniques used for autologous transfusion are preoperative blood donation, perioperative blood donation, and acute normovolemic hemodilution.

Preoperative blood donation is commonly recommended for patients scheduled for orthopedic surgery, which causes large blood loss. The donation period begins 4 to 6 weeks before surgery. The patient can donate blood at a rate of one unit every 7 days until 3 to 7 days before surgery. Beginning at least 1 week before the first donation, the patient takes ferrous sulfate or another iron preparation three times a day. Before donating blood, his hemoglobin level must be 11 g/dl or above and he should drink plenty of fluids to prevent hypovolemia.

Perioperative blood donation (sometimes called intraoperative or postoperative) is used in vascular and orthopedic surgery and in treatment of traumatic injury. Blood may be collected during surgery or up to 12 hours afterward. It's transfused immediately after collection or processed (washed) before infusion.

Blood obtained postoperatively may be collected from chest tubes, mediastinal drains, or wound drains (placed in the surgical wound during surgery). Commonly inserted during orthopedic surgery, wound drains can be used when enough uncontaminated blood is recovered from a closed wound to reinfuse.

Acute normovolemic hemodilution is used mainly in open-heart surgery. One or two units of blood are drawn immediately before or after anesthesia induction. The blood is replaced with a crystalloid or colloid solution, such as lactated Ringer's solution or 5% dextran, to produce normovolemic anemia. The blood is reinfused right after surgery.

Autologous transfusion is contraindicated in patients with malignant neoplasms, coagulopathies, excessive hemolysis, or active infections; in patients taking antibiotics, whose blood is contaminated by abdominal contents; and in patients who've recently lost weight because of illness or malnutrition.

Complications

Patients undergoing autologous transfusion risk developing such problems as coagulation, coagulopathies, emboli, hemolysis, sepsis and, rarely, citrate toxicity. The causes of these problems and appropriate interventions are listed below.

Coagulation

This complication may result if the blood doesn't contain enough anticoagulant or isn't defibrinated in the mediastinum. To correct the problem, add citrate phosphate dextrose (CPD) or another regional anticoagulant at a ratio of seven parts blood to one part anticoagulant. Keep blood and CPD mixed by shaking the collection bottle regularly. Check for anticoagulant reversal. Strip chest tubes as needed.

Coagulopathies

This problem occurs when platelet and fibrinogen levels are reduced, when platelets are caught in filters, and when levels of fibrin split products are increased. Patients receiving autologous transfusions of more than 4,000 ml of blood may also need transfusion of fresh frozen plasma or platelet concentrate.

Emboli

Caused by the presence of microaggregate debris or air in the blood, emboli can be prevented by not using equipment with roller pumps or pressure infusion systems. Always remove air from blood bags before reinfusion, and reinfuse with a 20- to 40-unit microaggregate filter.

Hemolysis

This problem results from trauma to the blood caused by turbulence or roller pumps. To prevent hemolysis, don't skim the operative field or use equipment with roller pumps. When collecting blood from chest tubes, keep the vacuum below 30 mm Hg; when aspirating from a surgical site, keep the vacuum below 60 mm Hg.

Sepsis

This complication may be caused by the lack of aseptic technique during the procedure or the use of contaminated blood. To intervene, give broad-spectrum antibiotics and use strict aseptic technique. Reinfuse blood within 4 hours. Don't infuse blood drawn from infected areas or blood with feces, urine, or other contaminants.

Citrate toxicity

A rare, unpredictable complication, citrate toxicity may result from the chelating effect on calcium of citrate in the CPD. Predisposing factors include hyperkalemia, hypocalcemia, acidosis, hypothermia, myocardial dysfunction, and liver or kidney problems. To intervene, watch for hypotension, arrhythmias, and myocardial contractility. Prophylactic calcium chloride may be administered if more than 2,000 ml of CPD-anticoagulated blood has been given over 20 minutes. Stop infusing CPD and correct acidosis. Measure arterial blood gas and serum calcium levels frequently to assess for toxicity.

Key steps

To perform autologous transfusion safely, follow these key steps.

For preoperative blood donation

• Check vital signs before blood donation.
• Help the patient into a supine position.
• Clean the needle insertion site (usually the antecubital fossa) with povidone-iodine solution and then with alcohol.
• Apply a tourniquet.
• Insert a large-bore needle into the antecubital vein. Have the patient squeeze a rubber ball while you collect blood.
• Recheck vital signs after the collection.
• Send a blood sample to the hospital laboratory to be tested.
• Before reinfusion, check vital signs again and make sure that the I.V. line is patent.
• Administer blood over 1½ to 4 hours, depending on the patient's cardiovascular status and hospital policy.

For perioperative blood donation using the Pleur-evac connected to a chest tube

• Establish underwater seal drainage. Following the steps printed on the Pleur-evac unit, connect the patient's chest tube. Inspect the blood collection bag and tubing, making sure that all clamps are open and all connections are airtight.
• Before collection, add an anticoagulant such as heparin or CPD if prescribed. With CPD, add one part to seven parts blood. The system is now ready to use. You should see chest cavity blood begin to collect in the bag.
• To collect more than one bag of blood, open a replacement bag when the first one is nearly full. Close the clamps on top of the second bag. Before removing the first collection bag from the drainage unit, reduce excess negativity by using the high-negativity relief valve. Depress the button; then release it when negativity drops to the desired level (watch the water seal manometer).
• Close the white clamp on the patient tubing. Then close the two white clamps on top of the collection bag.
• Disconnect all connectors on the first bag. Attach the red (female) and blue (male) connector sections on top of the autologous transfusion bag.
• Remove the protective cap from the collection tubing on the replacement bag. Connect the collection tubing to the patient's drainage tube, using the red connectors.

• Remove the protective cap from the replacement bag's suction tube and attach the suction tube to the Pleur-evac unit, using the blue connectors. Make sure all connections are tight. Open all clamps, and inspect the system for airtight connections.

• Spread the metal support arms and disconnect them. Remove the first bag from the drainage unit by disconnecting the foot hook.

• Use the foot hook and support arm to attach the replacement bag.

• To reinfuse blood from the original collection bag, slide the bag off the support frame; then invert it so that the spike points upward.

• Remember to reinfuse blood within 6 hours of the start of collection. Never store collected blood.

• Remove the protective cap from the spike port and insert a microaggregate filter into the port, using a twisting motion. Prime the filter by gently squeezing the inverted bag. A new filter should be used with each bag.

• Continue squeezing until the filter is saturated and the drip chamber is half full. Then close the clamp on the reinfusion line and remove residual air from the bag. Invert the bag and suspend it from an I.V. pole.

• After carefully flushing the I.V. line to remove all air, infuse blood according to your hospital's policy.

For acute normovolemic hemodilution

Acute normovolemic hemodilution is performed the same way as preoperative blood donation, and blood collected this way is reinfused the same way as any other transfusion.

Special considerations

Make sure that the patient isn't bacteremic when he donates blood. Bacteria can proliferate in the collection bag and cause sepsis when reinfused.

Be alert for signs and symptoms of a hemolytic reaction: pain at the I.V. site, fever, chills, back pain, hypotension, and anxiety. If any of these signs and symptoms occur, stop the transfusion and call the blood bank and doctor. The patient may have received the wrong unit of blood.

Monitor the patient closely during and after donation and autologous transfusion to prevent vasovagal reactions. Although vasovagal reactions are usually mild and easy to treat, they can quickly progress to severe reactions, such as loss of consciousness and seizures.

Check the patient's laboratory data (coagulation profile and hemoglobin, hematocrit, and calcium levels) after he donates blood and again after reinfusion.

Clearly label the collection bag: AUTOLOGOUS USE ONLY. This way, the blood won't be subjected to rigorous blood bank testing or be accidentally given to another patient.

Before reinfusion, identify the patient and make sure that the collection bag is clearly marked with his name, the hospital identification number, and an autologous blood label.

Document the amount of blood that the patient donated and had reinfused and how he tolerated each procedure.

For preoperative blood donation

Caution the patient to remain supine for at least 10 minutes after donating blood.

Encourage him to drink more fluids than usual for a few hours after blood donation and to eat heartily at his next meal.

Tell him to keep an eye on the needle wound in his arm for a few hours after blood donation. If some bleeding occurs, he should apply firm pressure for 5 to 10 minutes. If the bleeding doesn't stop, he should notify the blood bank or his doctor.

If the patient feels lightheaded or dizzy, advise him to sit down immediately and to lower his head between his knees. Or he can lie down with his head lower than the rest of his body until the light-headed feeling subsides.

Tell him that he can resume normal activities after resting 15 minutes.

───────────────── ❖

Respiratory procedures

Impaired respiration generally causes one or all of these physiologic dysfunctions: ineffective airway clearance, ineffective or abnormal breathing patterns, and impaired gas exchange. The respiratory procedures described here aim to establish an airway when all other attempts fail, to manually and mechanically ventilate a patient who can't breathe for himself, to provide oxygen, to suction secretions blocking the airway, and to restore negative pressure in the pleural cavity to keep the lungs expanded.

Mastering manual ventilation

In this procedure, oxygen or room air is manually delivered to the lungs of a patient who can't breathe on his own. The procedure uses a hand-held resuscitation bag – an inflatable device that can be attached to a face mask or directly to an endotracheal or tracheostomy tube. Manual ventilation is usually performed in an emergency but may also be used while a patient is temporarily disconnected from a mechanical ventilator – for example, during a tubing change, while being moved, before suctioning, or after each pass of the suction catheter. Using the hand-held resuscitation bag maintains ventilation. Oxygen administration with a resuscitation bag improves oxygenation.

Complications

Manual ventilation may result in complications, including gastric distention from air forced into the patient's stomach, that cause vomiting, aspiration, and pneumonia. Other possible complications include aggravated cervical injury and underventilation, leading to hypoxia and hypoxemia. Underventilation commonly occurs because it's difficult to keep the hand-held resuscitation bag positioned tightly on the patient's face while maintaining an open airway. What's more, the volume of air delivered to the patient varies with the type of bag used and the hand size of the person compressing the bag.

Key steps

To perform manual ventilation, follow these key steps:

• Connect a hand-held resuscitation bag to an oxygen source with a reservoir if possible. Reservoirs increase the concentration of inspired oxygen.

• Attach a face mask to the hand-held resuscitation bag.

• Position the patient's head using the head-tilt, chin-lift maneuver to open the airway. Then place the mask against the patient's face and, with your nondominant hand, exert downward pressure to prevent leakage of air and oxygen. Make sure that the patient's mouth is open underneath the bag.

• Alternatively, if the patient has an endotracheal or tracheostomy tube, attach the hand-held resuscitation bag directly to the tube.

• With the resuscitation bag in place, compress the bag once every 5 seconds in an adult patient or once every 4 seconds in an infant or child.

• Observe the patient's chest to ensure that it rises and falls with each compression of the hand-held resuscitation bag.

Special considerations

Observe for vomiting through the clear part of the mask. If vomiting occurs, stop the procedure immediately, lift the mask, wipe and suction the vomitus, and resume resuscitation.

Avoid neck hyperextension if the patient could have a cervical injury; instead, use the jaw-thrust technique to open the airway. If you need both hands to keep the patient's mask in place and maintain hyperextension, have another person compress the bag, or use the lower part of your arm to compress the bag against your side.

To guard against underventilation, have someone assist with the procedure if possible.   ❖

Managing tracheotomy

If all other attempts to create an airway have failed, the doctor may perform a tracheotomy at the patient's bedside. In this emergency procedure, an external opening in the trachea – called a tracheostomy – is surgically created and an indwelling tube is inserted to maintain the airway's patency.

Contraindications to tracheotomy include patient refusal and bleeding tendencies. The procedure can cause airway obstruction, which may occur at any time after tube placement. The obstruction may result from improper tube placement or from dry mucus secretions in the inner lumen of the tracheostomy tube. (See *Preventing a tracheostomy obstruction.*)

Preventing a tracheostomy obstruction

Help prevent a future obstruction episode by monitoring the patient for tenacious, blood-tinged tracheal mucus, a telltale whistling sound, and decreased airflow at the stoma during respirations.

Keep his secretions liquefied by ensuring that he's well hydrated and that any oxygen received is humidified. If he's not receiving oxygen, use an ultrasonic humidifier.

Have the patient routinely perform coughing and deep-breathing exercises to mobilize secretions and facilitate expectoration. If the exercises don't mobilize secretions, you can try routine chest physiotherapy.

Complications

Potential complications from surgery include hemorrhage, edema, a perforated esophagus, subcutaneous or mediastinal emphysema, infection, and lacerations of arteries, veins, or nerves. Removing a partially expelled tracheostomy tube may close the airway completely, and improperly reinserting an expelled tracheostomy tube may cause tracheal trauma, perforation, compression, and asphyxiation.

Neck swelling and constriction may also occur in the patient with a traumatic injury, radical neck dissection, or cardiac failure.

Key steps

To help the doctor perform a tracheotomy, follow these essential steps:
• Place the patient in a supine position with a pillow under his shoulders to help expose and hyperextend his neck.
• Shave a male patient's neck if necessary. Clean the skin with povidone-iodine solution. Inject a local anesthetic in the area where the incision will be made, and give the patient medication to calm and sedate him as ordered. A confused patient may need wrist restraints.
• Prepare a sterile field with the equipment needed for tracheotomy and tube placement.
• Inflate the cuff on the tracheostomy tube using sterile technique. Inspect the cuff to ensure that it has no leaks; then deflate it.
• Assist the doctor with the tracheotomy and insertion of the tube. (The tube may be sutured to the skin at the tab sites on the tube collar.) Inflate the cuff.
• Suction the patient regularly to maintain an open airway.
• Attach the patient to an oxygen source or a mechanical ventilator if needed.
• Apply a dressing and tracheostomy ties to secure the tube.
• Place an extra tracheostomy tube, an obturator, and a hemostat at the patient's bedside to facilitate replacement should the tube be expelled or dislodged.

Special considerations

If you're inflating the cuff using cuff pressure measurement, don't exceed 25 mm Hg. If the pressure exceeds 25 mm Hg, notify the doctor because you may need to change to a larger tube, use higher inflation pressures, or permit a larger air leak. A cuff pressure of about 18 mm Hg is usually recommended.

Check for a leak-free cuff seal. Even with minimal cuff inflation, you should feel no air coming from the patient's mouth, nose, or tracheostomy site, and a conscious patient shouldn't be able to speak.

Be alert for air leaks from the cuff itself. Suspect a leak if injection of air fails to inflate the cuff or increase cuff pressure, if you can't inject the amount of air you withdrew, if the patient can speak, if ventilation fails to maintain adequate respiratory movement with pressures or volumes previously considered adequate, or if air escapes during the ventilator's inspiratory cycle.

To prevent airway obstruction, frequently check that the tube is in place, and suction mucus secretions as needed in the inner lumen of the tracheostomy tube and under dressings. Ensure that suctioning equipment is on hand because the patient may need his airway cleared at any time. (See Managing tracheostomy tube obstruction.)

Have on hand a spare sterile tracheostomy tube and an obturator (used to insert the tracheostomy tube) that are the same sizes as those used in the procedure, in case the tube is expelled. Also have a tube and an obturator one size smaller than those used, in case the tube is expelled and the trachea begins to close. Have a spare sterile inner cannula available in case the cannula is expelled, and a spare sterile tracheal dilator or sterile hemostats to maintain an open airway if a new tracheostomy tube is being inserted. Review your hospital's policy for an expelled or blocked tube.

To avoid accidental tube dislodgment and expulsion, don't change tracheostomy ties unnecessarily during the immediate postoperative period until the stoma track is well formed (usually 4 days). Then, unless secretions or drainage is a problem, you can change ties once a day.

Don't change a single-cannula tracheostomy tube or the outer cannula of a double-cannula tube. Because of the risk of tracheal complications, the doctor usually changes the cannula as often as the patient's condition warrants.

Tube displacement may stimulate the cough reflex if the tip rests on the carina, or it may cause blood vessel erosion and hemorrhage. Just the presence of the tube can produce tracheal erosion and necrosis.

For the patient with a traumatic injury, radical neck dissection, or cardiac failure, check tracheostomy-tie tension frequently because his neck diameter can increase from swelling and cause constriction. Also check a neonate or restless patient frequently because this patient can loosen his ties, possibly dislodging his tube.

If the patient's neck or stoma is excoriated or infected, apply a water-soluble lubricant or topical antibiotic cream. Never use a powder or oil-based medication

Managing tracheostomy tube obstruction

Suspect tube obstruction by a mucus plug if the patient appears pale and diaphoretic and if you hear whistling with each breath. His labored respirations will be rapid and shallow, and you'll feel minimal airflow at the stoma. He may look cyanotic. If you hear a whistling sound and feel minimal airflow, the patient is receiving some air, but you must act quickly to remove the plug before he develops further respiratory distress.

Intervention
Call for assistance as you help the patient sit upright. Remove the tube's inner cannula and have him try to cough out the plug. (Because he won't be able to perform Valsalva's maneuver or cough with sufficient force, this may be difficult.)

If this doesn't work, quickly attach a hand-held resuscitation bag with supplemental oxygen to his tracheostomy tube and deliver several vigorous hyperinflations. If they don't dislodge the plug, or if you feel resistance to inflation, you'll need to suction.

Prepare a syringe of 2 ml of sterile isotonic saline solution (without preservatives). Instill the solution and vigorously suction for no longer than 10 seconds at a time.

Hyperinflate with the supplemental oxygen between each suctioning attempt.

If you still haven't been able to establish an effective airway, call the doctor immediately, cut the tracheostomy ties, and gently remove the entire tube. Keep the stoma open with a Kelly clamp and try to insert a new tube. If you can't get the tube in, insert a suction catheter instead and thread the tube over the catheter.

If you still can't establish an effective airway and you no longer detect a pulse, call a code. Then either ventilate with a face mask and a hand-held resuscitation bag or remove the Kelly clamp to close the stoma and perform mouth-to-mouth resuscitation until the doctor arrives. If air leaks from the stoma, cover the stoma with an occlusive dressing. Never leave this patient alone until you're certain that he has an effective airway and can breathe comfortably.

Once the patient has a new tracheostomy tube in place and can breathe more easily, provide supplemental humidified oxygen until he receives a full evaluation. Monitor his vital signs, skin color, and level of consciousness and, unless contraindicated, elevate the head of his bed.

on or around a stoma because their aspiration can cause infection and abscess.

——————————❖

Avoiding endotracheal intubation problems

In endotracheal (ET) intubation, a flexible tube is inserted orally (orotracheal intubation) or nasally (nasotracheal intubation) through the larynx into the trachea to control the airway and mechanically ventilate the patient. Performed by a doctor, an anesthesiologist, a nurse-anesthetist, a respiratory therapist, or a specially trained nurse, this procedure is usually done in emergency situations. However, this method bypasses normal respiratory tract defenses against infection, reduces cough effectiveness, and prevents oral communication.

Complications

ET intubation may cause bronchospasm; aspiration of blood, upper airway secretions, or gastric contents; tooth damage or loss; injury to the lips, mouth, pharynx, or vocal cords; laryngeal edema and erosion; and apnea caused by reflex breath-holding or interruption of oxygen delivery. Nasotracheal intubation can result in nasal bleeding, laceration, sinusitis, and otitis media. Traumatic injury to the larynx or trachea may result from manipulation of the tube, accidental extubation, or slippage of the tube into the right mainstream bronchus.

Other common complications of ET intubation are tracheal erosion, stenosis, necrosis, and dilation. And while low-pressure cuffs have significantly reduced the incidence of tracheal erosion and necrosis caused by cuff pressure on the tracheal wall, overinflation of a low-pressure cuff may negate this benefit. Aspiration of upper airway secretions, underventilation, or coughing spasms may occur if a leak is created during cuff pressure measurement.

Ventilatory failure and airway obstruction caused by laryngospasm and marked tracheal edema are the most serious complications of extubation.

Key steps

Follow these essential steps to reposition a dislocated tube, inflate a cuff, or remove a tube.

Repositioning the tube

Accidental dislocation from something as simple as the patient coughing is a very real danger and requires immediate repositioning. Call in a respiratory therapist or another nurse to assist you, as follows:
• Suction the patient's trachea through the ET tube to remove any secretions, which can irritate the bronchi and cause the patient to cough. (Coughing increases the risk of traumatic injury to the vocal cords and the likelihood of dislodging the tube.) Then suction the patient's pharynx to remove any secretions above the tube cuff and prevent aspiration of secretions during cuff deflation.
• Deflate the cuff before moving the tube because the cuff forms a seal within the trachea and

movement of an inflated cuff can damage the tracheal wall and vocal cords. Deflate it by attaching a 10-ml syringe to the pilot balloon port and aspirating air until you meet resistance and the pilot balloon deflates.

• Reposition the tube as necessary, noting new landmarks or measuring the length. Then immediately reinflate the cuff by telling the patient to inhale and slowly inflating the cuff using a 10-ml syringe attached to the pilot balloon port. With a stethoscope, listen to the patient's neck to determine whether an air leak exists.

• Once air leakage ceases, stop cuff inflation and, while still listening to the patient's neck with your stethoscope, aspirate a small amount of air until you detect a slight leak. This creates a minimal air leak, which indicates that the cuff is inflated at the lowest pressure possible to create an adequate seal. If the patient is being mechanically ventilated, aspirate to create a minimal air leak during the inspiration because the positive pressure of the ventilator during inspiration will create a larger leak around the cuff. Note the number of cubic centimeters of air required to inflate the cuff to achieve a minimal air leak.

Inflating a cuff
When inflating a cuff, use the minimal-leak technique, as follows, to avoid problems such as tracheal erosion and necrosis, which may result from overinflation of a low-pressure cuff.

• First, attach a 10-ml syringe to the port on the tube's exterior pilot cuff, and place a stethoscope on the side of the patient's neck. Inject small amounts of air with each breath until you hear no leaking around the cuff.

• Then aspirate 0.1 cc of air from the cuff to create a minimal air leak. Record the amount of air needed to inflate the cuff for subsequent monitoring of tracheal dilation or erosion. Once the cuff has been inflated, measure its pressure every 8 hours or according to your hospital's policy to avoid overinflation. Normal cuff pressure is 18 mm Hg.

• Keep the connection between the measuring device and the pilot balloon port tight to avoid an air leak that could compromise cuff pressure when measuring the pressure.

• Always record the volume of air needed to inflate the cuff. A gradual increase in this volume indicates tracheal dilation or erosion; a sudden increase indicates rupture of the cuff that requires immediate reintubation if the patient is being ventilated or if he requires continuous cuff inflation to maintain a high concentration of delivered oxygen.

Removing the tube
When you're authorized to remove the tube, get another nurse to assist you. This will help prevent traumatic manipulation of the tube when it's untaped or unfastened. Proceed as follows.

• Elevate the head of the patient's bed to approximately 90 degrees.

• Suction the patient's oropharynx and nasopharynx to remove any secretions that may have accumulated above the cuff and to help prevent aspiration of secretions when the cuff is deflated.

• Using a hand-held resuscitation bag or the mechanical ventilator, give the patient several deep breaths through the ET tube to hyperinflate his lungs and increase his oxygen reserve.

• Attach a 10-ml syringe to the pilot balloon port and aspirate air until you meet resistance and the pilot balloon deflates. If you fail to detect an air leak around the deflated cuff, notify the doctor and stop the extubation immediately. Absence of an air leak may indicate marked tracheal edema and can result in total airway obstruction if the ET tube is removed.

• If you detect the proper air leak, untape or unfasten the ET tube while the assisting nurse stabilizes it.

• Insert a sterile suction catheter through the ET tube. Then apply suction. Suctioning during extubation removes secretions retained at the end of the tube and helps prevent aspiration.

• Ask the patient to take a deep breath and to open his mouth fully and pretend to cry out. This causes abduction of the vocal cords and reduces the risk of laryngeal trauma during withdrawal of the tube.

• In one smooth outward and downward motion, simultaneously remove the ET tube and the suction catheter, following the natural curve of the patient's mouth.

• Give the patient supplemental oxygen. For highest humidity, use a cool-mist, large-volume nebulizer to help decrease airway irritation, patient discomfort, and laryngeal edema.

• After extubation, auscultate the patient's lungs frequently and watch for signs of respiratory distress. Be especially alert for stridor or other evidence of upper airway obstruction. If ordered, draw an arterial sample for blood gas analysis.

Special considerations

Never extubate a patient unless someone skilled at intubation is readily available. After extubation of a patient who has been intubated for an extended time, keep reintubation supplies readily available for at least 12 hours or until you're sure that the patient can tolerate extubation.

If you inadvertently cut the pilot balloon on the cuff, immediately call the person responsible for intubation, who will remove and replace the damaged ET tube. Don't remove the tube yourself before assistance arrives because a tube with an air leak is better than no airway.

When repositioning a tube, be especially careful in patients with highly sensitive airways. Sedation or direct instillation of 2% lidocaine to numb the airway may be indicated in such patients.

Administering transtracheal oxygen

In this procedure, oxygen is administered through a catheter inserted into the base of the neck and held in place with a chain necklace. Some patients find this more comfortable and less restrictive than oxygen therapy by nasal cannula. Transtracheal oxygenation doesn't interfere with eating or talking, doesn't dry mucous membranes, may easily be concealed by a shirt or scarf, and allows better oxygenation with lower oxygen flow. And because transtracheal delivery uses half the oxygen that's required with a nasal cannula, the cost of oxygen to the patient is cut in half.

But, because this form of oxygen therapy requires a minor surgical procedure, it shouldn't be used in patients at risk for bleeding; in patients with severe bronchospasm, uncompensated respiratory acidosis, or pleural herniation into the base of the neck; or in patients receiving high dosages of corticosteroids.

Transtracheal oxygenation is also contraindicated in patients with severe anxiety and in patients who aren't alert, who are unaware of their surroundings, who show a low level of compliance, or who are unable to sustain interest in intensive patient education.

Complications

Possible complications may include hematoma, pneumothorax, infection, and airway obstruction due to mucus plug accumulation. Also, the airway may close if the tracheal catheter is removed for more than a few minutes.

Key steps

Insertion of the transtracheal catheter first involves the insertion of a stent about 1 week prior to insertion of the catheter. The stent maintains the opening into the trachea while the body lines the opening with epithelial tissue. Once the catheter is in place, maintenance involves careful cleansing of the catheter.

Assisting with insertion of the transtracheal stent

• Make sure that the patient's nasal cannula is in place and functioning. Position the patient so that he's sitting upright in bed or in a chair. Assist the doctor as he cleans and anesthetizes the area, inserts the guidewire, dilates the opening, and inserts the stent into the trachea by passing the guidewire over it.
• Place a slit drain sponge lightly around the stent so that the slit points toward the patient's chin, and secure it with two small pieces of tape—one in each of the right and left upper corners.

Assisting with insertion of a transtracheal catheter

• Assist with removal of the stent and insertion of the catheter as necessary.
• Once the catheter is in place, attach the chain link necklace that comes with the catheter to the catheter's flanges to secure the transtracheal catheter in place.
• Connect the Spofford-Christian Oxygen Optimizing Prosthesis (SCOOP) oxygen hose adaptor to the catheter and then connect the oxygen tubing to the oxygen source. Turn on the oxygen and adjust the flow rate as prescribed. Remove the patient's oxygen cannula.

Maintaining a transtracheal catheter

• Using a cotton-tipped applicator, clean mucus crusts from the skin around the catheter. Blot the area dry with a tissue.
• Remove the oxygen source from the catheter and apply a nasal cannula.

Special considerations

Remind the patient never to remove or insert a tracheal catheter while oxygen is flowing through it. Instead, he should put on a nasal cannula, disconnect the catheter from the oxygen source, and then remove the catheter.

If the patient is using a SCOOP, don't use the SCOOP stent for oxygen delivery. Some doctors allow the other tracheal catheters to be used immediately for oxygen delivery. Others wait 1 week for the stoma to heal and to lessen the risk of subcutaneous emphysema.

If the patient is in respiratory distress and you suspect the catheter isn't working, give him oxygen with a nasal cannula.
_____❖

Suctioning tracheal secretions

In this procedure, secretions are removed from the trachea or bronchi by a catheter inserted through the mouth, nose, tracheal stoma, tracheostomy tube, or endotracheal tube. Besides removing secretions, tracheal suctioning also stimulates the cough reflex. The procedure helps maintain a patent airway to promote optimal exchange of oxygen and carbon dioxide and to prevent pneumonia from pooled secretions. Perform tracheal suctioning as frequently as the patient's condition warrants, always using strict aseptic technique; however, prolonged suctioning can cause tracheal or bronchial trauma.

Use extreme caution when you perform nasotracheal suctioning in patients with a history of nasopharyngeal bleeding or in those taking anticoagulants. Also be cautious with patients who have had a recent tracheotomy, who have a blood dyscrasia, or who have increased intracranial pressure.

Complications

Because oxygen is removed along with secretions, the patient may experience dyspnea and hypoxia. Cardiac arrhythmias may result from hypoxia and stimulation of the vagus nerve in the tracheobronchial tree. Patients with compromised cardiovascular or pulmonary status are at risk for hypoxia, arrhythmias, hypertension, or hypotension.

Other complications may include laryngospasm or bronchospasm (rare), and misplacement of the catheter into the right mainstem bronchus.

Key steps

To properly perform tracheal suctioning, follow these essential steps:
• Suction only when necessary, and then gently and briefly; never exceed a suction pressure of 120 mm Hg or a time span of 15 seconds to avoid traumatic injury. If you insert the catheter into a nostril and meet an obstruction, withdraw the catheter and try the other nostril or a smaller catheter.
• Keep the patient well hydrated and administer humidified oxygen and aerosol treatments, as prescribed, so that the mucosa won't dry and become prone to

60-SECOND SOLUTION

 ## Suctioning thick secretions

Standard suction catheters may not be able to suction thick and copious oral secretions. Try a Yankauer tonsil-tip catheter and frequently flush 0.9% sodium chloride solution or sterile water through the catheter and tubing to prevent clogging. For neonates and infants, use a tuberculin syringe. Remove the plunger and needle; cut off the wings at the plunger end. Now the syringe will fit into the suction tubing and will handle thick secretions.

injury. (See *Suctioning thick secretions*.)
• Monitor the patient's color, heart rate, and heart rhythm before suctioning to assess his risk of cardiopulmonary complications. If the patient shows evidence of sudden cardiac or respiratory difficulty during suctioning, stop, administer oxygen, and call the doctor immediately.
• Hyperoxygenate and hyperventilate the patient throughout suctioning.
• Always use aseptic technique, date solution bottles, and discard opened bottles after 24 hours to minimize the risk of infection. If you implement tracheal suctioning after oral suctioning, change the suction catheter between procedures.
• Encourage the patient to divert himself with relaxing activities. Relaxation decreases the airway's sympathetic tone, helping prevent bronchospasm.
• Avoid inserting the catheter too far down into the airway, which could trigger reflexive bronchospasm. Gagging or coughing can trigger bronchospasm; remove the catheter if they occur. Discuss using bronchodilators with

the doctor to reduce the risk of this complication.
• Make sure that the catheter is the right size for the patient's nostrils to prevent mucosal trauma and bleeding; try a smaller catheter if necessary. Also avoid nasotracheal suctioning in patients with coagulation disorders.
• To prevent increased intracranial pressure (ICP), try to keep the patient's neck in a neutral position while suctioning. If the patient experiences sudden cardiac or respiratory difficulty, stop suctioning, administer oxygen and, if appropriate, place the patient on a ventilator.
• Administer sedatives, as ordered, to relax the patient and reduce the risk of increased ICP.

Special considerations
Never allow the collection container to become more than three-quarters full to keep from damaging it.

Disconnect the suction catheter from the connecting tube and allow the catheter to act as an airway if laryngospasm or bronchospasm occurs. Also discuss using bronchodilators or lidocaine with the doctor to reduce the risk of these complications.

Raise the patient's nose to align the larynx and pharynx and facilitate passing the catheter during nasotracheal suctioning. If the patient's condition permits, have an assistant hyperextend the patient's head and neck and move his jaw up and forward, if necessary. If the patient is responsive, ask him to stick out his tongue so that he won't be able to swallow the catheter during insertion.

Use an angled catheter (such as a coudé or Bronchitrac L) to help guide the catheter into the left mainstem bronchus, if needed, to prevent its entry into the right mainstem bronchus. Rotating the patient's head to the right also seems to help, because the tracheobronchial structure deflects the catheter into the left mainstem bronchus.

———————————————— ❖

Conducting closed tracheal suctioning

A newer way to facilitate suctioning while reducing its complications, closed tracheal suctioning is used for patients on mechanical ventilation who require suctioning or who are being weaned with a T-piece. It poses a lower risk of suction-induced hypoxemia than open tracheal suctioning because the patient can maintain tidal volume, oxygen concentration, and positive end-expiratory pressure while being suctioned. And because the catheter remains in a protective sleeve, closed tracheal

suctioning reduces the risk of infection, even when the same catheter is used many times. However, gloves are required for this procedure.

Complications

Possible complications associated with this procedure include arterial oxygen desaturation, hypotension and arrhythmias (due to hypoxia), bronchoconstriction, and dehydration. Infection, bronchospasm, mucosal trauma and bleeding, and increased intracranial pressure also may occur.

Key steps

To perform closed tracheal suctioning, follow these key steps:
• Attach the closed tracheal suction system to the ventilator tubing and wall suction.
• Using your thumb, depress the suction control valve and keep it depressed while you set the suction pressure to the desired level (usually 80 to 120 mm Hg).
• Connect the T-piece adaptor to the ventilator breathing circuit. Then connect the T-piece adaptor to the patient's endotracheal or tracheostomy tube.
• Use the thumb and index finger of your other hand to advance the suction catheter through the tube and into the patient's tracheobronchial tree.
• While continuing to hold the T-piece with one hand, grasp the control valve with the other hand. Apply intermittent suction. Never apply suction for more than 10 seconds. Then withdraw the catheter with a straight motion.
• Continue to withdraw the catheter until it's fully extended within the sleeve and is clear of

the T-piece. You should see a mark in the sleeve, and the suction catheter lumens should be under the irrigation port.
• After you complete suctioning, flush the catheter.
• After flushing, release the suction catheter's control valve to discontinue the suction. Lock the catheter by lifting and turning the thumb piece on the control valve 180 degrees to the locked position.
• Turn off the suction machine and place that catheter and suction tubing alongside the ventilator tubing or disconnect the catheter from the suctioning tubing. Remove and discard your gloves and wash your hands. Document the procedure.

Special considerations
Before suctioning, hyperoxygenate the patient with 1 to 2 minutes of 100% oxygen, especially if the patient is prone to arrhythmias or hypotension.

Depress the suction control valve when setting the vacuum to achieve adequate suction.

Never use the tracheal suction setup for naso-oral suctioning. You'll need a separate suctioning setup. Use a Y-adapter at the suction canister to change the setup, and use a clean pair of gloves for the new setup.

Mastering mechanical ventilation

A mechanical ventilator moves air in and out of a patient's lungs by using positive or negative pressure. Although the equipment ventilates the patient,

it doesn't ensure adequate gas exchange. For mechanical ventilation to be effective, you may have to administer a sedative or a neuromuscular blocking agent to relax the patient and prevent spontaneous breathing, which can interfere with the ventilator.

Complications
Mechanical ventilation may lead to tension pneumothorax, decreased cardiac output, oxygen toxicity, infection, fluid volume excess caused by humidification, and such GI complications as abdominal distention or bleeding from stress ulcers.

Complications of weaning the patient from the ventilator may include respiratory muscle fatigue, respiratory alkalosis, and respiratory arrest. (See *Coping with problems of mechanical ventilation*, pages 352 to 355.)

Key steps
Follow these steps to start the patient on mechanical ventilation and to wean him from the ventilator when he can breathe on his own.

Starting mechanical ventilation
To start the patient on mechanical ventilation, follow these key steps:
• Plug the ventilator into the electrical outlet and turn it on. Adjust the settings on the ventilator as ordered. Make sure that the ventilator's alarms are set as ordered and that the humidifier is filled with distilled water.
• Put on gloves if you haven't already done so. Connect the endotracheal tube to the ventilator. Observe for chest expansion and auscultate for bilateral breath

(Text continues on page 356.)

Coping with problems of mechanical ventilation

Mechanical ventilation can save your patient's life, but it can also cause serious complications. The chart that follows will help you recognize and manage such problems.

PROBLEM	SIGNS AND SYMPTOMS
Acid-base, fluid, and electrolyte imbalances Results from positive water balance created by secretion of antidiuretic hormone; also caused by reduced insensible losses from respiratory tract	Probable change in arterial blood gas (ABG) measurements (decreased vital capacity), weight gain, ankle edema, moist crackles in lower lobes of lungs, pulmonary edema confirmed by X-rays
Airway obstruction Caused by secretions, incorrect tube position, or bronchospasm	Cyanosis, bradycardia or tachycardia, anxiety, increased airway pressures
Atelectasis Caused by insufficient deep breathing, pneumothorax, retained secretions, or a combination of these	Transient fine crackles, diminished breath sounds over the affected lung segment, bronchial sounds over the peripheral lung fields, decreased compliance, possible change in ABG values
Barotrauma Occurs as pneumothorax, subcutaneous emphysema, or mediastinal emphysema; usually caused when volume and pressure settings are too high or during administration of positive end-expiratory pressure (PEEP)	Sudden cyanosis, drop in blood pressure, and decrease in lung compliance; increased anxiety • With pneumothorax, diminished or absent breath sounds over the affected lung, acute pain on the affected side, and a trachea deviated away from the pneumothorax • With subcutaneous emphysema, crepitus of the face, abdomen, and extremities • With mediastinal emphysema, reduced cardiac output and crepitus over the heart

INTERVENTIONS

• Carry out the doctor's orders to restrict fluid intake and administer diuretics.	• Give medications (or, rarely, apply rotating tourniquets) to control pulmonary edema or to correct acid-base or electrolyte imbalance as ordered.
• Suction frequently. • Perform chest physiotherapy. • If the doctor orders bronchoscopy, prepare the patient for the procedure.	• Use a pulse oximeter to monitor the patient's oxygen level. • Adjust the endotracheal (ET) tube's position. • Administer nebulizer treatments as ordered.
• Turn the patient frequently. • Suction and hyperinflate the patient's lungs periodically. • Have the patient cough and take deep breaths every 2 hours.	• Perform chest physiotherapy as ordered. • Prepare the patient for bronchoscopy if ordered.
• Call the doctor immediately; he may insert a chest tube.	• Use pulse oximetry to monitor the patient's oxygen levels.

(continued)

Coping with problems of mechanical ventilation (continued)

PROBLEM	SIGNS AND SYMPTOMS
Cardiovascular impairment Occurs when positive intrathoracic pressure reduces venous return to the right side of the heart and compresses pulmonary circulation	Decreased blood pressure and cardiac output, possible decreased urine output, increased central venous pressure and pulmonary artery pressure, increased heart rate
GI distress Occurs as GI bleeding, gastric distention, paralytic ileus, or stress ulcer; usually caused by stress or swallowing air	Abdominal distention, steady decrease in hemoglobin and hematocrit values, positive Hematest results on nasogastric (NG) drainage and stools, tarry stools
Oxygen toxicity Caused by oxygen concentrations over 60% administered over prolonged period (8 hours or more); may cause fibrotic tissue changes in lungs, possibly leading to death	Retrosternal pain; sore throat; nasal congestion; burning chest pain on inspiration; dry, hacking cough; dyspnea; decreased compliance; decreased arterial oxygen levels despite the same oxygen concentration; decreased vital capacity; changes seen on X-rays
Respiratory tract infection Occurs from ventilator equipment bypassing the upper airway and thereby eliminating the body's natural defense mechanisms against infection; also caused by flawed aseptic technique	Elevated temperature and white blood cell count, increased respiratory secretions, change in secretion color or odor
Tracheal trauma Caused by constant pressure of cuffed ET tube or tracheostomy tube on the patient's trachea or by injury related to intubation	Decreased tidal volume (because of air leak), bleeding from trachea

INTERVENTIONS

• Carry out the doctor's orders to reduce intrathoracic pressure by decreasing PEEP, inspiratory flow rate, or tidal volume.

• Administer additional I.V. fluids or plasma expanders, such as albumin or colloidal substances, as ordered.

• As ordered, insert NG tube for drainage.
• Replace lost blood.

• Use NG tube to provide antacids or other medications to decrease acid production.

• Monitor oxygen levels carefully, and report signs of oxygen toxicity immediately.

• Notify the doctor.
• Change the patient's position frequently, and perform chest physiotherapy as indicated.

• Use aseptic technique for tracheostomy care and for suctioning.
• Administer prescribed antibiotics.

• Depending on the type of damage, help the doctor insert a new tracheostomy tube, which changes the position of the ET tube's cuff and allows the injured area to heal.

• Provide meticulous cuff care until you can remove the ET tube.

sounds to verify that the patient is being ventilated.

Weaning from the ventilator

To wean a patient from a mechanical ventilator, you'll first need to determine his readiness to breathe on his own. Weaning is contraindicated in any patient who doesn't meet the three basic criteria: spontaneous respiratory effort, a stable cardiovascular system, and sufficient respiratory muscle strength and level of consciousness (LOC) to sustain the breathing.

• Expect a decreased tidal volume, increased respiratory rate, and some decrease in partial pressure of arterial oxygen and increase in partial pressure of arterial carbon dioxide ($PaCO_2$) while weaning. Help the patient avoid activities that will cause fatigue during the weaning process.

• For the patient who's received mechanical ventilation for a long time, switch the ventilator to pressure support ventilation with or without intermittent mandatory ventilation. This way, each of the patient's spontaneous breaths is augmented by the ventilator. As the patient's own respirations improve, the intermittent mandatory ventilation and pressure support ventilation can be decreased.

• Use the T-piece weaning method for the patient who has received ventilation for a short time. This method progressively decreases the frequency and tidal volume of the ventilated breaths.

• Immediately return the patient to mechanical ventilation if he displays any of these signs: a blood pressure increase of more than 20 mm Hg systolic or more than 10 mm Hg diastolic, a heart rate increase of more than 20 beats/minute or a rate above 120 beats/minute, a respiratory rate increase of more than 10 breaths/minute or a rate above 30 breaths/minute, arrhythmias, reduced tidal volume, elevated $PaCO_2$, anxiety, dyspnea, and accessory muscle use or deteriorating breathing pattern.

Special considerations

Never turn off a ventilator alarm. If an alarm sounds and the problem can't be easily identified, disconnect the patient from the ventilator and use a hand-held resuscitation bag to ventilate him.

Also make sure that emergency equipment is readily available in case the ventilator malfunctions or the patient is accidentally extubated. Take extra steps to ensure the safety of a paralyzed patient, such as raising the bed rails during turning and covering and lubricating his eyes.

Unless contraindicated, turn the patient from side to side every 1 to 2 hours to guard against lung contraction and accumulation of secretions. If the patient's condition permits, position him upright at regular intervals to increase lung expansion.

Ensure that the patient receiving a neuromuscular blocking agent is also receiving a sedative. Neuromuscular blocking agents cause paralysis without altering the patient's LOC.

Performing thoracic drainage

A thoracic drainage system uses gravity and sometimes suction to restore negative pressure in the pleural cavity and keep the lungs expanded following chest trauma. In this procedure, one or more chest tubes are surgically inserted and connected to a thoracic drainage system that removes air, fluid, or both from the pleural space and prevents backflow, thus promoting lung reexpansion.

For pneumothorax, the second intercostal space is the most common site for chest tube insertion because air rises to the top of the intrapleural space. For hemothorax or pleural effusion, the sixth to eighth intercostal spaces are most common because fluid settles at the lower levels of the intrapleural space. For removal of air and fluid, a chest tube is inserted into a high and a low site.

Complications

Possible complications associated with this procedure include chest tube dislodgment, clots, and cracks, leaks, and filling of the drainage system. Tension pneumothorax resulting from excessive accumulation of air or drainage in the pleural cavity can eventually exert pressure on the heart or aorta and cause a drop in cardiac output.

Key steps

To perform thoracic drainage, follow these essential steps:
• Maintain sterile technique throughout the procedure and whenever you make changes or alterations to any part of the system.
• Keep two rubber-tipped clamps at the patient's bedside. Use these to clamp the chest tube if a drainage bottle breaks, the drainage system cracks, a tube disconnects, or you need to locate an air leak. Place the clamps close to each other near the insertion site; they should face in opposite directions to provide a more complete seal. Observe the patient closely for signs of tension pneumothorax while the clamps are in place; then replace the damaged equipment.
• Instead of clamping the tube, you may submerge the distal end of the tube in 0.9% sodium chloride solution to create a temporary water seal while you replace the bottle.
• Wrap a piece of petroleum gauze around the tube at the insertion site to make an airtight seal.
• Strip (or milk) the tubing when clots are visible, according to your hospital's policy. (See *When to strip tubing*, page 358.)
• Replace a filled drainage collection chamber by double-clamping the tube closest to the insertion site (using two clamps facing in opposite directions). Now exchange the system, remove the clamps, and retape the bottle connection. Never leave the tubes clamped for more than 1 minute; doing so could cause a tension pneumothorax.

Special considerations

Be prepared to immediately respond to ventilator alarms, which may signal potentially

When to strip tubing

When you strip tubing, you create high negative pressure that could suck viable lung tissue into the drainage ports of the tube, resulting in ruptured alveoli and a pleural air leak. So strip tubing only when clots are visible. Use a mechanical stripper or follow this manual procedure:

Use an alcohol sponge or lotion as a lubricant on the tube, and pinch it between your thumb and index finger about 2″ (5 cm) from the insertion site. Using the other thumb and index finger, compress the tubing as you slide your fingers down the tube. Release the thumb and index finger, pinching near the insertion site.

hazardous changes in the patient's status.

Watch for and immediately report any signs of tension pneumothorax (hypotension, distended neck veins, absent breath sounds, tracheal shift, hypoxemia, weak and rapid pulse, dyspnea, tachypnea, diaphoresis, and chest pain).

If the patient's chest tube comes out, immediately cover the site with petroleum gauze or 4″ × 4″ gauze pads and tape them in place; then call the doctor. Monitor the patient's vital signs every 10 minutes.

Locate a suspected leak by clamping the tube briefly at various points. Work down toward the drainage system, paying special attention to the seal around the connections. If any connection is loose, push it back together and tape it securely. The bubbling will stop when a clamp is placed between the air leak and the water seal unless the drainage unit is cracked.

❖

Gastrointestinal procedures

Gastrointestinal (GI) procedures have varied uses. For example, depending on the patient's problem, you may need to perform nasogastric intubation to establish and maintain a route for nutrients, esophageal intubation to control hemorrhage from esophageal or gastric varices, gastric lavage to cleanse the stomach of ingested poisons, or tube feedings to provide supplemental nutrition.

Inserting and removing a nasogastric tube

Inserted through the patient's nose and extending into the stomach, a nasogastric (NG) tube is used for emptying the stomach of gas or liquids or for administering liquids. NG tube insertion requires special measures to ensure that the tube doesn't move. Removing the tube can provoke injury and aspiration. Most NG tubes have a radiopaque marker at the distal end so that the tube's position can be verified by X-ray. (See *Measuring NG tube length*.)

NG intubation is contraindicated in patients with facial fractures or basilar skull fractures. If these fractures are unstable, tube insertion and manipulation can worsen them; the doctor will decide if the need for a tube outweighs the potential problems.

Complications

NG tubes can cause choking and breathing difficulties. Perforation may result from aggressive intubation, while prolonged intubation may provoke skin erosion at the nostril, sinusitis, esophagitis, esophagotracheal fistula, gastric ulceration, and oral infection.

If suction is applied to the NG tube, electrolyte imbalances and dehydration may result; vigorous suction may also damage the gastric mucosa and cause significant bleeding. Epigastric pain and vomiting may result from a clogged or improperly placed tube. Aspiration pneumonia may result from gastric reflux. Any NG tube—the Levin tube in particular—may migrate and aggravate ulcers or esophageal varices, causing hemorrhage. Bradycardia may also occur during insertion or removal because of vagal stimulation.

Key steps

To ensure proper NG tube placement and to irrigate and remove a tube, follow these essential steps.

Measuring NG tube length

To determine how much of a nasogastric (NG) tube to insert, hold the end of the tube at the tip of the patient's nose. Extend the tube to the patient's earlobe and then down to the xiphoid process, as shown below. Mark this distance on the tubing with tape. The average tube length for an adult ranges from 22″ to 26″ (56 to 66 cm).

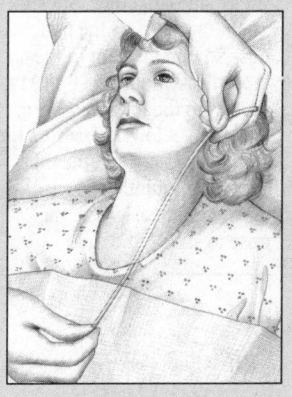

Ensuring proper tube placement

Use the catheter-tip or bulb syringe to inject 5 to 10 cc of air into the suction lumen of the tube. At the same time, auscultate for air sounds with your stethoscope placed over the patient's epigastric region.

• If you're working with a tube other than a Levin tube, move the syringe to the suction lumen of the tube and aspirate. Stomach contents should flow up the tube and into the syringe.

• After inserting the tube, ensure the tube remains properly posi-

Securing an NG tube

Take precautions to ensure that a nasogastric (NG) tube remains properly positioned after insertion. If you're not using a prepackaged product that secures and cushions the NG tube at the nose, secure the tube yourself.

Secure the NG tube to the patient's nose with hypoallergenic tape. You'll need about 4″ (10 cm) of 1″ tape. Split one end of the tape up the center about 1½″ (4 cm). Make tabs on the split ends by folding the sticky sides together. Stick the uncut tape end on the patient's nose so that the split in the tape starts about ½″ (1 cm) to 1½″ from the tip of her nose, as shown below. Crisscross the tabbed ends around the tube. Then apply another piece of tape over the bridge of the nose to secure the tube.

Alternatively, use a Coverlet dressing to anchor the tube in place. First swab the patient's nose with a liquid adhesive to help the dressing adhere. Then place the wide end of the dressing over the bridge of the patient's nose and wrap the smaller end around the tube, as shown below. The dressing won't irritate the patient's nose and is less expensive than a box of regular nasal tube fasteners.

Pin the tubing to the patient's gown to decrease tension on the tube.

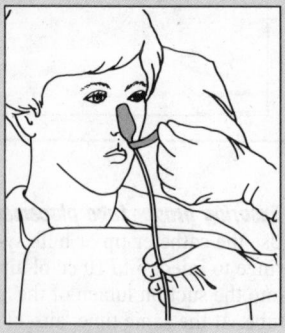

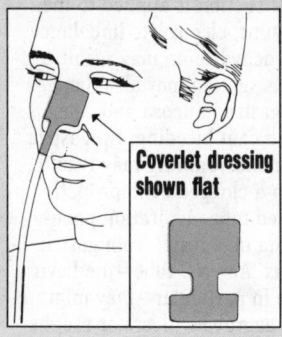

Coverlet dressing shown flat

tioned. (See *Securing an NG tube*.)

Irrigating the tube
First review the ordered irrigation schedule (usually every 4 hours), and check NG tube

placement using the method described previously. Then proceed as follows:
• Place a towel or linen-saver pad under the NG tube.
• Measure the ordered amount of irrigant (usually 30 ml) in the

bulb syringe or the 60-ml catheter-tip syringe to maintain accurate intake and output.

• Disconnect the tube from the suction equipment.

• Slowly instill the irrigant into the suction lumen of the NG tube.

• Gently aspirate the solution with the bulb syringe or the catheter-tip syringe to prevent excessive pressure on the delicate gastric mucosa or on a suture line.

• After completing the irrigation, reconnect the NG tube to the suction equipment.

• Note any difference between the amount of solution injected and the amount aspirated as intake on the intake and output record.

Removing the NG tube

• First, assess bowel function by auscultating for peristalsis or flatus.

• Help the patient into semi-Fowler's position. Then drape a towel or linen-saver pad across the patient's chest to protect his gown and bed linens from spills.

• Using a catheter-tip syringe, flush the tube with 10 ml of 0.9% sodium chloride solution to ensure that the tube doesn't contain stomach contents that could irritate tissues during tube removal.

• Untape the tube from the patient's nose, and unpin it from his gown.

• Clamp the tube by folding it in your hand.

• Ask the patient to hold his breath to close the epiglottis. Then withdraw the tube gently and steadily. When the distal end of the tube reaches the nasopharynx, which is evident when

the patient begins to gag, withdraw it quickly.

Special considerations

While advancing the tube, observe for signs that it has entered the patient's trachea, such as choking or breathing difficulties in a conscious patient and cyanosis in an unconscious patient or a patient without a cough reflex. Remove the tube immediately, allow the patient to rest a few minutes, and then try to reinsert the tube.

Never place the tube's end into a container of water when confirming tube placement. The patient could aspirate water if the tube is placed in his trachea. And never tape the tube to a patient's forehead; the resulting pressure on the nostril could cause necrosis.

Don't clamp the vent lumen on a Salem sump tube while suctioning because this will create a vacuum and pull the gastric mucosa against the end of the NG tube, causing mucosal trauma. Also, don't reposition any tube that was inserted during surgery; doing so can tear gastric or esophageal sutures.

❖

Assisting with esophageal intubation

Used to control hemorrhage from esophageal or gastric varices, an esophageal tube is inserted nasally or orally and advanced into the esophagus or stomach. A doctor usually inserts and removes the tube, but you may be asked to remove it in an emergency. All esophageal tubes have a gastric balloon, which, once the tube is in place, is inflated and drawn tightly against the cardia of the stomach. Most tubes also have an esophageal balloon that can be inflated to control esophageal bleeding.

Use of an esophageal tube is contraindicated in patients who have peptic ulcer disease, gastric or esophageal tumors, or gastric or esophageal perforation.

Complications

Acute airway obstruction may develop during tube placement, if the tube enters the trachea instead of the esophagus, or during gastric or esophageal balloon deflation if the gastric balloon moves up into the trachea. Pressure from prolonged balloon inflation can cause esophageal or gastric mucosal ulceration.

Esophageal rupture (indicated by sudden back pain, upper abdominal pain, unstable vital signs, and fluid in the mediastinum) may occur during intubation or esophageal balloon inflation or while an esophageal tube is in place.

Nasal irritation, erosion, and necrosis can result from tube pressure on the nose, and air leaks and aspiration of secretions are both constant dangers. Secretions may cause vomiting and pulmonary aspiration since swallowed secretions can't pass into the stomach if the patient has an inflated esophageal balloon in place.

Key steps

To insert and remove an esophageal tube, follow these essential steps.

Inserting the esophageal tube

• Before insertion, test all balloons for air leaks.
• Then, using the 60-ml syringe, inflate the gastric balloon with 300 cc of air and the esophageal balloon with 50 to 100 cc of air. Using aseptic technique, submerge the balloons in a basin of water. If no bubbles appear in the water, the balloons are intact. Remove them from the water and deflate them. Clamp the tube lumens or insert plastic plugs (included in the kit) so that the balloons stay deflated during insertion.
• Measure the length of tubing to be inserted by holding the balloon tip at the patient's ear and bringing the tube forward to his nose. Mark this point on the tube (usually the 50-cm mark) with a waterproof pen.
• To inflate the esophageal balloon on a Minnesota tube, the doctor attaches the mercury aneroid manometer directly to the esophageal pressure-monitoring outlet. Then, using the 60-ml syringe and pushing the air slowly into the esophageal balloon port, he inflates the balloon until the pressure is between 35 and 45 mm Hg.
• Set up esophageal suction to prevent accumulation of secretions. For a Linton or Minnesota tube, attach a suction source to the esophageal aspiration port. For a Sengstaken-Blakemore tube, advance a nasogastric tube through the other nostril into the esophagus to the esophageal balloon, and attach the suction source.

Removing the tube

The doctor deflates the esophageal balloon after 12 to 24 hours by aspirating all the air from the esophageal balloon port with a syringe. If bleeding does not recur within 6 to 24 hours, he'll remove the traction from the gastric balloon port.

Observe the patient for an additional 12 to 24 hours, as ordered, keeping the gastric balloon inflated without traction. If bleeding does not recur, the doctor will aspirate all of the air from the gastric balloon port with a syringe and remove the tube. He'll then deflate the gastric balloon just before removing the tube.

Special considerations

Be prepared to address immediately any special situations that may arise as complications of esophageal intubation.

Tape scissors to the head of the bed. If the patient then develops cyanosis or other signs of airway obstruction, cut across all lumens (ports) while holding the tube at the nose and then quickly remove the tube.

If using traction, release the tension before deflating any balloons. If weights and pulleys supply traction, remove the weights; if a football helmet is used for traction, untape the esophageal tube from the face guard before deflating the balloons.

Keep the gastric balloon port clamped at all times. Unclamp the esophageal balloon port on a Sengstaken-Blakemore or Minnesota tube only to check esophageal balloon pressures or to periodically relieve pressure from the mucosa as ordered.

Administering gastric lavage

After poisoning or drug overdose, gastric lavage flushes the stomach and removes ingested substances through a nasogastric (NG) tube. It's especially useful for patients with central nervous system depression or an inadequate gag reflex. For patients with gastric or esophageal bleeding, lavage with tepid water, iced water, or 0.9% sodium chloride solution may be used to stop the bleeding. However, some controversy exists over the use of iced lavage for this purpose because iced irrigating solutions stimulate the vagus nerve, which triggers increased hydrochloric acid secretion. This, in turn, stimulates gastric motility, which can irritate the bleeding site. Check your hospital's policy before using iced lavage.

Gastric lavage is contraindicated in patients who have ingested a corrosive substance (such as lye, ammonia, or mineral acids) because the NG tube may perforate the already compromised esophagus.

Complications

Vomiting and subsequent aspiration, the most common complications of gastric lavage, occur more often in groggy patients than alert ones. Also, the body's natural vagal response to intubation can depress the patient's heart rate or provoke bradyarrhythmias. After iced lavage especially, the patient's body temperature may drop, triggering cardiac arrest.

PROBLEMATIC
PROCEDURES

Key steps

To perform gastric lavage successfully, follow these key steps:
• Aspirate the contents of the patient's stomach with a syringe before instilling water. Save the aspirated material for analysis.
• Remove the syringe and attach a funnel to the tubing or use a 60-ml syringe to instill lavage solution into the stomach. If you're using a funnel, elevate the funnel high enough to facilitate gravity drainage into the stomach.
• To drain the instilled lavage solution, lower the funnel or aspirate contents into a collection container.
• Always place any aspirated poisons or drugs in a labeled container and send them to the laboratory for analysis.
• Repeat the above steps until the gastric aspirate is relatively clear of particulate matter.
• Leave the gastric cavity empty or instill an absorbent material (such as charcoal) through the tube and allow it to remain in the stomach.
• If charcoal is used, mix charcoal tablets with the irrigant after lavage and administer through the NG tube to absorb any remaining toxins as ordered. The tube may then be clamped temporarily, be allowed to drain via gravity, be attached to intermittent suction, or be removed.

Special considerations

Never leave a patient alone during gastric lavage. Observe him continuously for changes in level of consciousness, and monitor his vital signs frequently.

If the amount of drainage falls significantly short of the amount of lavage solution instilled, reposition the tube until sufficient solution flows out.

Keep tracheal suctioning equipment nearby, and watch closely for airway obstruction caused by vomiting or excess oral secretions. Be prepared to suction the oral cavity frequently during gastric lavage to ensure a patent airway and prevent aspiration. For the same reasons, and if he doesn't have an adequate gag reflex, the patient may require an endotracheal tube before the procedure.

When performing gastric lavage to stop bleeding, keep precise intake and output records to measure blood loss. If the patient is having large volumes of fluid instilled and withdrawn, you may also need to measure serum electrolyte and arterial blood gas levels during or after lavage.

❖

Giving tube feedings

In tube (or enteral) feeding, a liquid nutrient is administered directly into the stomach (known as gastric gavage), duodenum, or jejunum by continuous infusion. Duodenal or jejunal feedings decrease the risk of aspiration because the formula bypasses the pylorus. A patient receiving jejunal feedings may require an elemental diet because such feedings result in reduced pancreatic stimulation. As the patient's tolerance improves, or if the patient requires long-term feeding, he may start receiving intermittent gravity-drip feedings or syringe feedings.

Gastrostomy feeding buttons

For an ambulatory patient receiving long-term enteral feedings, a gastrostomy feeding button offers several advantages. This alternative feeding device reduces skin maceration and irritation, poses a decreased risk of dislodgment or migration, is more easily maintained, and is more cosmetically appealing than a gastrostomy tube.

The button has a mushroom dome at one end and two wing tabs and a flexible safety plug at the other end, as shown below.

reflux valve mounted just inside the mushroom dome prevents accidental leakage of gastric contents. The device must be replaced when the antireflux valve wears out—usually after 3 to 4 months.

If the button pops out during feeding, reinsert it, if you can, and continue feeding. If the patient feels nauseated or vomits during feeding, use the adapter and feeding catheter to vent the button, as shown below.

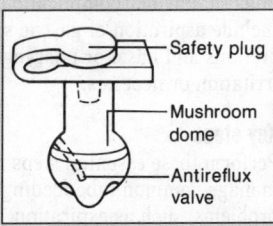

- Safety plug
- Mushroom dome
- Antireflux valve

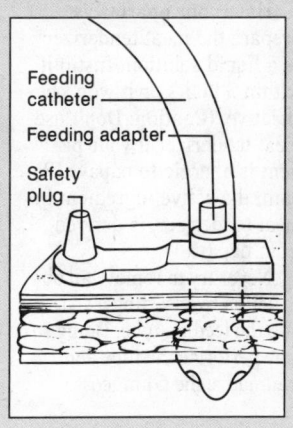

- Feeding catheter
- Feeding adapter
- Safety plug

When inserted into an established stoma, the button lies almost level with the skin, with only the top of the safety plug visible. A one-way, anti-

Liquid nutrient solutions come in various formulas for administration through a nasogastric tube, a small-bore feeding tube, a percutaneous endoscopic gastrostomy or jejunostomy tube, or a gastrostomy feeding button. (See *Gastrostomy feeding buttons.*)

While tube feedings are safe, convenient, and cost-effective and

preserve the physiologic integrity of the bowel, they're contraindicated in patients with complete or suspected gastric or intestinal obstruction or in those with questionable enteral access.

Contraindications for endoscopic placement include obstruction (such as esophageal stricture or duodenal blockage), previous gastric surgery, morbid

60-SECOND SOLUTION

Alternative declogging methods

To clear an obstructed feeding tube safely and quickly, try using actively fizzing colas or a meat tenderizer solution. Some nurses prefer cranberry juice, but colas and meat tenderizer solutions have proved more successful. These solutions may work better than water because of their alkaline or chemical properties. Instilling some of these substances may require a doctor's order, so check your hospital's policy.

Have your pharmacist prepare the meat tenderizer as a liquid solution. Instill it within 3 hours or it won't be effective. (Caution: Don't use meat tenderizer if your patient is allergic to papaya. Papain, the active ingredient in meat tenderizer, is derived from papaya.)

Never try to remove an obstruction by inserting a stylet into the feeding tube. Doing so may perforate the tube and traumatize the GI mucosa.

obesity, and ascites. These conditions would necessitate surgical placement.

Complications
Mechanical, metabolic, or GI complications may result from tube feedings. Mechanical complications include tube malposition or rupture, local trauma from tube insertion, and tube occlusion. Metabolic complica-

tions, such as prerenal azotemia, dehydration, electrolyte imbalance, hyperglycemia, and hypoglycemia, may result from improper formula selection, and infection may result from contaminated formula or administration equipment. GI complications include constipation, vomiting, bloating, diarrhea, or cramps.

The patient also may experience dumping syndrome, in which a large amount of hyperosmotic solution in the duodenum causes excessive diffusion of fluid through the semipermeable membrane, causing diarrhea. In a patient with low serum albumin levels, these symptoms may result from low oncotic pressure in the duodenal mucosa. Further complications include aspiration of gastric secretions and nasal or pharyngeal irritation or necrosis.

Key steps
Perform these essential steps to manage common tube feeding problems, such as aspiration, tube obstruction, constipation or diarrhea, and electrolyte imbalances:
• Check tube placement before feeding to prevent aspiration of gastric secretions.
• If the feeding solution won't flow through a catheter tip, attach a plunger or bulb and gently depress the plunger a short distance or squeeze the bulb to start the flow. Never use the plunger or bulb to force formula through the tube.
• To maintain patency, flush the feeding tube regularly with water. If the tube becomes obstructed, flush it with warm water. (See *Alternative declogging methods*.)

• If constipation occurs, give the patient additional fluids (if he can tolerate them), administer a bulk-forming laxative, and increase the fruit, vegetable, or sugar content of the feeding.

• If nausea or vomiting occurs, stop the feeding immediately. The patient may vomit if his stomach becomes distended from overfeeding or delayed gastric emptying.

• If electrolyte imbalance occurs, monitor serum electrolyte levels and notify the doctor, who may adjust the formula's electrolyte content.

• If hyperglycemia occurs, monitor blood glucose levels and notify the doctor, who may adjust the sugar content of the formula. Administer insulin if ordered.

• If nasal or pharyngeal irritation or necrosis occurs, provide frequent oral hygiene, using mouthwash or lemon-glycerin swabs, and apply petroleum jelly to cracked lips. Place the tube in another nostril, and replace the tube if encrusted or obstructed.

• If bloating, diarrhea, or cramps occur, reduce the flow rate, warm the formula, and administer metoclopramide to increase GI motility. Then position the patient on his right side with his head elevated for 30 minutes after the feeding to facilitate gastric emptying. Notify the doctor, who may want to reduce the amount of formula in each feeding or use a diluted or more isotonic formula.

Special considerations

If aspiration occurs, discontinue feeding immediately, and suction the patient's trachea of aspirated contents if possible. Notify the doctor, who may order prophylactic antibiotics and chest physiotherapy.

❖

Genitourinary procedures

Because the renal and urologic systems produce, transport, collect, and excrete urine, their dysfunction usually impairs fluid, electrolyte, and acid-base balance and the elimination of waste products. To restore or facilitate effective function of these systems, treatment usually involves temporary or permanent insertion of a urinary, peritoneal, or vascular catheter. Depending on your patient's condition, you may perform procedures that provide continuous urine drainage from the bladder with a catheter; ensure adequate drainage of the kidneys and bladder; remove impurities from the blood; filter fluid, solutes, and electrolytes; or infuse replacement solution.

Performing urinary catheterization

This procedure provides continuous urine drainage via an indwelling catheter that remains in the bladder. A balloon inflated at the catheter's distal end prevents it from slipping out of the bladder after insertion. An indwelling catheter is inserted only when absolutely necessary, however, because of its high rate of injury and infection, and should be removed when decompression is no longer necessary, when the patient can resume voiding, or when the catheter is obstructed.

Indwelling catheters are used most often to relieve bladder distention caused by urine retention and when the urinary meatus is swollen from childbirth, surgery, or local trauma. Other indications for an indwelling catheter include urinary tract obstruction (by a tumor or enlarged prostate), urine retention secondary to postoperative narcotic administration (especially through an epidural catheter), urine retention or infection from neurogenic bladder paralysis caused by spinal cord injury or disease, or any illness in which the patient's urine output must be monitored closely.

Complications

Among the complications associated with this procedure are urinary reflux (which promotes infection), injury to the urethra and bladder wall or mucosa caused by improper insertion and, most commonly, urinary tract infection. Bladder distention, acute renal failure, urinary stasis, and subsequent infection may also occur from an obstructed catheter.

Additional complications include hypovolemic shock, bladder atony or spasm (from rapid decompression of a severely distended bladder), and urinary sediment and calculi formation. Sediment, such as casts or mucus plugs, can occur anywhere in a catheterization system, especially in bedridden and dehydrated patients. When removing a catheter, watch for failure of

the balloon to deflate and balloon rupture.

Key steps

Follow these essential steps when inserting a urinary catheter:
• If you encounter resistance instilling the irrigating solution, stop the procedure and notify the doctor. Don't try to force the solution into the bladder.
• Never inflate a balloon without first establishing urine flow. Urine flow assures you that the catheter is lodged in the bladder, not the urethral channel.
• Hang the urinary drainage bag below bladder level to prevent urine reflux into the bladder, which can cause infection, and to facilitate gravity drainage. Make sure the tubing doesn't get tangled in the bed's side rails.
• Empty the drainage bag at least every 8 hours. Excessive fluid volume may require more frequent emptying to prevent traction on the catheter, which can cause the patient discomfort, and to prevent urethra and bladder wall injury. Also change catheters every 30 days, or according to your hospital's policy, for patients on long-term continuous drainage.
• Encourage patients with unrestricted fluid intake to increase their intake to at least 3,000 ml per day to flush the urinary system and reduce sediment, which may obstruct the drainage tube and be intensely painful. To prevent urinary sediment and calculi, some patients are placed on an acid-ash diet (cranberry juice, for example) to acidify the urine.

Handling difficult insertions

Follow these additional steps for difficult catheter insertions:
• Tell a female, elderly, or disabled patient (such as one with severe contractures) to lie on her side with her knees drawn up to her chest during catheterization to facilitate insertion.
• Never force a catheter during insertion. Maneuver it gently as the patient bears down or coughs. If you still meet resistance, stop the procedure and notify the doctor. Strictures, sphincter spasms, misplacement in the vagina, or an enlarged prostate may all cause resistance.
• If you can't see the urinary meatus in a female patient, reposition your nondominant hand and separate the labia outward and upward.
• If the catheter is apparently inserted into the vagina, leave the catheter in place. Obtain another sterile catheter and repeat the procedure.
• If you can't insert the catheter into the meatus because of spasm or obstruction, tell the patient to take a deep breath and slowly exhale. If spasm or obstruction persists, discontinue the procedure and notify the doctor.
• If no urine returns from the catheter, insert it further and wait for urine return. This may take several minutes if the patient voided recently or has oliguria. If you are absolutely confident of placement and still have no urine return, ask the doctor for further instructions.

Special considerations

If an indwelling catheter becomes totally obstructed, obtain an order to remove and replace it. Bladder distention, acute renal failure, urinary stasis, and subsequent infection may all result from an obstructed catheter.

Avoid injecting a catheter with air. This makes identifying leaks, and maybe balloon deflation, more difficult.

Also avoid removing excessive residual urine, which may trigger hypovolemic shock. Clamp the catheter at the first sign of shock, and notify the doctor. Check your hospital's policy to determine the maximum amount of urine you may drain at one time. Some hospitals limit the amount to 700 to 1,000 ml, but whether there should be limits at all is controversial.

Use strict aseptic technique to avoid introducing bacteria into the bladder, which may cause urinary tract infection.

Don't pull on the catheter while cleaning it because this can injure the urethra and the bladder wall and expose a section of the catheter that was previously inside the urethra. This potentially contaminated section will then introduce potentially infectious organisms into the urethra.

If you're irrigating the catheter and encounter resistance when instilling the irrigating solution, stop the procedure and notify the doctor. Don't try to force the solution into the bladder.

Attach a leg bag to allow the patient greater mobility, where practical. Mobility prevents sediment buildup. If the patient will be discharged with an indwell-

PROBLEMATIC
PROCEDURES

ing catheter, teach him how to use a leg bag.

If fluid can't be aspirated from the balloon with a syringe, cut the balloon catheter stem with bandage scissors. The fluid should then flow freely from the tube, draining and deflating the balloon.

When the catheter must be removed but the balloon won't deflate or is ruptured, cystoscopy is usually performed to ensure its removal and removal of any balloon fragments.

Avoid too-rapid decompression of a severely distended bladder to prevent bladder atony or spasms.

———————————————❖

Performing peritoneal dialysis

In patients with acute or chronic renal failure, peritoneal dialysis performs the kidneys' function of removing impurities from the blood. Dialysate, the solution instilled into the peritoneal cavity by a catheter, draws waste products, excess fluid, and electrolytes from the blood across a semipermeable membrane.

A surgeon inserts the peritoneal catheter in the operating room or at the patient's bedside. A specially trained nurse may then perform peritoneal dialysis, either manually or using an automatic or semiautomatic cycle machine.

Peritoneal dialysis is usually contraindicated in patients who have had extensive abdominal or bowel surgery, or extensive abdominal trauma. Its most common complication is peritonitis.

Complications

Peritonitis usually results from a break in the integrity of the closed system or from contamination during an exchange or tubing change. Peritonitis may also develop if dialysate leaks from the catheter exit site and flows back into the catheter tract. Protein depletion, as much as ½ oz (15 g) daily and even more in patients with peritonitis, may result from the diffusion of blood protein into the dialysate through the peritoneal membrane.

Respiratory distress may result when dialysate in the peritoneal cavity increases pressure on the diaphragm, thus decreasing lung expansion. Constipation is a major cause of inflow-outflow problems, and excessive fluid loss from the use of dialysate with 4.25% dextrose concentration may cause hypovolemia, hypotension, and shock. Excessive fluid retention may lead to hypertension, peripheral edema, pulmonary edema and, ultimately, congestive heart failure. Other possible complications include electrolyte imbalances and hyperglycemia (which can be identified by frequent blood tests), exit site or subcutaneous tunnel infections, catheter malfunction, increased intra-abdominal pressure, and pain and cramping from cold dialysate.

Key steps

To perform peritoneal dialysis safely and reduce the risk of complications, follow these essential steps:

• To reduce the risk of peritonitis, use strict aseptic technique during catheter insertion, dialysis, and dressing changes. Everyone in the room should wear masks whenever the dialysis system is opened or entered.

• Change the dressing every 24 hours or whenever it becomes wet or soiled; doing so will also help prevent skin excoriation caused by any leakage.

• To prevent respiratory distress, turn the patient frequently and encourage him to do deep-breathing exercises to promote lung expansion. If the patient suffers severe respiratory distress during dialysis, drain the peritoneal cavity and notify the doctor. Monitor any patient on peritoneal dialysis who's being weaned from a ventilator.

• To ensure regular bowel movements and prevent constipation, give the patient a laxative or stool softener as needed.

• To prevent protein depletion, give the patient a high-protein diet or protein supplements, as ordered, and monitor serum albumin levels.

• Dialysate is available in three concentrations: 4.25% dextrose, 2.5% dextrose, and 1.5% dextrose. The 4.25% dextrose solution usually removes the largest amount of fluid from the blood because its glucose concentration is highest. If your patient receives this concentration of solution, monitor him carefully to prevent excess fluid loss.

• Also be prepared to inject or add insulin to the dialysate because some of the glucose in the 4.25% dextrose solution may enter the patient's bloodstream and cause severe hyperglycemia.

• As ordered, add antibiotics to the dialysate solution of patients with peritonitis, or add potassium for patients with low serum potassium levels (especially those on hourly exchanges) to prevent further losses.

• Warm dialysate to prevent pain and cramping and increase urea clearance. To warm dialysate, apply dry heat, such as a heat lamp or heating pad, to the fluid for 2 hours before administration.

Special considerations

When warming dialysate, avoid using moist heat, which increases the risk of contamination. Also avoid using a microwave oven, which may distribute heat unevenly. A bag of dialysate warmed in a microwave oven may feel tepid in one spot but be overheated in another; this overheated solution may injure the patient. If you must use a microwave, mix the solution after heating and then manually measure the temperature.

Carefully monitor effluent color. Only clear or pale yellow effluent is normal. Amber fluid suggests occult blood or even a bladder perforation; brown fluid indicates a perforated bowel; milky or opaque fluid suggests peritonitis; and bloody fluid signals abdominal bleeding. Notify the doctor immediately of any of these abnormal findings. ❖

Providing continuous arteriovenous hemofiltration

This procedure filters fluid, solutes, and electrolytes from the patient's blood and infuses a replacement solution. Continuous arteriovenous hemofiltration is used to treat patients who have fluid overload but who don't require dialysis. It's contraindicated in patients who have a mean arterial pressure of less than 60 mm Hg.

Complications

Procedure complications include bleeding, hemorrhage, infection, hemofilter occlusion, and thrombosis. Further complications include clotting and membrane leaks in the hemofilter; the latter leaves the blood compartment open to contamination.

Key steps

Follow these essential steps to avoid complications:
• Anticoagulate the blood in the hemofilter by infusing heparin in low doses (usually, 500 units/hour to start) into an infusion port on the arterial side of the setup. Then measure thrombin clotting time or activated clotting time (ACT). Keep ACT between 100 and 300 seconds during the procedure, depending on the patient's clotting times. If ACT is too high or too low, the doctor will adjust the heparin dose accordingly or write parameters.
• Another way to prevent clotting in the hemofilter is not to infuse medications or blood through the venous line. Use this line only in emergencies to infuse I.V. fluids.
• A third way to prevent clots in the hemofilter and to prevent kinks in the catheter is to make sure the patient doesn't bend the affected leg more than 30 degrees at the hip. The patient may logroll from side to side with assistance, however. When helping the patient turn, move the patient and the hemofilter as a single unit.
• Inspect the ultrafiltrate during the procedure. It should remain clear yellow, with no gross blood. Pink-tinged or bloody ultrafiltrate may signal a membrane leak in the hemofilter. If you suspect a leak, notify the doctor and have the hemofilter replaced.
• Calculate the right type and amount of filter replacement fluid every hour or according to your hospital's policy. Infuse this through the infusion pump into the arterial side of the circuit. (See *Calculating the right amount of filter replacement fluid.*)

Special considerations

Clamp the ultrafiltrate line only after checking your hospital's policy. Pressure may build up in some hemofilters, clotting them and collapsing the blood compartment. ❖

Mastering colostomy and ileostomy care

A patient with an ascending or transverse colostomy or ileostomy must wear an external pouch to

Calculating the right amount of filter replacement fluid

To calculate the amount of filter replacement fluid needed to infuse a patient undergoing continuous arteriovenous hemofiltration, you need to determine:
• the amount of ultrafiltrate produced during the previous hour
• the patient's other outputs during the previous hour, such as urine, feces, and nasogastric or chest drainage
• the patient's I.V. intake during the previous hour, including total parenteral nutrition, lipids, I.V. drips, medication boluses, heparin infusion (if applicable), and tube feedings
• the net desired hourly fluid loss as determined by the doctor.

Calculations
Once you've obtained these figures, subtract the patient's I.V. intake and desired fluid loss from the total of his ultrafiltrate production and other outputs. The equation reads:

(ultrafiltrate + other outputs)
− (I.V. intake + fluid loss)
= filter replacement fluid

Say your patient's ultrafiltrate production during the previous hour was 750 ml, and his other outputs amounted to 60 ml, for a total of 810 ml of output. And let's say that his I.V. intake for the previous hour was 130 ml and his doctor wanted him to lose 100 ml of fluid every hour. The equation for determining the amount of filter replacement fluid you'll need reads:

(750 + 60)
− (130 + 100)
= 580

So, over the next hour you'd want to infuse a total of 580 ml of filter replacement fluid. If the patient had received an unusually large amount of I.V. fluids or medications during the previous hour, or if his ultrafiltrate production was very low because of clotting in the hemofilter, the equation might yield a minimal or negative amount of filter replacement fluid. In that case, skip the filter replacement fluid infusion for the next hour or simply continue it at a keep-vein-open rate of 10 ml/hour.

collect fecal discharge (unless the surgeon has created a continent internal or magnetic ring fecal diversion). Besides collecting waste, the pouch helps to contain odor, and the appropriate skin barrier protects peristomal skin from emerging fecal matter.

Complications
Failure to fit the pouch properly over the stoma or using a belt improperly can injure the stoma. (See *Modifying a stoma appliance*, pages 374 and 375.)
Additional complications in-

(Text continues on page 376.)

Modifying a stoma appliance

If your patient's stoma appliance often leaks and overflows, he may quickly develop chronic peristomal excoriation. Perhaps the position of his stoma adds to the problem; his abdominal folds may tend to twist the belts, lifting the bag from the flange and allowing leakage when he sits. Contact with the highly acidic effluent also causes wafers and appliances to deteriorate rapidly.

You may be able to solve your patient's problem by using a hydrocolloid dressing to modify the stoma appliance. The hydrocolloid dressing should allow the skin around the patient's stoma to heal within 72 hours.

These are the basic steps you'll take.

1 Obtain a 1½″ (3.8-cm) two-piece appliance, such as Sur-Fit. Cut away the outside wafer, leaving only the flange or ring.

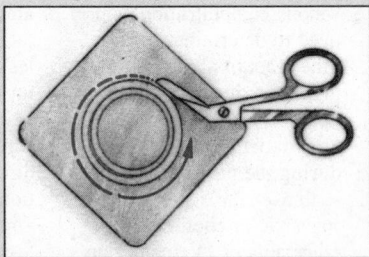

2 Using the measuring guide from the wafer box, determine the stoma's size and shape. Cut out the center of the wafer to fit your patient properly.

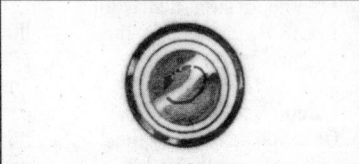

3 Using an 8″ × 8″ or 8″ × 12″ sheet of hydrocolloid dressing, measure and mark the location of of the stoma. Place the wafer over the stoma marking on the hydrocolloid dressing. Mark the outer circle of the ring in ink on the exterior surface of the hydrocolloid dressing.

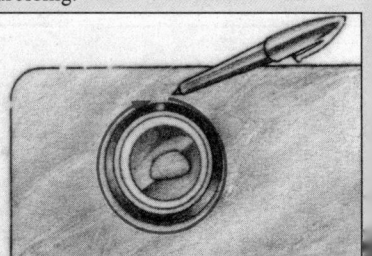

4 Lift the wafer off and cut out the opening ¾″ (2 cm) smaller than marked on the hydrocolloid dressing, to leave a ledge for the wafer to rest on.

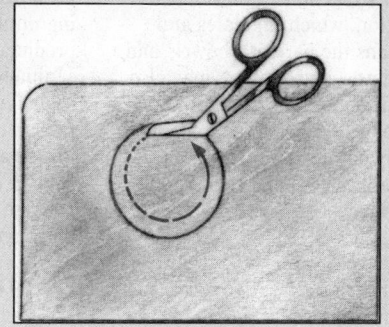

5 Cover this ledge with a skin bond element, place the wafer on it, and set the hydrocolloid dressing aside to dry.

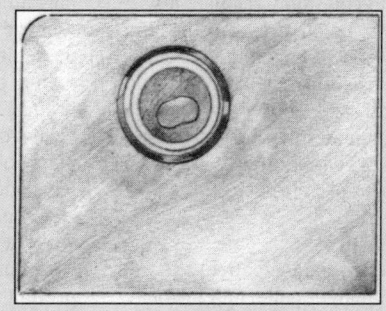

6 Prepare the patient's skin by treating any excoriated areas with warm water compresses and patting dry; sprinkle karaya-based powder on any deep (bleeding) areas. Peel off the back of the hydrocolloid dressing and press it into place around the patient's stoma. Then snap a new pouch onto the flange.

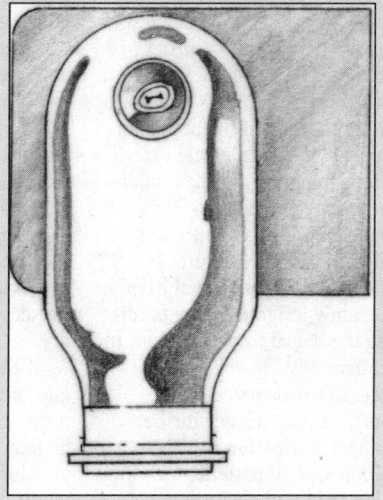

clude leaks, causing burning and itching; epidermal stripping with tape removal; and irritation of the patient's skin, or hypersensitivity reactions. Colostomy irrigation, which regulates and cleans the patient's bowels and relieves constipation, may also cause bowel perforation and prolapse. As well, the patient may develop an allergic reaction to adhesives and other ostomy products.

Key steps

Colostomy irrigation lets a patient with a descending or sigmoid colostomy regulate his bowel function; cleans the large bowel before and after diagnostic tests, surgery, or other procedures; and can relieve constipation on an infrequent, as-needed basis. To determine whether you should perform colostomy irrigation and, if so, when, review these steps:

• Determine the patient's bowel elimination pattern. A history of a regular bowel elimination pattern or of constipation suggests greater success than a history of diarrhea. Irrigation may not work if the patient has had radiation therapy to the abdomen or pelvis, has used certain medications long-term, or has inflammatory bowel disease.

• Determine the patient's suitability for this procedure. In a patient with a peristomal hernia, colostomy irrigation may predispose the bowel to perforation. In a patient with bowel prolapse (excessive protrusion at the stoma), it may trigger further prolapse. Irrigation is also contraindicated in patients with unstable fluid and electrolyte balance or any condition that con-

traindicates vagal stimulation.

• Colostomy irrigation may begin as soon as the postoperative patient regains bowel function, but most experts recommend waiting until bowel movements are predictable.

• Initially, you or the patient should irrigate the colostomy at the same time every day, recording the amount of output and any spillage between irrigations. Encourage the patient to assume as much responsibility as possible.

Special considerations

If a leak develops, change the pouching system immediately. Remove the pouching system if the patient reports burning or itching beneath it, if purulent drainage appears around the stoma, or if the patient complains of unexplained episodes of fecal odor (which may result from undetected contact of feces with the skin).

A liquid skin sealant helps prevent epidermal stripping with tape removal. Most skin sealants must be completely dry before you can apply additional products. Be sure to closely follow the manufacturer's directions.

Use adhesive solvents and removers only after patch-testing the patient's skin. Some products may irritate the skin or cause hypersensitivity reactions.

Because charcoal filters are ineffective when wet, use protective devices to keep the filters dry.

If the patient has severe allergies or sensitive skin or prefers not to use adhesive components, he may choose a nonadhesive pouching system. One such system (Cook VPI) consists of a reusable vinyl pouch with a silicone ring sized to fit around the stoma. An elastic belt secures the pouch.

Never make a pinhole in a pouch to release gas. This will destroy the odor-proof seal.

Use commercial pouch deodorants if desired. However, be aware that most pouches are odorless and that odor should be obvious only when the pouch leaks or is emptied. (Never use aspirin in the pouch to reduce odor because this could induce stomal bleeding.)

❖

Skin and wound procedures

The skin protects internal structures, regulates body temperature, controls homeostasis, and acts as a sensory and excretory organ. When the skin is compromised through wounds, burns, ulcers and other lesions, the procedures you'll perform aim to prevent infection, protect the skin from further trauma, and promote regrowth.

❖

Caring for surgical wounds

When caring for a patient with surgical wounds, your main goal is to prevent infection caused by pathogens entering the wound. To do this, you'll perform procedures to promote patient comfort, to protect the patient's skin from maceration and excoriation

caused by contact with irritating drainage, and to measure wound drainage so that fluid and electrolyte balance can be monitored. Certain wound care procedures are especially problematic, such as irrigating wounds in the limb and thigh, caring for wounds with a wide opening or deep wounds with a small opening, and caring for an amputated body part that will be reattached.

Complications

The major complication of surgical wounds is infection, introduced at the time of wound formation or during your care. Changing dressings may provoke friction and allergic reactions to antiseptic cleaning agents, topical medications, or adhesive tape that may lead to skin redness, rash, excoriation, or infection. Excessive exudate and copious drainage may also damage the skin. To promote healing, most wounds should be irrigated; however, conditions unique to the wound may make this impossible.

Key steps

Dressing a wound requires sterile technique and sterile supplies to prevent contamination. Use the color of the wound to determine which type of dressing to apply. Follow these essential steps to dress a wound with a drain, pouch a wound, and irrigate difficult wounds.

Tailoring wound care to wound color

If your patient has an open wound, assess how well it's healing and take appropriate action according to its color.

Red wounds. The color of healthy granulation tissue, red wounds indicate normal healing. When a wound begins to heal, a layer of pale pink granulation tissue covers the wound bed. As this layer thickens, it becomes beefy red.

Cover a red wound, keep it moist and clean, and protect it from trauma. Use a transparent dressing (such as Tegaderm or Op-Site), a hydrocolloid dressing (such as DuoDerm), or a gauze dressing moistened with sterile 0.9% sodium chloride solution or impregnated with petroleum jelly or an antibiotic.

Yellow wounds. Yellow is the color of microorganisms' exudate in an open wound. When a wound heals without complications, the immune system removes microorganisms. But if there are too many microorganisms to remove, whitish yellow, creamy yellow, yellowish green, or beige exudate accumulates.

Clean a yellow wound, and remove exudate using high-pressure irrigation; then cover it with a moist dressing. Use absorptive products (for example, Debrisan beads and paste) or a moist gauze dressing with or without an antibiotic. You may also use hydrotherapy with whirlpool or high-pressure irrigation.

Black wounds. Black signals necrosis. Dead, avascular tissue slows healing and provides a site for microorganisms to proliferate.

Debride a black wound, and apply a dressing to keep the wound moist and guard it against external contamination. As ordered, use enzyme products (such as Elase or Travase), hy-

drotherapy with whirlpool or high-pressure irrigation, or a moist gauze dressing.

Multicolored wounds. If you note two or even all three colors, classify the wound according to the least healthy color present. For example, if your patient's wound is both red and yellow, classify it as a yellow wound.

Dressing a wound with a drain

Certain wounds may require a drain to help siphon off exudate. Here's how to dress a wound with a drain:
• To save time performing this procedure, use precut tracheostomy pads or drain dressings instead of custom-cutting gauze pads to fit around the drain.
• If your patient is sensitive to adhesive tape, use paper or silk tape because these are less likely to cause a skin reaction and will peel off more easily than adhesive tape.
• Use a surgical mask to cradle a chin or jawline dressing; this provides a secure dressing and avoids the need for shaving the patient's hair.

Pouching a wound

If a sump drain isn't adequately collecting wound secretions, reinforce it with an ostomy pouch or other collection bag.
• Use waterproof tape to strengthen a spot on the front of the pouch near the adhesive opening; then cut a small "X" in the tape. Feed the drain catheter into the pouch through the "X" cut. Seal the cut around the tubing with more waterproof tape; then connect the tubing to the suction pump.
• Record the volume of drainage.

Irrigating difficult wounds

Flushing a wound with irrigating solution removes exudate and keeps the wound clean. Your technique will vary according to the wound's size and location.

• Irrigate a wound with a wide opening with irrigating solution in a syringe, using slow, continuous pressure. Hold the syringe tip 1" (2.5 cm) above the upper edge of the wound and make sure the solution flows from the clean to the dirty area of the wound so that exudate won't contaminate clean tissue.

• Irrigate a deep wound that has a small opening with a filled irrigating syringe, also using slow, continuous pressure. Attach a sterile, soft rubber catheter to the syringe, and gently insert the tip until you feel resistance; then pull out the catheter about ½" (1 cm) to remove the tip from the fragile inner wall of the wound. Pinch off the catheter just below the syringe to prevent aspirating drainage and contaminating the equipment.

• You may soak an arm or leg wound in a large basin of warm irrigating fluid, such as water, 0.9% sodium chloride solution, or an appropriate antiseptic. If necessary, use an agitator to dislodge bacteria and loosen debris. Rinse the wound several times, if possible, and carefully dispose of the infected liquid.

• To irrigate trunk and thigh wounds, you may want to try a special device that uses Stomahesive and a plastic irrigating chamber applied over the wound. You may run warm solution through an infusion set and collect it in a drainage bag.

• For a hard-to-reach wound, try performing syringe irrigation at the time of dressing. Where possible, direct the flow at right angles to the wound and allow the fluid to drain by gravity. You'll need to position the patient carefully, either in bed or on a chair. He may need analgesia during this procedure.

• If irrigation isn't possible, you'll have to swab-clean the wound, which is time-consuming. Swab away exudate before using an antiseptic or 0.9% sodium chloride solution to clean the wound, taking care not to push loose debris into the wound. If your hospital's policy permits, use sharp sterile scissors to snip off loose, dead tissue. Never pull it off.

Special considerations

Always practice strict aseptic technique for all wound care.

If the patient has two wounds in the same area, cover each wound separately with layers of sterile 4" × 4" gauze pads. Then cover both sites with an abdominal pad secured to the patient's skin with tape. A single pad may become quickly saturated, promoting cross-contamination.

Don't pack a wound too tightly because this compresses adjacent capillaries and may prevent the wound edges from contracting. The packing should be moist, but avoid using overly damp packing because it slows wound closure from within and increases the risk of infection.

Use a moisture- and contaminant-proof collodion spray or similar topical protectant instead of a gauze dressing if ordered. This covering dries in a clear, impermeable film that leaves the wound visible for observation and avoids the friction caused by a dressing.

If your patient has suffered a traumatic amputation, wrap the amputated body part in dry, sterile gauze. Place the part in a plastic bag or other waterproof container. Then place this container on a bed of ice, and rush it to the doctor or the appropriate department.

❖

Caring for pressure ulcers

Lesions caused by unrelieved pressure on skin, pressure ulcers impair circulation, depriving tissues of oxygen and other life-sustaining nutrients and damaging the skin and underlying structures. Most pressure ulcers develop over bony prominences, where friction and shearing forces combine with pressure to break down skin and underlying tissues. Common ulcer sites include the sacrum, coccyx, ischial tuberosities, and greater trochanters. Pressure ulcers also commonly develop over the vertebrae, scapulae, elbows, knees, and heels in bedridden or immobile patients. Your expert assessment is crucial in identifying and then solving the specific problems placing such patients at risk.

Complications

Untreated, pressure ulcers can lead to serious infection. Other complications include breakdown of healthy skin around a wound, circulatory compromise and, in a deep wound, abscess

formation. Ischemia may be exacerbated by a wound that's packed too tightly. External mechanical forces, such as pressure, friction, and shearing, may also exacerbate an ulcer. Guard your patient against allergic reactions and dried skin.

Key steps

To properly care for your patient with pressure ulcers, you need to know which topical agent best cleans which type of wound. You must be able to assess the ulcer stage to ensure proper care. (See *Staging and dressing a pressure ulcer*, pages 382 and 383.) Perform these essential steps:
• Turn and reposition the patient every 1 to 2 hours unless contraindicated. For a patient who can't turn himself or who is turned on a schedule, use pressure-relieving and pressure-reducing devices, such as a static air-mattress overlay or a low-air-loss or air-fluidized bed.
• Implement active or passive range-of-motion exercises to relieve pressure and promote circulation. To save time, combine these exercises with bathing if appropriate.
• Teach the patient to avoid heat lamps and harsh soaps because they dry the skin. Instruct him to apply lotion after bathing to keep his skin moist. Also tell him to avoid vigorous massage because it can damage capillaries.

Cleaning with topical agents

Using the appropriate topical agent more efficiently promotes healing, whereas using improper cleaning solutions may inadvertently cause injury.

Antibiotics. Use antibiotics, such as bacitracin (Neosporin Ointment and Polysporin Ointment), only for early-stage ulcers. These agents may not penetrate sufficiently to kill deeper bacterial colonies.

Antiseptics. Use antiseptics only as irrigating solutions, not for packing. Dilute standard 3% hydrogen peroxide solution to half-strength or quarter-strength.
• Avoid using hydrogen peroxide after granulation tissue develops because its foaming action may cause blistering. Also avoid using it to clean deep or tunneled wounds because the wound may retain and absorb oxygen bubbles, creating air emboli.
• Avoid using povidone-iodine on open wounds because it may damage granulation tissue, retard collagen synthesis, and irritate surrounding skin.
• Apply diluted sodium hypochlorite, as directed, only for initial wound debridement.
• Avoid multiple applications of sodium hypochlorite because it inhibits granulation tissue growth, delays epithelialization, and irritates surrounding skin.

Circulatory stimulants (Granulex, Proderm). Use these agents to promote blood flow. Both contain balsam of Peru and castor oil. However, Granulex also contains crystallized trypsin, an enzyme that promotes debridement.

Enzymes. Apply collagenase in thin layers after cleaning the wound with 0.9% sodium chloride solution. Avoid concurrent use of collagenase with agents that decrease enzymatic activity, including detergents, hexachlorophene, antiseptics with heavy-metal ions, iodine, or such acidic solutions as Burow's solution.
• Use collagenase cautiously near the patient's eyes. If contact occurs, flush his eyes repeatedly with 0.9% sodium chloride solution or sterile water.
• Use fibrinolysin only after surgical removal of dry eschar.
• Apply sutilains ointment first if using concurrently with a topical antibacterial agent. Avoid applying sutilains to ulcers in major body cavities, to areas with exposed nerve tissue, or to fungating neoplastic lesions. Don't use sutilains in women of childbearing age or in patients with limited cardiopulmonary reserve.
• Store sutilains at a cool temperature (35.6° to 50° F [2° to 10° C]). Also use sutilains cautiously near the patient's eyes. If contact occurs, flush the eyes repeatedly with 0.9% sodium chloride solution or sterile water.

Exudate absorbers. Clean but don't dry the secreting ulcer before applying dextranomer beads. Discontinue use when secretions stop, removing gray-yellow beads (which indicate saturation) by irrigating with sterile water or 0.9% sodium chloride solution. Don't use in tunneling ulcers.

Use exudate absorbers cautiously near the eyes. If contact occurs, flush the eyes repeatedly with 0.9% sodium chloride solution or sterile water.

Special considerations
Always check your hospital's policy concerning cleaning pressure ulcers. Some experts recommend using only physiologic solutions,

(Text continues on page 384.)

Staging and dressing a pressure ulcer

Assessing the stage of your patient's pressure ulcer helps ensure appropriate care. For instance, the type of dressing you'll use on a pressure ulcer depends on the ulcer stage. Use these descriptions recommended by the Agency for Health Care Policy and Research as a guide.

Stage I

In this stage, the skin lesion is erythematous, nonblanching, and intact—the heralding lesion of skin ulceration. *Note:* Reactive hyperthermia normally occurs for a period lasting one-half to three-fourths as long as the pressure-occluded blood flow to the area. Don't confuse this phenomenon with a stage I pressure ulcer.

Stage II

The ulcer is superficial and appears as an abrasion, blister, or shallow crater. Expect to assess partial-thickness skin loss involving the epidermis, dermis, or both.

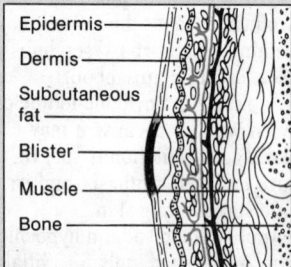

Dressing

A *film dressing* (such as Tegaderm, Bioclusive, Op-Site, or UniFlex) guards against shearing. It may be left in place for up to 7 days if the occlusive seal remains intact. A film dressing allows wound assessment, however. A *hydrocolloid dressing* (such as DuoDERM, Comfeel, or IntraSite Absorbent) also may be left in place for up to 7 days if the occlusive seal remains intact.

Dressing

A *composite dressing* (such as Viasorb or a film dressing over Telfa) provides an absorbent, nonadherent layer over the wound, with an occlusive cover. A *hydrogel dressing* (such as Vigilon, Geliperm, or J & J Gel Dressing) absorbs an ulcer's drainage. It usually requires a gauze dressing cover. A *burn dressing* (such as EXU-DRY) is absorbent, nonadherent, nonocclusive, and protects against shearing. It may also be used with a topical agent. A *hydrocolloid dressing* may also be used for a stage II ulcer.

Stage III

The ulcer resembles a deep crater, with or without undermining of adjacent tissue. Expect full-thickness skin loss involving damage to or necrosis of S.C. tissue, which may extend to – but not through – underlying fascia.

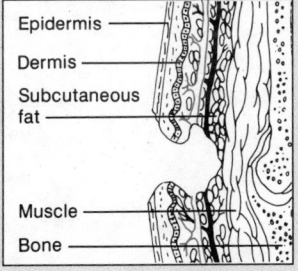

Dressing

A *hydrocolloid dressing* increases absorbency and wear time but is not preferred because it may cause tissue damage if removed frequently (daily or more often). A *hydrogel dressing* or *burn dressing* may be used as a carrier for topical agents.

Stage IV

The ulcer involves full-thickness skin loss with extensive destruction, tissue necrosis, or damage to muscle, bone, or supporting structures (such as tendons or joint capsules). *Note:* Undermining and sinus tracts are also associated with stage IV pressure ulcers.

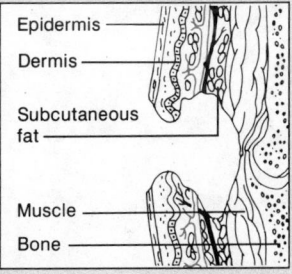

Dressing

A *gauze dressing* (such as a Kerlix dressing) is absorbent, nonocclusive, and usually must be changed every 8 to 12 hours. A *hydrogel dressing* or *hydrocolloid dressing* can also be used. However, a hydrocolloid dressing may be contraindicated because of ulcer location, exposed bone, or the amount of drainage.

such as 0.9% sodium chloride solution because other solutions (such as povidone-iodine, hexachlorophene, sodium hypochlorite, and hydrogen peroxide) may injure cells and retard healing.

Don't use tincture of benzoin compound as a skin sealant because it triggers an allergic reaction in some patients.

Avoid using elbow and heel protectors that fasten with a single narrow strap. The strap may impair neurovascular function in the involved hand or foot. ❖

7 Correcting Equipment Problems

Cardiovascular monitors and devices

Cardiac and hemodynamic monitoring provides you with valuable information about your patient's cardiovascular status. For various reasons, though, the devices can produce inaccurate readings and set off malfunction alarms. Consequently, you need to know how to anticipate, spot, and correct these potential problems.

Automated vital signs monitors

An automated vital signs monitor measures a patient's vital signs independently, freeing you to carry out other patient care activities. A noninvašive device, the monitor measures pulse rate, systolic and diastolic blood pressures, and mean arterial pressure at preset intervals. Some models also monitor the patient's temperature.

Troubleshooting problems

Occasionally, an automated vital signs monitor may display an inaccurate reading. Some common problems follow, along with possible causes and appropriate nursing interventions.

No value or error message

A value may fail to appear if the patient is experiencing a cardiac arrhythmia. After confirming an arrhythmia, check the patient's clinical status (for example, blood pressure, pulse rate, and mental status) and take measures to stabilize him. In the absence of an arrhythmia, check the patient's heart rate. If it's below 40 beats/minute, use an alternative method to determine blood pressure, such as a Doppler ultrasound stethoscope.

Other possible causes of no value appearing or an error message being displayed are kinked or occluded tubing, a leak in the tubing or cuff, and patient movement, including shivering or seizures. To solve the problem, unkink the tubing or reposition the patient if he's leaning against the tubing, replace the cuff set, and remind the patient not to move his arm. If the patient is chilled, warm him with blankets. Also give medication, as ordered, to decrease seizures.

Extremely high blood pressure value

This reading may occur if the cuff is too small or if it's positioned below heart level. To remedy the problem, always use the right-sized cuff (as described in the operating manual or inside the cuff) and place the cuffed limb at heart level.

Extremely low blood pressure value

This problem typically results from a cuff that's too large or that's positioned above heart level. Again, use the right-sized cuff and place the cuffed limb at heart level. A low pressure value may also result from faulty internal calibration. If this is the cause, replace the monitor and call for service.

No value or only mean blood pressure value

This reading may be triggered by rapid blood pressure fluctuation caused by cardiac arrhythmia or vasoactive drugs; patient movement, shivering, or seizures; or an excessively low heart rate. In all of these instances, use an alternative method to determine blood pressure such as a Doppler ultrasound stethoscope. This problem may also occur if the patient's weight is under 20 lb (9 kg). If your patient weighs less than 20 lb, use an appropriate pediatric or neonatal cuff and tubing or an alternative device as mentioned above.

No heart rate or blood pressure value for a stable patient

This situation may occur because of inadequate circulation to a limb or a faulty cuff or sensor. Respond to the problem by using a different limb to monitor vital signs. Also try using another cuff; if that doesn't help, change the entire unit.   ❖

ECG monitors

Electrocardiogram (ECG) monitors provide a picture of the heart's electrical activity. They may do this continuously (as with a single-lead monitor) or intermittently (as with a 12-lead ECG). Or the monitor may be used to discern specific abnormalities such as ST-segment elevations.

Single-lead (continuous) monitor

Although single-lead monitoring doesn't give you a complete picture of the heart's electrical activity, it does give you a continuous one. You can monitor a single lead using either hardwire monitoring or telemetry (wireless monitoring). The choice depends on several factors, including whether the patient is ambulatory and which particular lead you want to monitor.

The leads in single-lead monitoring approximate those in 12-lead monitoring. But the electrode positions for the limb leads differ. With single-lead monitoring, you place the limb lead electrodes on the chest.

Careful electrode placement is essential to proper ECG function and accurate readings. What seems to be a strange reading may reflect improper electrode placement. (See *Placing electrodes for single-lead ECGs*, pages 388 and 389.)

Troubleshooting problems

As with any piece of technical equipment, a cardiac monitor may occasionally malfunction. Following are some of the most common problems you may encounter, along with their possible causes and appropriate interventions.

False high-rate alarm. This spurious alarm may occur if the monitor is interpreting large T waves as QRS complexes, which doubles the rate. If you think this may be the cause, reposition the electrodes to a lead where QRS complexes are taller than T waves. The alarm may also sound because of skeletal

(Text continues on page 390.)

Placing electrodes for single-lead ECGs

This chart shows the correct electrode positions for some of the electrocardiogram (ECG) monitoring leads you'll use most often. For each lead, you'll see electrode placement for a five-leadwire system, a three-leadwire system, and a telemetry system.

In the two hardwire systems, the electrode positions for one lead may be identical to the electrode positions for another lead. In this case, sim-

ply change the lead selector switch to the setting that corresponds to the lead you want. In some cases, you'll need to reposition the electrodes.

In the telemetry system, you can create the same lead with two electrodes that you do with three, simply by eliminating the ground electrode.

The chart uses these abbreviations: RA, right arm; LA, left arm; RL, right leg; LL, left leg; C, chest; and G, ground.

FIVE-LEADWIRE SYSTEM	THREE-LEADWIRE SYSTEM	TELEMETRY SYSTEM

Lead I

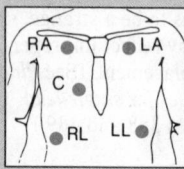 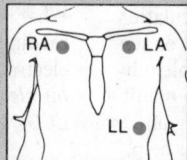 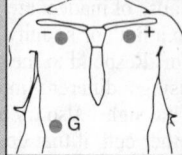

Lead II

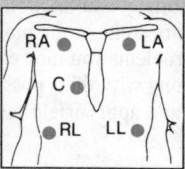 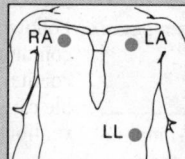 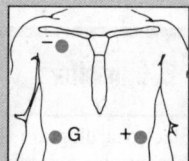

Lead III

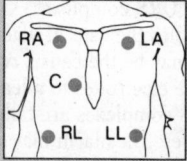 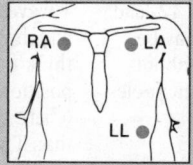 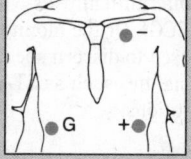

FIVE-LEADWIRE SYSTEM	THREE-LEADWIRE SYSTEM	TELEMETRY SYSTEM

Lead MCL₁

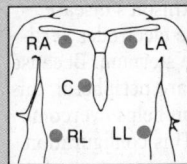 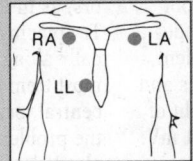 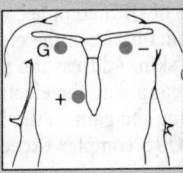

Lead MCL₆

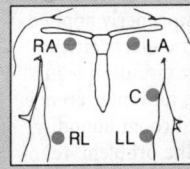 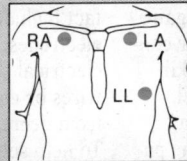 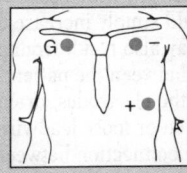

Sternal lead

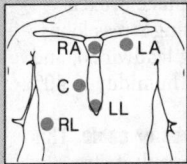 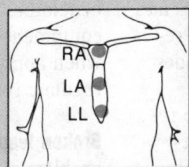 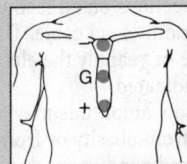

Lewis lead

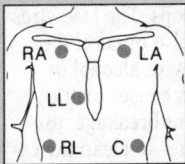 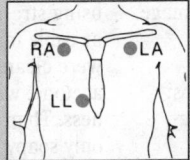 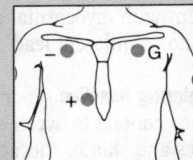

muscle activity. To solve this problem, place the electrodes away from major muscle masses.

False low-rate alarm. Possible causes include a shift in electrical axis from patient movement (making QRS complexes too small to register), a low amplitude of QRS complex, or poor contact between the electrodes and skin. Address the problem by reapplying the electrodes and setting the gain so the height of the QRS complex exceeds 1 mV.

Low amplitude. This problem may occur if the gain dial is set too low, in which case you should simply increase the gain. It may also result from poor contact between the patient's skin and the electrodes, dried gel, broken or loose leadwires, a poor connection between the patient and the monitor, or a malfunctioning monitor. To remedy these situations, first check the connections on all leadwires and the monitoring cable. Then replace or reapply the electrodes as indicated.

Low amplitude may also result from obesity or from decreased conduction due to irreversible myocardial damage. For an obese patient, move the electrodes closer to midline. For a patient with myocardial damage, monitor a different lead.

Wandering baseline. Poor position or contact between electrodes and skin or thoracic movement with respirations may cause a wandering baseline. To solve the problem, reposition or replace the electrodes.

Artifact (waveform interference). If the patient is experiencing seizures, chills, or anxiety, an erratic waveform may result. Notify the doctor and intervene as ordered. Reassure the patient and keep him warm.

Similarly, artifact can occur in a patient experiencing tremors, as in Parkinson's disease. Try placing the electrodes vertically along the sternum. Because most tremors are peripheral, this central location helps overcome the problem. This configuration also helps when movement of soft (breast) tissue causes artifact.

Other possible causes of artifact include improperly applied electrodes, static electricity, an electrical short circuit in leadwires or cable, and interference from decreased room humidity. To help solve the problem, reapply the electrodes, make sure the cable doesn't have exposed connectors, change static-causing bedclothes, replace broken equipment (using stress loops when applying leadwires), and regulate room humidity to 40%.

Broken leadwires or cable. This problem may result if stress loops were not used on leadwires. In this situation, replace the leadwires and retape them, using stress loops. The leadwires or cable may also break if they were cleaned with alcohol or acetone, which causes brittleness. To prevent breakage, use only soapy water to clean the cable and leadwires. *Don't allow cable ends to become wet.*

60-cycle interference. Also known as a fuzzy baseline, this problem may result from electrical interference from other equipment in the room, or from the patient's bed being improperly grounded. Remedy the problem by attaching all electrical equipment and the patient's bed to the room's common ground. Check plugs to make sure the prongs aren't loose.

Twelve-lead ECG

The 12-lead ECG provides a dozen different views of the heart's electrical activity, with each lead transmitting information about a particular area. That's why one lead may clearly show an abnormality that another lead omits.

The 12 leads include 3 bipolar limb leads (I, II, and III), 3 unipolar augmented limb leads (aV_R, aV_L, and aV_F), and 6 unipolar precordial, or chest, leads (V_1, V_2, V_3, V_4, V_5, and V_6). As with the single-lead ECG, careful electrode placement is essential to proper ECG function and accurate readings. (See *Placing electrodes for 12-lead ECGs*, pages 392 and 393.)

Troubleshooting problems

The 12-lead ECG contains a margin for error. The most common problem you'll encounter is electrical interference.

Electrical interference. While the 12-lead ECG monitors the heart's electrical activity, it may also pick up electrical activity from other sources, such as skeletal and respiratory muscles. Additional sources of electrical interference include high-frequency power lines, electrodes, and amplifiers.

Although modern ECG machines can override the interference from electrical equipment and power lines, they're powerless against interference from muscles. For most patients, this doesn't present a significant problem. The changes are slight and don't hinder diagnosis. Occasionally, however, the extra signals generated by the muscles may mask subtle changes in the ECG. As a result, you and others won't have a complete picture of the patient's cardiac status, and this may lead to a misdiagnosis.

You can avoid interference problems by using a signal-averaged ECG. This test involves transferring ECG impulses into a computer, which averages the waveforms into one complex. In the process, the computer amplifies the voltage of the QRS complexes as much as 1,000 times, and sometimes more.

ST-segment monitoring

A relatively new technique, ST-segment monitoring helps detect myocardial ischemia, electrolyte imbalances, coronary artery spasm, and hypoxic events by showing ST-segment changes as they occur. The ST segment represents early ventricular repolarization, and any changes in this waveform component reflect alterations in myocardial oxygenation. Subtle changes in the patient's ST segment may be precursors to major changes in his condition. But individual ST-segment values are less important than the changing trend in the ST segment.

Any monitoring lead that views an ischemic heart region will reveal ST-segment changes, and these ST-segment patterns of ischemia are patient specific. A deviation of more than 1 mm

Placing electrodes for 12-lead ECGs

The illustration shows how 5 electrodes (4 limb, 1 chest) record the heart's electrical potential from 12 different electrocardiogram (ECG) views (leads).

To record the six limb leads, you'll place electrodes on the patient's right arm, left arm, and left leg, with a fourth on the patient's right leg to serve as a ground. You'll also place the six precordial electrodes at key locations across the patient's chest as follows:
V_1 – fourth intercostal space, right sternal border
V_2 – fourth intercostal space, left sternal border
V_3 – midway between V_2 and V_4
V_4 – fifth intercostal space, left midclavicular lane
V_5 – fifth intercostal space, left anterior axillary line
V_6 – fifth intercostal space, left midaxillary line

The standard bipolar limb leads (I, II, III) rely on two electrodes, detecting variations in electrical potential at the negative pole and the positive pole and recording the difference.

The unipolar augmented limb leads (aV_R, aV_L, aV_F) rely on only one electrode, representing the positive pole. (The negative pole is computed by the ECG machine.) These leads measure electrical potential between the lead and the electrical midpoint of the remaining two leads.

By monitoring the heart's electrical activity from above and below and from the right and left sides, the six limb leads give a two-dimensional view of the heart's frontal plane.

In contrast, the six unipolar chest leads (V_1 through V_5) view electrical potential from the horizontal plane, helping to locate abnormality in the heart's lateral and posterior walls.

---

from the original baseline is considered significant and may indicate myocardial ischemia.

Because chest pain may not always accompany ischemia, ST-segment monitoring is especially important in detecting asymptomatic ischemia. ST-segment monitoring allows prompt assessment and immediate treatment, which can prevent myocardial necrosis. It also helps evaluate the effectiveness of treatments by showing the ST segment's return to baseline. ST-segment monitoring is contraindicated in a patient with ventricular pacing because pacing alters the ST segment.

As with ECGs, electrode placement is essential to proper readings. (See *Placing electrodes for ST-segment monitoring,* pages 394 and 395.)

Troubleshooting problems

Following are two of the most common problems associated with ST-segment monitoring, along with possible causes and

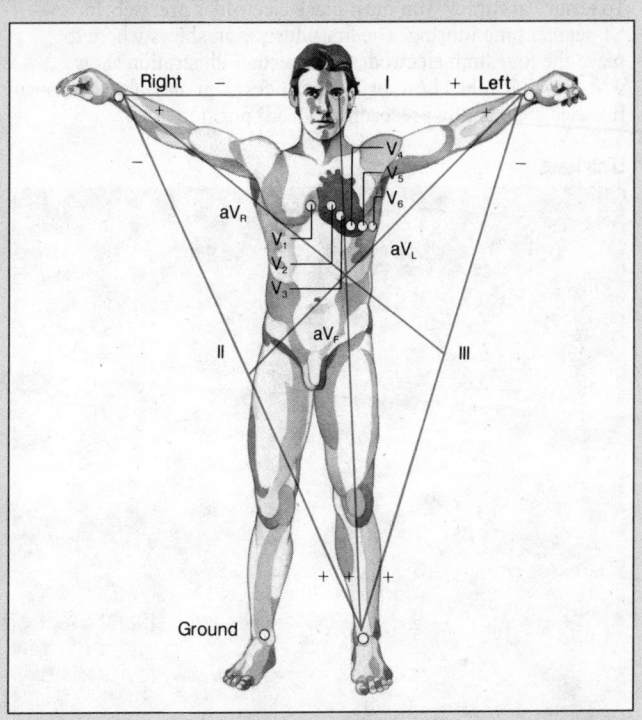

the appropriate nursing interventions.

False alarm. Dramatic changes in heart rate or ECG patterns from arrhythmias may alter the monitor's measurement points and sound an alarm. Check the measurement points and readjust if necessary, or select an alternate lead.

Inexplicable alarm. If an alarm sounds and you can't determine a reason, the problem may be a faulty electrode or poor contact between the electrode and the patient's skin. Replace or reposition the electrodes to ensure a clear signal.

Placing electrodes for ST-segment monitoring

To ensure accuracy, you must place electrodes precisely for
ST-segment monitoring. The first illustration shows where to
place the four limb electrodes. The second illustration shows
where to place the chest, or V, electrodes. You may place the positive electrode at any precordial (V-lead) position.

Limb leads

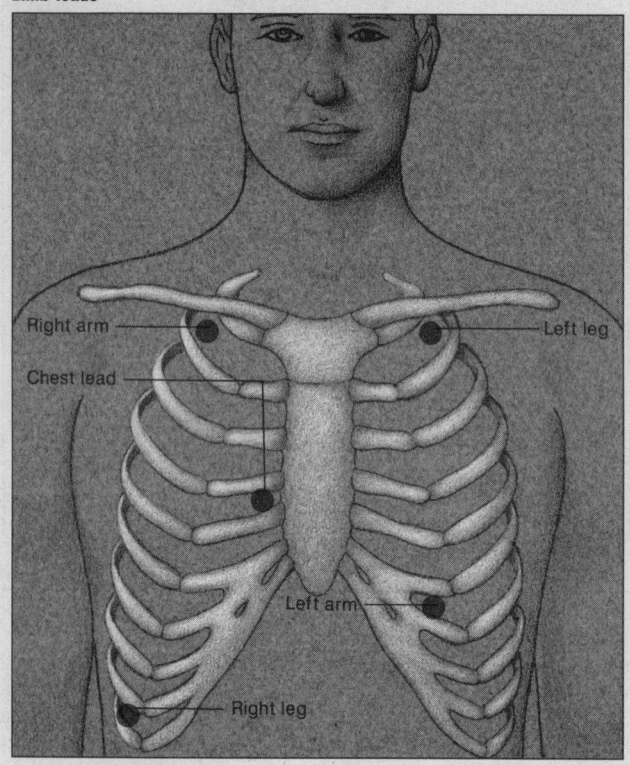

Pacemakers

A battery-operated generator, the
pacemaker emits timed electrical
signals that trigger contraction
of the heart muscle and control
the heart rate. A pacemaker may
be either temporary or permanent.

V leads

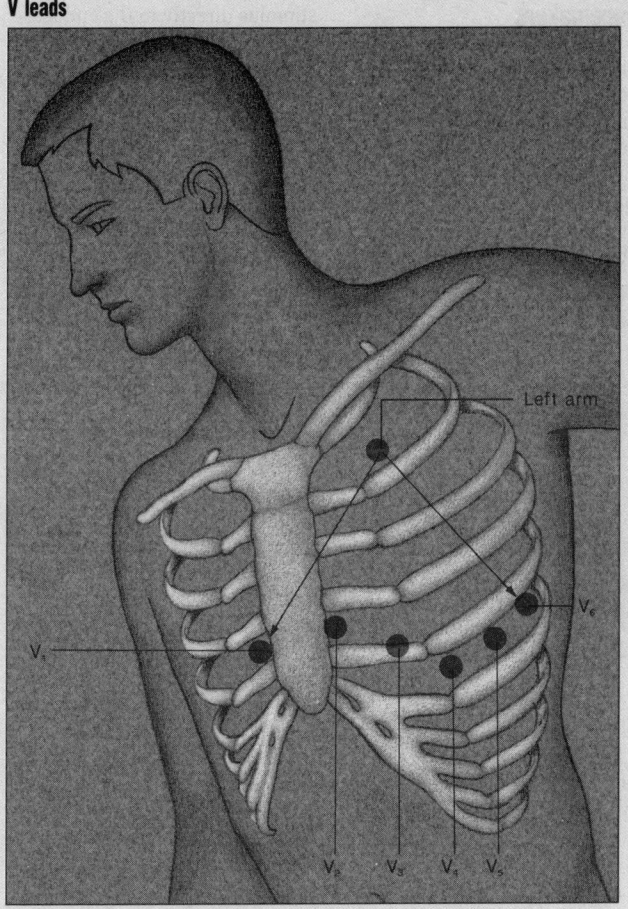

Temporary pacemakers

Usually inserted in an emergency, a temporary pacemaker consists of an external battery-powered pulse generator and a lead or electrode system. Four types of temporary pacemakers exist: transcutaneous, transvenous, transthoracic, and epicardial.

In a life-threatening situation, when time is critical, a *transcutaneous pacemaker* is the best choice. This device quickly

Placing electrodes for noninvasive temporary pacemakers

Place the electrodes for a noninvasive temporary pacemaker at heart level, with the heart lying between the two electrodes. This placement ensures the shortest distance that the electrical stimulus must travel to the heart.

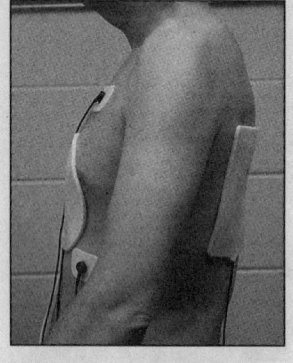

and effectively sends an electrical impulse from the pulse generator to the patient's heart by way of two electrodes, which are placed on the front and back of the patient's chest. (See *Placing electrodes for noninvasive temporary pacemakers.*) Transcutaneous pacing is used only until the doctor can institute transvenous pacing.

Besides being more comfortable for the patient, a *transvenous pacemaker* is more reliable than a transcutaneous pacemaker. Transvenous pacing involves threading an electrode catheter through a vein into the patient's right atrium or right ventricle. The electrode then attaches to an external pulse generator. As a result, the pulse generator can provide an electrical stimulus directly to the endocardium. This is the most common type of pacemaker.

As an elective surgical procedure or as an emergency measure during cardiopulmonary resuscitation, a doctor may choose to insert a *transthoracic pacemaker.* To insert this type of pacemaker, the doctor performs a procedure similar to pericardiocentesis, in which he uses a cardiac needle to pass an electrode through the chest wall and into the right ventricle. This procedure carries a significant risk of coronary artery laceration and cardiac tamponade.

During cardiac surgery, the surgeon may insert electrodes through the epicardium of the right ventricle and, if he wants to institute atrioventricular sequential pacing, the right atrium. From there, the electrodes pass through the chest wall, where they remain available if temporary pacing becomes necessary. This is called *epicardial pacing.*

Troubleshooting problems
Following are some of the problems you may encounter with different types of pacemakers, along with their possible causes and appropriate interventions.

All pacemakers. When caring for a patient with a pacemaker, continuously monitor the electrocardiogram reading, noting capture, sensing, rate, intrinsic beats, and competition of paced and intrinsic rhythms. If the pacemaker is sensing correctly, the sense indicator on the pulse generator should flash with each beat. On some models, both the sense and pacer indicators on the pulse generator flash with each beat. (See *Handling temporary pacemaker malfunction*, pages 398 and 399.)

Closely monitor the sensitivity setting on the pulse generator. Excessive sensitivity (oversensing) may cause the pulse generator to interpret P or T waves or artifact as QRS complexes and fail to pace. On the other hand, insufficient sensitivity (undersensing) may cause the generator to deliver a pacing stimulus at the wrong time, resulting in a lethal arrhythmia.

You'll also need to take care to prevent microshock. This includes warning the patient not to use any electrical equipment that isn't grounded, such as telephones, electric razors, televisions, or lamps. (See *Preventing microshock*, page 400.)

Other safety measures include placing a plastic cover supplied by the manufacturer over the pacemaker controls to avoid an accidental setting change and insulating the pacemaker by covering all exposed metal parts (such as electrode connections and pacemaker terminals) with nonconducting tape or placing the pacing unit in a dry, rubber surgical glove. If the patient is disoriented or uncooperative, use restraints to prevent accidental removal of pacemaker wires. Check that the batteries are still functioning before using the pulse generator, and change them as needed, according to the manufacturer's instructions. If the patient needs emergency defibrillation, make sure the pace-

maker can withstand the procedure. If unsure, disconnect the pulse generator to avoid damage.

Transcutaneous pacemaker. Don't place the electrodes over a bony area because bone conducts current poorly. Keep in mind that, if the patient is diaphoretic, you'll need to change the electrodes frequently. Also, with female patients, place the anterior electrode under the patient's left breast but not over her diaphragm. Placing the electrode over the diaphragm could cause the diaphragm to be paced, resulting in shortness of breath and increased patient anxiety.

Use the lowest amount of pacing current to produce capture to decrease the incidence of skeletal muscle stimulation, which can be painful.

Transvenous pacemaker. During insertion, expect to see temporary ventricular ectopy or tachyarrhythmias. Treat these arrhythmias, as indicated, with lidocaine. If bradyarrhythmias occur, administer atropine. If the doctor inserts the electrode through the brachial or femoral vein, immobilize the patient's arm or leg to avoid putting stress on the pacing wires.

Transthoracic pacemaker. Loss of capture and an elevated ST segment are two potential problems. Usually, loss of capture results from an inability to produce electrical stimulation, which is caused by poor positioning of the pacing wire, insufficient electrical output from the pacemaker generator, or myocardial necrosis or ischemia at the pace-

Handling temporary pacemaker malfunction

On occasion, a temporary pacemaker may fail to function appropriately. When this occurs, you'll need to take immediate action to correct the problem. Study the following chart to learn which steps to take to correct pacemaker malfunctions.

Failure to pace
This happens when the pacemaker either doesn't fire or fires too often. The pulse generator may not be working properly or it may not be conducting the impulse to the patient.

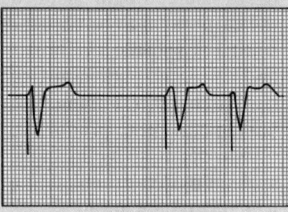

Nursing interventions
• If the pacing or sensing indicator flashes, check the connections to the cable and the position of the pacing electrode in the patient (by X-ray). The cable may have come loose, or the electrode may have been dislodged, pulled out, or broken.
• If the pulse generator is turned on but the indicators still aren't flashing, change the battery. If that doesn't help, use a different pulse generator.
• Check the settings if the pacemaker is firing too rapidly. If they're correct, or if altering

them (according to hospital policy or the doctor's order) doesn't help, change the pulse generator.

Failure to capture
Here you see that the pacemaker spikes but the heart doesn't respond. This may be caused by changes in the pacing threshold from ischemia, an electrolyte imbalance (high or low potassium or magnesium levels), acidosis, an adverse reaction to a medication, a perforated ventricle, fibrosis, or the position of the electrode.

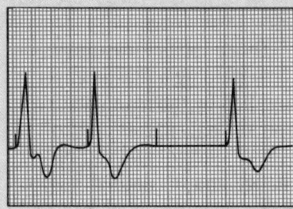

Nursing interventions
• If the patient's condition has changed, notify the doctor and ask him for new settings.
• If pacemaker settings are altered by the patient or others, return them to their correct

maker site that can't respond to stimulation. If this problem occurs, first check the connections at the pacemaker generator; then notify the doctor and try slowly

increasing the pulse generator output while observing the monitor to see if capture occurs. If the problem is caused by poor positioning of the pacing wire, positions. Then make sure the face of the pacemaker is covered with a plastic shield. Also tell the patient or others not to touch the dials.

• If the heart is not responding, try any or all of these suggestions: Carefully check all connections; increase the milliamperes slowly (according to hospital policy or the doctor's order); turn the patient on his left side and then on his right (if turning him to the left didn't help); reverse the cable in the pulse generator so the positive electrode wire is in the negative terminal and the negative electrode wire is in the positive terminal; schedule an anteroposterior or lateral chest X-ray to determine the position of the electrode.

Failure to sense intrinsic beats
This could cause ventricular tachycardia or ventricular fibrillation if the pacemaker fires on the vulnerable T wave. Failure to sense intrinsic beats could be caused by the pacemaker sensing an external stimulus as a QRS complex, which could lead to asystole, or by the pacemaker not being sensitive enough, which means it could fire anywhere within the cardiac cycle.

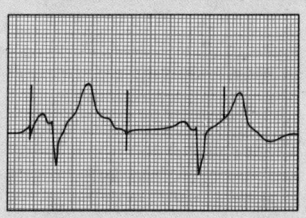

Nursing interventions
• If the pacemaker is undersensing, turn the sensitivity control completely to the right. If it's oversensing, turn it slightly to the left.
• If the pacemaker isn't functioning correctly, change the battery or the pulse generator.
• Remove objects in the room causing electromechanical interference, such as razors or radios. Check the ground wires on the bed and other equipment for obvious damage. Unplug each piece and see if the interference stops. When you locate the cause, notify the hospital engineer and ask him to check it.
• If the pacemaker is still firing on the T wave and all else has failed, turn off the pacemaker. Make sure atropine is available in case the patient's heart rate drops. Be prepared to call a code and institute cardiopulmonary resuscitation if necessary.

the doctor will reposition the wire.

An elevated ST segment precedes cardiac arrest in a patient experiencing cardiac tamponade after puncture of the right ventricle with the pacing wire. Patients with cardiac tamponade rapidly become acutely distressed and lapse into cardiac

PREVENTIVE PRACTICE

 Preventing microshock

The patient with a temporary pacemaker is at risk for microshock—minute electrical charges delivered to the heart through the pacing electrode. These charges can't be felt, but they can cause lethal ventricular fibrillation if delivered straight to the heart. Here's how you can prevent microshock and protect your patient:
• Protect the tips of the epicardial pacing electrode wires by covering them with finger cots or gloves if they aren't connected to the pulse generator. You could also insert them into plastic foam or needle caps.
• Wear gloves whenever you're touching the uninsulated ends of the pacing electrodes.

• Keep the dressing dry and intact.
• Make sure that a defibrillator is nearby when the pacemaker wire is inserted. The pacemaker lead may trigger ventricular ectopy or fibrillation.
• Don't let ungrounded, unchecked electrical equipment (such as the patient's own radio) come in contact with the patient or be used in the patient's immediate area.
• Don't forget to touch a grounded area when you're entering the patient's room. This will discharge any static electricity before you touch the patient or lean against his bed.

arrest. When the ST segment is elevated, blood can be seen in the introducer sheath.

Epicardial pacemaker. Potential problems include under- and oversensing. Undersensing can result from low-voltage P or R waves secondary to a poorly positioned lead, myocardial ischemia or necrosis, or electrolyte disturbances. Correct the problem by lowering the sensitivity level on the pacemaker pulse generator to make the pacing wire more sensitive to the R waves.

In oversensing, the pacing wires identify artifact or T waves as P or R waves and inhibit pulse generator output. Over-

sensing is identified when pacing wires fail to fire the electrical stimuli required to pace the heart as set on the pulse generator. On the monitor this appears as prolonged episodes without P waves or QRS complexes and with pacing spikes occurring throughout the heart's electrical cycle. Correct the problem by increasing the sensitivity level to make the pacing wires less responsive to lower voltage artifact.

When a pacemaker fails to sense accurately, the patient usually experiencies dizziness, fatigue, shortness of breath, chest pain, and hypotension.

If the patient is symptomatic and adjusting the pacing sensi-

tivity levels doesn't correct un-
der- or oversensing, the doctor
may have to place a temporary
transvenous pacing wire.

Permanent pacemakers

Electronic devices implanted in
a pocket beneath the skin, permanent pacemakers are used for
long-term management of arrhythmias and bradycardia.
They're usually inserted in the
operating room under local anesthesia. They're implanted
transvenously into either the
atrium or ventricle or both
chambers (as with the atrioventricular sequential, dual-cham-
ber pacemaker) or into the epicardium (during cardiac surgery).

Troubleshooting problems

Following are some of the most
common problems that can arise
with permanent pacemakers.
(See *Detecting pacemaker problems*, pages 402 and 403.)

**Failure to discharge (pace), cap-
ture, or sense.** A failed pacemaker battery and a dislodged
electrode wire are two possible
causes for pacemaker malfunction.

Watch the patient for the following signs and symptoms: dizziness, fatigue, light-headedness,
syncope, chest pain, shortness of
breath, undue fatigue, and fluid
retention. Take the patient's
pulse daily as soon as he awak-
ens, and notify the doctor if the
rate is 4 to 6 beats/minute below
the preset rate or if his resting
heart rate is 120 beats/minute or
more. If he has a demand pacemaker, an irregular rhythm
without accompanying physical
symptoms may be normal be-

cause the intrinsic rate and the
pacer rate are working together
to maintain adequate cardiac
output.

Caution the patient to avoid
activities—for example, contact
sports—that put stress or pressure on the insertion site. Because the pacemaker lead takes
a few weeks to become secure
within the endocardium, tell the
patient not to lift anything heav-
ier than 5 lb (2.3 kg) or to extend the arm on the affected side
laterally or over the head for 2 to
3 weeks following insertion to
avoid strain on the leadwire
placed in the heart.

**Asynchronous or high-rate pac-
ing.** Magnetic resonance imaging
(MRI) can cause these pacemaker malfunctions and thus is
contraindicated for pacemaker
patients. The large magnetic
field can produce asynchronous
pacing (the pacemaker paces but
doesn't sense) and radio frequency interference from the
MRI can cause high-rate pacing
(up to 400 beats/minute).

Inaccurate sensing. During surgery, electrocautery can inhibit
the pacemaker, causing it to
sense the signals and mistake
them for cardiac signals. It can
also change the pacemaker's
programming or cause it to lose
its ability to deliver a stimulus.

So patients undergoing electrocautery must be monitored
closely. Be alert for dizziness,
shortness of breath, light-headedness, fatigue, or fluid retention. Assess for inappropriate
pacing and sensing or a heart
rate less than the programmed
lower rate.

Detecting pacemaker problems

After the doctor attaches the catheter to the pulse generator, check the cardiac monitor. If the pacemaker isn't pacing and sensing appropriately, you may see one of these problems on the screen.

Loss of atrial capture (DDD mode)

A DDD (or atrioventricular sequential) pacemaker senses the atrium and ventricle and delivers an impulse when normal electrical activity doesn't occur. In this rhythm strip, the atrial (A) and ventricular (V) pacer spikes are initially followed by atrial and ventricular capture.

Suddenly, atrial capture is lost. The pacemaker's atrial electrode still senses that normal atrial activity isn't occurring and continues to deliver an impulse, but the impulse doesn't cause atrial activity or capture as it should. The ventricular electrode is still sensing and pacing properly.

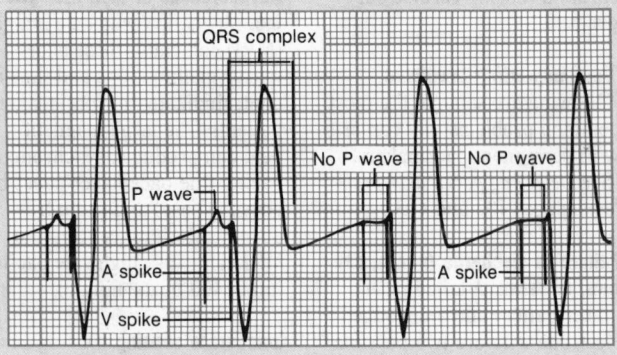

Notify the doctor of any findings. The pacemaker can be programmed to the original settings unless the generator is damaged and needs replacing.

Failure to pace or inappropriate sensing. Radiation therapy can have a cumulative effect on the pulse generator's circuitry, changing the molecular structure of the silicone chip and causing pacemaker failure. So be sure to cover the pacemaker with a lead shield during the procedure and then check it for proper functioning afterward. ❖

Ventricular assist devices

A ventricular assist device (VAD) can temporarily sustain the life of a patient with acute ventricu-

Loss of ventricular capture and sensing (VVI mode)

A VVI (or ventricular demand) pacemaker delivers an impulse to the ventricle when it doesn't sense a normal ventricular impulse. In this rhythm strip, the pacemaker delivers an impulse but doesn't capture the myocardium, so you'll see a V pacer spike but not a QRS complex. Also, the pacemaker isn't sensing normal ventricular activity and is inappropriately delivering an impulse, so you'll see the QRS complex, and then a pacer spike.

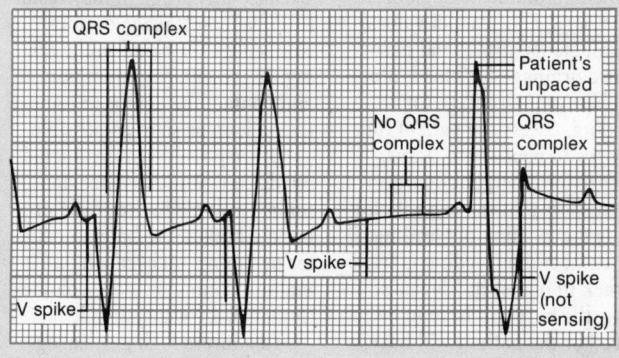

lar failure when maximum medical and surgical intervention are unsuccessful. It provides support to the heart and circulation, allowing the heart to recover from any type of insult. With its pump, a VAD augments cardiac output just enough to allow tissue and organ perfusion while the heart rests and recovers.

Troubleshooting problems

The doctor inserts the VAD during surgery, and the pump perfusionist is usually responsible for the VAD's postoperative function. Following is a sign of several problems you may note in your monitoring of the patient.

Bleeding from systemic anticoagulation

Bleeding can be caused by dislodgment at cannulation sites, stress ulcers (GI bleeding), coagulopathy from prolonged use of a VAD, or a crack in the mechanical parts of a VAD. Patients can bleed from any site when this problem occurs. Check the patient's gums for bleeding. Look for petechiae, melena, and skin ecchymosis. Check I.V. sites and all other cannulation sites for bleeding, including chest tube sites. The patient may vomit blood or have it in his nasogastric tube drainage, or the secretions from his endotracheal tube may be bloody. Epistaxis and hematuria may occur. Cerebrovascular bleeding may also occur. Notify the doctor of a bleeding problem. Monitor hemoglobin, hematocrit, and platelet values. Test all stools, urine, and nasogastric drainage for blood. Monitor chest tube drainage for bleeding. Assess the patient for changes in neurologic status. Prepare for emergency surgery if you suspect that the cannulation site is the location of bleeding. If you suspect the bleeding is from a crack in one of the device's parts, the part will have to be replaced or the patient will have to undergo emergency surgery to replace the VAD.

❖

Intra-aortic balloon counterpulsation devices

Providing temporary support for the heart's left ventricle, intra-aortic balloon counterpulsation (IABC) mechanically displaces blood within the aorta by means of an intra-aortic balloon attached to an external pump console. When used correctly, IABC

increases the supply of oxygen-rich blood to the myocardium and decreases myocardial oxygen demand.

Troubleshooting problems

When your patient undergoes IABC, you must respond immediately to any equipment problems. Following are the problems most often encountered in the Model 700 IABC Control System, a commonly used device, along with possible causes and nursing interventions.

High gas leakage (automatic mode only)

Because this problem may result from balloon leakage or abrasion, check for blood in the tubing. If present, stop pumping and contact the doctor to remove the balloon as soon as possible.

Other possible causes include condensation in the extension tubing, volume limiter disk, or both; a kink in the balloon catheter or tubing; tachycardia; a malfunctioning or loose volume limiter disk; or a system leak.

To address high gas leakage, straighten the tubing, tighten all connections, and perform a leak test. Also remove any condensation in the tubing and volume limiter disk, and replace or tighten the volume limiter disk if necessary. Afterward, refill, auto-purge, and resume pumping.

Tachycardia may also trigger high gas leakage. If this is the cause, change the wean control to 1:2 or operate in the manual mode. Be aware, though, that gas alarms are inoperable when the IABC device is in the manual mode. While in this mode, auto-purge the balloon every 1 to

2 hours, and monitor the balloon pressure waveform closely.

Balloon line block (automatic mode only)

Line block may result if the balloon catheter or tubing kinks, if the balloon is not unfurled, or if the sheath or balloon is positioned too high. In this situation, check the catheter and tubing for kinks, and then refill and resume pumping. If indicated, contact the doctor to verify placement. The balloon may have to be repositioned or inflated manually.

Condensation in the tubing or volume limiter disk or a malfunctioning volume limiter disk may also cause a balloon line block alarm. In this instance, remove condensate from the tubing and volume limiter disk and replace the volume limiter disk if indicated. Then refill, autopurge, and resume pumping. If the balloon is too large for the aorta, the alarm will also sound. To solve this problem, decrease the volume control percentage by one notch.

No ECG trigger

This may result from an inadequate signal, a disconnected lead or electrode patch, or the improper selection of the electrocardiogram (ECG) input mode. Respond to the problem by adjusting the ECG gain and changing the lead or trigger mode, replacing the lead or electrode patches (especially if they've been in use for an extended time because the gel dries out and loses conductivity), and adjusting the ECG input to

the appropriate mode (skin or monitor).

No arterial pressure trigger

If the arterial line is damped or the patient is hypotensive, you should flush the line. Also check all connections on the arterial line to make sure none are open to the atmosphere.

Trigger mode change

This alarm may sound if the trigger mode changed while pumping, in which case you should resume pumping.

Irregular heart rhythm

If the patient has an irregular rhythm (such as atrial fibrillation or ectopic beats), change to R or QRS sense (if necessary) to accommodate the irregularity.

Erratic AV pacing

If demand for paced rhythm occurs while in atrioventricular (AV) sequential trigger mode, change to the pace reject trigger or QRS sense.

Noisy ECG signal

This may result from malfunctioning leads or electrical or muscle artifact. Replace the leads and check the ECG cable. The use of electrocautery may also cause a noisy signal; during use, switch to the arterial pressure trigger.

Internal trigger

This results if the trigger mode is set on internal 80 beats/minute. Be aware that the internal trigger should be used only during cardiopulmonary bypass surgery or cardiac arrest. Select an alternative trigger if the patient has a heartbeat or rhythm.

Purge incomplete
This will occur if the OFF button is pressed during autopurge, which interrupts the purge cycle. To solve the problem, initiate autopurge again or initiate pumping.

High fill pressure
This may result from a malfunctioning volume limiter disk or an occluded vent line or valve. In this situation, replace the volume limiter disk, refill, autopurge, and resume pumping. If this fails to correct the problem, contact the manufacturer.

No balloon drive
Disconnected tubing or the absence of a volume limiter disk may trigger the no balloon drive alarm. Make sure a volume limiter disk is locked securely in place and that all tubing is appropriately connected. Refill, autopurge, and resume pumping.

Incorrect timing
This will result if the inflate and deflate controls are improperly set. To solve this problem, place the inflate and deflate controls at set midpoints. Then reassess the timing and adjust as necessary.

Low volume percentage
This results if the volume control percentage is not set on 100%. You should assess the cause of the decreased volume and reset if necessary.

❖

Hemodynamic monitoring systems

Hemodynamic monitoring systems provide valuable information about a patient's cardiovascular status. All such systems consist of certain components:
• a catheter, with one- to four-way stopcocks for flow control and blood sampling
• pressure tubing
• a flush device for system patency
• a transducer, which converts physiologic signals to electrical signals
• an amplifier, which enhances the electrical signals and filters out unwanted background signals
• a bedside monitor, which displays the symbols on an oscilloscope.

To obtain accurate readings, you must zero the transducer to atmospheric pressure because physiologic pressures are relative to atmospheric pressure. Zeroing establishes atmospheric pressure as the baseline, preventing it from affecting pressure readings. You'll do this at least once every 24 hours (or according to hospital policy), each time you use a disposable transducer, and after patient transport. Crucial to zeroing is identifying the phlebostatic axis consistently for all readings. (See *Where to place the transducer.*)

Troubleshooting problems
If a problem occurs when your patient has a hemodynamic monitoring system in place, ask yourself the questions that follow

Where to place the transducer

When zeroing a pressure transducer before taking a pressure reading, place the transducer on the phlebostatic axis, which bisects two thoracic planes. Using this intersected point allows the head of the bed to be raised or lowered.

To identify the phlebostatic axis, locate the patient's fourth intercostal space; then draw an imaginary line that extends down the lateral thoracic area. Next, identify a second point at the midpoint between the anterior and posterior chest walls. The site at which these two reference points bisects is the phlebostatic axis.

Some nurses use the mid-axillary line rather than the midpoint between the anterior and posterior chest walls as the lateral plane. However, this line doesn't always coincide with the midheart level. Also, one caregiver may identify the midaxillary line differently than another. For reproducibility and accuracy, regard the midpoint as being more accurate.

Keep in mind that the key to ensuring accurate pressure values isn't just *locating* the phlebostatic axis precisely but identifying it *consistently* for all readings. Therefore, be sure to make a reference spot on the patient's torso to ensure a consistent leveling point.

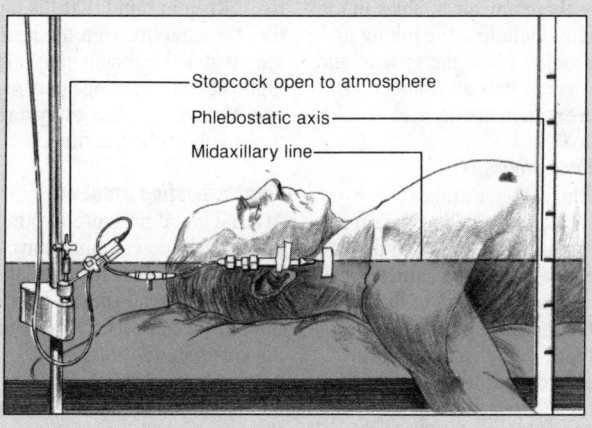

Stopcock open to atmosphere
Phlebostatic axis
Midaxillary line

o help pinpoint the cause, and hen take appropriate actions to orrect the situation.

Monitor problems
• Is the monitor plugged into the wall outlet and turned on?
• Is the pressure module plugged in?

• Does the monitor show the right scale?
• Are all cable connections dry and tight?
• Is the viewing contrast knob turned up so the wave form and values can be seen clearly?
• Is the correct channel being used?

Transducer problems
• Is the zeroing port at the correct level?
• Has the zeroing port been turned on to the patient and off to air, as it should be during monitoring?
• Has the transducer been rezeroed in the last 24 hours or more recently? If the patient was disconnected from the system or the pressure tubing was changed, the transducer should have been rezeroed.
• Are all stopcock connections tight?
• Are there any air bubbles in the system, including the tubing and stopcocks? Flush the system, and then verify that all connections in the system are secure.

Patient problems
• Is the catheter kinked?
• Has a clot formed at the tip of the catheter? If you can't aspirate blood from the catheter, call the doctor; don't try to flush the system because pulmonary or systemic embolism may result.
• Has the patient's clinical status changed? Reassess the patient and verify the arterial blood pressure on the monitor by taking a cuff pressure.

Arterial pressure monitoring
Arterial pressure monitoring permit continuous measurement of systolic, diastolic, and mean

pressures and allow arterial blood sampling. Direct monitoring is indicated when highly accurate or frequent blood pressure measurements are required—for example, in patients with low cardiac output and high systemic vascular resistance. It also may be used for hospitalized patients who are obese or have severe edema, if these conditions make indirect measurement hard to perform. What's more, it may be used for patients who are receiving titrated doses of vasoactive drugs or who need frequent blood sampling.

Usually the arterial catheter is inserted in a radial or brachial artery, although the radial artery's distance from the heart may produce false-high pressure readings. If these sites are unsuitable, the femoral and dorsalis pedis arteries are alternatives. Keep in mind that the farther the artery is from the heart, the greater the chance that false high-pressure readings may occur. Most of the sites carry a risk of thrombosis or bleeding.

Troubleshooting problems
Arterial blood pressure monitoring can lead to complications, such as air embolism, arterial bleeding, arterial spasm, infection, or thrombosis. (See *Managing complications of arterial pressure monitoring*.)

Additional problems may interfere with proper functioning of the setup or your ability to interpret a waveform. Causes and solutions to some of the most common problems follow.

Damped waveform. Appearing as a small waveform with a slow

Managing complications of arterial pressure monitoring

Insertion of an arterial line may cause various complications, some of them life-threatening. This chart lists possible causes for each complication, along with preventive and corrective measures.

COMPLICATION AND POSSIBLE CAUSES	NURSING MEASURES
Air embolism Entry of air into system, such as during initial setup and priming, catheter insertion, catheter dislodgment, accidental disconnection of pressure setup, open stopcocks, or inadvertent emptying of flush solution bag	• Check entire system for secure connections during each shift. • Remove all air from line during initial setup. • Immobilize insertion site to prevent accidental catheter dislodgment. • Make sure all stopcocks are in proper position. • Check I.V. bag for remaining I.V. flush solution. • Assess patient for signs of air embolism, such as decreased blood pressure; weak, rapid pulse; cyanosis; and loss of consciousness. If these signs occur, turn patient onto left side so air entering heart is absorbed in pulmonary artery. Notify doctor and implement standing orders as appropriate.
Arterial bleeding • Loose connections • Oozing around catheter insertion site • Catheter dislodgment	• Check entire system for secure connections during each shift. • Assess for oozing around catheter insertion site every hour. • Immobilize catheter insertion site to prevent accidental catheter dislodgment. If catheter dislodges, immediately apply direct pressure, assess vital signs, follow standing orders for fluid administration, and notify doctor. • Notify doctor of any ecchymosis or hematoma. With a femoral line, assess for these problems lateral and posterior to insertion site as well as over the site itself.

(continued)

Managing complications of arterial pressure monitoring *(continued)*

COMPLICATION AND POSSIBLE CAUSES	NURSING MEASURES
Arterial spasm or thrombosis • Arterial trauma • Improper maintenance of flush solution or pressure system • Patient history of hypercoagulability	• Immobilize insertion site to prevent arterial wall irritation. • Every hour, check extremity distal to insertion site for color, pulses, sensation, movement, and temperature. Notify doctor of any changes. • If arterial spasm occurs, administer lidocaine as ordered. • If thrombosis occurs, discontinue arterial line as ordered and permitted. Prepare for arteriotomy and Fogarty catheterization if ordered.
Infection • Failure to maintain aseptic technique during arterial line insertion, setup or maintenance of pressure system, tubing changes, or blood sample withdrawal • Failure to change components of pressure system as often as required • Contamination of multidose heparin vial	• Use careful aseptic technique during all procedures involving monitoring system or insertion site. • Assess for signs of local infection every hour. Report suspicious signs to doctor. • Assess patient's vital signs and evaluate for signs and symptoms of systemic infection. Notify doctor if vital signs change or if signs or symptoms of infection occur. • Cover all stopcocks with dead-end caps. Change tubing, flush solution, and dressing according to hospital policy. The Centers for Disease Control and Prevention recommends changing pressure tubing every 48 hours and changing the flush solution bag every 24 hours. • Use only single-dose heparin vials.

rise in the anacrotic limb and a reduced or nonexistent dicrotic notch, a damped waveform may result from interference with transmission of the physiologic signal to the transducer.

Common causes of this problem include air in the system, a loose connection, a clotted catheter tip, a catheter tip resting against the arterial wall, kinked tubing, or an inadequately inflated pressure infuser bag. Also a change in the patient's condition, such as rapid onset of hypotension resulting from hypovo lemia or shock, can result in decreased pressures that mimic a damped waveform.

Corrective measures include checking the patient's blood pressure, pulses, and neurologic status, and notifying the doctor of any changes. Also, check the system for air, paying particular attention to the tubing and the transducer's diaphragm. If you find air, aspirate it or force it from the system through a stopcock port. Never flush any fluid containing air bubbles into the patient. Also check and tighten all connections, and unkink the tubing if necessary. If you suspect a clotted catheter tip, attempt to aspirate the clot. If you're successful, flush the line. If you're not successful, avoid flushing the line; you could dislodge the clot. If you think the catheter tip may be resting against the arterial wall, reposition the catheter insertion area— usually the wrist—and flush the catheter. (If the wrist is the insertion site, remember not to hyperextend it for radial artery lines because doing so may lead to radial nerve damage.) Or reposition the catheter by carefully rotating it or pulling it back slightly. Finally, make sure the pressure infuser bag has been inflated to 300 mm Hg.

Drifting waveform. A drifting waveform is when the waveform floats above and below the baseline. This may result from a temperature change in the flush solution or a kinked or compressed monitor cable.

To solve this problem, allow the temperature of the flush solution to stabilize before infusing

it. Also check the cable and relieve the kink or compression.

Inability to flush the arterial line or to withdraw blood. This problem may occur because of incorrectly positioned stopcocks, kinked tubing, an inadequately inflated pressure infuser bag, a near-empty infuser bag that needs refilling, a clotted catheter tip, a catheter tip resting against the arterial wall, or the position of the insertion area.

To intervene, properly reposition the stopcocks if necessary; check to make sure the tubing is unkinked and the pressure infuser bag inflated to 300 mm Hg. If you suspect that the catheter tip is clotted or resting against the arterial wall, take the corrective steps outlined previously. Finally, check the position of the insertion area, and change it as indicated. For radial and brachial arterial lines, use an armboard to immobilize the area and avoid hyperextending the wrist. With a femoral arterial line, keep the head of the bed at a 45-degree angle or less to prevent catheter kinking.

Artifact. Erratic or unrecognizable waveform tracings may result from electrical interference, patient movement, or catheter whip or fling (excessive catheter tip movement).

Respond to the problem by checking the equipment in the room and by asking the patient to lie quietly while you try to read the monitor. If the artifact continues, try shortening the tubing if possible.

False-high pressure reading. If the patient's arterial pressure exceeds normal values without a significant change in baseline clinical findings, first recheck the system to make sure the reading is accurate. Then recalibrate the system, and try releveling the transducer on the phlebostatic axis. Make sure that the catheter is unkinked and, if necessary, take measures to unclot or reposition the catheter tip. Also remove any air bubbles in the tubing close to the patient, and shorten the pressure tubing if it appears too long.

False-low pressure reading. If the patient's arterial pressure drops below his normal pressure without a significant change in baseline clinical findings, recheck the system to ensure that the reading is accurate before responding to the low pressure reading. First recalibrate the system and reposition the transducer on the phlebostatic axis. Check and tighten all connections and unkink the catheter if necessary. If indicated, take measures to unclot or reposition the catheter tip. Shorten the pressure tubing if it appears too long. Also check for, and remove, any large air bubbles close to the transducer.

No waveform. A waveform may not appear on the monitor for any one of several reasons, including the lack of power supply, a loose connection, a stopcock turned off to the patient, or a transducer disconnected from the monitor module. An occluded catheter tip, a catheter tip resting against the arterial wall, a displaced arterial line, or severe hypotension may also interfere with the waveform display.

Correct the problem by checking the power supply and tightening all connections. Make sure the stopcocks are set properly, that the transducer is open to the catheter, and that the transducer is connected to the monitor module. If you feel the catheter tip may be occluded or resting against the arterial wall, take the appropriate steps outlined earlier. If the catheter is displaced or pulled out, take immediate steps to avert hypovolemic shock. (See *Managing a displaced arterial line*.)

Pulmonary artery monitoring

Pulmonary artery (PA) monitoring can help you learn about a patient's cardiovascular and pulmonary status, obtain blood samples, and infuse solutions. The basic PA catheter allows you to measure intracardiac pressure, pulmonary artery pressure (PAP), and cardiac output. This kind of catheter has two to five lumens, a balloon-inflation valve, and a thermistor.

Troubleshooting problems

When your patient has a PA catheter, you'll need to know how to respond to uncharacteristic waveforms and pressures on the monitor. Some of the most common problems follow.

No waveform on monitor. A waveform may fail to appear on the monitor for several reasons—for example, if the transducer is not open to the catheter, the transducer or monitor has been set up improperly, the monitor scale is incorrectly set for the pressure

Managing a displaced arterial line

Your patient is in danger of hypovolemic shock from blood loss if his arterial line is pulled out or otherwise displaced. Follow these steps to avert serious complications.

Initial care
• Immediately apply direct pressure at the insertion site, and have someone summon the doctor. Because arterial blood flows under high intravascular pressure, be certain to maintain firm, direct pressure for 5 to 10 minutes to encourage clot formation at the insertion site.
• Check the patient's I.V. line and, if ordered, increase the flow rate temporarily to compensate for blood loss.

After the bleeding stops
• Apply a sterile pressure dressing.
• Reassess the patient's level of consciousness (LOC) and offer reassurance.

• Estimate the amount of blood loss from your observations of the blood and from the changes in the patient's blood pressure and heart rate.
• Assist the doctor as he reinserts the catheter. Ensure that the patient's arm is immobilized and that the tubing and catheter are secure.
• Withdraw blood for a complete blood count and arterial blood gas analysis as ordered.

Ongoing care
• Frequently assess the patient's vital signs, LOC, skin color and temperature, and circulation at the insertion site and beyond.
• Watch for further bleeding or hematoma formation at the insertion site.
• Once the patient's condition stabilizes, reduce the I.V. flow rate to the previous keep-vein-open level.

that's being monitored, or the catheter is occluded by a clot.

Corrective measures include checking the stopcock, calibration, or scale mechanisms; setting the correct scale for PAP measurements; tightening connections; rezeroing the setup; or replacing the transducer.

Overdamped waveform. If air bubbles, blood clots, or a catheter tip lodged in the vessel wall cause an overdamped waveform

to appear on the patient's monitor, you may correct the problem in several ways.

Try removing any air bubbles observed in the catheter tubing and transducer. (See *Preventing air embolism*, page 414.) Try restoring patency to an occluded catheter by aspirating the clot with a syringe. (*Never* irrigate the line as a first step.) Or try moving a lodged catheter by repositioning the patient or by having him cough and breathe

PREVENTIVE PRACTICE

 ## Preventing air embolism

One way to prevent air embolism in your patient during hemodynamic monitoring is to use a closed arterial blood sampling system.

Unlike an open arterial blood sampling system, a closed system has a reservoir, which doesn't allow air to enter the system during blood collection. It eliminates the use of needles and permits reinfusion of collected but unused arterial blood.

After the reservoir has been filled with blood, a syringe with an attached cannula is connected to the blood sampling site. Blood is withdrawn into the syringe. Once the syringe and cannula have been removed, the blood in the reservoir can be slowly reinfused into the patient.

deeply. If you need to move the catheter itself, do so only according to hospital policy. (See *Correcting an overdamped tracing.*)

Changed waveform configuration. Noisy or erratic tracings may result from arrhythmias or from an incorrectly positioned catheter, loose connections in the setup, or faulty electrical circuitry.

Respond to this problem by repositioning the patient (or the catheter if necessary), arranging for a chest X-ray to verify arrhythmias or catheter location,

or checking and tightening connections in the catheter and transducer apparatus.

Catheter fling. An erratic waveform may also result from catheter fling, which reflects excessive catheter movement (possibly caused by an arrhythmia or excessive respiratory effort). In such a case, you may need to reposition the catheter according to hospital policy.

False pressure readings. If the monitor records pressures that are inaccurately too high or too low, try recalibrating the system, repositioning the transducer (level with the phlebostatic axis), or rezeroing the monitor setup.

Ventricular irritability. An electrocardiogram (ECG) tracing indicating an arrhythmia may result from the catheter irritating the ventricular endocardium or the heart valves.

After confirming this arrhythmia on the patient's ECG, notify the doctor and administer antiarrhythmic drugs as ordered. (The doctor may prevent this problem during insertion by keeping the balloon inflated when advancing the catheter through the heart.)

Right ventricular waveform. A PA catheter migrating into the right ventricle will produce a ventricular tracing.

In this situation, inflate the balloon with 1.5 cc of air to move the catheter back to the pulmonary artery. If this measure fails, notify the doctor immediately so that he can reposition the catheter.

Correcting an overdamped tracing

If you see an unintended wedge tracing (as shown in the second tracing below) or an overdamped tracing on your patient's pulmonary artery (PA) pressure monitor, assume the catheter is wedged. With partial wedging, the tracing will be unclear; PA systolic pressure may be lower than baseline and PA diastolic pressure may be higher. With complete wedging, you'll see a typical wedge tracing.

To correct the problem, detach the syringe to verify that air has been removed from the balloon. If the tracing still shows a wedge, attempt to reposition the catheter. For instance, turn the patient (or ask him to turn), ask him to cough, or aspirate and then flush the distal port. If these measures don't restore a PA tracing, notify the doctor immediately.

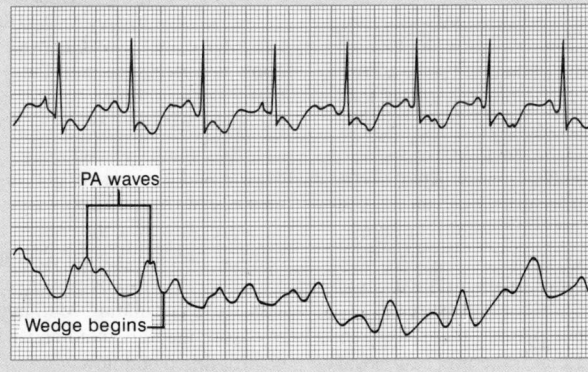

PA waves

Wedge begins

Continuous PAWP waveform. In obtaining the pulmonary artery wedge pressure (PAWP) to evaluate ventricular function, the catheter may migrate or the balloon may remain inflated. Either situation may cause a continuous PAWP waveform to appear.

To correct this problem, reposition the patient or have him cough and breathe deeply. Keep the balloon inflated no longer than two respiratory cycles or 15 seconds. Notify the doctor if the continuous PAWP waveform persists, as a chest X-ray may be necessary. Pulmonary infarction can occur with a prolonged wedged catheter. Prepare to have the doctor pull back the catheter or to do this yourself if hospital policy permits.

Missing PAWP waveform. The monitor may fail to record a PAWP waveform—possibly because of a malpositioned catheter, insufficient air in the balloon

tip, or even a ruptured balloon. To intervene:
• reposition the patient (don't aspirate the balloon)
• reinflate the balloon adequately (remove the syringe from the balloon lumen, wait for the balloon to deflate passively, and then instill the correct volume of air)
• assess the balloon's competence (note resistance during inflation, feel how the syringe's plunger springs back after the balloon inflates, and check for blood leaking from the balloon lumen)
• if the balloon has ruptured, turn the patient onto his left side, tape the balloon-inflation port, and notify the doctor.

Any patient who has a PA catheter in place is at risk for several complications. Besides observing the patient's electrocardiogram, waveform pattern, and pressure values on the bedside monitor, watch for signs and symptoms of the complications that follow. Implement appropriate care measures to resolve or prevent them. Keep in mind that these procedures vary according to each state's nurse practice act.

Bacteremia. If your patient has an elevated temperature, chills, warm skin, headache, and malaise, he's showing signs and symptoms of an infection such as bacteremia. Administer antibiotic medications as ordered. To prevent such an infection, maintain sterile technique. Also be sure to maintain and change the monitoring setup according to hospital policy. To ensure that no infection exists, send the PA catheter tip to the laboratory for culture and sensitivity testing when the catheter is removed or changed.

Blood backflow. Caused by leaks in the PA catheter apparatus or a pressure bag that's inflated below 300 mm Hg, blood backflow is easily seen in the pressure tubing. To intervene early, be sure to tighten connections in the monitoring setup. Preventive measures include returning stopcocks to their proper position after use and keeping the pressure bag adequately inflated.

Bleeding at the insertion site. If the patient has prolonged oozing or frank bleeding at the insertion site after catheter withdrawal, apply firm pressure until the bleeding stops. To prevent this problem, maintain pressure on the site during catheter withdrawal and for at least 10 minutes afterward, and apply a pressure dressing over the site. At a femoral site, apply a sandbag for 1 to 2 hours. (Also be sure to assess distal circulation routinely to ensure that a hematoma isn't obstructing blood flow.)

Pulmonary embolism. A thrombus that migrates from the catheter into pulmonary circulation or a catheter tip clotted from inadequate flushing may cause a pulmonary embolism. To prevent an embolus, administer anticoagulants as ordered, and use a continuous flush system.

If prevention fails and your patient shows signs and symptoms of a pulmonary embolism, such as sharp and stabbing chest pain, anxiety, cyanosis, dyspnea, tachypnea, and diaphoresis, try to aspirate blood (don't irrigate if you suspect an embolus). If you can't aspirate blood, a pulmonary embolus may be obstructing the line. Notify the doctor at once.

Ruptured pulmonary artery. PA rupture results from pulmonary hypertension, thrombus, catheter migration into the peripheral branch of the artery, or improper inflation or prolonged wedging of the catheter's balloon. In PA rupture, the patient will experience restlessness, tachycardia, hypotension, hemoptysis, and dyspnea. In such a situation, notify the doctor immediately.

Keep in mind several preventive measures:
• Slowly inflate the balloon only until the PAWP waveform appears on the monitor, and then let the balloon deflate passively.
• Never overinflate the balloon.
• Reposition a migrating catheter (if permitted).

Pulmonary infarction. Chest pain, hemoptysis, fever, pleural friction rub, and low arterial oxygen levels point to pulmonary infarction, possibly caused by the catheter migrating into a wedged position in the blood vessel. Don't flush the catheter if you suspect that it has migrated. Do monitor PAP continuously and notify the doctor.

Never allow the balloon to be inflated for more than two respiratory cycles or 15 seconds.

Cardiac output monitors
Measuring cardiac output – the amount of blood ejected by the heart – helps evaluate cardiac function. The most widely preferred method for calculating this measurement is the bolus thermodilution technique.

To measure cardiac output, a quantity of solution colder than the patient's blood is injected into the right atrium via a port on the PA catheter. This indicator solution mixes with the blood as it travels through the right ventricle into the pulmonary artery, and a thermistor on the catheter registers the change in temperature of the flowing blood. A computer then plots the temperature change over time as a curve and calculates flow based on the area under the curve.

Troubleshooting problems
Some of the most common problems that may occur with cardiac output monitors follow, along with their consequences and appropriate interventions.

Injectate loss. This problem may occur when injectate is warmed after the injectate temperature is measured, or when injectate leaks from the delivery system. Because cardiac output is calculated using a known amount of solution at a known temperature, any warming or loss of injectate will affect the computed cardiac output and thus the accuracy of the cardiac output measurement. Loss of the indicator will produce false-high cardiac output readings – a 1% error for every 0.1 ml (of a 10-ml volume) lost. To prevent injectate loss, carefully check for loose connections at the injection site where injectate may leak.

Indication of injectate loss may also result from inaccurate measurement of the injectate or from changes in injectate temperature after the injectate has been registered by the cardiac output computer. Always measure the injectate volume carefully and make sure the syringe is free of air bubbles. Avoid handling the barrel of the syringe, especially with a bath injectate setup.

Certain conditions, such as right-to-left shunts and severe tricuspid regurgitation, may cause injectate loss between the injection port and where the temperature measurement is taken within the pulmonary artery.

Incorrect catheter placement. Correct catheter placement is essential for accurate cardiac output measurements. The tip of the PA catheter must be positioned in the right, left, or main pulmonary artery. To verify correct placement, make sure the PA waveform isn't damped before making measurements. A damped tracing may mean that the thermistor isn't free-floating and therefore can cause incorrect cardiac output values.

Improper injection technique. To prevent errors in measurement, complete the injection within 4 seconds using a single, smooth motion. Irregular injections cause multiple peaks in the washout curve, resulting in inaccurate estimation of the area under the curve and thus an error in measurement.

If the injectate lumen of the catheter is blocked, boluses may be injected through other lines such as the venous infusion port on the PA catheter, introducer side port, or through any catheter that exits into a central vein or the right atrium. The injection port must be located beyond the introducer sheath to avoid retrograde flow and injectate loss.

Incorrect computation constant. The computation constant accounts for the gain of heat from the catheter tubing as injectate travels through the catheter into the blood. With some older monitors, the computation constant must be entered as a numerical value, whereas newer equipment calculates the value internally when you enter the injectate volume and catheter size. If you mistakenly use an incorrect computation constant, you can calculate the correct cardiac output by using a correction formula. (See *Correcting an inaccurate computation constant.*)

Inadequate signal-to-noise ratio. The *signal* (the temperature change induced by a cold injection) must be distinguished from *thermal noise* (the normal temperature changes in the pulmonary artery) in order to produce accurate bolus thermodilution measurements. Thermal noise is created when blood returns to the heart from the superior and inferior vena cavae and is affected by muscle movement and ventilation.

To strengthen the signal, you can either increase the volume or lower the temperature of the injectate. Because an 18° F (10° C) difference between injectate temperature and blood temperature is recommended, you may need to give iced injectate to hypothermic patients for accurate cardiac output measurement.

Correcting an inaccurate computation constant

When using a cardiac output monitor, you may inadvertently enter an incorrect computation constant. Suppose, for example, you are using 5 ml of room-temperature injectate with a #7.5 French catheter. The computation constant as specified by the manufacturer is .294.

However, suppose the nurse before you was using 10 ml of room-temperature injectate and the cardiac output computer was set for a constant of .607. If you didn't change the constant and used 5 ml of injectate, the measured cardiac output (CO) would be 4 liters/minute, when the patient's actual CO is 1.9 liters/minute.

The following formula allows you to correct the CO value without making more injections:

$$\text{Correct CO} = 4 \text{ liters/minute} \times \frac{.294}{.607}$$

$$= \frac{1.18}{.607}$$

$$= 1.9 \text{ liters/minute}$$

Respiratory monitors and ventilators

You're sure to encounter many patients with respiratory problems in your nursing practice. Many of these patients will require specific monitors to help you track their oxygen status. The most common respiratory monitors include pulse oximeters, mixed venous oxygen saturation monitors, and mechanical ventilators.

Pulse oximeters

A noninvasive procedure, pulse oximetry measures arterial oxygen saturation (SaO_2) by determining the amount of hemoglobin that's carrying oxygen within the arterial bed. A sensor containing a photodetector and light sources is placed on either the finger, toe, nose, hand, or forehead. (See *Choosing the right pulse oximetry sensor*, pages 420 and 421.) The photodetector measures the relative absorption of red and infrared light within the arterial bed and then relays this data to a monitor, which displays the SaO_2 value with each heartbeat and shows the pulse rate measured at the sen-

Choosing the right pulse oximetry sensor

Selecting the correct sensor can promote accurate pulse oximetry results. Keep in mind that the weight limits for sensors overlap, which will allow you to use a sensor appropriate for the patient's size and activity level. You could use the pediatric sensor for a small adult, for example.

After you've chosen the appropriate sensor, position it correctly. Place the pediatric and adult adhesive sensors and the finger-clip sensor for adults on the index, middle, or ring finger. You can also place the infant, pediatric, and adult adhesive sensors on a toe, but don't put the finger-clip sensor there. Also, avoid the toe if your patient has compromised circulation in the lower extremities. Avoid a finger-tip or toe-tip sensor if the patient has peripheral edema.

Place the neonatal sensor on either a neonate's foot or hand or on an adult's finger. Put the nasal sensor on the cartilaginous portion of the nose, just below the bridge.

Adhesive neonatal sensor
Less than 3 kg (6.6 lb)

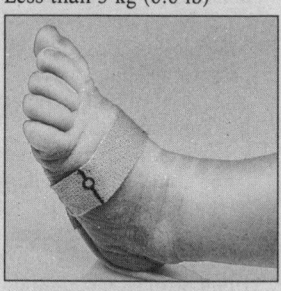

Adhesive infant sensor
1 to 20 kg (2.2. to 44 lb)

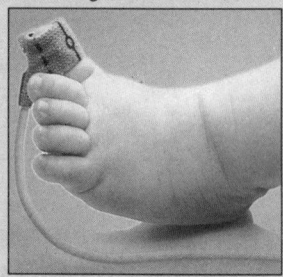

Adhesive pediatric sensor
10 to 50 kg (22 to 110 lb)

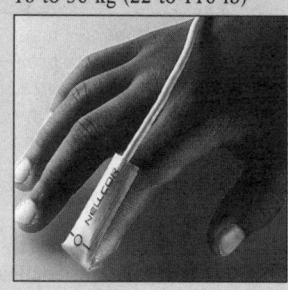

sor site. An arterial oxygen saturation measurement provided by a pulse oximeter is commonly referred to as SpO_2.

Some monitors also display a waveform, called a plethysmogram, and a pulse amplitude bar. Because blood volume changes constantly, the plethys-

Adhesive adult sensor
More than 30 kg (66 lb)

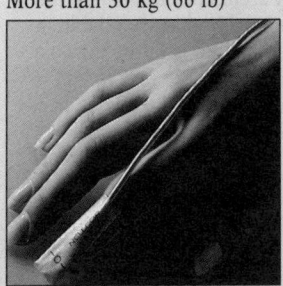

Adhesive adult nasal sensor
More than 50 kg (110 lb)

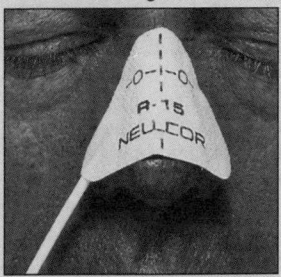

Finger-clip sensor
More than 40 kg (88 lb)

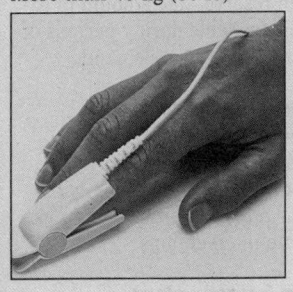

mogram shows variations in the amount of light absorbed by the arterial bed during systole or diastole. (Motion or weak pulse signals may cause the plethys-mogram to deviate from its normal appearance, rendering pulse oximetry measurements unreliable.)

Troubleshooting problems
Accurate readings depend on the type of sensor used and how appropriate it is for the expected duration of monitoring, the patient's activity level and weight, and infection concerns. An adhesive sensor, designed for single-patient use, is appropriate for either short- or long-term SaO$_2$ monitoring. For a highly active patient, an adhesive sensor provides a stabilizing, "second-skin" fit. Its light sources and photodetector are more likely to remain securely positioned, allowing it to move with the patient and provide more reliable readings. A sterile adhesive sensor is preferred for the patient with an increased risk for infection, such as a neonate or an immunosuppressed patient.

If your patient is being monitored by pulse oximetry, you'll maintain a continuous display of the SpO$_2$ value. Here are some factors that commonly affect pulse oximetry readings and measures you can take to prevent or correct false readings.

Poor skin contact
To prevent this problem, apply an adhesive sensor with fresh adhesive.

Movement
If the patient is moving the finger or toe to which the sensor is attached, the pulse oximeter may identify the motion as arterial pulsations, causing an inaccurate SpO$_2$ value. To minimize motion artifact, use an adhesive

sensor or stabilize the sensor by immobilizing the monitoring site.

You can also try connecting the oximeter to an electrocardiogram (ECG). The ECG will tell the sensor to work only when blood pulsation results from heart contractions (called ECG synchronization).

Low perfusion
Only small amounts of blood may flow through the finger's arterial bed if the patient has poor perfusion (such as results from peripheral vascular disease or vasoconstrictive drugs if the patient has peripheral edema). That means the oximeter won't identify the arterial pulse and may not display an SpO_2 value. To prevent low perfusion, use a nasal sensor or place a reflectance sensor on the patient's forehead.

Venous pulsation
Normally nonpulsatile, venous blood may pulsate from right ventricular heart failure, a tight sensor, or any tourniquet-like effect. Because the oximeter looks for pulsating blood, it will detect both pulsating venous blood and pulsating arterial blood, producing a false SpO_2 value. Usually you can avoid this problem simply by making sure the sensor isn't too tight.

Outside light
The SpO_2 value may be inaccurate if the photodetector senses large amounts of outside light (such as direct sunlight, procedure lamps, or bilirubin lights in the nursery). You can easily correct this problem by covering the sensor with a sheet or towel.

Anemia
Always double-check the patient's hemoglobin level. Even if he's anemic with a hemoglobin value of 5 g/dl, his SpO_2 value may seem normal because the hemoglobin that's available to carry oxygen is fully saturated. Yet he may have insufficient oxygen to meet his metabolic needs. To correct this problem, be prepared to administer red blood cells or whole blood.

❖

Mixed venous oxygen saturation monitors

An invasive procedure, mixed venous oxygen saturation ($S\bar{v}O_2$) monitoring reveals the balance between oxygen supply and demand. A special fiber-optic catheter placed in the pulmonary artery continuously measures the oxygen saturation of hemoglobin in mixed venous blood. The resulting $S\bar{v}O_2$ value represents oxygen reserve – the amount of oxygen available during periods of increased oxygen demand.

Troubleshooting problems
Common problems that may arise during continuous $S\bar{v}O_2$ monitoring follow, along with their possible causes and appropriate interventions.

Low-intensity alarm
Inadequate blood flow past the catheter tip or damaged fiber-optic filaments may cause this alarm to sound. To intervene, look for and straighten any obvious kinks in the catheter, follow hospital procedure to ensure

patency of the distal lumen, and check for proper connection between the optical module and the computer. If necessary, replace the catheter.

Damped waveform or erratic intensity

A blood clot over the catheter tip or wedging of the catheter tip will cause the waveform to damp. Correct the problem by ensuring patency of the distal lumen (according to hospital procedure) and repositioning the catheter.

High-intensity alarm

If the catheter tip presses against the vessel wall or the catheter floats distally into a wedge position, this alarm will sound. To address the problem, reposition the catheter and check the balloon status. Confirm proper position by examining the pressure waveform.

Low-light message

This message will flash if a poor connection exists between the catheter and optical module or between the optical module and computer. Damaged fiber-optic filaments or a defective optical module may also trigger a low-light message.

To check the connection between the catheter and optical module, disconnect the catheter from the optical module, close the lid, and place the optical module out of direct light. If the low-light message disappears, the problem lies with the catheter. Check the connection and reattach as needed. To check the connection between the optical module and computer, check all connections, and reconnect as

needed. Turn off the computer for a few seconds and turn it back on. You'll hear two beeps if the computer is functional and connections are secure.

If the low-light message persists, gently manipulate the catheter, particularly around the insertion site. If this doesn't solve the problem, replace the catheter. Then, if necessary, replace the optical module.

Calibration failure (CAL FAIL) message

This message results from unsuccessful preinsertion calibration. If this problem occurs, verify a correct attachment between the catheter and the optical module; then repeat calibration. If the CAL FAIL message still appears, replace the optical module.

Dashes in oxygen saturation display

The lack of an oxygen saturation display may occur because of improper preinsertion calibration, optical module malfunction, catheter damage, an improperly positioned catheter tip, or the loss of electronic memory.

To remedy the problem, first verify a correct attachment between the catheter and the optical module; then repeat calibration. If dashes continue to appear, replace the optical module and repeat calibration. You may also need to gently manipulate and reposition the catheter. If the monitor does not compute a range, replace the catheter and repeat calibration.

If a power failure caused the problem, determine the cause of the failure and then repeat calibration.

❖

Mechanical ventilators

Mechanical ventilators come in four basic types: negative-pressure, volume-cycled, pressure-cycled, and high-frequency. You'll usually work with volume-cycled or pressure-cycled ventilators.

Negative-pressure ventilators alternately remove and replace gas from a chamber that encloses either the entire body except for the head (the Drinker respirator, or iron lung) or just the front and sides of the chest and upper abdomen (the chest shell). As the machine drives gas from the chamber, the resulting negative pressure forces the chest wall to expand, pulling gas into the lungs. Then the machine's diaphragm returns to its normal position, allowing the chest wall to fall, thereby causing exhalation.

Volume-cycled ventilators stop inspiration after delivering a preset tidal volume of gas, despite increased airway resistance as in adult respiratory distress syndrome or bronchospasm. Then they allow passive expiration. As ordered, you can set the tidal volume, respiratory rate, inspiratory-expiratory ratio, inspiratory time, and oxygen concentration. These unique ventilators have an automatic sigh mechanism, a pressure limit alarm to alert you to high peak airway pressures that can damage lungs, and a high-pressure relief valve to relieve excessive pressure when high pressure is needed to deliver a preset volume.

Pressure-cycled ventilators deliver a preset volume of gas, as do volume-cycled ventilators, but at a preset airway pressure. When the preset airway pressure is reached, inspiration stops to allow passive expiration.

High-frequency jet ventilators are the newest type of positive-pressure ventilators. They prevent fluctuation of pressure within the lungs and don't cause the detrimental effects on the cardiovascular system that other positive-pressure ventilators do.

These ventilators were developed for use when high peak-airway pressures or large intrapleural air leaks preclude conventional mechanical ventilation. They employ a narrow injector cannula to deliver short, rapid bursts of oxygen to the airways under low pressure. The combination of high rate, low tidal volumes, and low pressure enhances alveolar gas exchange without elevating peak inspiratory pressures and compromising cardiac output – the major drawback of conventional high-volume, high-pressure mechanical ventilation.

Thus, high-frequency jet ventilators are valuable for patients with hemodynamic instability and those at high risk for pulmonary barotrauma, such as young children. They're also useful for ventilating patients during bronchoscopy, laryngoscopy, and laryngeal surgery because the narrow cannula doesn't obstruct the operating field. And because the cannula can be inserted directly into the trachea through a cricothyrotomy, these ventilators may be used when upper airway trauma or obstruction precludes intubation, such as in emergency respiratory situations.

Troubleshooting problems

Common problems that may arise with mechanical ventilators follow, along with their possible causes and appropriate interventions.

Low-pressure alarm

A simple reason for this alarm may be that the tube is disconnected from the ventilator. More complicated causes include the displacement of the endotracheal (ET) tube above the vocal cords (or the extubation of a tracheostomy tube), leaking tidal volume from low cuff pressure (from an underinflated or ruptured ET cuff or a leak in the cuff or one-way valve), a ventilator malfunction, or a leak in ventilator circuitry (from a loose connection or hole in tubing, loss of a temperature-sensing device, or a cracked humidification container).

To address the problem, make sure all connections between the tube and ventilator are intact. Also check the humidification container and the tubing for holes or leaks, and replace them if necessary. If extubation or displacement has occurred, manually ventilate the patient and call the doctor. If these problems don't appear to be causing the alarm, listen for a whooshing sound (an air leak) around the tube, and check cuff pressure. If you can't maintain pressure, the doctor may insert a new tube. If the ventilator appears to be malfunctioning, disconnect the patient and manually ventilate him if necessary. Replace the ventilator if needed.

High-pressure alarm

This alarm may result from increased airway pressure or decreased lung compliance caused by worsening disease. Other causes include the patient biting on the ET tube; the patient coughing, gagging, or trying to talk; secretions in the airway; condensate in large-bore tubing; intubation of the right mainstem bronchus; chest wall resistance; bronchospasm, pneumothorax, or barotrauma; or a malfunctioning high-pressure relief valve.

Begin to address the problem by auscultating the patient's lungs for evidence of increasing lung consolidation, barotrauma, wheezing, absence of breath sounds (such as with right mainstem intubation or a mucus plug). At the same time, check the tube's position. Call the doctor if indicated.

Other appropriate interventions include suctioning the patient or having the patient cough and inserting a bite guard if needed. Remove any condensate in the tubing. If the patient is fighting the ventilator in any way, he may need sedation or a neuromuscular blocker as ordered. Reposition the patient if his position limits chest expansion. If repositioning proves ineffective, give a prescribed analgesic. Finally, have the faulty equipment replaced.

Spirometer or low exhaled tidal or minute volume alarm

An interruption of power, a loose connection, or a leak in the delivery system may trigger this alarm. Other possible causes include a leaking cuff or inadequate cuff seal, a leaking chest tube, increased airway resistance in a patient on a pressure-cycled ventilator, a disconnected spirometer, or a malfunctioning volume measuring device. Also any change that sets off high- or low-pressure alarms and prevents delivery of full air volume may also trigger this alarm. (See the sections on high- and low-pressure alarms for interventions.)

Respond to the alarm by auscultating the patient's lungs for signs of an airway obstruction, barotrauma, or lung consolidation. If the patient is stable, check all electrical connections. Then make sure that all connections in the delivery system are secure and free from leaks and that the spirometer is connected. Use a stethoscope to check the cuff for leaks. If necessary, reinflate or replace the cuff according to hospital policy. If the patient has a chest tube, check all chest tube connections. If the tube is leaking, make sure that the water seal is intact and then notify the doctor. If the volume measuring device appears to be malfunctioning, alert the respiratory therapist to replace it.

High respiratory rate alarm

If the patient is anxious, in pain, or has secretions in his airway, this alarm may sound. If so, assess the patient for the cause. Suction the patient if necessary. If he's anxious, dispel his fears as much as possible and sedate him if necessary. If the patient is in pain, position him comfortably. Administer medication for pain as ordered.

Low PEEP-CPAP alarm

A leak in the positive end-expiratory pressure and continuous positive airway pressure (PEEP-CPAP) system will set off this alarm. Respond by checking that all connections are secure. Check for holes in the tubing and replace it if necessary.

Another possible cause of this alarm is a mechanical failure of the PEEP mechanism. In this instance, discontinue PEEP and call the respiratory therapist. ❖

Neurologic monitors

When caring for a neurologic patient, you'll need to use all your skills to help preserve and restore optimal nervous system function. As part of your care, you'll no doubt use sophisticated equipment, such as an intracranial pressure monitor or a cerebral blood flow monitor.

Intracranial pressure monitors

Continuous intracranial pressure (ICP) monitoring has become common practice in intensive care units. It's most often used for monitoring trauma patients, who are susceptible to cerebral edema. Other likely candidates include patients with subarachnoid hemorrhage, tumors that obstruct the ventricular system, cerebral aneurysm, intracranial hemorrhage, or Reye's syndrome. ICP is also used for monitoring patients in the first 24 hours after surgery.

All ICP monitoring systems share three basic components: a sensor, a pressure transducer, and a recording device. The sensor can be placed in the ventricle, subarachnoid space, epidural space, subdural space, or brain parenchyma. It transmits ICP changes to the transducer, which converts the impulses to electrical or light signals. A recording device converts the signals to visible tracings, which appear on an oscilloscope or are transferred to graph paper.

Troubleshooting problems

Most hospitals use a direct pressure monitoring system for evaluating ICP. Following are some of the most common problems that may arise with ICP monitors, along with their probable causes and appropriate interventions. As needed, consult the manufacturer's instruction manual.

No reading on monitor

A waveform may fail to appear if the circuit breaker switch is in the down position, or if the battery power is too low. To solve the problem, make sure the circuit breaker switch is in the up position. Also verify that the battery is charged.

Low-battery (LOW BATT) indicator

A failing battery charge is the typical cause for this indicator to light up. Corrective measures include fully recharging the battery by connecting the monitor to an AC power source for about 12 hours. Also confirm that the

circuit breaker switch is in the up position.

Catheter connection warning message

A loose connection in the system will produce this message: CHECK CATHETER CONNECTION +350 or more, −99. Appropriate interventions include checking the connections between the catheter and the preamp cable, the preamp cable and the preamp extension cable, and the preamp extension cable and the V420 preamp extension cable receptacle. As necessary, replace equipment components, such as the preamp cable, preamp extension cable, V420 monitor, or catheter.

Improperly sized waveform

An overly large or overly small waveform may result from incorrect scale selection. To solve the problem, press the SCALE key to change the scale selection. ❖

Cerebral blood flow monitors

Traditionally, caregivers have estimated cerebral blood flow (CBF) in neurologically compromised patients by calculating cerebral perfusion pressure. However, modern technology permits continuous regional blood flow monitoring at the bedside. A sensor surgically placed on the cerebral cortex calculates CBF in the capillary bed by thermal diffusion. Thermistors within the sensor measure the temperature ferential between two metallic plates—one heated, one neutral.

The CBF monitor yields continuous real-time values for CBF, which are essential in conditions where compromised blood flow may put the patient at risk, such as ischemia and infarction.

Troubleshooting problems

Some of the most common problems that may arise with the CBF monitor follow, along with their probable causes and appropriate interventions.

Unusually low or high CBF value

A sudden 20% increase or decrease from the patient's baseline CBF value may be caused by the sensor's incomplete contact with the cerebral cortex. A low CBF value may also be caused by a fluid layer (a small hematoma) between the sensor and the cortex. Check the patient's neurologic status. If you detect a change, notify the neurosurgeon. If there is a 20% increase or decrease from the patient's baseline CBF value and no change in the patient's neurologic status, turn the patient toward the side of the sensor or gently wiggle the catheter back and forth (using a sterile gloved hand). Observe the CBF value on the monitor as you perform these maneuvers. The value should return to the patient's baseline level.

8 Overcoming Barriers to Patient Teaching

How to hone your teaching skills

With so many responsibilities and so little time, thorough patient teaching can be a challenge. But you can meet the challenge – not by attempting to teach faster but by streamlining your teaching techniques.

Teaching within time constraints

Streamlining your patient teaching involves two key processes: staying organized and learning to recognize patient attitudes that impede learning.

Getting organized
One way to simplify patient teaching is to break it down into manageable steps. (See *Four steps to better patient teaching.*)

As you work with each patient, keep in mind that learning styles and rates vary. A person's intelligence and educational level have an influence – and so do personal preferences. To get the most out of each session, determine which of these learning styles best matches your patient:
• Visual learners learn best by seeing or reading what you're trying to teach.
• Auditory learners learn best by listening to what you're teaching.
• Tactile, or psychomotor, learners learn best by doing. Play to your patient's learning style, but don't restrict your teaching to that one style. Research indicates that

learning increases when it involves more than one sense.

Assess your patient's learning style by watching him or simply asking him how he learns best. You can also experiment with different teaching tools, such as printed material, illustrations, videotapes, and actual equipment. One caution: Never assume that your patient can read well.

Setting teaching priorities
When you find yourself with too much to teach your patient and too little time to do it, the following method will help you set priorities, distinguish the patient's learning needs from his nursing care needs, and help you organize your time. You will also get back on track more easily after interruptions if you have:
• listed the patient's learning needs
• ranked these needs in order of importance
• written your "teaching to-be-done" list based on this ranking.

Of course, your hardest task is ranking your patient's learning needs. To make this easier, classify each learning need as:
• either *immediate* – one that must be met promptly, such as teaching the patient who's being discharged in 2 hours – or *long-range*
• either *survival* – life-dependent, such as teaching the warning signs of adrenal crisis – or *related to well-being* – nice to know but not essential
• either *specific* – related to the patient's disorder or treatment, such as preparing him for an upcoming cholecystectomy – or *general* – teaching done for every patient, such as explaining hospital visiting hours.

Four steps to better patient teaching

Before you teach your patient, you need to take four important steps. The first step is to set standards for what the patient should learn, and the next two steps are collecting and evaluating data. The last step is to formulate a statement of the patient's readiness to meet those standards—in effect, your teaching diagnosis.

Along the way, you'll probably uncover other topics you need to teach, based on what your patient and his family want to learn about his condition. If so, you'll need to reassess the patient or modify your teaching standards to create the best possible teaching plan.

Set teaching standards
• What does the patient need to learn?
• What does the health care team want the patient to learn?
• When does teaching need to take place?

Collect data
• What do interviews with the patient and his family tell you about learning needs and goals?
• What does the patient's chart reveal?
• What information can other members of the health care team provide?

Evaluate data
• What does the patient want to learn?
• Do his goals conflict with those of his family or the health care team?
• Are there any barriers to learning?
• Are there any factors that can promote learning?

Establish a teaching diagnosis
• What is the patient ready, willing, and able to learn?
• Do the patient, family, and health care team confirm your findings?
• Do you need to set new teaching standards?

After you've classified the patient's learning needs, establish priorities. For instance, an immediate survival need would top your list.

Deciding if your patient is ready to learn
Sometimes, a patient has difficulty accepting his illness, especially if it's serious. And because patients use different coping mechanisms, you can't predict how each one will react. (See *Recognizing how your patient copes*, pages 432 and 433.)

If the patient hasn't come to terms with his condition, he won't want to learn about it. By recognizing and understanding the coping mechanisms your patient is using, you can avoid teaching him something he's not ready to learn.

Recognizing how your patient copes

Coping mechanisms aren't always harmful. But they can interfere with a patient's learning, so you need to recognize and understand them. Here are the coping mechanisms patients commonly use.

COPING MECHANISM	BEHAVIOR TRAITS	REASONS FOR USE
Denial (refusing to recognize some aspect of reality)	Denies known facts or reality of illness, refuses responsibility for learning self-care	Protects patient from painful reality
Rationalization (justifying behavior by using a plausible excuse)	Intensely defends own position	Maintains patient's self-respect and wards off guilt feelings
Displacement (redirecting an emotion or impulse toward another person or object)	Focuses on teaching inconsistencies of health care team	Allows patient to express repressed feelings
Conversion (translating psychological problems into physical complaints)	Claims physical problems that have no clinical cause, requests self-care information about the physical problems	Helps patient avoid anxiety-producing situation because he's "ill," gives patient legitimate reason for seeking help, or removes focus from psychological problems
Regression (returning to a previous, immature way of behaving)	Refuses to participate in learning, performs previously learned tasks at a lower level of ability	Lets patient avoid anxiety of real situation

Recognizing how your patient copes *(continued)*

COPING MECHANISM	BEHAVIOR TRAITS	REASONS FOR USE
Projection (transferring unwanted thoughts and tendencies to others)	Minimizes own guilt by making others feel guilty, blames others for own problems, makes others responsible for learning tasks or for own failure to learn	Provides an outlet for patient's repressed thoughts and tendencies

Stage 1: Disbelief
Your patient thinks:
• "There's nothing wrong with me."
• "This can't be happening to me!"
His actions:
• deny the existence or seriousness of illness
• show disregard for prescribed activity or restrictions and for attempts to teach him self-care.

Stage 2: Developing awareness
Your patient thinks:
• "Why me?"
• "If only I'd been more careful, maybe I wouldn't have gotten sick."
His actions:
• place blame for illness on himself or others
• involve striking out at others to relieve pent-up hostilities.

Stage 3: Reorganization
Your patient thinks:
• "How does my family see me now?"
• "I'm beginning to see how my life is changing."
His actions:
• show avoidance of discussing his condition or changes with family
• include asking more questions about his condition.

Stage 4: Resolution
Your patient thinks:
• "I see how my life has changed."
• "Other people with my condition seem to get along all right."
His actions:
• include seeking out others with the same condition
• convey a more open expression of emotions.

Stage 5: Identity change
Your patient thinks:
• "I've changed, and my life is going to be different from now on."
His actions:
• include seeking out information about his condition
• show attempts at greater independence.

Stage 6: Successful adaptation

Your patient thinks:
• "I accept the way my life has changed."
• "I want to make each moment count."
His actions:
• show compliance with the health care regimen
• involve openly discussing his condition with his family.

Expressing clear learning goals

To clearly express your patient's learning goals, focus on his behaviors that need to be modified. His learning behaviors, and your goals for him, fall into three learning domains: cognitive, psychomotor, and affective.

Your patient may have learning goals in all three categories. For example, understanding dietary changes would fall into the cognitive domain; complying with these changes, the affective domain; taking his blood pressure, the psychomotor domain.

With these domains in mind, you can write clear and concise learning goals for your patient, based on his needs.

Review the two sets of sample learning goals for a patient with chronic renal failure. (See *Writing clear goals.*)

The goals in the poorly phrased set include many tasks and describe learning that is difficult or even impossible to measure. But the well-phrased goals start with a precise action verb, limit themselves to one task, and describe learning that is measurable and observable.

Making standard forms work for you

If your hospital has standard teaching plans for some common disorders, you can easily adapt them to each patient's specific learning needs. Simply follow these steps.

First, determine your patient's learning needs; then decide if he's ready for patient teaching. Choose the tools you'll use.

Next, using the standard teaching plan as your guide, assess your patient's knowledge and skills in the areas listed. This will tell you which points to delete from the teaching plan, which ones to include, and which ones to modify. You can now design individualized learning goals and determine your teaching priorities.

If your patient isn't emotionally ready to discuss his illness, you might simply discuss his concerns and dispel any misconceptions.

You can leave some pamphlets for the patient to look over. Laying some groundwork might help make future teaching sessions more productive. Before you meet again, reevaluate to determine what else you might want to use from the standard teaching plan.

Giving feedback

Effective patient teaching depends on helpful feedback. The patient tells or shows you what he's learned, and you point out his successes and weak spots. This exchange of information should help build the patient's confidence and improve his skills.

Writing clear goals

POORLY PHRASED LEARNING GOALS	WELL-PHRASED LEARNING GOALS
Cognitive domain	

The patient with chronic renal failure will be able to:

• state his medication schedule	• state when to administer each drug
• identify when his blood pressure is elevated	• describe symptoms of elevated blood pressure
• realize his dietary restrictions.	• list allowed and prohibited foods on his diet.

Psychomotor domain	

The patient with chronic renal failure will be able to:

• take his blood pressure	• take his blood pressure accurately, using a stethoscope and a sphygmomanometer
• use a thermometer	• read a thermometer correctly
• bring in a urine sample for laboratory studies.	• collect a urine sample, using sterile technique.

Affective domain	

The patient with chronic renal failure will be able to:

• appreciate the relationship of diet to renal failure	• comply with his dietary restrictions to maintain normal electrolyte values
• adjust successfully to limitations imposed by chronic renal failure	• describe adjustments needed in the home environment
• realize the importance of regular doctor visits.	• keep scheduled doctor appointments.

To ensure that your feedback is effective, keep your comments helpful, not hurtful. Share information and present alternatives, rather than dictate rules. And avoid using absolute words, such as "always" and "never."

Be sure to focus on the patient's behavior, not on his progress or personality. And discuss his current behavior, not his past.

Give the patient positive feedback to reinforce desired behavior. Then discuss the points that he still needs to master.

Offer constructive criticism as soon as possible after observing an incorrect action. The longer the patient continues with an undesirable behavior, thought, or attitude, the more comfortable he'll become with it and the greater difficulty he'll have changing it.

Offer specific suggestions for improvement along with the rationale. If the patient understands why something needs to be done, he'll more easily remember to do it — and do it correctly. And make sure the patient understands the feedback you've given him.

Be sure to comment on situations that the patient can change, not ones beyond his control. And remember to move at the patient's pace, not yours. Keep in mind his needs and abilities and the amount of information he can handle.

Relying on timesavers
A little advance preparation goes a long way toward speeding up your patient teaching. Before you begin a session, have the patient review written materials, audiocassettes, or videotapes to gain a basic understanding of his illness. Use diagrams, charts, and other visual aids to speed comprehension.

Be sure to involve the family, especially if they'll participate in the patient's home care. Schedule your teaching sessions during their visits. And combine patient teaching with routine nursing care. Let the patient's questions guide your teaching.

If you're teaching a short-stay patient who'll be visited by a home health nurse, emphasize major points in your teaching and leave less immediate points for the home health nurse. Document your teaching to avoid duplication of instruction.

When you've developed a teaching plan for a specific disorder, file it for reuse or adaptation. Then you can give the patient copies of preprinted information and instructions to take home, rather than writing new ones yourself.

Constantly evaluate your teaching to find the methods that work best for you. Then use them.

Facilitating group teaching
Use group teaching sessions for patients with similar teaching needs, such as instruction in diabetes, hypertension, cardiac rehabilitation, and postnatal care. However, be aware that many people feel uncomfortable in group situations, and this can interfere with your teaching. To enhance the learning process, help your patients develop a group identity and cohesiveness. Here are some useful techniques.

Create a comfortable setting
• Hold the meeting at a round table, or arrange chairs in a circle. This increases interaction by making participants feel equal to each other and to the teacher.
• Limit the group to between five and seven patients to allow for maximum personal exchange and discussion.
• Check the temperature and lighting of the meeting room to make sure neither is uncomfortable or distracting.
• Arrange for coffee, tea, or soft drinks to be served to keep the atmosphere informal and relaxed.

Be gracious
• Introduce yourself.
• Ask patients to introduce themselves and to share a bit of personal information.
• Explain the meeting's purpose.

Using checklists

Checklists provide a roster of learning needs. For instance, the checklist below helps you know if a patient can draw up insulin.

Drawing up insulin

Yes	No	
☐	☐	Disinfected top of vial thoroughly
☐	☐	Inserted needle into vial without contamination
☐	☐	Injected air into vial
☐	☐	Withdrew proper amount of insulin
☐	☐	Expelled air from syringe
☐	☐	Retained exact dose of insulin in syringe
☐	☐	Replaced cap on needle without contamination

• Invite the group to set up the meeting's goals and ground rules.
• Encourage everyone's participation, and be gracious about allowing anyone to leave who isn't comfortable or willing to participate.

Lead the group effectively
• Use a light rein, yet keep the group close to the topic of discussion.
• Act as a resource, providing information and clarification when necessary.
• Summarize at the end of the discussion, and lead the group to agree on what has been learned.

Creating effective checklists
Checklists give you and the patient clear evidence of which learning goals he's achieved and which goals need further work. (See *Using checklists*.) To devise a helpful checklist, follow these tips:
• Make the list concise but wide-ranging enough to cover all aspects of the skill or activity you're evaluating.
• Limit the items on the checklist to a group of related activities, such as the steps in the tracheostomy plan of care or the facets of a cardiac rehabilitation plan. Arrange the items in a logical order—sequentially, chronologically, or in order of importance.
• Identify the essential steps of the activities or behavior you're evaluating.
• Make the checklist items relate to the patient's learning goals and to your teaching methods.
• Use only one idea or concept in each item.
• Phrase each item concisely and accurately.
• Test your checklist on at least two patients before adopting it.
• Use the checklist along with other evaluation tools to avoid giving it undue importance.

Streamlining teaching with clinical pathways of care

If you're like many nurses, you want to tailor a plan of care to your patient's specific needs, but you don't have the time. Ideally, you'd set goals and expected outcomes with the patient, evaluate the effectiveness of care, and document the patient's progress throughout his stay. In reality, though, using a plan of care documentation system can be a challenge when patient acuity is high or staffing is low.

But you can streamline the process and still ensure continuity of care by integrating the principles of case management into both nursing documentation and patient care. Instead of using a Kardex and nursing care plan, use a multidisciplinary plan of care form (known as a clinical pathway or critical path in some hospitals). Be sure to involve your patient right from the start. (See *Using a plan of care form*, pages 440 and 441.)

The plan of care format identifies the patient's diagnosis, his expected length of stay, care guidelines, and expected outcomes. Care guidelines and outcomes, which are specified for each day of the patient's stay, are organized into five categories: activity, nutrition, treatments, teaching, and other focal areas, including code status. Using this format, you can evaluate patient outcomes every day and keep goals on track.

Involving the patient

As each patient is admitted, give him his own plan of care form if he hasn't already received one from his doctor. That way, he'll be involved in his care right away, which will help teach him about his condition.

The patient's copy includes the same information as the nursing staff's copy, but is written in layperson's language. Make sure the patient's version explains his diagnosis, reviews the care he'll receive, lists tests or procedures he'll undergo, outlines his expected length of stay, and informs him about activity restrictions, diet, medications, and home care services.

Also give the patient typed teaching and discharge sheets and review all teaching information with him daily, documenting what you covered and how well he understood it. Review discharge instructions with him before he leaves the hospital. ❖

Simplifying postdischarge plans

The trend toward shorter hospital stays means patients need more care after discharge. That means you have to plan your patients' postdischarge care and ensure that those plans are carried out. The easiest way to proceed is to establish a postdischarge care program. As you set up the program, keep in mind these guidelines:
• Tailor postdischarge care to fit each patient's situation.

• Work closely with other facilities and community service organizations, such as outpatient clinics, hospices, home health care agencies, and Meals On Wheels.
• Ensure continuity of care for patients scheduled for future hospital treatment.
• Help terminally ill patients and their families cope during the grieving process after discharge.

Planning for patient transfer

If a patient is being transferred to another hospital or facility, write a discharge summary and a nursing plan of care detailing medication regimens and feeding schedules. Include your name and the phone number of your unit. After reviewing the plan of care with the patient and family, call the other facility to discuss with the admitting nurse the patient's hospital stay and the plan of care.

If appropriate or if expected by your hospital, call a family member a week or two after the transfer to see how the patient is doing. If possible, visit the patient and assess his condition to determine whether the plan of care is working.

This approach to postdischarge care can also benefit a terminally ill patient. The primary nurse has to help such a patient and his family deal realistically with his prognosis. Only then can the nurse guide the patient and family through the grieving process.

Making an ongoing commitment

Emphasizing postdischarge care will likely lead to important changes on your unit. For instance, you'll probably start inserting possible discharge needs into a patient's care plan within 48 hours of his admission. And you might decide to hold interdisciplinary planning rounds once a week, including the patient's primary nurse, charge nurse, visiting nurse, doctor, social worker, physical therapist, occupational therapist, and dietitian.

To foster everyone's commitment, encourage primary nurses to accept responsibility for staffing and setting priorities. Flexible schedules will help you and your coworkers allow each other time for planning postdischarge care and visiting patients. During primary nurse conferences and staff meetings, share information obtained from visits, phone calls, and letters.

After using the program for a year, evaluate it to see whether the original goals are being met. You'll probably find that discharge teaching is usually appropriate for each patient; the primary nurse gets to know him and his family well enough to recognize their strengths and limitations. Because you start patient teaching early, you can anticipate certain problems before they arise. And because patients may call you after discharge, you can handle problems that develop later.

By getting in touch with other facilities and community services, you learn more about the care they offer—and that can help you plan a patient's discharge better. For instance, if you know that no such services are available near a patient's rural home, you can plan on giving him and his family the detailed teaching and hands-on practice

Using a plan of care form

The following sample shows the teaching portion of a plan of care, designed for a patient with congestive heart failure. When you compare the nursing staff's copy with the patient's copy, you'll find that they both contain the same information but are written in different language.

NURSING STAFF COPY

Teaching

DAY OF ADMISSION	DAY 2	DAY 3	DAY 4
• Review plan of care with patient. • Explain medications to patient. • Give copy of plan of care to patient. • Give information sheet on congestive heart failure to patient. • Home health referral needed? • Home oxygen needed?	*Expected outcome* • Patient can verbalize understanding of present medications.	• Discharge medication sheets given. • Home health referral arranged if needed. • Home oxygen arranged if needed.	*Expected outcomes* • Patient can verbalize understanding of present medications. • Discharge medication sheet reviewed and patient can verbalize understanding. • Discharge instructions reviewed and patient can verbalize understanding. • Patient can verbalize understanding the need for follow-up visit and of when to call doctor.

they need for certain self-care procedures.

Expanding the role of the primary nurse beyond the hospital walls can help ease the transition from hospital to home or another facility for many patients. Of course, detailed plans

are necessary for successful discharges—but they're not enough. True continuity of care means continuing to care for the patient after discharge.

PATIENT COPY

Patient Information

DAY OF ADMISSION	DAY 2	DAY 3	DAY 4
• You'll need to understand what's going on with your body. Please ask questions if you don't understand something. • You'll be given a sheet to explain what congestive heart failure is. • Ask about your medications if you're unfamiliar with them.		• You'll be given information sheets that explain the medication you'll take at home. • You should know about the right foods to eat and what types of food you should avoid. • Your doctor may order a follow-up visit by a home health nurse.	• You'll need to follow up with your doctor. Make sure you know when your appointment is. • Know which problems may require medical attention.

How to prevent teaching missteps

When teaching seems to be consuming too much precious time, or when patients or family members become difficult, the problem often is poor communication between you and your patient or between your patient and the staff. Here are ways to prevent misunderstandings.

Avoiding communication problems

You can help keep the lines of communication open through patient care conferences. In fact, you should regularly schedule these meetings, even when you don't have a specific problem to discuss. Doing so can help prevent unnecessary confusion and frustration for patients, families, and health care workers.

Anyone taking part in the patient's care—even the patient himself or a family member—can request a patient care conference. The first step toward arranging the conference is to designate a conference leader. This could be the primary nurse or any health care worker who's familiar with the needs of the patient and his family. The conference leader plans and conducts the conference and notifies others about any decisions reached.

Planning the conference

When planning a conference, first establish its objectives. These usually center around meeting the patient's treatment needs and planning his discharge.

After setting objectives, make a list of the participants. An ideal number is 10 or fewer and includes only those people directly involved with meeting the conference objectives. If appropriate, invite the patient and his family.

Next, after checking with everyone, pick a convenient date, time, and place. Try to schedule the meeting in a room that's

comfortable, conducive to good eye contact, and away from busy areas. Arrange for coverage beforehand to avoid interruptions and, finally, choose a conference recorder.

Conducting the conference

Start the meeting by reviewing the objectives, and briefly go over the patient's history. Next, ask each caregiver to summarize her involvement to date with the patient and his family as well as her treatment and anticipated discharge objectives. Common discharge objectives might including ensuring that the patient knows how to:
• safely administer his medications
• perform self-care
• reduce his risk of infection
• contact appropriate health care team members if a problem arises.

Following up

At the end of the conference, review the important points discussed, and then schedule another meeting to determine whether the objectives have been met. Document in the patient's chart the decisions and plans made at the conference. You should also incorporate these into the nursing plan of care.

Next, discuss the outcome of the conference with the patient and his family. Document their responses in the patient's chart. After meeting again for a progress report, conference members can decide if a follow-up conference is necessary.

A well-planned patient care conference can help you communicate better with your patient and his family. And that benefits everyone—the patient, his family, and the health care workers involved in his care.

❖

Avoiding common errors

Patient teaching is a skill. The information you're teaching is familiar to you, so you can easily forget it's confusing to someone hearing it for the first time.

Here are some common mistakes that nurses make when teaching their patients. Guard against these errors, and you'll be one step closer to better patient teaching:

• Failing to negotiate goals. Acknowledge any discrepancy in goals, and recognize that the patient's goals supersede yours.

• Duplicating teaching effort. Although repetition can be a useful teaching device, it should be planned, not done haphazardly.

• Giving too much detail to patients who are clearly unable to understand it.

• Overloading the patient with information. Keep teaching sessions short. Shorter sessions will let the patient integrate new information and formulate questions for the next teaching session—something he couldn't do if you taught everything in one long session. Watch for signs that a patient is saturated: inability to answer questions regarding the material, fidgeting, yawning, and glazed, staring eyes. When you see these signs, tell the patient to prepare questions for the next session and, if appropriate, leave printed information with him.

• Not confirming that the patient has understood the information given to him. For example, make sure that printed material is not given to an illiterate patient.

• Using materials that you haven't reviewed or using media exclusively. Don't rely solely on media for patient education. This makes it impossible to individualize patient teaching, answer the patient's questions, or gather feedback from him.

• Exhibiting territoriality or "owning" the patient. You can fall into this trap when you invest a lot of time and effort in teaching patients. Remember, the patient is responsible for his own behavior.

• Denying or overlooking the patient's right to change his mind. This mistake occurs when you've overinvested yourself in the patient and his progress.

• Demonstrating an inability to learn from your mistakes. Don't be task-oriented and insist there's only one way to do things.

• Refusing to work within the restrictions of the patient's situation. Consider the patient's lack of family support, his educational level, his financial situation, and his cultural or ethnic background.

• Exhibiting poor timing and inattention to the patient's stress level. This problem is usually caused by focusing on your needs, not the patient's. Just as patients under stress aren't good candidates for teaching, neither are patients in denial. Also, the length of the patient's stay is too short sometimes for adequate teaching.

• Failing to reassess the patient throughout his hospitalization.

BARRIERS TO
TEACHING

 The liability of patient teaching

When deciding a nurse's legal responsibility for patient teaching, the court will likely examine the question under the general category of the patient's right to know (*Gerety v. Demers*, 1978; *Canterbury v. Spence*, 1972). Health care requires the patient's participation and cooperation; therefore, the right to know is an inherent part of successful treatment. If that right is crucial to the patient's health, the court will probably see patient teaching as a health care provider's legal duty and will determine whether you have met or breached it.

• Failing to arrange for feedback and evaluation. Ask for a return demonstration or verbal feedback; you might be surprised by how little the patient has actually absorbed. Be sure to allow time for patients to ask questions and encourage them to do so. Also, set aside time for skill-building. In order to master tasks requiring physical manipulation, patients need to practice these skills alone and in your presence.

――――――――――❖

Avoiding medical jargon

Communicating in medical terminology is second nature to you and your coworkers, but it's a foreign language to most patients. To make sure you're getting your message across, keep these guidelines in mind:
• While well-educated patients might understand some medical terminology, research shows that even these patients misunderstand some common terms. To avoid confusion, don't use clinical terms when you talk to patients.
• Give patients a list that explains commonly used terms. And arrange for workshops with your peers to discuss ways to improve communication with patients so you're sure everyone is on the same wavelength.
• Assess your patient's level of understanding, use only words he recognizes, and watch for signs that he's having difficulty grasping your meaning. Otherwise, unnecessary anxiety and poor compliance can result.

――――――――――❖

Avoiding legal liability

When it comes to patient teaching, do you realize that sharing information with your patients isn't enough? You also need to document that you did so to protect yourself legally. Regularly using patient-teaching plans when you teach can also help protect you. (See *The liability of patient teaching.*)

LEGAL LESSON

 Why document?

Accurate and detailed documentation helps ensure continuity in teaching. It tells the other health care team members what's been planned for the patient, what's already been carried out, and what remains to be done. It ensures that no one duplicates teaching efforts.

Careful documentation also protects you legally. If the patient claims he was harmed because you supplied inadequate instructions or provided none at all, your legal protection rests on documentation of your teaching and the patient's response. Documentation can support your judgment in setting priorities for learner needs, selecting teaching methods, and evaluating learned tasks.

BARRIERS TO TEACHING

Documenting when you teach

Kyslinger v. United States (1975) addresses the nurse's liability for patient teaching. In this case, a Veteran's Administration (VA) hospital sent a hemodialysis patient home with an artificial kidney. He eventually died (apparently while on the machine), and his wife sued the federal government because a VA hospital was involved. She alleged that the hospital and its staff had failed to teach either her or her late husband how to properly use and maintain a home hemodialysis unit.

After examining the evidence, the court ruled against the patient's wife. During the 10 months that the husband underwent biweekly hemodialysis treatment on the unit at the VA hospital, the nurses' notes showed that both the husband and his wife were taught how to operate, maintain, and supervise such treatments. The court found no reason to conclude that they had not been properly informed on the use of the hemodialysis unit.

The proof was in the documentation. (See *Why document?*) The lesson, of course, is that giving and documenting patient teaching—and patient response to teaching—can protect you, and not doing so could be grounds for a successful suit against you.

When deciding issues involving patient teaching, the court considers prevailing standards—both national and local. Most nurse practice acts in the United States and Canada contain wording about promoting patient health and preventing disease. But they don't specify a nurse's responsibility for patient teaching. This information is established in the practice standards developed by professional organizations, in statements about nursing practice from national commissions, in hospital procedure manuals and policies, in written job descriptions, and in the testimony of expert witnesses.

Documenting what you teach

Typically, standards for patient teaching include the following responsibilities:

• discussing the plan of care and interventions with the patient and his family

• assessing what the patient and his family want or need to know

• identifying goals that you and the patient want to reach

• choosing teaching strategies that will help you reach the goals

• incorporating teaching-learning principles into the plan of care and stating learning objectives in behavioral terms

• teaching the patient and his family with help from other staff members as needed, or assisting other staff members in teaching as needed

• evaluating the effectiveness of teaching in objective, measurable terms

• documenting the results of patient teaching.

In addition to the teaching you do, you should document when you delegate teaching to another staff person. To protect yourself legally, document your referral, the staff person's name and position, and the subject matter you intend that person to teach the patient.

When planning to refer a patient for teaching, be careful in your selection. For example, remember that licensed practical nurses aren't allowed to teach but they can reinforce what you've already taught.

Some patients may do their own delegating, requesting that you teach a relative instead of them. In this situation, document the patient's exact words, and then describe what you taught the relative and how he responded.

Documenting when you don't teach

Most state nurse practice acts require patient teaching. But sometimes you may encounter a doctor who wants to do the teaching himself or a patient who doesn't want to listen because too much information upsets him. If a patient repeatedly balks at your teaching attempts, chart his refusal, tell his doctor, and inform other health care team members. If a doctor asks you not to do any teaching, talk to him about what he plans to teach, and then chart his request and your conversation. Also arrange to talk with nursing administrators to review the hospital's policy: This may produce acceptable guidelines that protect legal and professional nursing practice.

❖

How to teach patients with special needs

Communication is the key to successful patient teaching. Yet, some patients, just by the very nature of their illnesses, have special communication needs. Talking with a person who is dysphasic will require your utmost patience and skill, while communicating with a dying patient calls for warmth and sensitivity. The guidelines that follow will help you get your points across effectively in a variety of challenging situations.

Cutting through language barriers

Today, roughly 15% of the population in North America speaks a language other than English at home, up from 11% a decade ago. This growing population is forcing more and more caregivers to face the challenges of overcoming language barriers and understanding cultural differences.

Although communicating with someone who doesn't speak English or whose culture is drastically different from ours might seem a daunting task, these guidelines can help you bridge the gap.

Reaching across cultural boundaries

Illness, pain, and healing are perceived differently from culture to culture. These perceptions directly affect a person's behavior and personal health practices. For example, many Hispanic girls learn that showering or bathing while they're menstruating can cause *pasmo* (body chills). And women who've given birth may not shower for 7 to 10 days for the same reason.

A patient's response to pain is culturally ingrained as well. In Japan, for example, displaying pain in public isn't acceptable. So for women to express pain during labor is considered a sign of weakness. In contrast, an American woman may convey her true feelings about the intense pain of labor.

By being open to your patients' beliefs, you can begin to understand their habits and behaviors. Then you can respond appropriately and, if necessary, teach them a better approach.

Start by respecting each patient's history and personal experiences — and don't stereotype or make assumptions. For example, don't presume that a patient who doesn't speak English is uneducated. And don't think that every non-English-speaking patient is a foreigner. Many people born in the United States don't speak English well, and some immigrants become naturalized citizens before mastering our language. Also, in some areas of North America, people speak French, Spanish, Chinese, or another language almost exclusively.

Communicating creatively

To successfully assess and treat a non-English-speaking patient, you'll need to learn effective ways to obtain and convey important information without frustrating him — or yourself. Here are some tips for communicating effectively:

• If you don't know what language your patient speaks, address him in English initially. Speak in a slow, gentle, and respectful tone at a normal volume. Remember, speaking louder won't make your words any easier for the patient to understand. If he doesn't respond, try repeating your question.

• If you determine that your patient doesn't understand English, call for an interpreter — but make sure you continue to address the patient, not the interpreter. If you have a choice of interpreters, be sensitive to your patient's sex and age when selecting one. If an interpreter isn't immediately available, find out if the patient has a bilingual dictionary. If he doesn't, try gesturing or writing down some simple words or phrases. Many people learn to read a new language before they become conversational with it.

To obtain specific information from a patient, such as dates or medications, use visual cues, such as a calendar or medication bottles. You could also draw a picture. For example, if you're asking about measles or a rash, draw a face with dots on it. Or use photographs or illustrations from medical books.

• At some point, you'll need your patient to perform a task, such as disrobing and putting on a gown. You might have to act out or pantomime the steps involved (use your hands, arms, body, and facial expressions). But be aware that nonverbal communication, such as eye contact, certain hand or finger gestures, and physical touch may be considered offensive, disrespectful, or sexually suggestive in some cultures.

• After you've demonstrated the task, nod your head and ask your patient, "Do you understand?" or "Okay?" Then wait to see if he performs the task correctly.

• Be prepared to spend a little extra time working with the patient. Remember, he can't understand you, ask questions, or convey his thoughts or concerns, so he'll probably need more of your attention, not less.

Adjusting your teaching for children and adolescents

Teaching youngsters demands ingenuity. You'll need to adjust your teaching style to fit their physical, emotional, and intellectual levels. Children have a short attention span and a thirst for support and nurturing, so keep teaching sessions short and frequently offer praise and show affection.

Tips for teaching children

Because children learn more easily through active participation, using play to teach them about their condition can help them grasp the information. This tactic is especially effective when used before a procedure or when explaining a disease. You can also use it after a procedure to help children understand what happened. This follow-up will let them work through unresolved feelings and questions.

When teaching children, invite parents to join you, so they can offer emotional support during the session and can later reinforce what you taught.

Allow plenty of time for children to absorb information and ask questions. Meet with parents alone to give them more detailed information and answer their questions.

Tips for teaching adolescents

Youngsters develop the ability to think abstractly and to reason deductively around age 12. Adolescents' thought processes are similar to adults', so teach them much the same as grown-ups.

However, adolescents differ from adults in two main aspects: their social development and the importance of their peers. Adolescents develop their identity in relation to their peers and in opposition to their parents. So it may be inappropriate to teach them with their parents present. And don't assume that they have more knowledge about their anatomy and physiology than they actually do. Use illustrations as much as possible to reinforce what you teach.

Finally, be honest with adolescents. If their body image will change because of surgery or disease, prepare them for that change. Because adolescents want to blend in with the crowd, those who face a change in appearance feel especially threatened. They'll need your help to hide or camouflage the change whenever possible.

Tips for helping children cope with surgery

Facing surgery can be scary for children and their parents. As the child's primary nurse, your mere presence provides some much-needed continuity. Yours may be the one face he and his parents recognize throughout his hospital stay. You want the parents to see you as a competent, concerned substitute for them as caregiver. And you want the child to trust and accept you.

To build rapport, speak to the child as well as to his parents during your initial interview. The older the child, the more questions and information you can direct to him, but even a very young child will want attention—and resent being ignored. Be sure to find out what the

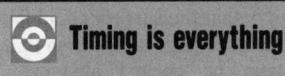

RULE OF THUMB

◎ Timing is everything

When teaching children about their surgery, keep in mind that older children need time to develop coping mechanisms, but younger children will worry if they have too much time to fantasize. In general, use the following guidelines:
• Prepare children ages 4 and younger on the morning of (or just before) surgery.
• Prepare children ages 4 to 7 the day before surgery.
• Prepare older children and adolescents up to 1 week before surgery.

child likes to be called, and address him that way.

Whatever his age, try to assess the child's emotional readiness. (See *Timing is everything.*) Keep in mind that children understand (and fear) much more than they verbalize: Silence may indicate terror, not calm.

Understanding fears

Just what the child fears about the surgery will depend on his age and level of development. An infant or toddler is usually more anxious about the separation from his parents than about the surgery itself. But a preschooler also can conceptualize—and worry about—bodily injury and pain.

In a school-age child, fears of pain and injury are compounded by the stress from his loss of control and forced dependency. An adolescent may feel the stress

BARRIERS TO TEACHING

of the situation more, too, and worry that the surgery could mutilate or change his body so that it won't be "normal" anymore. In fact, for the adolescent, this situational stress and worry about body image may be greater than the fear of pain. And although the adolescent may appear to shrug off the separation from his parents, he may dread this separation as well as separation from his peer group.

To help determine what the child fears, ask if he's had any experience with hospitals and surgery. Listen to the emotional content of what he says. Is the child grappling with the fear of the unknown or the memory of a bad experience? Or does he simply miss his familiar routines? You can help minimize the child's loss of control and forced dependency by giving him as many choices as possible.

Fear of the unknown. The unknown is frightening, especially for youngsters. So your patient teaching becomes particularly important when the child is facing surgery for the first time. It also gives you a chance to build rapport.

Your youngest patients may present the greatest challenge. You'll need to stress that they aren't being punished for their injury or illness. Children ages 4 to 8 sometimes have trouble separating a body part from its function and many also have active imaginations. In fact, children raised on Saturday morning cartoons may fear the worst when they hear the term "laser surgery." Careful teaching will help convince them that laser surgery won't "blast" them but

will help them heal with less scarring.

"Magical thinking" can be another problem. Some children believe their thoughts have the power to make things happen, so they end up suffering needless guilt. For example, 4-year-old Jennie refused to talk after her emergency surgery. She'd been injured in a car accident that had killed both her parents. A child psychologist discovered that Jennie was struggling not only with grief but also with tremendous guilt. Because her mother repeatedly abused her, Jennie had sometimes wished her dead.

Fighting fear with knowledge

You can reduce a young child's fears by telling him both what will happen and the sensations he'll feel.

Let him put on a surgical mask and cap. This "play" will help him understand that the nurses and doctors won't change into someone (or something!) else when they're masked.

Give the child a tour of the operating room or a picture book describing the surgery. Use puppets or dolls as teaching aids. Give a favorite doll or stuffed animal an injection first, for example. Or, if the child will be bandaged after surgery, bandage the toy. Some children fear that a bandaged limb will fall off. By using the toy, you can demonstrate that this isn't so.

Also, make sure the child understands what's expected of him. Have him practice any procedures that require his cooperation. For example, you might give a child older than age 3 a balloon so he can practice breathing into the anesthesia mask.

When teaching an older child, you can include more cognitive terms, but explain words not usually in a youngster's vocabulary—for example, "anesthesia is a special kind of sleep." Choose words that don't have double meanings; say, "we'll help you go to sleep" rather than, "we'll put you to sleep."

Whatever the child's age, honesty is the best policy, even if it's uncomfortable for you. One small lie can destroy days of work in developing trust. If you can't answer a question truthfully, redirect or distract the child.

But make sure you address the question after you've had a chance to think through your response and to choose the right time to discuss both the question and your answer.

Remembering the parents
Try to schedule your teaching sessions for times that are conducive to learning and coping, such as after rest or play. Ask the child's parents what's best.

As you plan your teaching, don't forget that the parents might have their own fears. And because children have sensitive antennae when it comes to their parents' feelings, explain to the parents how important their emotional stability is during this time. Also, teach the parents nondrug, pain-relief techniques, such as distracting the child with games, lullabies, and imagery or massage.

Stay alert to family dynamics, too. Is there anything in the situation that might complicate the child's recovery? Observe how the parents interact with each other and with the child. Do they talk with or at him? Are they oversolicitous?

Pampering a child at a time like this is only human nature. However, if parental spoiling threatens to slow the child's recovery, you should politely intervene.

With younger children especially, try to reduce separation from the parents. Ask yourself—and the administration—if the separations are really necessary, or if they're based solely on "those are the rules" thinking. If you can't avoid the separations, try to soften their effects.

Allow the parents to stay with the child as much as possible, and encourage them to sleep in the room with him. In fact, have his parents go with him to the patient waiting area before surgery. If the child is very young, allow his parent to carry him to the patient waiting area. Once there, the parent might hold or rock the child. If the parents remain composed, the child may be less anxious.

If the parents wait outside the operating room during the surgery, you can alleviate their tension by keeping them informed about the child's progress.

Handling postsurgical care
Of course, you might not be there when the child awakes in the postanesthesia care unit (PACU). But seeing your familiar face could greatly reduce his anxiety. As soon as he's awake, you or the PACU nurse should call his parents in. A rocking chair makes a nice addition to the room; giving the child a

comforting "rock" can get the postsurgical period off to a good start.

For both the child and his parents, surgery can be an anxious time. Not only may your preparation set the stage for a smooth recovery, it may also influence the child's lifelong attitudes about hospital care.

—————————————❖

Adjusting your teaching for older adults

If you're like most nurses, you sometimes feel as if you've hit a brick wall when trying to teach an older patient. A few of these bad experiences could prompt you to stereotype all older people as unteachable and unmotivated. And that attitude may come across in the way you teach elderly patients. Think about the last time you gave instructions to an older patient:
• Did you talk to his family and ignore him when you described home care?
• Did you tell him not to worry when he asked questions – just to trust the doctor?
• Did you leave out information you would have given a younger patient?

If you said "yes" to any of these questions, don't be too hard on yourself. Your behavior stems from some very real frustrations in teaching older adults. But the frustrations aren't a given. Elderly patients are motivated and can learn – but their abilities and needs differ from those of younger patients. If you tailor your style to fit older pa-

tients' learning, motivational, and social differences, teaching them will be more rewarding. (See *Teaching elderly patients.*)

Understanding aging's toll

Aging affects intellectual ability, sensory perception, and psychomotor function in a variety of ways. While an older patient might appear to be disoriented or confused, he might actually be suffering from slowed reflexes or hearing or vision loss.

Loss in mental capacity

Intellectual ability changes with age. Most of us think of intellectual decline when we think of aging, but we're only half right. People have two kinds of intelligence, fluid and crystallized.

Fluid intelligence enables us to perceive relationships, to reason, and to perform abstract thinking.

Crystallized intelligence is the wisdom we absorb during our lives: vocabulary and general information, understanding of social situations, math reasoning, and the ability to evaluate experiences. Because this kind of intelligence increases as people age, you can enhance older patients' learning ability by:
• using concrete examples
• asking them what they know about the subject before starting
• asking them for examples from their own lives.

As degenerative changes occur, fluid intelligence declines, causing the changes that follow.

Slowed processing time. Older patients need more time to process and react to information, especially if you're asking them

RULE OF THUMB

 Teaching elderly patients

Teaching older patients sometimes requires patience and flexibility. Follow these guidelines to help make your patient teaching effective.

Be supportive
Positive reinforcement increases confidence and self-worth.

Ask probing questions
Your patient might have several chronic conditions and may not recall the specifics about each one. He may mention only what's bothering him at the moment and fail to mention other diagnoses.

Be a detective
Find out if your patient is illiterate. Some clues might be unmarked menus or the inability to operate the bed or television, even with simple written instructions. Or you might hear complaints such as, "They never send anything I like" or "I forgot my glasses." These excuses might be honest, but they could also indicate an inability to read.

Think of everything
Look at the number and type of medications your patient takes and assess for possible adverse reactions. Overmedication may explain why he seems drowsy or forgetful.

Be flexible
After demonstrating a procedure, ask the patient if he'd like to adapt the method to his own way of dealing with everyday situations.

Go above and beyond
Contact the occupational therapy department for tools that can help your patient. Also ask for input on how to improve muscular strength, endurance, and motor skills.

---

to see relationships between an action and a result. Adapt your teaching by avoiding long lists.

For example, you might tell a young adult with diabetes: "You should eat the food on menu A if you're not active, menu B if you're moderately active, and menu C if you're very active." A young adult can see these relationships quickly. But an older adult may not, so divide the series into three discrete messages and wait for his response after each one, as follows.

NURSE: You should eat the food on Menu A if you're not very active.
PATIENT: That's what I should eat if I'm not very active?
NURSE: That's right. And if you're moderately active...

Stimulus persistence or "after image." Older people sometimes confuse the word or symbol you've just taught with the word or symbol you're introducing—for example, hypoglycemia and hyperglycemia. Again, wait for a

response before you introduce a
new concept or definition.

Decreased short-term memory.
Give older patients more time to
comprehend what you've said
and repeat your demonstrations.
You might also want to devise
clues to help them remember.
Don't be surprised if older people need coaching to remember
a procedure you've explained
just hours before. Let them help
you devise ways for them to remember steps to a procedure or
the need to perform a procedure
at a certain time.

Test anxiety. As a reaction to
their decrease in fluid intelligence, older people are especially anxious about making
mistakes on tests—and especially
frustrated when they do. Because of their anxiety, they may
take an inordinate amount of
time to answer questions, particularly on written tests. Help
them relax before testing and, if
possible, give oral rather than
written tests.

Hearing loss
Sensory deficits are common, especially hearing loss. A patient
who routinely fails to respond to
you (or who responds inappropriately) may not be confused—
he may have trouble hearing.

The ability to discriminate
high-frequency sounds diminishes around age 50 and declines greatly after age 65. Because hearing loss progresses
slowly with age, your patient
may not be aware of the loss. If
the impairment is severe,
though, it could make him feel
isolated, suspicious, or even paranoid.

If your patient speaks loudly
or tilts his head when listening,
assess him carefully for deafness. Check his ears for excess
cerumen—a common, reversible
cause of hearing loss.

If he has a chronic hearing
problem, make sure he uses his
hearing aid, if he has one, during teaching sessions. Face him
when you talk so he can watch
your mouth. Speak slowly,
clearly, and in a normal tone.
Don't raise your voice, or he
may have even more trouble distinguishing your words.

Keep in mind that if your patient has suffered a loss in hearing, he might not benefit from
audio teaching aids. Instead,
give him written material to
reinforce your oral instructions.
(See *Overcoming vision and
hearing loss*.)

Vision loss
Cataracts and presbyopia prevent many older people from
reading small print or glossy
pages. Yellowing of the ocular
lens produces color distortion.
Consider the consequences if an
elderly patient can't read the
small print on his medication
bottles or distinguish differently
colored pills, which he's supposed to take at different times
of the day, because they all look
gray to him.

Take note of the drugs your
patient is taking and how they
might affect his sight. For example, phenylbutazone, an anti-inflammatory agent, may cause
blurred vision.

Impaired vision could prevent your patient from learning
from videos, closed-circuit TV,
or filmstrips. He may not be able
to read written instructions or

PREVENTIVE PRACTICE

 Overcoming vision and hearing loss

These do's and don'ts will help you avoid problems caused by vision and hearing loss among elderly patients.

Vision loss
• Do use nonglare butcher paper on an easel to help overcome patients' visual deficits while you're teaching. Print in large letters with a broad-tipped felt pen. To make sure patients can read what you're writing, ask them to read something back to you. Keep a magnifying glass handy to help them read smaller print.
• Don't refer to medications by color. Instead, encourage the patient to read each label, using his glasses or a magnifying glass if necessary. Print dosage schedules for your patients in a size they can read.

Hearing loss
• Do keep your voice pitched as low as possible. Speak slowly and don't drop your voice at the end of words or phrases. Ask the patients to repeat oral instructions, and reinforce them with written instructions, which you give to the patients.
• Don't teach in a busy spot. Instead, choose a private office or classroom to reduce visual and auditory distractions.

handle equipment such as medication syringes. To teach him, make sure he has access to his glasses, contact lenses, or other devices, and make sure they're clean. Plan to use large teaching aids with oversized print.

The colors used in any patient-teaching aids must be easily distinguished and have contrast to help the patient differentiate between print and background. Warm shades — reds, oranges, and yellows — are best. Avoid blues and greens. Make sure reading lights are bright but diffused and properly placed.

Loss in flexibility
Aging causes gradual loss of muscular strength and endurance. This can limit flexibility and prevent your patient from completing tasks requiring fine motor skills.

In fact, many older people can't turn a dial or knob. Check for such limitations before giving patients a videocassette, tape recorder, and audiocassette for self-paced learning, or before showing them how to perform a procedure. Otherwise, you may misinterpret a lack of motor skills as a lack of motivation.

If your patient has severe musculoskeletal impairment, work with his primary caregiver from the beginning.

Keeping older patients motivated
Motivation is as important to learning as ability. To increase an older patient's motivation, try these tactics:

• Schedule teaching sessions at a time when your patient is ready to learn. Make an appointment with your patient, and let him set the time if you can. Make sure he hasn't just taken medication that will affect his ability to concentrate. If he tires easily, break the skill he'll be learning down into steps and teach just a few in each session. Avoid sessions right after breakfast and bath, which have probably sapped his energy. Find out if your patient has other immediate concerns and try to address them. For example, if he's in pain or hungry, trying to teach foot care may be useless. Teach when the patient is alert—at a time of day when he usually reads the paper. And keep the sessions short. Motivation is tricky enough without fatigue.

• Determine your patient's values and note the activities and lifestyle he wants to maintain when he returns home. This will allow you to present information so that he views it as important—people tend not to do well when learning tasks they judge to be unnecessary.

• List the nursing diagnoses that teaching can correct. Identify these problems for the patient and ask him if he wants to overcome them. Explain the relationship between the techniques or procedures you're teaching him and his desire to overcome his health problems.

• List health habits that will help keep him well. Ask him whether he's interested in learning some techniques that'll help him stay well. And explain how the things you're teaching will help him.

Gaining your patient's confidence

You might have to convince your patient his illness is a problem. Some elderly people adapt to their conditions so well that they don't consider them problems and don't want to learn about them.

Convincing older patients that you're teaching them something useful is only half the motivation battle. You may also have to convince them that the methods you're teaching them are in their best interest.

• To make this job easier, ask older patients about their sleeping, eating, and other health habits. For example, many were taught as children that they needed a daily bowel movement. If you don't find this out before you tell them to give up their daily laxatives, you'll never win them over.

• Make a list of their health beliefs that will reinforce or hinder your teaching efforts. Discuss these beliefs before you try to teach something new.

• Ask them what they know about a technique or health care tip before you explain it. Don't patronize by repeating things they already know.

Enlisting family support

An important part of your preteaching assessment is analyzing a patient's relationship with his family. Is he financially and emotionally dependent on them? Will family members reinforce the lessons you're teaching, or will they withdraw? Will they try to help the patient function independently, or will they foster dependency?

Here's an example that demonstrates that teaching without family support is probably doomed to failure. Mrs. Mc-Ilwaine, a 57-year-old woman with right-sided weakness after her stroke, resisted all efforts at rehabilitation. Finally, she told a nurse why: Her husband had promised never to abandon her as long as she was "helpless." As soon as she recovered, he planned to divorce her.

Lack of other resources can also sabotage a teaching plan you think is unbeatable. Can the patient afford the diet or equipment you're recommending? If not, will an agency help? Does he have a ride to the therapy sessions you're telling him about? If not, will a transportation service or family member help?

Get answers to all these questions before you teach the older patient. Include his family or friends in the teaching sessions (with his permission, of course) and enlist their support.

If you're teaching the patient techniques for self-care, enlist the family's support during hospitalization. Let them see and understand the need for him to act in his own behalf, so they don't take over later just because they can do it faster.

By keeping these points in mind, you'll not only be able to make the most of patient teaching, but you'll also send your elderly patient home with confidence in his ability to care for himself.

❖

Getting through to patients with Alzheimer's disease

When a patient with Alzheimer's disease is hospitalized for an acute illness, he'll need to adjust to his new surroundings. You can help reduce his confusion by incorporating these teaching guidelines into your patient care.

Communicating effectively

• Approach a patient with Alzheimer's disease from the front and move slowly so you don't startle him. Never touch him without speaking first.
• Be sure he's wearing his glasses and hearing aid if he needs them.
• Begin conversations by identifying yourself, calling the patient by his name, and explaining what you're going to do or want him to do.
• Talk with him at his level of ability – without patronizing him – and use a calm and gentle tone.
• When giving him instructions, use short, simple sentences with clear and familiar words. Be sure to give only one direction at a time, and allow time for him to respond.
• Give him a sense of personal control and allow him to maintain his self-esteem by offering realistic choices whenever possible. Praise him when he completes a task successfully. Provide comfortable surroundings.
• Place identifying labels on the patient's room, bathroom, and closet doors.
• Ask the family to bring in some familiar personal items, such as

a bedspread, slippers, and family pictures.

• Provide structured routines, based as closely as possible on the patient's normal daily routine. (You may need to ask family members for input.) ❖

Helping diabetic patients adjust

You'll need to teach patients diagnosed with Type II (non-insulin-dependent) diabetes mellitus a vast amount of information in a short time. You'll have to teach them how to control their condition by making some lifestyle changes, such as eating right and exercising. Plus, you'll instruct them about monitoring their blood glucose levels and recognizing the adverse effects of oral antidiabetic drugs. The amount of information can be overwhelming. You can help your patients by first telling them about the very nature of their disease.

Clearing up any confusion

When your patient hears the word "diabetes," the first thing he'll probably think of is insulin injections. Explain to him that often blood glucose levels can be controlled with diet and exercise, and that oral antidiabetic agents may be used as well. Also tell him that if he remains hyperglycemic despite all of these interventions, insulin therapy may be required.

Explain to your patient that he might have one or more of the following problems contributing to persistent hyperglycemia: diminished insulin sensitivity, delayed insulin secretion, diminished insulin binding to receptors, decreased islet cell sensitivity to glucose, increased hepatic glucose production, or beta cell dysfunction.

If your patient is a woman of childbearing age, advise her to normalize her blood glucose levels before conceiving and suggest that she see a diabetes pregnancy specialist if conception occurs.

Explaining diet therapy

When you discuss diet therapy with a patient who has been newly diagnosed with Type II diabetes, try to help him understand why he should control his weight. When he accepts the need for change, you can talk about the specifics of his diet. Also, during your discussion, keep in mind that sticking to a diet isn't easy. Help the patient set realistic goals. He doesn't have to maintain his ideal body weight to control his glucose levels. Plus, he's more likely to meet a modest goal and to maintain a body weight that he feels is reasonable.

The patient's diet should consist of 55% to 60% carbohydrates, less than 30% fat, and 0.8 g/kg of body weight of protein. He should cut down on foods high in cholesterol and saturated fats, such as eggs, cream, whole milk, and fatty beef.

Because the patient's ability to secrete insulin in response to hyperglycemia is delayed, he should avoid rapidly absorbed simple sugars, such as honey, molasses, cake frosting, or regular soda. Tell the patient that he should eat plenty of fiber, which decreases glucose levels by slowing GI absorption of carbohydrates.

The patient should also limit his salt intake to no more than 3,000 mg/day. Ideally, a patient with Type II diabetes shouldn't drink alcohol, especially if he's taking oral antidiabetic agents or insulin. If your patient drinks regularly, ask a dietitian to work a small amount of alcohol into his meal plan.

Arrange for a dietitian to teach your patient how to plan his meals. Reinforce the teaching as necessary and, if he's taking an oral antidiabetic agent or insulin, make sure he understands that meal timing is as important as food types and amounts. Teach him to space meals (including snacks, if ordered) evenly throughout the day. The dietitian may recommend the food exchange system. This widely used method, based on the carbohydrate, fat, and protein content of six basic food groups, allows greater flexibility in meal planning. Exchange groups include milk products, vegetables, fruits, breads, meats, and fats.

Teach the patient how to adjust his diet when he engages in extra activity or exercise. If he eats many meals out, have the dietitian show him how to select a restaurant meal that fits his diet plan; if appropriate, tell him how to obtain nutrient composition lists from fast-food restaurants.

For an overweight patient, implement weight reduction measures, as ordered, and explain the reduced-calorie diet.

Suggest a support group, such as Weight Watchers or Overeaters Anonymous, if necessary.

Explaining exercise guidelines

When you're teaching the patient about dietary changes, be sure to explain the importance of exercise and have him talk with his doctor about guidelines for starting a workout program. He should begin with a 10- to 15-minute warm-up period. For the next 20 to 30 minutes, he should do exercises that will sustain his pulse rate at 75% of his maximum heart rate. He might perform low-impact aerobics, run, or take a brisk walk, for example. Then he'll need a 15- to 20-minute cool-down period.

If a patient doesn't enjoy strenuous exercise, recommend walking or swimming. A patient who has hypertension or proliferative retinopathy should avoid exercises that may involve the Valsalva maneuver—weight lifting, isotonics, and the like. A patient with hypertension should also avoid intense exercise of the arms and upper body because it produces sharper increases in blood pressure than exercise of the legs. Rhythmic exercises in which the patient uses his legs—such as walking, jogging, and cycling—are generally preferred.

Explaining oral antidiabetic agents

For some patients with Type II diabetes, diet and exercise alone don't control their glucose levels. These patients must take oral antidiabetic agents. Currently, six such drugs, also known as sulfonylureas, are available—acetohexamide, chlorpropamide, glipizide, glyburide, tolazamide, and tolbutamide.

If the starting dose of an oral antidiabetic agent isn't effective, the patient's doctor may increase the dose at 1- to 2-week intervals. If the drug still isn't effective at its maximum dose, one of several things can happen. The doctor may switch to another antidiabetic agent, he may prescribe insulin (temporarily or permanently) instead of the oral antidiabetic agent, or he may prescribe both insulin and the antidiabetic agent.

Explaining complications

Teach the patient the complications of diabetes and diabetic therapy, especially hyperglycemia. Tell him to be alert for vagueness, slow thinking, dizziness, weakness, pallor, tachycardia, diaphoresis, seizures, and coma. Also tell him to be alert for signs of diabetic ketoacidosis—acetone breath, dehydration, weak and rapid pulse, and Kussmaul's respirations—and hyperosmolar nonketotic syndrome—polyuria, thirst, neurologic abnormalities, and stupor.

Hypoglycemia alert

If your patient will be taking an oral antidiabetic agent, explain its potential adverse effects, the most common of which is hypoglycemia. Make sure he knows the signs and symptoms of hypoglycemia—hunger, nausea, sweating, tremors, anxiety, lethargy, confusion, agitation, headache, and diplopia. If your patient is elderly, explain that he may have difficulty recognizing hypoglycemia. That's because aging alters a person's reaction to many drugs, including oral

antidiabetic agents. So the usual signs and symptoms may be absent or difficult to detect. Encourage him to check his blood glucose level if he suspects hypoglycemia.

When a patient with Type II diabetes detects hypoglycemia, he'll need to raise his blood glucose level by taking an oral form of glucose. Within 10 to 15 minutes, he can raise his blood glucose level by 40 to 50 mg/dl if he consumes either 4 oz of orange juice, 8 oz of skim milk, 1 tbs of jelly, 6 oz of cola, 2 packets of sugar, 5 hard candies, or 4 sugar cubes. Any of those sources will give him about 10 g of glucose in a hurry. You can also suggest that he buy glucose in chewable tablets or gel form to keep on hand so he can raise his blood glucose level quickly.

Be sure to explain that these sources produce only a temporary improvement, and a recurrence of hypoglycemia can follow. To prevent that, the patient should also consume longer-acting carbohydrates—crackers, milk, or high-fiber fruit, for example.

Other adverse effects

Several skin reactions are associated with oral antidiabetic agents. These reactions include pruritus, urticaria, exfoliative dermatitis, and Stevens-Johnson syndrome. A patient may also develop photosensitivity, predisposing him to severe sunburn. Be sure to tell a patient with this problem to use a sunscreen.

The syndrome of inappropriate antidiuretic hormone (SIADH) has been associated with chlorpropamide and, rarely, tolbutamide. Apparently, elderly patients and those taking diuretics are more prone to drug-induced SIADH. Teach your patient the signs and symptoms of SIADH – nausea, anorexia, dizziness, confusion, and depression – and tell him to report them immediately. Usually, treatment for SIADH includes discontinuing the oral antidiabetic drug and restricting fluid intake to about 1,000 ml daily.

Oral antidiabetics may produce mild thyroid abnormalities or hematologic conditions such as leukopenia or thrombocytopenia. A patient may also develop nausea, vomiting, heartburn, indigestion, abdominal pain, or a metallic taste in his mouth. To prevent those GI problems, advise your patient to take his antidiabetic drug at mealtime – unless it's glipizide. That drug should be taken 30 minutes before a meal.

If a patient drinks alcohol while taking an oral antidiabetic drug, he may experience hypoglycemia or hyperglycemia. Alcohol may affect hepatic metabolism of the drug and inhibit hepatic glucose production during hypoglycemic episodes. When combined with chlorpropamide or glyburide, alcohol can cause a reaction similar to (though milder than) an Antabuse (disulfiram) reaction.

Teaching self-monitoring

You should teach a patient with newly diagnosed Type II diabetes how to monitor his blood glucose measurements. Explain that he can have a laboratory measure his blood glucose levels, but it'll be easier for him to do it himself. Self-monitoring also

gets the patient more involved in managing his condition.

There are two ways your patient can monitor his blood glucose levels – with glucose test strips that he reads visually or with an automatic glucose meter that reads test strips mechanically. Most insurance companies will reimburse patients for these meters.

If a patient can't use a glucose meter, he should be able to use the test strips. A patient whose diabetes is well controlled doesn't really need a glucose meter. The test strips will suffice if he doesn't have a vision problem such as color blindness. The well-controlled patient may have to check his fasting blood glucose levels only three times a week and obtain a complete profile (levels before and after meals, at bedtime, and possibly during the night) one to three times a month.

No matter which measurement method your patient uses, he'll have to learn to perform fingersticks. Don't overlook the importance of teaching him to stick himself as painlessly as possible. Good teaching may make the difference between compliance and noncompliance. (See *Tips for teaching blood glucose monitoring,* page 462.)

Also, remember to show your patient how to use his meter or test strips. Don't assume that he'll read and understand the product instructions.

Suggest that the patient attend a diabetes education program to optimize his self-monitoring skills.

Remember, the key to helping a patient recently diagnosed with Type II diabetes is effective

Tips for teaching blood glucose monitoring

Teach your patient these techniques for obtaining blood samples and testing his glucose levels.

• To enhance blood flow:

— Use your ring finger or thumb because blood flows more easily to them.

— Hold your finger under warm water before sticking it.

— Place your hand below your heart and milk the blood toward your finger.

— Stick the finger just to the side of the finger pad (where there are more blood vessels and fewer nerve endings).

• To prevent a deep puncture, don't press the lancet device too hard and don't steady your finger against a hard surface.

• To ensure an accurate reading, place a large drop of blood on the reagent pad at the end of the test strip. You don't have to cover the four corners of the pad, but you should cover all four sides.

• Use a watch with a second hand to make sure the blood is exposed to the reagent pad for the proper amount of time. The reading will be inaccurate if the blood is on the pad too long or isn't on it long enough.

• Read your visual test strip in natural light, preferably sunlight; fluorescent light distorts the color of the pad.

teaching. When your course is completed, your patient will have learned an invaluable lesson—how to live well with Type II diabetes mellitus.

——————————————❖

Reaching dysphasic patients

Dysphasia is hindered speech brought on by a brain lesion, while aphasia is the inability to communicate due to damaged brain centers. (Some aphasic patients also have hindered speech.) Both conditions are common after a stroke. In addition, neurologic disorders such

as Parkinson's disease may cause speech problems. And dysarthria, caused by an impaired tongue or other muscles essential to speech, results in unclear speech. Communicating with patients who have one of these conditions is challenging, not only for you but for friends and family members as well.

Minimizing frustration

Communication is tied to a person's identity, so when someone can't participate in an open exchange of ideas, he often feels as if he's lost his sense of self. Because their speech is blocked, patients with dysphasia often feel extremely frustrated, helpless, and hopeless. These feelings can lead to depression, so early treatment is paramount. If the patient can't communicate, he's likely to become angry and bitter. He'll probably resist treatment, impeding his rehabilitation and recovery. By establishing a way for him to communicate, you will help ease his feelings of isolation and, more importantly, restore his hope and self-worth.

Using communication aids

A dysphasic patient has trouble encoding messages and could also experience decoding problems. Fortunately, a variety of devices are available to assist such patients. The easiest to use are letter, word, or picture boards, which you might have in your hospital. If not, they're simple to make. Just cut out pictures or words for the patient to place on a flat surface. For example, the patient might hold up a picture of a TV if he wants the television turned on or the word "walk" if he wants to take a stroll. He can use a letter board to spell out more complex messages.

The patient can also send messages on a magic slate or computer if he's able to do so. Or he can use computer-aided devices such as scanners to help him stop at appropriate responses. Of course, the ultimate goal, if possible, is to restore normal speech. In the meantime, these tools provide a way for the patient to communicate.

❖

Orienting visually impaired patients

Grasping a person's meaning sometimes depends more on nonverbal messages than verbal ones. If a patient can't see your nonverbal communication cues, he's at an immediate disadvantage. And that poses obstacles for both you and your patient.

Keep in mind that if your patient is visually impaired, he probably will speak only when he's addressed because he's not sure about the presence or location of other people. He'll limit his gestures because he fears knocking something over. If several people are in the room, he may speak loudly because he's confused about where others are located, and silence might make him uncomfortable because he won't know if others are in the room.

Carefully orienting

When you familiarize a visually impaired patient with the hospital, warn him of any obstacles in his surroundings. Also, explain everyday sounds that he'll hear because strange noises can be frightening to someone who can't determine their source.

At mealtimes, use the face of a clock as a reference point to tell your patient where food is located on his plate. For example, say, "Your chicken is at 3 o'clock, your potatoes are at 6 o'clock, and your string beans are at 9 o'clock." Guide his hand in the proper direction to locate each item.

To make your patient feel comfortable, identify yourself every time you enter his room and speak in your usual tone of voice. Explain all procedures, describing each step and its accompanying touch. Touch is just as important to a person who's visually impaired as it is to a sighted person.

You might be tempted to give more help than usual to a patient who's visually impaired, but remember he must remain independent. If his blindness is recent, he'll need to replace skills that disappeared as a result of losing his sight. Be sure to allow him private time to practice.

❖

Getting through to hearing-impaired patients

Learning to communicate with a patient who is hearing impaired will take plenty of practice and tolerance from both of you. Because he won't be able to hear you enter his room, lightly touch him on the arm whenever you approach.

While many people with hearing impairments know sign language, this isn't something you can learn quickly, so don't try. If your patient can speech-read or lip-read, communicating with him will be easy if you follow these guidelines:
• Make sure that the room is well lit and that you're fully facing the patient.

• Speak slowly and deliberately, slightly exaggerating as you form each word.
• Gesture as much as possible.

If your patient can't lip-read, or if you're having trouble getting your points across, try writing notes to each other. While this method can be a time-consuming way to communicate, it is effective.

Showing tolerance

Often, people who can't hear are lonely. They also can be paranoid, frequently looking over their shoulders to determine if someone – or something – is behind them.

Don't be surprised if your patient becomes stubborn or angry. This often happens out of the frustration of not being able to understand what you want him to do.

Remember, too, that many people who can't hear can speak. But because they can't hear themselves, they often speak in either a low monotone or very loudly.

❖

Supporting terminally ill patients

Some people are uncomfortable talking about an impending death, while others need to discuss it. That makes knowing what to say – or not to say – difficult for you. By taking your lead from your terminally ill patient and his family, you won't find yourself in an awkward situation.

Encouraging conversation

Sometimes, family and friends don't talk with their dying loved one because they're afraid of saying the wrong thing. But the patient needs to say goodbye and also might want to talk about fears he has. If he can't express himself, he could become angry and withdrawn, making his last hours emotionally painful for everyone.

Don't fall into the trap of using small talk and standard responses to avoid talking about death and dying. Encourage your dying patient to discuss his fears about death so he can feel more peaceful. And help the family say goodbye to the patient.

Encourage the patient's family and friends to talk in normal tones. They can tell him what's happening in the family and let him know they care. Allow them to participate in aspects of his care, such as applying ointment to his lips or wiping perspiration from his brow. This interaction might help the family accept his death.

Make sure you stop in often to check on both the patient and his family. And make sure that coffee or other refreshments are available.

Recognizing coping tactics

Often, people who are dying deny that death is near. If you suspect your patient is coping with his impending death by denying it, don't force him to face reality. If, on the other hand, your patient wants to talk about his death, you should listen.

Dying patients aren't the only ones who cope through denial. Sometimes, health care workers see death as a failure. Because they view themselves as healers, when a patient dies, they think their efforts have been futile. Of course, your work isn't in vain. You fill a great need by providing comfort and support during someone's last days.

Respecting cultural differences

Naturally, there are individual preferences within every race and ethnic culture. As a general rule, though, African-Americans and Mexican-Americans want to be with a dying loved one, while Japanese-Americans and Native Americans usually prefer to die alone. Most Anglo-Americans are less in contact with death than many other cultures. Southeast Asians follow a variety of rituals when a loved one dies, but many of these are frowned upon in the United States. If the family's traditions aren't followed, their grieving process could be extended.

In addition to respecting your patient's cultural traditions, you should ask if he would like to talk with a religious representative. If so, you should call the appropriate clergy.

Keeping the patient comfortable

Obviously, you'll administer competent physical care to your dying patient. But you should also make sure that his pain is properly managed.

Help him keep his individuality while he's conscious and make sure other staff members respect his decisions, even if they're unpopular.

If your patient is comatose, remember that he is still an individual. Talk to him directly, and don't discuss his condition in front of him. Assume he can still hear.

Whenever possible, don't let patients die alone. In fact, ensuring this should be a top priority.

Helping to tie up loose ends

Patients who are terminally ill might look to you for help in various areas such as business affairs, wills, and funeral details. Naturally, you can't take care of these details, but you should get in touch with those who can.

Your dying patient might not be able to talk freely about his death with family and friends because they become too upset. He might turn to you for support. Assure him that you or someone else will be available.

Be ready to discuss any topic your patient throws out. Some dying patients plan long trips or picture themselves in new occupations. Others joke about death. However your patient deals with his impending death, you should accept his attitude without judgment.

Helping with closure

Allow your dying patient to make choices and remain in control until the very end. When available, offer alternatives such as home care for the patient who doesn't want to die in the hospital. Answer questions honestly, but don't feel compelled to give information that's not requested.

Help the patient and his family discuss any unanswered questions; some are better resolved before death. Encourage the family to bring in the patient's favorite items from home. Suggest the family keep a diary detailing what the patient talked about during his last days. This can be a comfort after the patient dies.

Caring for a dying patient can put you at emotional risk. You might become attached to the patient and feel grief and loss after he dies. But knowing that you gave comfort and support during his last days can be extremely rewarding.

——————————❖

9 Managing Difficult Patients and Colleagues

468

Handling coworkers

Handling staff

DIFFICULT PERSONS

Handling yourself

Understanding your own and others' responses and learning how to be flexible, handle criticism, listen better, and face conflict will help you become a better nurse and a better person. To help yourself grow professionally, you also need to know how to appreciate agency nurses, how to float safely, when to call in sick, and how to care for yourself while caring for a patient with acquired immunodeficiency syndrome.

Flexibility

Difficult people come in countless varieties, and each may provoke you in a different way. One may sit back and simmer and never really tell you what she thinks or feels. Another may whine and complain endlessly or be loud and self-centered and unwilling to let you work together in any cooperative or productive way. Still another might talk too much, getting little accomplished and interfering with your work. At times, you may be left fuming, yelling, or speechless.

The difficulty may stem from the two of you trying to meet your needs in different ways. Maybe you have different opinions, attitudes, goals, or values. You may want different things from the relationship or the situation you're in. What usually separates you from the other person is an unwillingness to

yield, accept feedback, or confront issues. Expect no more from other people than you expect from yourself—a willingness to try to change behavior, not personalities.

Effective communication depends on two things:
• acknowledging, appreciating, and productively using the differences in people
• developing a personal strategy for dealing effectively with people you find difficult to work with. These insights might help.

Separating the people from the problems

The first step in dealing with difficult people is to remember that the problem is the *relationship*, not the people themselves. Many interpersonal conflicts arise simply because one person is inflexible to another's viewpoint or work style. This stress diverts both people's energy in unplanned directions.

Some people can get so caught up in their work that they get oversensitive about their personal viewpoints and don't recognize that a differing opinion or approach isn't necessarily better or worse than their own—it's simply different. Every one of us is hard to get along with in some way, sometimes, with some people. And in most cases, these natural, inherent differences become difficulties only when we let them.

Appreciating the differences

When you're trying to make sense out of something that seems illogical, look for a difference in thinking styles. According to communications researchers, there are two, broad, basic

thinking styles in the workplace:
• *Vertical thinkers* detect and manipulate differences, methodically finding distinctions and making separations. They look at end points, identify the route, pinpoint problems, eliminate the unnecessary, and then break up the task into small, discrete steps.
• *Horizontal thinkers* detect and manipulate commonalities, methodically finding constants and making novel, unpredictable associations among unrelated items, ideas, or events. They focus on a common thread that all points share and organize their thoughts according to significance to an underlying purpose or theme.

Neither style is better, and most people don't fall exclusively into one style. But the useful point is that there are a variety of ways to approach job challenges.

You should take care not to affix negative labels to behavior that's unexpected or different from your own. If you catch yourself starting to label someone or getting upset, pause and ask yourself if it's simply a difference in thinking style. If so, look for new ways to clarify things and work together.

Remaining flexible
To be successful in today's world, you need to think creatively, invent options for mutual gain, and deal with competing demands and different values among your work team. In any situation, recognize your preferences and perspective, and then step back so you're more open to consider alternative viewpoints and methods.

Remind yourself that successful organizations focus on results. Various choices and methods of doing things are merely a means to the end; their value is determined by how much they help achieve the desired results.

Weighing risks against rewards
Coping with difficult people takes considerable effort. Before you plunge ahead with a plan to change behavior – your own or someone else's – decide what it will take to change it, what it's worth to you, what kind of payoff you can expect, and what the chances are that you'll get it accomplished. How will a positive or negative change in behavior influence your stress, interpersonal relationships, and productivity? What are the risks?

Accepting the inevitable
Some people are extremely stubborn about change. At times, their behavior is so disruptive that you need special self-defense tactics. You may even be forced to go over someone's head to seek a solution. But be certain you have sufficient grounds for the person up the line to take action on your behalf.

When it's not worth this kind of effort, either remove yourself from the situation or resign yourself – temporarily, at least – to the status quo and improve your stress-management skills. Either way, shift your attention away from the problem itself and onto those work areas where you can create progress.

Criticism

Being on the receiving end of criticism is an inevitable part of your job. If it's delivered in a positive way, you'll recognize it as a sincere desire to help you grow. Unfortunately, not all managers are skilled in handling criticism.

If your manager doles out criticism ineffectively or insensitively, you can become angry, discouraged, offended, or hurt, causing you to respond inappropriately. Here are several techniques to help you maintain your perspective.

Responding professionally

If the person criticizing you is sarcastic, accusatory, or blaming, your first reaction might be to attack her. Instead, calmly express your feelings or even sidetrack the conversation if you want some time to calm down.

For example, suppose your manager stops you in the hallway to tell you that your coworkers have complained that you don't communicate or cooperate with them. Although tempted to blow up at her for delivering such news in the hallway, you'd be better off with a calm, professional response: "I'd like to understand the specific complaint and your suggestions for remedies. But I'm embarrassed to be talking about it in the hallway. I'd like to meet with you later so we could talk about it in private."

Identifying the problem

Make sure you understand the behavior or activities your manager is criticizing. If the problem seems vague (a "bad" attitude, "inappropriate" behavior, "poor" teamwork), ask her for specifics. For instance, if your manager says you're disorganized, ask for examples that will help you understand what you do that appears disorganized. Ask her how often the problem occurs.

Clarify the source of the problem. Does it involve a deficiency in knowledge, skills, attitude, or behavior? Does it boil down to inefficient time management? Lack of experience? Do other staff members share the same problem? If appropriate, ask your manager to identify a coworker who has mastered it. Determine if your problem involves unsafe practice or if it violates hospital policy. If either is true, take corrective action immediately.

Initiating change

When you understand the problem, think about how you can solve it. Let your manager know you want to improve, and ask for her help. For instance, if you need to learn new skills, tell her you'd like to attend some staff-development classes on the subject. Establish a behavioral contract with measurable goals and outcomes.

As you work to correct the problem, document your improvement with a clear list of positive behaviors. Set up a time to meet with your manager to review *your* perception of progress—and *hers*.

Considering personal style

Your response to criticism probably is rooted in values and rules you learned as a child and to

DIFFICULT PERSONS

your own interpersonal style. You might react assertively, aggressively, or passively. Similarly, your manager has her own leadership style. Democratic leaders respect and encourage staff input; autocratic leaders inform staff of their decisions; laissez-faire leaders wait to see what happens without much structure.

Conflicts arise when your style isn't compatible with your manager's and when values, expectations, and personal styles differ from those of the people you work for. For example, your manager might expect you to know what to do to improve, and you might expect more concrete direction. Some leaders inspire teamwork, soften criticism with praise, and motivate nurses to improve; other leaders believe negative feedback enhances performance.

Reduce the potential for conflict and criticism by understanding your manager's expectations and leadership style. Think about how they mesh with your own. You may value spending time with your patients but have to rush and work overtime to get your charting finished. If your manager looks for neat charting at the end of the shift, the two of you will be on a collision course. You'll feel stressed and so will she, but it's your job to follow her style or to work with her on a compromise that satisfies both of you.

Correcting unjust criticism

If your perspective on a situation or problem differs from your manager's, don't be afraid to say so. For example, suppose your nurse-manager mistakenly accuses you of violating profes-

sional standards. If you typically respond submissively to criticism and you're too embarrassed or upset to contradict her, she might see your silence as an admission of guilt. If you can't respond on the spot to unjust criticism, request a chance to meet with your manager later to clarify what happened. In preparation for that meeting, document the facts of the incident from your point of view.

Remember that reports of formal counseling sessions become part of your personnel file, so documenting the facts from your viewpoint is in your best interest. For example, what if your manager claims you've been uncooperative because you've refused to follow a doctor's order to give a narcotic injection? If you felt the order was incorrect or unsafe, document your actions (you informed the doctor, charge nurse, and your manager of your judgment) and attach your explanation to your manager's report.

Anticipating criticism

Don't wait for your manager to review your performance. Instead, ask her for informal feedback before your performance evaluation or annual review takes place. This will give you extra time to correct any weaknesses she points out in your meeting. Go prepared with a written self-evaluation, including a list of your strengths and the ways you've improved your practice. Remember that your manager has the responsibility to provide feedback and counseling to improve your nursing practice. Your role is to accept her comments, turning what may feel like negative feedback into positive change.

━━━━━━━━━━━━━━━ ❖

Listening

Speaking is only half of your communication with a patient. The other half is listening. The better your listening skills, the better your communication will be.

Being a good listener isn't an inborn talent. You can train yourself to "hear" your patient's *unspoken* as well as spoken communication—the embarrassed or hesitant tone of voice, the uneasy stance or clenched fist, or the look in the eye. You can also train yourself to listen in a patient and nonjudgmental way, giving other people time to express their thoughts without correction or assistance. And you'll explore with questions instead of presuming you know what the other person is trying to say.

Like most people, you probably half-listen as you plan what you want to say next. Or you listen to the first few words and assume the rest or finish the sentence for your patient. This type of conversation can only leave your patient feeling bored, depressed, or helpless. To improve your communication with others, consider changing your listening style.

Overcoming barriers

Start by looking at the ways you typically block good communication. Which of the following traits apply to your communication style?

• *Judging*. Do you fail to hear people because you're busy mentally criticizing what they've just said? You'd do better to withhold your judgment until you fully understand what someone is saying.
• *Interrupting*. Do you finish sentences for people or add details to their stories? If you're trying to show you understand, make sure you understand by letting them finish speaking first. As they speak, compare your unspoken assumptions with what's being said; a wide gap between the two may stop you from jumping to conclusions in the future.

If they're talking too much and you're getting impatient or losing track of the conversation, ask them to summarize. Then continue to listen.
• *Listening selectively*. From time to time, we all use some form of selective listening, hearing only what we expect to hear—or what we need or want to hear. For example, if you haven't been feeling very confident, you might filter everything so you hear only the negative: "I'm not a good clinician." Or you might hear only the *positive* because anything critical is too threatening. Become familiar with your own selective tendencies and the way they block listening.
• *Giving advice*. Do you rush to answer every question, feeling you have to offer advice that solves every problem? Other people may simply need to think out loud or may just be looking for support. Unless they specifically ask for your help or advice, just listen.
• *Daydreaming*. Does your mind sometimes wander during a con-

versation? Do you let noises or your own thoughts distract you? Don't be embarrassed to admit this to the person who's speaking. Perhaps fatigue, anxiety, or a pressing appointment can account for a lapse in careful listening. However, if the cause is boredom, the antidote may be making an effort to get more involved in the conversation. Ask questions. Ask for examples. Summarize your understanding of what the other person is saying. Or make an appointment for a time when meetings or work duties won't prevent you from giving him your full attention.

Becoming a better listener

Recognizing the listening blocks that you typically use is the first step in changing them. Next, think about when you use them, with whom, and why. Choose one block and one person, and then practice listening differently to that person. During the conversation, be aware of each time you revert to the listening block—and of each time you manage *not* to revert. You can actually tally the numbers, if that helps, and watch the pattern change in future conversations. Writing about the experience can also help you become a more active listener.

_____❖

Conflicts

Working in a hospital promotes conflicts. It brings together intelligent, highly skilled people with strong personalities, puts them under pressure 24 hours a day,

and makes them answer to others who are short on time or patience. It places demands on them that are sometimes unclear and contradictory. Conflict is bound to result.

But conflict isn't bound to be destructive. Handled well, it can produce fresh, innovative approaches and prevent mistakes. But handled poorly, conflict can impair communication, motivation, and relationships. In many cases, your behavior makes the difference. There are three secrets to handling conflict well: understanding the dynamics of conflict, concentrating on conflicts that matter, and learning to manage conflicts well.

Understanding conflict dynamics

To manage conflict effectively, you first have to accept your responsibility for it and understand the other person's motivation. Don't take the easy way out by blaming your hospital, the other person, or the world. Unless you have overwhelming evidence to the contrary, assume the following:

• You are at least 50% responsible for causing and resolving any conflict that involves you.
• Most people aren't evil. Rather, they behave in a way that annoys you because they don't know how their behavior is affecting you or because they have a strong need to do what they're doing.
• Most conflicts can be resolved successfully—and many can be prevented—with the right approach.
• You can't change other people. The best you can hope to do is change your own behavior.

Focusing on what's important

If you analyze your conflicts, you'll probably find that they fit the 80/20 principle: 80% of your conflicts are with 20% of the people in your life. And 20% of those conflicts are causing 80% of the negative consequences in your life.

Obviously, you can't resolve all the conflicts around you. You have to concentrate on the ones that matter. If an isolated conflict isn't likely to affect your long-term relationships or motivation, ignore it. Instead, concentrate your energy on the few conflicts that are causing 80% of your problems.

Managing conflicts

Your next step is to analyze what's causing your major conflicts, so you can resolve them. Here's advice on how to avoid or handle four common causes of conflict.

Avoid misunderstandings

Have you ever listened to two people who thought they were talking about the same thing, but who were really carrying on two separate monologues? Given their assumptions, biases, blind spots, distractions, and inattentiveness, most people at best hear only 50% of what someone says. To avoid misunderstandings or reduce their destructive effect, try the following:

• Maintain a healthy skepticism about your ability to understand people. When you find a calm discussion getting heated, stop concentrating on your point of view and start clarifying any opinions you may have misunderstood. Repeat or paraphrase what the other person has said.

And compare his words with his tone of voice, facial expression, posture, and other nonverbal clues to make sure you're hearing what he means.

• Assume innocence until you can prove guilt. Remember times when you intended to do something noble but others misunderstood your intentions? You could be doing the same thing to others.

• Speak clearly. When you need to explain something, follow the standard advice: Tell the person what you're going to say; say it; then tell him what you said. And be specific. If you need results of a laboratory test by the end of the shift, don't say, "I need those results back as soon as possible." Instead, say, "I need those results by 3 p.m."

• Put your thoughts in writing if a conversation has left you confused and disorganized. Written communication gives you more time to compose your thoughts and the other person more time to digest them.

Don't become defensive

Many destructive conflicts arise because people let their insecurity or fear spark defensiveness. For example, Carolyn, a nurse on a medical-surgical unit, tells her nurse-manager that Dr. Jones has ordered morphine by I.V. drip, an unusual order on the unit. Her manager suggests she call an oncology nurse and ask about morphine drips. Defensive and angry because the suggestion calls attention to her inexperience, Carolyn says she doesn't need any help. Then, having rejected the chance to find out how to handle the problem, she has to start the morphine drip through trial and error. She and her manager feel angry for the rest of the shift.

To control your own defensiveness, adopt the following rules:
• Check your feelings frequently. When you notice yourself getting defensive, figure out why. The best way to handle feelings of inadequacy is to admit to yourself that you're not perfect – and give yourself permission to learn. You'll be able to accept others' help, and you'll reduce your ignorance and inexperience.
• Train yourself to respond instead of react. If a patient accuses you of being late with a medication, respond to her feelings: "I know you're ready for that pain pill, Mrs. Murphy. Let me see if I can make you more comfortable while you wait for it to take effect."

Such a response to the other person's feelings and needs shifts your attention away from any defensiveness you feel for causing those needs – or being accused of causing them.

Reacting with denial has the opposite effect. You obviously inflame your own anger and Mrs. Murphy's if you ignore her feelings and try to defend your behavior with something like "I have a lot of patients sicker than you are. I'll get your pill when I can."
• Face situations that make you feel defensive before they create open conflict. For example, Mary, an inexperienced surgical nurse, did a slow burn every time her coworker Holly offered advice and help. Seeing that the situation was getting out of

hand, Mary decided to risk the relationship and tell Holly that she felt Holly was flaunting her own experience. Holly was amazed; she had only wanted to help. Mary realized that Holly's desire to help was genuine. Both nurses came away with a clearer understanding of themselves and their working relationship. Their growing conflict was resolved.

Acknowledge conflicting viewpoints

Many people get embroiled in a conflict over *who* is right, rather than *what* is right. This is a common cause of destructive conflicts. Each person becomes so determined to prove his position that he can't see the big picture: He and the other person have very different points of view.

If you find yourself falling into such situations over and over, remember these tips:
• Maintain a healthy skepticism about the validity of your position. To avoid getting backed into a corner defending your decision on something, don't say no. Give yourself time to get the whole story – and a chance to change your position.
• Make sure you fully understand the other person's point of view. After you've won a delay, ask questions and listen carefully to the other person's side of the story.
• State your opinions in a nonchallenging, nonthreatening way.
• Don't let yourself be drawn into an argument about who's right. Instead, suggest consulting a source you both respect so you can concentrate on *what's* right.

The source can even be a book. If a new staff nurse insists that she can give I.V. digoxin because she gave it at another hospital, consult your procedures manual. Let her read that only intensive care nurses are allowed to perform that procedure at your hospital.

Concentrating on shared goals

Too often, conflicts escalate because people think all differences of opinion have to produce a winner and a loser – and because no one wants to be the loser.

Instead of concentrating on differences the next time you have a conflict, look for goals you and the other person share. When you start trying to resolve the conflict by looking at your shared goals, you and the other person will develop the trust you need to work through the problem together. To avoid a win-lose situation, do the following:
• Make your own goals clear, and ask what the other person's goals are. If doctors' rounds occur at the busiest time on your unit – during new admissions, for example – tell each doctor your goal: "I need to get new patients admitted right away and still be available to make rounds with you. Is there any special reason why you make rounds at that time every day?"
• Be open-minded when you and the other person look for ways to solve your clash of needs. You may be the one who needs to yield.

❖

Floating

No doubt you work with float nurses at times – and do your share of floating as well. Or maybe you work on an as-needed basis. In either case, you're probably sent to one of the busiest units in the hospital under the most difficult circumstances. To help make your floating easier and more effective, try the tips outlined below.

Asking for an orientation

If it's not possible for you to receive a basic orientation to the unit you'll be working on, take the initiative to learn your way around. Arrive early and explore the unit's basic layout, including the location of emergency equipment such as crash carts and fire extinguishers. Introduce yourself to the charge nurse and ask her to review the unit's routine. Also ask her to review your patient assignment with you. Here are two good questions to ask: "Are any of the patients having special problems that might not have been documented?" and "Do you have any tips for working well with these patients?"

Communicating clearly

Make note of patients with special needs or problems that developed during the previous shift. If you aren't qualified to care for certain patients, tell the charge nurse. Be sure she's aware of your limitations as well as your level of expertise. Communicate in a positive way by conveying your concern for the patients' best interest and, if needed, ask the charge nurse to assign you a buddy – someone who usually works on the unit and who is willing to help.

Checking all orders

Check medication orders, care plans, and the Kardex as soon as possible after receiving your patient assignment to see what your patients will need and how you can organize your day. The way you start the day will set the tone for the rest of it; assess each patient as early as possible so you have a baseline for comparison during the shift and can set priorities.

At the same time, make a list of things you might easily overlook or forget. This will help keep you on track, even if you're distracted and interrupted many times during the day. You might include medications that are due at odd times or that are unavailable from the pharmacy at the required times. Cross off tasks as you complete them, and report any unfinished ones to the oncoming shift.

Asking for help

If in doubt, ask questions. Reading your own internal warning signs helps avoid mistakes. If you're uneasy about a medication order or if a procedure doesn't seem quite right – STOP! Pay attention to your intuition. Investigate the accuracy and validity of the order; you may have misread it or someone may have transcribed it incorrectly. The patient's condition may even have changed so much that the order is no longer appropriate.

Don't make assumptions about your patients. If you pick up something abnormal in a patient's condition, don't assume it was always there. Check with a staff member who has been on duty for the past few days and is familiar with the patient, or consult the patient's chart for prior entries concerning the abnormality.

Developing a support system

One of the drawbacks to floating is the lack of a support system. On your regular unit, you're familiar with each other's strengths and weaknesses and can support each other. As an outsider on another unit, you may need that kind of support more than anyone. Develop it by introducing yourself to each nurse in the unit.

Although getting to know all the different nurses well is difficult, you'll probably find that a few of them are more open and helpful to outsiders. Take breaks and lunches with them when possible. Making this effort every time you float to a different unit can help you develop a support network throughout the hospital. Learn the strengths and weaknesses of the nurses you work with; each nurse has some area in which she shines. Seek advice from the experts in your own weak areas.

Also, as you float, expect to be evaluated. The nurse-manager will be evaluating your competence and expertise. The staff nurses will weigh your willingness to do your part and carry your share of the load. Don't be offended by their watchful eyes. Any suspicions they may have will fade as you demonstrate a professional, caring attitude and quality work. Your presence during a busy day will be welcomed.

Keeping anecdotal notes

Some days, everything will seem to go crazy and your best efforts to organize won't be enough to keep up with the pace and volume of work that needs to be done. Ask your charge nurse for help if you're overwhelmed. Jot down notes about any problems that arise so you can refresh your memory later if needed. Include brief facts about the situation, the date, and the time, and remember to take care to protect patients' identities and maintain confidentiality.

Double-checking everything

At the end of your shift, make rounds one last time. Check your documentation, especially about medications given. Review your list to ensure that you've completed each task. If someone was particularly helpful, let her know.

_____❖

Sick calls

If you feel ill or have been exposed to someone with a contagious disease, should you take a chance on infecting your patients and coworkers, or should you stay home and leave your unit short-staffed?

Weighing the illness

Researchers have quizzed infection control nurses and hospital administrators on this question, and here are their recommendations:
• _Sore throat and fever._ The obvious danger is streptococcal (strep) infection, which is highly contagious. Usually, when you get a strep throat, you don't feel like working for a day or so. The problem is, you feel better after a few days and you return to work, but you're still contagious.

Instead, see a doctor and ask him to take a culture if he suspects strep throat. If it isn't strep, go back to work whenever you feel well enough. If it is strep, stay home for a few days after you start treatment; this will reduce the risk of transmitting the infection and give you a chance to regain some strength.
• _Cold with sneezing and coughing._ The American Hospital Association recommends continuing with work. Don't bother with a mask; it doesn't keep the virus away from patients because you carry the virus on your hands and clothes and many viruses are small enough to pass through a mask. Wash your hands frequently, use a tissue when you sneeze, and avoid coughing or sneezing directly toward others.
• _Boil on your finger._ Stay home. The boil may be caused by strep or staphylococcal (staph) infection. If it's staph, it's not an innocent strain; the fact that it's causing a boil shows that it's virulent.
• _Boil in your axilla._ Stay home. A boil in the axilla is just as dangerous as one on the finger because bacteria don't stay in the boil. They colonize in the entire body, including hands, nose, and hair. The fact that a patient may not come into direct contact with the boil doesn't mean there's less danger of infection. A boil anywhere on your body

should keep you home until it's no longer draining. Then, avoid caring for susceptible patients until your culture tests negative.

• *Diarrhea controlled by medication.* Stay home, unless you know that your diarrhea is caused by a noninfectious condition like ulcerative colitis, irritable colon syndrome, or regional enteritis. If it's caused by a bacteria or a virus (usually indicated by fever), you're still infectious even though the diarrhea is under control. Check with your doctor to find out when you can return to work.

• *Exposure to chicken pox.* If you've already had chicken pox, you're immune to it, so exposure poses no risk. If you haven't had chicken pox (or don't know if you have), you can continue to work with patients for 7 days after exposure. After the seventh day, you'll begin shedding the virus if you've become infected, so ask to work in an area, such as staff development, that doesn't include patient contact for 10 to 14 days. Make doubly sure you avoid all contact with immunosuppressed patients.

• *Exposure to meningitis.* Go to work. You can count on one hand the documented cases of meningitis spread in a hospital. Chances are slim that you'll get meningitis from a patient and even slimmer that you'll transmit it to another patient when you're not infected. If you *are* infected, stay home and seek medical help; meningitis can be life-threatening if untreated.

• *Exposure to active tuberculosis.* Go to work. Tuberculosis (TB) is slightly more contagious in the hospital than meningitis. Even so, the chance of your carrying the TB bacillus from one patient to another is so remote, you should disregard it. But if you've had close contact with a TB patient who's a transmitter, you should have a skin test immediately. If it's negative, you should have another one in 10 weeks to ensure that you haven't been infected.

Understanding hospital policy

Many nurses believe they'll lose pay if they stay home. Instead of risking unpaid sick leave, they'll probably make the decision themselves. The fact is, though, that few hospitals penalize nurses for missing work if they have a contagious disease or are asymptomatic carriers. If you're still unsure about whether to stay home or go to work, consult your employee health service if your hospital has one. Better yet, take the following steps before becoming ill so that you'll know how to make a decision when the time comes.

Be informed

Find out whether your hospital has a policy on employee illness and infection prevention. If so, the person appointed to advise nurses about infection control should be familiar with the current recommendations about hospital employees and must have the authority to tell you to stay home. Nurse-managers are ideal for the job: Since they administer the floor's activities, they should make the staffing decisions.

Know your rights

Hospitals must let employees with potentially contagious diseases take time off without any penalty, financial or otherwise. Hospitals should consider giving sick pay above and beyond the normal limits if a nurse has an infection that's potentially transmissible to patients.

Naturally, hospitals are reluctant to allow extra sick days because that costs money. However, they should realize that a nurse who's infecting patients and other nurses can end up costing them a lot more than a few days' sick pay.

❖

Remembering your patients

Taking care of patients who are going to die can be daunting. One way to keep your patient from becoming just another statistic is to keep a log of those who've died on the unit.

As the list grows ever longer, you might feel overwhelmed by the task of keeping up with it. However, the names and the memories they evoke could also help to bring solace.

DIFFICULT PERSONS

Self-care while treating AIDS patients

The physical and emotional stress of caring for patients with acquired immunodeficiency syndrome (AIDS) is often complicated by their situations. Along with being ravaged by a terminal disease, many patients with AIDS die shunned by family and friends. Others have been forced to go on welfare, even though they had good incomes at one time. Still others are homeless.

In addition, the patient population itself has been undergoing a major shift from gay males to heterosexual I.V. drug users, females, and children. The shift to I.V. drug users in particular has made nursing care even harder. While gay men (who are generally well educated) have been knowledgeable about the disease, I.V. drug users aren't as receptive to teaching, and they tend to be more manipulative.

More patients are showing up with severe neurologic deficits. Some of them need total nursing

care, including bathing and feeding. And worst of all, you know that your patients, most of whom are in their twenties and thirties, are doomed to die. (See *Remembering your patients.*)

All of these factors add to an already stressful job. That stress can catch up with you, leading to burnout or even physical illness. That's why you need to take measures to ensure your emotional health.

Taking care of yourself

Because AIDS is such a misunderstood and socially unacceptable disease, you might find that your family, friends, or even other health care workers have trouble relating to you or can't understand what you're going through. They might give you a hard time, saying such things as "You're going to get AIDS there," or "Take a shower before you come home," or "Wash your uniform there."

And even though health care professionals know that the disease isn't casually transmitted, coworkers might distance themselves from you. In fact, they may think you're weird: "You've got to be crazy," they might say, or "You must have your own personal agenda to be doing this."

Alleviate your stress

Because of the unique pressures involved in caring for AIDS patients, you need to be able to vent your stress with people you can trust.

If you don't have family or friends who will listen about your work, maybe you can confide in your coworkers or nurse-manager. If not, you might want to consider therapy. Or perhaps you can suggest that your hospital initiate a voluntary support group for the AIDS unit nurses.

Whether you go to a group or rely on family, friends, or colleagues, the important thing is to discuss your feelings in a supportive atmosphere. In addition, there are a number of things you can do on your own:

• *Take time off.* This means more than simply taking days off or going on vacations – which, of course, are musts. If anyone questions you about AIDS when you're off duty, tell them you prefer not to talk about AIDS in your free time. And use the time to do what you really enjoy.

• *Learn to say no.* People who have jobs that are dedicated to AIDS are in great demand to do other things, such as speak to other nurses about AIDS education or participate on committees. While lecturing about prevention can be therapeutic, be realistic about your time constraints. If you overbook yourself, you'll burn out.

• *Maintain a realistic sense of responsibility.* Don't take responsibility for things that are out of your control. For instance, if a patient is noncompliant, don't assume it's because of something you didn't do or say right.

With AIDS patients, you have to accept – not just intellectually but emotionally – what you can and can't do. You can't cure AIDS. But you *can* help the patient feel better.

• *Assess yourself.* Keep an eye on your own mental health. Ask yourself: How much time have I spent with my children this week? Have I been home before 8 o'clock at night? How many hours have I worked this week? Have I read a book for pleasure? If you don't like your answers, remedy the situation the following week.

• *Develop outside activities.* Make time for exercise and hobbies. ❖

Handling special patients

Throughout your practice, you encounter patients who have special needs. For example, your patient may be depressed or even suicidal. Or perhaps your patient is delirious, morbidly obese, or afflicted with a chemical dependency. These are just a few of the special needs you need to be able to respond to when providing care.

Depressed patient

Sometimes, hospitalized patients become depressed in response to illness or surgery. Most likely, you've cared for patients suffering from this type of depression, which differs from clinical depression.

Although this depression may not last longer than the time needed for the patient to recover, it can seriously affect his response to treatment and his ability to plan for his future. That's why you need to know how to recognize this depression in its many forms—and how to help your patients cope with it.

Recognizing depression

Each patient is vulnerable to depression because he faces some kind of crisis: a life-threatening emergency, an acute or chronic illness, or surgery. Of course, when a patient's depressed, your job is to help him handle it; but first you have to recognize it.

Some depressed patients are easy to recognize. They cry readily, wring their hands, pick at their food, aimlessly turn the pages of a magazine, and lie awake most of the night. These patients make no secret of how unhappy they feel. And they're exhibiting the classic signs of depression—a sadness and a loss of interest and pleasure in usual activities or pastimes.

But other depressed patients act out their depression in seemingly contradictory ways. They might even disguise it. For example, a man who's well enough to shave and bathe himself but just doesn't have the energy to do it may not be indifferent to personal cleanliness; he may be depressed. And a woman who keeps her shades drawn, sleeps too much, and turns her back on you when she's awake may be depressed, too.

Here's another familiar example of disguised depression: the patient who refuses his medication, demands special food, complains all day, and can't be satisfied no matter what you do. Or the patient who simply doesn't make the progress he's supposed to, puzzling you *and* the doctor. He may complain of gastric problems and headaches that have no apparent cause; he may not want to leave the hospital. Very possibly, he isn't malingering; he's depressed.

Responding to depression

When you realize your patient is depressed, you should respond immediately. (See *Reacting quickly to depression*, page 484.) Use the six steps that follow.

Listen to your patient

A depressed patient may not be able to say exactly how he feels about his illness, so listen closely for clues. If his chief topic of conversation is *your* work, *your* family, or *your* interests, he'd probably rather not talk about himself. If he avoids topics such as work, family, or friendships, he could be worried about how his illness will affect them.

And don't forget to take note of his mannerisms. If he consistently looks away, fidgets, or frowns whenever a particular subject comes up, that could be the one that's bothering him.

If you're able to identify the cause of his depression, don't

RULE OF THUMB

 Reacting quickly to depression

As soon as you discover that your patient is depressed, tell his doctor and other staff members. This will help you revise care plans as needed to address the patient's problem. Then follow these guidelines:

• Assess a depressed patient for suicide risk on an ongoing basis. This will help you stay alert for self-destructive behaviors, allowing you to provide for your patient's safety.

• Ask for a clinical nurse specialist-liaison consultation. This can provide an objective assessment of the patient and staff situation. A clinical nurse specialist has the expertise in depression that's needed, and she'll be a sounding board for the staff's anxiety.

• Don't allow a history of substance abuse to interfere with assessing the patient for depression. Biased reactions can interfere with your ability to provide objective patient care and may further alienate the patient.

• Remember to document your conversation with the doctor and other staff members, along with what you did for the patient. If the patient attempts suicide and his family sues you, you'll need to prove you recognized his problem and took steps to treat it.

press him to talk about it. Being a good listener means being able to endure long silences without feeling an urgent need to talk. Even if the patient isn't ready to share his feelings, he'll find comfort knowing that you're available and that you understand.

Reflect his feelings

When your patient expresses negative feelings about his condition or future prospects, paraphrase his message, thereby acknowledging and emphasizing the feelings he has expressed.

For example, you might tell a patient who's having trouble coping with his recent diagnosis of testicular cancer: "You sound like you feel that you'll never be able to adjust to this illness or enjoy life anymore." Or you might tell a patient who can't see an end to his depression: "I hear you saying that, because you're so blue now, you're afraid you'll always feel this way."

Be kind but firm

When dealing with a depressed patient, apply the principle of "kind firmness." This means to communicate empathy for the patient's feelings while communicating your firm belief that he can *act* contrary to the way he *feels*.

For instance, if your patient refuses to attend his regular occupational therapy session, say, "I know you don't feel like going to therapy, but you can force yourself to go for an hour, even if you don't feel like it. Some activity will be good for you." By saying this, you're acknowledging the patient's depressed feelings *and* firmly directing him toward attending therapy. Chances are he *will* feel better after being involved in structured physical activity, even for a short time.

Help him set realistic goals

Apathy is probably the most common mood of the depressed patient. His illness or injury has crushed his confidence in his ability to control his own life. If he can't do anything about his condition, he reasons, why should he do anything at all? And his role as a passive, dependent hospital patient isn't doing much to shake him out of this mood.

You can help by encouraging your patient to establish realistic short-term goals that he can readily achieve. These can be as simple as shaving himself or sitting up with the shades open for a half hour.

Suggest the goal, but let the patient decide whether or not he'll meet it and when. Then, leave it up to him. These must be the patient's accomplishments, not yours.

Show him his choices

A depressed patient tends to see the world in only one way—negatively. He may feel stuck with this one way of viewing things or one way of behaving.

To help him see the world more positively, try to instill in him the idea that he can *choose* to view the world differently. Help him see his problems as a challenge to adapt positively to a new set of conditions. Show him

that he has many choices in living—maybe more than he realizes.

For example, a patient who has lost both legs in an automobile accident will naturally be grief stricken at first. After that, help him see that he has choices: He can continue to view his accident as a tragedy from which he'll never recover. Or he can learn to view the accident as a serious loss but one that won't shatter his life forever. Help him understand that, after he weeps over the activities he'll never again enjoy, he can go on to focus on the things in his life that can still bring him pleasure. He can still see, for example, so he can take up new reading interests. He can still hear, so he can listen to new types of music.

Help your patient see his depression as temporary

Your depressed patient's despair or apathy may seem overwhelming and never-ending to him. But you can truthfully tell him that depression generally doesn't last. Assure him that, with time, his emotional balance and energy will return, and new solutions to old problems will appear. Explain that, with time, he'll learn to change his views as he encounters new people and new experiences.

Make sure he understands that feeling helpless and hopeless *now* doesn't mean that he'll feel helpless and hopeless in the *future.*

Offering hope

The best antidote for depression is hope. You can give hope to a depressed patient by communicating this positive message whenever you care for him. Remind him that even the most well-adjusted people have problems to cope with. Even though the patient's problems may seem insurmountable to him now, ensure him that he has the skills he needs to cope with them.

————————————❖

Suicidal patient

You don't have to work in a psychiatric hospital to be faced with a suicidal patient. Many people who try to kill themselves receive their initial care in medical-surgical or critical care units. That means you could be called on to care for a patient who has attempted suicide.

Protecting the patient
As a nurse, you're in the best position to assess the moods and gain the trust of a suicidal patient. This advantage will help you reach your two most important goals:
• to keep him from harming himself again
• to encourage him to accept psychiatric treatment.

To help you meet these goals, follow these 10 guidelines.

Ensure safety
Safeguard the patient's room before he even gets to your unit. Remove objects that he could use to hurt himself – including metal coat hangers, cords, soft drink cans and, of course, glass objects and scissors.

Remember to move equipment carts out of arm's reach of the bed. Remove unused monitoring cables, and run essential tubing under the bed. These precautions should also be taken if you're working in an intensive care unit.

Try to arrange for a private room for the patient. If he must share a room, ask his roommate to keep potentially dangerous objects out of the patient's sight and reach. (The nature of a suicidal patient's illness should be kept confidential, but safety is your primary concern.)

When the patient arrives, remove all personal belongings that he might use to hurt himself. Most of these are quite obvious – sharp objects, matches, belts, and medication. But be sure to check *everything*. Let the patient know where these items will be (with his family or with hospital security). Tell food service to send plastic utensils at mealtime, and make sure that every piece is returned with the food tray.

Keep a watchful eye
If possible, make arrangements for continuous observation before the patient arrives on your unit. You could enlist the help of students or nursing assistants to serve as attendants in the patient's room. You may be tempted to have a family member monitor the patient, but you should be aware that having a family member present often adds to the patient's distress.

Even with an attendant present, you'll need to monitor the patient regularly – usually every 15 or 30 minutes, depending on his mental state. Remember that *you* are responsible for the patient. Ensure that his room is as near the nurses' station as possible, even if it means moving another patient.

Take a history
After the patient has been admitted, assess his physical and general emotional status. Ask him if he knows why he's been admitted.

Ask him how he's been feeling, if he's been under pressure recently, how he's been sleeping, and if he's been withdrawing from friends. Don't just rely on what he tells you. Look for signs of stress, agitation, or confusion.

While taking the patient's history, don't be afraid to talk with him about suicide—that's why he's there. Talking about it, contrary to what many people believe, isn't going to push him into trying it again. Gently ask him such questions as "Did you really want to die? Do you still want to? Are you still planning to hurt yourself? How?"

Other questions you may want to ask the patient include: Has he ever attempted suicide before? Does he take drugs or drink alcohol and, if so, how much? Has he ever received psychiatric counseling? Has anyone in his family ever tried to commit suicide?

Contact the doctor
Immediately call the patient's doctor, who may recommend that you call a psychiatrist who has previously worked with the patient. The doctor may also be familiar with any other suicide attempts or relevant details in the patient's history.

Arrange a psychiatric evaluation
Check your hospital's policy for the proper way to arrange a psychiatric evaluation. You might need to ask for an immediate assessment by an on-call psychiatrist. Or you might be expected to do the initial history taking and assessment, laying the foundation for a psychiatrist's follow-up evaluation.

Provide a controlled environment
The patient shouldn't leave his room during his evaluation. Visitors are allowed—but only if he wants to see them. Remember that even though the waiting room may be crowded with loving members of his family, all of them deeply distressed, the patient might be afraid or ashamed to face any of them.

You can help him make a plan for visitors, including putting a sign on his door that directs people to the nurses' station. You and the other nurses can then screen visitors according to the patient's wishes. Upon admission, review a form letter with the patient that sums up hospital policies regarding room restrictions, constant observation, and psychiatric evaluation.

Maintain patient confidentiality
Let the patient know you're going to keep the nature of his illness confidential. (Remember, though, that a roommate must be informed of special precautions.) Don't give any information to visitors or people calling on the phone.

Document everything
Write down *everything* – the patient's use of plastic utensils, his reactions and behavior, and the consultations you've had with other nurses and doctors.

Encourage discussion
Allow the patient to talk without interruption – or to be silent for long periods. Don't break in to challenge, advise, or criticize. But don't support denial or unrealistic ideas. Share with him how *you* see things. For example, you might say, "This is what I hear you saying," or "This is what I think is happening."

At the same time, avoid probing too deeply into his motivations. Leave that to the specialists. Express warmth, honesty, and concern so the patient understands that you recognize his suffering.

Arrange follow-up care
Psychiatric follow-up care may be given on an outpatient basis or your patient may need to be transferred to an inpatient unit. If a transfer is planned, make sure the patient knows where and when he'll be going. (Usually, psychiatrists discuss this with the patient and the patient's family.)

———————————❖

Delirious patient

Delirium is an acute, reversible change in behavior that's characterized by clouded consciousness, mental incoherence, and difficulty maintaining concentration and attention. It affects up to 13% of the general hospital population and up to 16% of elderly patients. (See *Who's at risk?*)

Even though delirium is prevalent, you might not know what to do when your patient becomes delirious. Or you might not be sure it's delirium and not dementia or some other disorder. The tips that follow will help you take better care of these difficult patients.

Recognizing signs and symptoms
A delirious patient has a short attention span, which is caused by a lack of awareness or a tendency to be distracted. You can assess awareness by seeing if the patient is dull, drowsy, or able to pay attention to you when you rouse him.

When a patient is delirious, he can't remember new information. And he may not know where he is, let alone what time or day it is. Keep in mind, though, that a patient may not know the date or time simply because he hasn't seen a newspaper or a clock and has no other way of orienting himself.

A delirious patient may speak incoherently. But even when he's coherent, what he tells you may not be accurate. For instance, a patient may say he's just returned from a movie when in fact he's been in the X-ray department. Such a patient is trying to make sense out of a confusing environment. He'll sometimes use the wrong words to describe things, making it difficult for you to follow what he's saying. He may also hallucinate – usually visually, but sometimes through what he hears and feels.

You may also find patients with sleep pattern disturbances, including nocturnal restlessness and daytime drowsiness. Some delirious patients may pull out catheters or I.V. lines. Yet others may be in a stupor, drifting in and out of consciousness.

Some neurologic signs associated with delirium are postural or action tremors, myoclonus (sudden, sporadic muscular contractions), asterixis (flapping tremors), and slurred speech. EEG results will usually be abnormal, showing signs of diffuse slowing.

Remember that delirium is a reversible condition, even if some of the underlying causes aren't. Don't confuse it with irreversible conditions (for example, organic brain diseases, such as Alzheimer's disease, or functional psychoses, including schizophrenia and psychotic depression). Mistaking delirium for an irreversible condition would deny the patient appropriate treatment.

Providing required care
A delirious patient can't take care of himself—emotionally or physically. Your job is to keep him safe and help him regain the control he's lost. You can meet this responsibility most effectively by anticipating his needs.

Make sure he can see and hear properly. If he usually wears glasses or a hearing aid, for example, ask the family to bring them to the hospital and make sure he uses them. If he becomes agitated or appears to feel threatened, reassure him in a calm voice: "I know you feel afraid. I won't harm you. I'm here to help you."

Who's at risk?

Elderly patients are at high risk for delirium because they're particularly sensitive to changes in their metabolic status and fluid and electrolyte balance.

Hypnotics, sedatives, and minor tranquilizers must be used cautiously with elderly patients because these drugs can have toxic effects on the brain and precipitate withdrawal reactions.

Patients most likely to become delirious are those with chronic cognitive impairments, such as Alzheimer's disease, and those who can't manage their own activities of daily living.

Also, patients with abnormal sodium levels, elevated blood urea nitrogen levels, leukocytosis, or leukopenia have been known to become more delusional than those without these problems.

Knowing whether to restrain
Many delirious patients lose control and sometimes require tranquilizers or restraints. (See *Restraints and the delirious patient*, page 490.) Usually, you should resort to these measures when your assessment tells you the patient may do something to hurt himself, such as pulling out an I.V. line or falling out of bed.

The patient's doctor might prescribe a low dose of a major tranquilizer, such as 0.5 mg of haloperidol or 10 mg of thioridazine, several times a day. One

RULE OF THUMB

 ## Restraints and the delirious patient

Avoid using restraints unless they're absolutely necessary. Even then, use the least restrictive method needed. For example, if the patient is pulling out his I.V. lines, you can avoid tying him down by putting mitts on his hands. This is an effective method, yet one that's rarely used.

If you have to use restraints, remember that wrist restraints are used to protect I.V. lines, dressings, and catheters. Vest restraints prevent falls by keeping patients in their beds or chairs. When restraining a patient, tell him you understand how upsetting it must be for him, but explain that the restraints are necessary to help keep him safe.

Tell the patient with wrist restraints that you'll remove them as soon as possible – at least every 1 to 2 hours. When you do remove them, even temporarily, perform range-of-motion exercises with the patient's affected limbs, and assess skin condition at the area covered by the restraint to prevent skin breakdown. When the restraints are in place, frequently assess neuromuscular status in the affected hand and assess for a pulse to prevent injury from the restraints. Afterward, encourage a family member to sit with him.

When using any type of restraint, remember to give emotional support to the patient's family members. Whenever possible, tell the family that you're using restraints and explain the reasons why *before* they see the patient. They'll most likely be upset and embarrassed by the patient's behavior.

Remind the family members that their loved one's medical condition – not some quirk in his personality – is responsible for his behavior. Assure them that he should eventually return to normal.

important point to remember is that these medications can actually make some delirious patients even more confused and agitated. You'll have to observe carefully to decide whether the drugs are helping or hurting.

The use – and abuse – of physical restraints has prompted a lot of negative comment, much of it focusing on institutionalized elderly patients. But few experts address the use of restraints on medical-surgical patients, even though an estimated 1 in 10 patients needs to be physically restrained at least once during hospitalization. (And this figure is climbing with the aging of the patient population.)

You should also realize that restraints, like tranquilizers, make some patients even more agitated. For instance, a vest restraint can contribute to a fall if the patient tries to untie it and climb over side rails.

Caring for delirious patients on a busy unit can be difficult. These patients need more of your time than most patients and they usually resist your care. Remember to stick to your major nursing goal—to protect and take care of the patient until he's able to take care of himself.

—————————————

Confused elderly patient

Elderly, confused patients feel disconnected from the world. Often, they call out to no one in particular or stare off into space. Communicating with these patients is frustrating because you're not sure if you're getting through. Still, you have to try. You could be the only link between your patient and reality.

As a nurse, you strongly influence the emotional world of the elderly, confused patient. With liberal use of empathy, sincere affection, and touch, you can help satisfy your patients' most basic needs for feeling positive and related to the world. In doing this, you also help prevent behavioral complications, extended hospital stays, and unnecessary placement in short- or long-term facilities.

Communicating effectively

The secret to getting through to elderly, confused patients lies in the ability to establish a meaningful relationship with them. Accept these patients as they are

and communicate with them on their own level. Here are ways to achieve this.

Speak evenly and concisely

Resist the urge to raise the pitch of your voice when talking with an older person as you might when talking with a child. Instead, lower your voice pitch to compensate for presbycusis, the hearing loss associated with aging.

And don't ooververbalize. Use as few words as possible and keep your directions simple and concrete. You can use conversation as a way to anchor a person by talking about what is familiar to him—his past, for example. Rather than remind him what day it is, talk about the weather, his family, or any other information that would stimulate interest in the external world.

Remember, accepting your patient is important. He may sense that he's losing his faculties, and this awareness must be devastating. So you need to respect his attempts to defend himself against this realization. The old gentleman who gives you an elaborate explanation of how the bathroom pipes are leaking may be using confabulation; that is, he may be fabricating his own truth to explain the puddle of urine on the floor, a result of his incontinence.

Use reassuring nonverbal communication

Effective nonverbal communication is a powerful tool. Even brain-damaged patients respond on this primitive and universal level that we all share.

You know the power of nonverbal communication from your

own experiences: Your patient will clasp your outstretched hand, return your warm smile, or respond positively when you put your arm around his shoulder. However, a threatening action, such as an attempt to remove clothing, can result in a combative response. Or a hurried, anxious attitude on your part can create feelings of anxiety and even panic.

Establish a slow pace

A confused patient needs time to process what's happening. When the world moves too fast for him, he may have no choice but to "put the brakes on" by being noncompliant or combative. Stubborn refusals to take medications or striking out at a caregiver may be the only way for him to control the situation.

Trying to hurry such a patient will only leave you feeling frustrated and behind schedule, so you might as well resign yourself to the inevitable. Use this time as an opportunity to relax with your patient.

Perhaps one of the most threatening situations for the patient is when someone invades his body space – for example, trying to take his clothes off for a bath. You'll need to repeat your explanations in a calm, reassuring voice. Don't use singsong tones, as though you were trying to manipulate a child.

Keep the patient as fully covered as possible during the bath, and use a heat lamp to keep him warm. Allowing him to keep a bath blanket on in the tub may be helpful, too.

Creating a familiar environment

The type of environment you create for your patient can affect how well he functions. Strive for a predictable, consistent, and familiar world amid the chaos of the hospital environment. Even in the hospital, the patient's room should make a statement about who he is in relation to the world. Family pictures, religious articles, holiday decorations, and so on will create a more secure environment.

Familiar rituals also help. For instance, try to determine the patient's usual bedtime routine, and write the specifics in the plan of care or post them on the wall so everyone will follow them.

Involving the family

Whether the patient lives at home or in an institution, his relationship with his family is another crucial part of his world. However, the family may need your help to *stay* involved with the patient.

Educate the family

Most people don't know how to act around someone who's confused and unable to carry on a conversation. Their loved one may act as though he's oblivious to their presence. Family members want to stay involved but may give up and stop visiting out of a sense of helplessness and despair.

If this is the case, you need to give them some positive reinforcement for visiting. By teaching them how to communicate with their loved one, you'll help them feel they have a purpose and an important role in the patient's life.

You can teach them the value of reminiscing with the patient. Families need to know that even though Grandma repeats the same story over and over, their listening to her is important and helpful.

Family members who are uncomfortable with the patient's condition may act unnaturally, which confuses the patient even more. These families need your support to be more comfortable and honest in their interactions.

Prod the patient's memory
Sometimes a patient with an attentive family will complain that "no one visits." He may simply not remember the last visit, even if it was a week ago. Keeping a record on a visiting board will help the patient's memory and prevent the family from becoming alienated by his "ungrateful" attitude.

Use a calendar or erasable marking board for family members to record their names, the day and date of their last visit, and planned future visits. Staff members can then use the board to orient the patient between visits. Advise family members to write down only the future visits they're sure to keep. ❖

Demented patient
Caring for patients with dementia can be challenging. Your first inclination is to force reality on them, and their inclination is to resist this.

In these cases, you should forget the textbooks and respond

Provocative questions about dementia
If you find yourself locking horns with a confused patient, ask yourself if your approach is:
• encouraging better behavior or diminishing his sense of well-being
• relating to him in his world or sowing the seeds of potentially difficult behavior in your world
• allowing him to enjoy familiar, safe, pleasant thoughts or feeding his anxiety.

intuitively. You may even have to suspend rational thought and ease up on reality orientation. By affirming your patient's fear, however irrational, and supporting him, you can produce a positive outcome. (See *Provocative questions about dementia*.)

Going with the flow
When caring for a patient with dementia, a creative approach can be far more therapeutic than textbook-style reality orientation, as the following stories illustrate:
• A woman continually sets the table and cooks for her dead parents. When her family gently reminds her that her parents are dead, she wails in grief. But when the family switches strategies, saying, "You must miss your parents very much," the patient becomes calm and nods, comfortable with that assessment. Everyone benefits from the arrangement.

• A nurse is driving her neurologically impaired father, who prides himself on his knowledge of cars. He compliments her on her new Buick. "It's a Chevrolet, Dad," she says, hoping to orient him. Her father's face falls in disappointment. Although well-meant, her comment embarrassed him. Yes, she oriented him to reality, but a simple acceptance of her father's compliment would have worked better.

• An agitated man claims that bugs are climbing all over the furniture and walls of the room. "There are no bugs in this room—you're seeing things," his wife keeps saying, infuriating him. Finally, in desperation, she takes out the vacuum cleaner and vacuums the furniture and walls with dramatic flair. Her husband relaxes.

Avoiding frustration

In each of these examples, the caregiver is frustrated because the patient can't see "reality." Unless someone gives in, a counterproductive and sometimes fierce struggle inevitably develops.

Think of the perennial lament of the confused patient, "I want to go home"—even when he *is* at home. Explaining this fact rarely satisfies him. Instead of arguing, try acknowledging his desire to feel secure. You could say, "You must be lonely for your home and family. Can you tell me about it?" Chances are this response will calm him—and perhaps thwart an impending break for the door.

You've been taught to orient patients to their environment and the people around them. But you're inviting trouble if you try

to force your reality on a patient who can't accept it.

❖

Pediatric patient

If you've ever worked with children, you know they all have distinctive needs. You've probably also discovered that you sometimes have to play detective to determine what those needs are. You can eliminate the guesswork and make hospitalization easier for your patients by remembering these five concepts: trust, autonomy, curiosity, industry, and identity.

These concepts correspond to five stages of childhood—infant, toddler, preschool age, school age, adolescent. During each stage, a child tries to understand a different concept, and as he does, predictable changes in behavior occur. Some of these are outlined below.

Gaining an infant's trust

During infancy, a child needs to develop trust in the people around him. If his caregivers keep changing, everyone will seem like a stranger and he'll withhold his trust. To create a bond with the infant, ask to be his primary caregiver. Then gain his trust by focusing first on his parents. Try to reduce the parents' anxiety through friendly conversation and reassuring pats. Encourage a smile that the baby can observe. As the parents' trust in you increases, so will your patient's.

You can also try this trick. Before examining the infant, lay your stethoscope beside him and continue talking with his parents. If the child becomes curious about the stethoscope, use that curiosity as a chance to start exploring its use together.

Giving a toddler autonomy

A toddler (ages 1 to 3) wants autonomy. When he can't do things for himself, he may cry, struggle, or throw a temper tantrum. And when his daily routine is disrupted, he may feel threatened. To help restore his sense of control in a strange place, incorporate his everyday rituals into his plan of care as much as possible. For instance, let him feed himself, put on his slippers, and do whatever he can for himself, even if he takes longer than you would. If he has special words for things, learn and use them.

If the toddler hasn't brought some of his own toys with him, keep a few at his bedside. Appropriate toys for a child this age include ones he can push or maneuver. Also encourage his parents to bring a photograph album for the child's crib. In addition to family photographs, suggest including pictures of his pets, playmates, and favorite playground.

Using a preschooler's curiosity

A child age 3 to 5 develops an intense curiosity – and a seemingly inexhaustible store of questions about everything. You can anticipate curiosity about the hospital setting and help ease your patient's fears by answering some questions before they're even asked.

If a child is scheduled for surgery, invite him and his parents to tour the unit, operating room, and postanesthesia room. Afterward, the child can try on surgical masks and gloves and experiment with tongue blades and a stethoscope.

Satisfying a youth's industriousness

A child age 6 to 12 is usually industrious, motivated, and intent on proving his intellect and physical prowess. When caring for a child in this age bracket, explain all procedures to him. Don't be surprised if each time you repeat a procedure, his questions change and he wants to learn more.

Offer him hands-on activities, such as puzzles or model building. If possible, give him a task that helps you as it fills his need to be industrious. For example, he might carry juice to other patients, read to a younger patient, or put together admission packets.

Establishing an adolescent's identity

An adolescent (ages 12 to 18) is working to create a personal identity. To help your adolescent patient do this, encourage him to think positively about himself and to do as much as he can without your help. Don't allow your patient to think of himself as a helpless sick person.

By letting the developmental concept for each age-group trigger your imagination, you can gain a better understanding of each pediatric patient and develop a plan of care to meet his needs.

DIFFICULT PERSONS

Visually impaired patient

A patient who is visually impaired is bound to feel disoriented when he enters any new setting, especially one as confusing as a busy hospital. You can help your patient feel safe and comfortable by orienting him to his hospital environment. Here are the methods you can use.

Orienting the patient

Let your visually impaired patient feel the length, width, and height of his hospital bed. Using the bed as a focal point, guide him along the walls so he can locate the bedside table, window, bathroom, closet door, and hall door. Then return him to the bedside.

Next, let him feel his way into the hallway; help him find specific areas he may need, such as the nurses' station or patient's lounge. This hands-on orientation will help him develop a mental image of his room and the surrounding environment.

Inspecting the room

Carefully inspect the patient's room and remove any obstacles. Make sure the lighting is appropriate: bright for patients with dimming vision and subdued for those with photophobia.

Keep the furniture and the contents of his bedside table in the same place. He'll become accustomed to their locations and always expect them to be there. Place the bed and side rails in the low position, but instruct him to ask for assistance if he wants to get out of bed.

Identifying common sounds

Sounds are especially important to a visually impaired patient. Learning to identify certain sounds – the noise of traffic, for instance – helps him protect himself against hazards.

In the hospital, certain sounds can help orient him to the time of day. Identify the sounds he might hear, such as, "That rumbling noise is the laundry cart. It usually arrives about 9 a.m." Or, "Dinner is served at 6 p.m. You'll hear the rattling of the trays."

Explain other hospital routines in detail, such as the times for medications, personal care, and visiting hours.

Providing emotional support

Schedule a time to discuss his feelings about his vision problem. Explore any alterations in his self-image. If he feels that he needs to change his lifestyle, support and encourage this effort.

In cases of sudden, total blindness, as in optic neuritis, use crisis intervention techniques. The patient's high stress level will prevent him from accurately interpreting what he hears. So give clear, simple directions. Empathize with him to gain his trust. Discuss his past coping behaviors and use them to help him adjust to his blindness.

Informing hospital staff

Note the patient's visual impairment on the Kardex. Instruct all staff members to identify themselves when they enter the room; they should also tell him when they're leaving. You may want to put a sign in the room to inform other hospital personnel of the visual impairment.

—————————————————❖

Patient who refuses to eat

You've no doubt come across more than one patient who desperately needs nutrition but refuses to eat. Three times a day—or more—you face defeat, and the frustration mounts. You may think there's nothing you can do to get your patient to eat. But there is. You can start by determining why the patient won't eat.

Identifying a physical reason

If a physical problem makes eating unpleasant or difficult, offer routine, practical support. For example, if the patient has trouble chewing or swallowing, tell him to order food that's easy to chew, to cut his food into bite-size pieces, and to take his time.

Perhaps the trouble is mechanical—he has difficulty holding utensils. If so, ask the occupational therapist for special equipment, such as swivel spoons or universal cuffs.

Recognizing an emotional reason

If you've ruled out physical causes, you need to start exploring the patient's feelings about eating and why he's choosing not to eat. Consider these common reactions:
• *Control.* Hospitalization robs patients of their independence; your patient may be looking for a way to control what's happening to him. Claims of nausea or poor appetite give him some sense of making his own decisions.
• *Anger.* Your patient may be displacing his anger on you or his family. Using mealtime as a battle arena, he can easily draw opponents into the ring.
• *Depression and despair.* Your patient, like so many others, may temporarily be depressed and have lost his appetite. Or he may be in deep despair about an overwhelming illness or long-term rehabilitation plans. Refusing food is one way of throwing in the towel.

By getting your patient to talk about these feelings, you can help him understand them. Such a discussion can provide him with insights that decrease his anxiety and increase his confidence, particularly if you acknowledge and accept any fears he expresses. Sometimes, just explaining his treatment will help.

Employing alternative methods

If you've exhausted conventional means of persuading a patient to eat, total parental nutrition or tube feeding may be necessary. Don't be surprised if your patient resists these alternatives as much as he's resisted eating; counseling may be needed.

Remember, however, that if the patient is in possession of his faculties, his decision to eat remains his. You may feel frustrated and defeated if he won't eat, and you may question his rejection of your help: "Why didn't he like me well enough to eat for me?" or "Why couldn't I make him feel life was worth living?" These are very human reactions, but recognize that you did all you could, that you let the patient know you wanted him to eat and to live. After that, the decision was his.

At this point, the only other thing you can do is alert other members of the health care team. When a patient is depressed or despondent, counseling or even drug therapy may be in order; you're the one who must intervene and make the connection.

❖

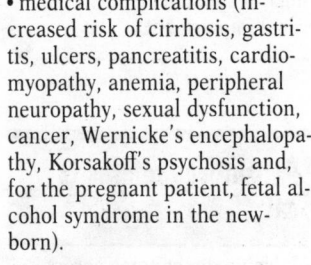

Alcohol abuser

Alcohol abuse refers to regular use of alcohol that depresses the patient's central nervous system and causes behavioral changes. It follows a pathologic course, impairs social or job function, and lasts at least 1 month. It may lead to dependency, in which the patient can't control use of alcohol and develops withdrawal symptoms if he attempts to stop or reduce intake.

Understanding the risks of abuse

Drinking alcohol excessively can produce these temporary or long-term effects:
• slowed brain function (impaired judgment, alertness, coordination, and reflexes)
• attitude and behavioral changes (hostility, aggression, life-threatening actions, taking risks)
• blackouts (loss of short-term memory with retention of remote memory; the patient may function effectively during a blackout, yet have no memory of his activity, unrelated to how much he drinks)

• medical complications (increased risk of cirrhosis, gastritis, ulcers, pancreatitis, cardiomyopathy, anemia, peripheral neuropathy, sexual dysfunction, cancer, Wernicke's encephalopathy, Korsakoff's psychosis and, for the pregnant patient, fetal alcohol symdrome in the newborn).

Assessing for alcohol abuse

Asking the patient the following questions may help uncover more information on his drinking pattern:
• How often do you drink?
• What kinds of liquor do you drink? How much of each? How much each day?
• For how long have you consumed alcohol at this rate?
• How have your drinking habits changed over time?
• When was your last drink?
• Have you ever experienced blackouts, tremors, delirium tremens, or seizures? When and for how long?
• Have you ever experienced auditory, visual, or tactile hallucinations? Were you drinking heavily at the time? Describe the experience.

Recognizing signs of abuse

Signs of alcohol abuse may include loss of inhibitions, disorganized thoughts, poor coordination, and unstable moods. Other signs include flushed face, slurred speech, prolonged reaction time, reduced visual acuity, blackouts, nystagmus, and disturbed sleep patterns (decreased rapid-eye-movement sleep). Signs and symptoms of a post-drinking hangover include accentuated feelings of anxiety, malaise, nausea, vomiting, sweating, thirst, and flushing.

Recognizing withdrawal signs

Signs of alcohol withdrawal may include tremors, anxiety, diaphoresis, diarrhea, tachycardia, tachypnea, hyperpnea, vomiting, and fever. Onset occurs several hours after the patient's last drink and usually peaks in 24 to 48 hours.

The patient may experience alcohol seizures 7 to 48 hours after his last drink. Complications during withdrawal may cause death, especially if the patient suffers from pneumonia, liver failure, subdural hematoma, or other problems. In alcohol withdrawal delirium (delirium tremens), the patient experiences confusion, disorientation, paranoid delusions, or visual or tactile hallucinations along with other signs and symptoms of withdrawal.

Helping the patient to recover

Your patient may be intoxicated, hungover, or experiencing withdrawal. He may also be asking others to sneak alcohol to him in the hospital. One of your greatest challenges may be to prevent personal feelings from interfering with the way you treat your patient. You can best help him by treating him objectively and by avoiding any expressions of judgment or reproach.

If your patient is intoxicated, you'll also need to take safety precautions, monitor his vital signs, and watch for signs of withdrawal. If he's in withdrawal, maintaining a calm environment may help prevent delirium tremens or ease the effects. To maintain a calm environment:

• Keep intrusions to a minimum.
• Move slowly and deliberately.
• Speak slowly and calmly, and call the patient by his name.
• Keep lighting balanced to prevent shadows and soft enough to prevent glare.
• Encourage a friend or family member to sit quietly with the patient and instruct the visitor to call you if a problem arises.

Continue to monitor vital signs and behavior. Try to keep the patient oriented. If he hallucinates, reorient him.

❖

Cocaine abuser

The cocaine and crack epidemic has created an unprecedented health crisis. That means some of *your* patients could be cocaine or crack abusers, even if they've been admitted to the hospital with another diagnosis. Before you can effectively treat such a patient, you'll need to recognize the signs and symptoms of abuse. Knowing what to look for when you assess these patients is becoming an important part of your job.

Recognizing signs of abuse

A cocaine or crack user could be dirty and unkempt, but he could also be wearing a three-piece suit. If you suspect that your patient uses crack or cocaine, try asking him. If he says yes, ask how long he's been using it, how frequently, and how he consumes it.

If he denies using the drug, there are ways to find out if he's telling the truth. Three of the most common methods of taking the drug—snorting, smoking, and injecting—produce characteristic signs. However, two other routes —ingesting the drug or applying it to the genitalia— reveal no visible signs.

Signs of snorting cocaine
Many users consume the powdered form of the drug by snorting it, achieving cortical numbness within 90 seconds. This is soon followed by feelings of euphoria as the drug affects the mesocortical areas (pleasure pathways). The high lasts up to 90 minutes.

To detect these users, look for nasal or sinus irritation and nasal bleeding. You may see changes in the mucosal lining of the nostrils (such as drying or perforations) caused by chronic snorting, which can lead to septal erosion and loss of the sense of smell. But keep in mind that not all users will have these signs and symptoms.

Signs of freebasing cocaine
This is the term for smoking cocaine, the deadliest form of consumption. Freebase users heat a mixture of cocaine and water with ammonium hydroxide or sodium bicarbonate (baking soda) to remove the water, then cool it into a hard chunk that contains a very high concentration of cocaine.

Smoked cocaine flashes and crackles (this is how crack got its name) before blitzing through the body, crossing the pulmonary vascular beds and entering

the brain within 5 seconds. The resulting high lasts about 5 minutes.

Smoking cocaine may not produce telltale external signs. But many freebase users have burns on their fingertips and singed eyebrows and eyelashes from leaning over a lighted pipe.

Signs of injecting cocaine
Some addicts prefer injecting a flame-heated, pasty form of cocaine into their veins, achieving an hour-long high within 60 seconds.

An I.V. user may have ecchymotic spots, I.V. tracks, or scars from previous injections on his extremities. He may also have cellulitis, necrotic skin, or abscesses.

Taking a thorough history
If you suspect, or can confirm, that the patient is a cocaine user, obtain a thorough history of his past surgical and medical problems. Keep in mind that cocaine is particularly threatening to people with a deficiency of cholinesterase, an enzyme that helps metabolize the drug in the liver. This enzyme deficiency can develop congenitally, but it may also appear in older men, children, pregnant women, and patients with liver dysfunction.

Understanding the risks of abuse
To appreciate the tragedy of the cocaine epidemic, you need to know how the drug devastates the body.

Vasospasm
The adrenergic response produced by cocaine includes pupil dilation and increased heart

rate, respiratory rate, myocardial contractility, glucose production, and peripheral vasoconstriction. The drug's most widespread effects result from transient vasospasm, which can occur in any of the major body systems. Vasospasm can lead to angina, myocardial infarction, hypertensive crisis, cerebrovascular accident, and other neurologic complications.

Always keep in mind the sympathomimetic effects of cocaine – specifically, increased myocardial contractility, heart rate, and blood pressure – when dealing with a suspected user. A checklist of possible cardiovascular problems will prove helpful – for example, coronary artery vasospasms, angina, myocardial infarction, hypertension, supraventricular tachycardia, ventricular tachycardia, and ventricular fibrillation, all of which can lead to asystole and cardiac arrest.

In addition, myocarditis is diagnosed in 20% of all chronic users.

Respiratory problems
A cocaine user may develop a chronic cough, pulmonary congestion, pulmonary infiltrates, and severe bronchiolitis. In addition, cocaine use may produce respiratory distress and precipitate respiratory distress syndrome.

If you suspect a patient is a cocaine addict, auscultate for adventitious breath sounds (gurgles, crackles, or wheezes). Use a pulse oximeter to help monitor his arterial oxygen saturation. If his respiratory status deteriorates, notify the doctor, draw

blood for arterial blood gas analysis, and administer oxygen.

Neurologic complications
Cocaine can cause catastrophic neurologic complications, primarily as a result of severe vasoconstriction. Researchers have found cases of subarachnoid hemorrhages and cerebral infarctions caused by cocaine-induced vasospasms. The hemorrhages are believed to result from sudden surges in blood pressure set off by adrenergic stimulation.

———————————— ❖

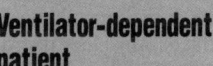

Ventilator-dependent patient

Focusing on the technical aspects of ventilator care is understandable whether you've been assigned to your first ventilator-dependent patient or your hundredth. But, while physical care is important, don't lose touch with the person at the other end of the tubing. Here are some tips to help you treat the patient with respect, dignity, and compassion.

Breaching the communication barrier
You've probably seen some health care professionals speaking slowly and loudly with a ventilator-dependent patient. But the patient isn't deaf or unaware. He simply can't talk because an endotracheal (ET) tube has been passed through his vocal cords. (A patient with a tracheostomy can talk if the tube is plugged so that air passes

through the vocal cords.) Try using some of the methods that follow to achieve effective communication.

Ask yes-or-no questions

Determine how the patient wants to respond: nodding his head for yes and shaking it for no, moving his eyes up for yes and down for no, or wiggling his hands. Avoid blinking, though, because a reflexive blink could be confused with an answer.

Provide tools for writing

If the patient can write, give him plenty of paper and a felt-tipped marker or pencils. Or try an erasable marking board (heavy cellophane over a smooth, black, waxy surface). Any blunt instrument can be used for a "pen," such as a tongue blade, needle cap, or an applicator with the wooden end wrapped in silk tape so it won't rip the cellophane.

Use a letter board

A letter board is another alternative for a patient who isn't strong or coordinated enough to write. These are available in stores, but you can make one yourself by printing the alphabet on a piece of heavy poster board and covering the board with clear plastic paper. The patient can point to the letters to spell words or you can point to each letter and the patient can nod or move his eyes if it's correct. On the back of the board, draw pictures or write the words for some common needs (bedpan, glass of water, and so on). Some hospitals have preprinted instruction boards of commonly used sentences, such as "I'm having pain" or "I want my

family." The patient can point to what he wants without spelling out a lot of words.

Inform the staff

No matter what method you use, it won't help unless others use it too. Pass the word in report and hang a sign over the patient's bed or on the door to his room.

Building a relationship

Most patients on a ventilator need to be assured that someone will respond if they have a problem. They also want to regain some control over their lives.

Unfortunately, when a patient tries to fulfill these needs, he can unwittingly become difficult by putting extra demands on your time. You can alleviate this problem by building a solid, trusting relationship with the patient and giving him some control.

Gain trust

Establish a rapport with your patient by going into his room at the beginning of each shift and saying hello. Chat with him for a few minutes, then ask if he needs anything before you go. He probably will.

After you help him, tell him that you have things to do but that you'll be back at a certain time. Keep your promise. If something comes up, poke your head into the room and tell him that you're dealing with a critical situation but that you'll stop in later. (Be sure to specify what you mean by "later.")

Give control

Allow your patient to take some responsibility for his care. For example, if he has a strong cough, show him how to disconnect the ventilator and cough into a tissue. He might be surprised that you're letting him do that, but it will help make him feel more secure because he can help keep his own airway patent. He's also spared the risk of infection and trauma from suctioning.

If the patient can't cough effectively, teach him how to suction himself. Have him sit upright in bed and disconnect the ventilator. As he watches in a mirror, teach him how to hyperventilate himself, pass the suction catheter down his airway, and suction.

Some patients can contribute to their own care by doing things such as washing their upper body. But don't allow them to do more than they can. They may become short of breath and weak if pushed past the limits of their endurance.

Avoiding self-extubation
A patient who wants to pull out his ET tube presents another challenge. Self-extubation, of course, is very dangerous. The patient loses his airway and he's at risk for anoxia until he's reintubated.

Also, he could traumatize his airway when he pulls the inflated balloon up and out of the trachea. If he damages the tracheal mucosa and vocal cords, he may develop edema that could make reintubation more difficult. Or he could permanently damage or paralyze his vocal cords.

Offer explanations
A simple explanation about the need for the tube and a warning about the risks of self-extubation would be enough for a patient

who's alert and oriented. You can also try various local measures to make him more comfortable—mild sedation (if you aren't trying to wean him from the ventilator), anesthetic spray alongside the tube, or diversional activities.

Use restraints
For a patient who's confused or uncooperative, you may have to use hand restraints and get an order for a sedative. Make sure you assess circulation and skin condition in the restrained hand about once an hour. Also assess the patient's mental status: He may be confused at night but fine during the day, so he may need hand restraints only at night.

Consider alternatives
Here's something else to consider: Is the patient really trying to pull out the tube? If the ventilator tubing is tugging on his nose or trachea, he may be trying to support the ET tube with his hands to feel more comfortable. A nurse could easily misinterpret his actions. Without asking him to explain what he's doing, she might give him a lecture about self-extubation while restraining his hands unnecessarily.

Coping with sensory overload and deprivation
Sensory overload and deprivation can add to a mechanically ventilated patient's confusion—and lead to attempts at self-extubation. The patient has few, if any, ways to screen out noises and disturbances. On most medical-surgical units, he'd be placed near the nurses' station so he

could be easily observed; but that's also the noisiest area on the unit.

Also, he may experience sensory overload and confusion from having his sleep constantly interrupted for procedures and medications. And sensory deprivation can occur simultaneously if he's denied meaningful stimuli, such as a clock, calendar, window, or newspaper.

Decrease confusion
You can decrease your patient's confusion by trying a few simple things. First, to minimize noise, you can have the patient wear a portable headset, watch television, or use a white-noise device (such as a fan). Second, place a clock and calendar where he can see them. Third, try to group nursing activities (medication administration, procedures, and so on) to allow for longer periods of uninterrupted sleep at night.

Administer sedatives as needed
If all else fails, you might ask the doctor to order a sedative – such as diazepam, 5 mg I.V. every 4 hours, with the dosage adjusted to the patient's response. The patient may not respond to sedation alone, though. As a last resort, the doctor might consider pancuronium bromide, a neuro-muscular blocking agent that causes general paralysis, at 0.01 mg/kg every 30 to 60 minutes. (This can be administered only on critical care units, so the patient will be transferred if he isn't already on one.)

He'll be paralyzed by the pancuronium, but he'll still hear and feel everything so he'll be frightened. All procedures should be explained to minimize his fears. A sedative will also be ordered, usually I.V. morphine.

❖

Angry patient

Like most nurses, you probably face a barrage of angry people on a daily basis: the patient who blames you because he didn't sleep well, the family member who says her loved one can't eat the awful food, or the patient who says you took too long to answer the call light.

When responding to these complaints, your natural inclination might be to rattle off excuses – or become angry yourself. Or you might try to change the subject or even get out of the room as quickly as possible. While these responses might make *you* feel better, they won't help the patient or family member. What's more, they tend to keep him angry – and that might cost you more aggravation in the future. To help ease a difficult situation, try making the following four steps a part of your normal response.

Listening actively
This is the most critical step, yet few people take the time and effort to *really* listen.

When you listen "actively," your whole body should say you're listening. Make good eye contact, lean forward slightly, and nod. If your patient's sitting or lying down, you might sit down to be on his level.

Give the person time to talk out his problem without interrupting him or leaping to conclusions. *Concentrate* on what he's saying. Because you want him to know his problem is important to you, don't let anyone interrupt your talk. If you know something unavoidable will interrupt you, warn him about it. Reassure him, however, that you'll get right back to him.

To be sure you've understood the problem, paraphrase what he tells you. And don't hesitate to ask questions. This tells him you're truly interested and may help clarify the problem for you.

Very often, just letting the person talk out his grievance is enough to resolve it. But be alert to the possibility that he's telling only a small part of the problem. You might get at the heart of it with just a few words: "Tell me more about it" or "You still look upset."

Identifying feelings

You need to understand not only *what* the problem is but also *why* it's making the person angry. This can be difficult to do when someone has insulted you, but it does get easier with practice.

Basically, you have to ask yourself what the other person is feeling—then try to put it into words: "It must be frustrating to wait so long for someone to answer your call light." Or simply say, "How do you feel about that?"

This type of response helps pave the way for the person to sort out his feelings. Even he might not know exactly why he's angry. Sharing some of your own feelings might help, too. For example, "I feel bad that I can't spend more time with you" or "I

feel guilty when I have to serve food that's not appetizing to you."

Exploring options

When confronted with an angry patient or family member, many nurses jump in and "fix" the apparent problem. But if you skip the first two steps, you might miss the *real* problem.

There may be more than one possible solution, too, so look at the options. Brainstorm with the person; getting him to help choose which solution to try will give him a sense of being in control again.

For instance, to the patient disturbed by his roommate's snoring, you might suggest, "Do you think earplugs would help?" Or to the wife of a noncompliant diabetic patient who is angry because her husband doesn't follow his diet, you might say, "Maybe you'd like the dietitian to speak with both of you."

If you can't help the person resolve the problem immediately, explain what you plan to do, how long it will take, and when you'll get back to him. *Do* get back to him on time, even if only to report that you're still working on the problem.

Sometimes, of course, you can't do anything to eliminate the problem. But knowing that you've listened and that you care will help appease the angry person.

Increasing the person's self-esteem

Compliment the patient or family member and remember to do so often. You don't need to say anything phony or flattering— just look for things someone does well. Many patients and

DIFFICULT PERSONS

their families feel helpless; a little pat on the back can be reassuring and may be just what they need to know that you respect them.

Compliments can be as simple as "I know you've been patient with us" or "Your father is lucky to have a daughter who cares so much about him."

This might sound like a lengthy process when your time is short. But helping an angry patient can make your job easier and more satisfying in the long run.

❖

Demanding patient

There's one on every unit. The crotchety patient who demands so much of your time that you end up neglecting your other patients. How can you meet his demands without becoming overly frustrated? The following practical tips can help you satisfy the most demanding of patients.

Putting yourself at ease
Take 10 deep breaths or meditate or do whatever you have to, but try to be relaxed when you walk into the patient's room.

Giving him the big picture
Introduce yourself and reinforce your role and the responsibilities of your day: "Hi, Mr. Bolten. I'm Ms. Davister and I'm the nurse caring for you on this shift. I also have five other patients on this unit."

Finding out the cause
When you find out your patient

has been giving others a rough time, say to him, "I understand you had a tough morning and needed the nurses quite often. What was the problem?" The form of these questions is important. Starting the question with "I" instead of "you" is less intimidating; starting with "what" instead of "why" will result in a less defensive answer.

A demanding patient is usually frightened or angry; your questions will help you find out which. He may be frightened about his illness or dying, loss of control, or isolation from family and friends or he may be concerned about his job. He may be angry about his treatment, medical costs, or his increasing dependency.

Defining your expectations
After you know why your patient is so demanding, set limits on his behavior and help him deal with his problem. Tell him that you and the other nurses on the unit are specialists in treating his type of illness. Say that you'll visit him every 40 minutes during the shift and that he can tell you then if he has any problems. If he does, you'll help him resolve them. If the patient's actions are simply unacceptable, tell him. Then find a way to help change the behavior.

Reinforcing his compliance
As you get to know your patient's needs, you'll figure out how to use your visits to meet them. An angry patient may use every opportunity to vent his anger. You don't have to agree with his complaints. Just hold your temper, ask questions to show you're listening, and otherwise

stop talking. Your role is to be a sponge, soaking up the patient's anger. That will give him a feeling of power and control.

A patient who's frightened is more likely to use you as a security blanket. He may not want to talk much, but he's likely to be reassured by contact care, such as back rubs, position changes, or just hand-holding.

At the end of the visit, reinforce your expectations: "I'm going to take care of my other patients now. I'll be back in 40 minutes, and you can tell me then how your medication is working. I appreciate the way you waited to talk to me last time. I'll see you at 4:10."

Giving it a chance
A patient who's been getting away with his demands for several days may take at least that long to accept the new system. A patient who's agitated or confused may take weeks. During the trial period, note the times the system works. With some patients, getting any 40-minute break is a victory.

Knowing when you're licked
You can't possibly cope with all the frustrations some patients cause. When all your efforts fail, look for other alternatives. ❖

Violent patient

You probably think that violent patients are out of control. But control is what violence is all about. Patients (and their fami-

lies) have little control over the hospital environment, and that sense of powerlessness can spark a violent act. Violence is a sure way to get the staff's attention.

When you're on the receiving end of aggression, you might feel angry, hurt, and violated. While understandable, these feelings can impair your handling of violent situations. That's why the first step to managing violence is understanding and governing your own feelings.

The next step is uncovering the violence *before* it strikes. To do that, you'll need to understand that violence is a progressive cycle. By recognizing the three stages of this cycle, you can help avert disaster.

Understanding the three stages of violence
Violence typically progresses through three stages: anxiety, defensiveness, and then aggression.

Acknowledge anxiety
The first signs of cracks in the calm may sneak up on you: A patient is pacing, perspiring, breathing fast, or showing other signs of anxiety. When trying to help, remember that the cause of this free-floating anxiety is generally unknown or made up of many smaller causes.

Don't ask, "Are you okay? What's wrong?" If the patient knew the answer to that, he wouldn't be anxious. In most cases, the patient responds poorly to this type of fact-finding question, perhaps with an angry "I don't know what's wrong! Leave me alone!"

Instead, simply acknowledge his emotions. Statements such as "You look anxious" or "Sounds as if you're upset" tell him you're listening and you care, but whether he responds is up to him. Chances are, if you respect the patient's privacy and dignity, you'll get more information from him.

Calm defensive behavior
If the patient's anxiety isn't noticed or managed, or if it's further provoked, he'll move to defensive behavior. He may threaten you, raise his voice, refuse to answer your questions, or insist that "nothing's wrong." The "last chance" to avoid violence, this phase usually escalates quickly to aggression. Now is the time to set limits in a nonthreatening manner. Here are some examples of limit-setting statements:
• "Sir, there *has* to be quiet here. How can you help me keep things quiet?"
• "Ms. Jones, we have to put these restraints on you. How can you help us?"

The right words alone aren't enough—your tone of voice and body language are vital. Always speak calmly and softly. Keep your arms comfortably at your sides, hands outside your pockets. Folded arms convey a message of "I'm not listening." Besides, your hands aren't free if you need to defend yourself.

Maintain good eye contact and, as the saying goes, "Never let 'em see you sweat." You can admit you're scared, but a calm facade will tell the patient that you're still in control. Remember, though, that many patients

move as quick as lightning from defensiveness to aggression.

Respond to aggression
Rage is the last phase in the cycle. This is the blind, animal-like fury seen in the physical attack, hurling of furniture, or breaking of windows—which, of course, requires immediate intervention.

Handling violent situations
When the patient lashes out in fury, the need for physical restraint is obvious. By following some basic guidelines, you'll not only make the situation safer, you'll also help the patient realize the therapeutic value of applying restraints.

Applying restraints should *always* be a therapeutic action, never an attempt to assert authority or to avenge an emotionally provocative gesture.

To underscore the restraints' therapeutic value, assure the patient that you'll begin removing them as soon as he regains control. For instance, you might say, "Mr. Smith, you've maintained control for 15 minutes. If you can maintain control for another 15 minutes, then we can take one restraint off." Then be sure to fulfill your end of the bargain.

Use teamwork
The key word in applying restraints is teamwork. Managing an emotional emergency, like a medical one, depends on cooperation among staff members.

Establish a unit policy. If any staff member feels restraints are necessary, that decision must be followed. Don't voice disagreements about this clinical decision in front of the patient—save them for the lounge or another private area. Decide ahead of time who will call for help and which staff member will lead the restraint effort.

To immobilize the violent patient with the least number of people and with maximum safety and comfort for everyone, try this: Apply gentle but firm pressure to the major joints, most notably the knees and shoulders. The two people holding the patient's shoulders should, with their other hands, hold his forearms halfway between the elbow and wrist. One or two other people should hold the patient's knees down.

Protect the patient
Whatever form of restraint you use, don't leave the patient alone. A restrained patient is as vulnerable as any other patient who's recently undergone a traumatic experience.

Remember, too, that other confused or unstable patients in the area might hurt an unobserved and restrained patient who can't defend himself. At the very least, place the patient in a room where he can be observed by someone on the staff.

Protect the patient further by checking for impaired circulation at least every 15 minutes. Also, perform complete range-of-motion exercises every 2 hours, or more often. You may need several people's help to free one limb at a time and to guide it through the movements.

Don't forget to protect yourself, too. When using restraints, be sure to document why and how they were used. (See *Protect yourself when applying restraints*, page 510.)

Remove restraints as indicated
As the patient's condition improves, consider removing the restraints. Do it progressively, closely watching his response. If he seems calmer and doesn't seem to want to harm himself or anyone else, you might try loosening or even removing one of the restraints. For example, if you've released the patient's left wrist and you notice that he remains calm 30 minutes later, you could then remove the restraint from the right ankle. "Alternate removal" prevents the patient from throwing himself over the side of the bed or from turning the stretcher over.

If the patient maintains control, remove the two remaining restraints. *Never* leave one limb restrained. The patient could use the stretcher as a weapon, or he could forget that one limb is immobile and injure himself trying to get out of bed.

Dealing with weapons
Although you'll rarely encounter a violent patient with a weapon, you should be prepared for this scenario. In these situations, your most valuable protection is your ability to avoid panic.

If the patient has a knife, maintain eye contact while slowly wrapping your hand and arm in a towel, lab coat, or pillow case. This will help protect you if he lunges at you and you can't escape. If the patient has a gun, speak very clearly and calmly, keeping both hands in sight.

No matter what the weapon is, clear any unnecessary people from the area. Make sure the patient has room to maneuver; cornering him will only increase the

LEGAL LESSON

 Protect yourself when applying restraints

What's your next step after restraining the patient? Document, document, document. Be specific when you explain *why* you restrained a patient. In the eyes of the law, a statement such as "Patient hostile to staff" wouldn't be sufficient grounds to apply restraints. A statement that more clearly reflects the actual incident might be "Patient tore I.V. from site and hit nurse with right arm."

Specific documentation like this will refresh your memory if you have to discuss the incident in court 2 years later. It also clearly indicates the patient was a danger to himself and others, thus diminishing doubt about the need for restraints.

One common pitfall in documenting a restrained patient's progress is an entry like this: "Patient sedated and resting quietly. Difficult to arouse. Restraints intact." If the patient is sleeping that soundly, why is he restrained?

Further, be sure to document *how* the restraints were applied and *by whom*. And don't forget to document range-of-motion exercises, restraint rotation, and each check for impaired circulation.

tension. Assure him that he will get whatever he wants and that he need not hurt anyone.

Whatever you do, don't be a hero. Don't try to jump someone holding a gun. That usually works only in the movies.

❖

Dying patient

When caring for dying patients, you might find yourself caught between wanting to offer support and being afraid of saying the wrong thing. Yet saying nothing can have the same results as saying the wrong thing. The key to talking with dying patients is to be open and honest. All patients need the facts about their illness so they can make decisions for themselves. Dying patients are no exception.

Finding the time

Even if a doctor's order doesn't prevent you from talking freely to the patient, you may feel confounded by another obstacle: not having enough time. Many nurses say the pressure of too little time stops them from really talking to the terminally ill patient. They feel guilty about it.

One way you can handle the stress of not having more time is to visit before or after your shift. Most patients know how busy nurses are without having to be told. They don't "impose" unless they're in need of reassurance or confirmation.

If you have to, make time to talk. When you're having a good exchange with a patient, trust your coworkers enough to ask one to cover your assignments briefly (say, for 20 minutes) while you finish your talk. You can "owe her one."

Avoiding being caught in the middle

Unfortunately, some doctors still withhold information from patients. They may even blatantly lie about the progression of the patient's disease. So you may find yourself torn between your obligation to follow a doctor's order and your reluctance to evade your patient's questions.

But if the doctor wrote an order for the wrong dosage, you wouldn't give it without first discussing it with him. It's the same thing. When a doctor's order and a patient's question put you in the middle, try talking to the doctor. It usually works.

If it doesn't, talk to the patient next. Of course, the doctor might report you to administration, but you shouldn't face any legal repercussions if you haven't volunteered unrequested information (such as metastasis sites), but have merely answered your patient's questions honestly. A doctor may still try to sue for interference with the patient-physician contractual relationship, but this rarely happens.

If the doctor must give the patient bad news, you might offer to go with him. The patient's high anxiety level may lead to selective listening; he may hear only what he wants to hear. By "being there" for the patient, you can clarify information and answer questions long after the doctor has left.

Taking risks

Caring for dying patients is all about risk – risking grief and loss because you've risked feeling love and attachment. The rewards are there, but you have to take a few chances to get them.

If a patient seems agitated and irritable, or depressed and withdrawn, take the chance that he might want to talk. But don't try to second-guess a patient. Ask him directly.

Dying dyspneic patient

More than 60% of lung cancer patients suffer attacks of dyspnea. Other patients are at risk, too. For example, many patients dying of heart disease and other forms of lung disease besides lung cancer experience increasing dyspnea during their final months. And dyspnea occurs in almost 25% of all terminal cancer patients, even those who don't have underlying heart or lung disease.

Dyspnea is an acute (and scary) awareness of a difficulty involved in breathing. Because it's subjective, simply understanding the physical causes of a patient's dyspnea won't tell you how severe the dyspnea is. Neither will his arterial blood gas (ABG) levels, breath sounds, or X-rays. There's no correlation between such objective findings and the severity of a patient's dyspnea. To accurately assess dyspnea, you must evaluate the patient's discomfort and fear.

Gauging an attack

When evaluating a patient's complaints of dyspnea, pay attention to both verbal and nonverbal messages. And ask him to grade his breathing difficulty from 0 to 10, with 0 being "no difficulty" and 10 being "unable to breathe." You can use this scale to evaluate the patient's acute episodes of dyspnea as well as his history of breathlessness. Then you'll have an ongoing record of the patient's discomfort.

To alleviate discomfort during an attack, position your patient upright and administer oxygen at 2 liters/minute. If the doctor has ordered 10-mg tablets of S.L. morphine to be given as needed, give the patient the morphine at this time. You could also encourage a family member to sit with him until his respirations slow down and his anxiety lessens.

Preparing the family

Naturally, family members will want to know how to handle an attack at home. To help prepare them, you'll need to teach them what to expect and how to intervene calmly when the patient becomes breathless. You should begin these lessons as soon as possible after admission.

Tell family members that they must make arrangements so someone will always be available to monitor the patient's condition. That way, they can detect the early indications of breathlessness and respond quickly.

During an attack of dyspnea, a home caregiver should stay with the patient. Stress the importance of not abandoning a patient who feels as though he's suffocating. But give family members fair warning: Tell them that staying with the patient will be difficult because they'll have to listen to him gasp for breath.

Explain that when dyspnea occurs, the caregiver should have the patient sit up and lean forward. Ideally, he should be in a high-backed chair or a bed with the head elevated. This position increases diaphragmatic excursion and reduces the use of accessory muscles. Because of discomfort or disability, some patients won't be able to assume this position. They will, however, assume *their* best position for breathing, so caregivers shouldn't try to make them move.

Administering oxygen

Frequently, administering oxygen makes the patient feel as though he can breathe more easily. Remember, you're dealing with a subjective problem. A patient may feel he's in great distress even though his ABG levels don't indicate that he's hypoxic. And he may feel tremendous relief when you administer oxygen even though his ABG levels don't change.

If family members don't have access to oxygen at home, they should improve air circulation by turning on a fan or opening windows. If these measures don't work, the family might want to investigate obtaining oxygen. You might tell them that sometimes just having it available helps allay a patient's anxiety.

Relying on drugs

Narcotics can help control dyspnea and may even prevent it if administered regularly. These drugs relieve breathlessness by reducing the patient's anxiety, decreasing his awareness of muscle exertion, suppressing ventilatory drive (thus lowering demand on respiratory muscles), and easing vascular resistance (thus reducing pulmonary edema).

Conventional wisdom holds that narcotics shouldn't be given to patients with advanced respiratory disease because of the risk of respiratory depression. Yet hospice nurses regularly administer narcotics to relieve dyspnea. And experience has shown that narcotics, when carefully administered, are not a cause of death in these cases. (See *Narcotics and the dying patient.*)

To reduce a patient's dyspnea, a doctor may order a narcotic to be given S.L., I.V., I.M., or S.C. S.L. morphine is easy to give and is absorbed directly into the bloodstream. Remember, though, that when giving morphine by any route, you should begin with small amounts—2 to 5 mg, depending on the degree of breathing difficulty.

Several drugs that have a sedative effect can also be used to ease dyspnea in a terminally ill patient. These include diazepam; phenothiazines, particularly promethazine; and antihistamines, especially hydroxyzine and diphenhydramine.

Diazepam controls the anxiety associated with breathlessness, but it may also depress the patient's respiratory rate. Promethazine, hydroxyzine, and diphenhydramine are probably ef-

---

RULE OF THUMB

Narcotics and the dying patient

Giving narcotics to a patient with advanced respiratory disease is an ethical question. You'll have to determine if the patient's comfort is worth the risk of respiratory depression. The President's Commission for the Study of Ethical Problems has concluded that giving narcotics to relieve the suffering of a terminally ill patient is acceptable—even when the drugs may suppress breathing. The paramount moral responsibility is to ease the terminally ill patient's suffering.

---

fective because they reduce anxiety, not because they directly affect the patient's breathing. Regular doses of these drugs may be helpful. When given I.M. during acute episodes of dyspnea, they provide striking relief.

Easing the final hours

Terminally ill patients with dyspnea are usually given 0.4 to 1 mg of atropine or 0.4 to 0.6 mg of scopolamine either S.L. or S.C. These anticholinergics dry profuse pulmonary and pharyngeal secretions, which produce a sound commonly called the "death rattle."

Actually, these drugs are more for the family's comfort than the patient's. Suppressing the death rattle helps ease family members' distress. And because death is so close, the adverse reactions caused by atropine or scopolamine (diminished smooth muscle tone, increased heart rate and blood pressure, and excitability) are irrelevant.

Encourage family members to do whatever brings peace to the patient and to themselves. You can teach the patient relaxation and meditation techniques, which may help slow down his respiratory rate and allay his fears. And caregivers can help him visualize open spaces and tranquil scenes. Depending on the patient's beliefs, prayer and pastoral care may also be appropriate.

Handling families

Along with caring for patients comes the additional responsibility of dealing with the patient's family. Many times, these families are in crisis. On other occasions, you may have to break bad news to a family, or ask an unreasonable family to leave. All of these situations require special skill and understanding on your part.

Visitors who overstay

Having visitors can really lift a patient's spirits and even hasten his recovery. But there are times when visitors can do more harm than good. Asking visitors to leave is clearly a judgment call. Here are some guidelines to help you do the right thing.

Considering the patient's condition

Are the visitors endangering the patient's condition? Some visitors become emotional, even hysterical, when they see their loved one hooked up to a ventilator or other equipment. Their reactions can frighten the patient, causing him to fight the equipment. In these cases, you should ask the visitor to leave until he can control his emotions.

Also, are the visitors interfering with the patient's rest? Your patient may be tired, but he doesn't have the heart to ask his family to go. So it's up to you to do it. Keep in mind, though, that some patients prefer napping while their loved ones stay in the room. And as long as they're quiet, why not let them stay?

Check in periodically, however. If the visitors aren't letting the patient get enough rest, they'll have to leave. You might direct them to a waiting area and tell them you'll get them as soon as the patient is awake.

Considering the patient's schedule

Is the patient undergoing an intimate or invasive procedure? If your patient's rectal temperature is being taken, he may not object to the company of his wife or a close relative. Of course, if he wants privacy, ask the visitor to step out into the hallway for a few minutes.

If the doctor is performing a medical procedure, he may want the visitors out of the room. But if the patient prefers company—and the doctor agrees—let the patient choose one person to remain with him. Show this support person where to stand, and explain what he should or shouldn't do. If the procedure upsets him, escort him to the other visitors. Reassure them that the patient is okay and that they can see him when the doctor is finished.

If visitors are keeping you from getting your job done either because they're in the way or they're disrupting successful communication with your patient, ask them to step out until you're finished with the patient. Realize, though, that hovering may be their style of coping. This trait, in fact, may comfort the patient. So don't banish the visitors because you find their behavior offensive.

Considering the visitor's health
Your patient is exposed to enough contagions in the hospital. The last thing he needs is an infection from a family member or friend. Tell any visitor who's obviously ill and whose presence isn't critical that he might help the patient more by staying home until he's well.

Sometimes, however, family members are so distraught over the patient's condition that they, in a sense, become patients themselves. You may end up giving them almost constant reassurance and attention. This is the time to call in the clergy or someone from social services to meet with the family and allow you more time to care for the real patient.

Considering the roommate's needs
Are the visitors disturbing the patient's roommate? If the roommate complains that they're loud or disruptive, ask the visitors to be more quiet. If that doesn't work and the patient is unable to meet them in a waiting area, the visitors will have to go.

Using diplomacy
When asking visitors to leave, be sure to stress that their departure will benefit the patient. If the visitors feel you're being fair and have the patient's best interest at heart, few will argue. Before the visitors go, give them a report on the patient's condition and, if possible, tell them when they can return.

❖

Family in crisis

You routinely meet families in varying stages of response to a loved one's illness. Because family members are emotionally attached to the patient, the stress of his illness can make them unreasonable and demanding.

Although all families are unique, most follow certain predictable stages during the struggle. Recognizing the stages will help you better understand, assess, and interact with your patient and their families.

Recognizing signs of denial
Denial is a common reaction to a harsh or painful reality. Most people learn this avoidance tactic in childhood and continue to use it as a natural defense mechanism against emotional pain and conflict throughout life. When someone becomes ill, the other family members typically react with shock and disbelief. This denial leads to various behaviors, such as rationalizing

away symptoms and resisting treatment.

Clinging to unrealistic expectations is an offshoot of denial. Not to be confused with hope, denial can become destructive if family members refuse to accept the implications of their loved one's illness.

A young mother who rejects the diagnosis that her child has diabetes, for example, may seem uninterested in learning how to give insulin injections. Actually, she may be feeling so overwhelmed or frightened that she's simply unable to cope with the situation.

Although denial usually is transitory, you can't "push" the family out of denial and on to the next stage. Acknowledging this defense as a normal part of the adjustment process is crucial. Your empathy and support can then guide the family to a deeper level of understanding.

Identifying disorganization
Out of denial comes a sense of disorganization. No longer able to deny the obvious, family members may fall into many negative behaviors.

As the crisis of illness disrupts their daily lives, some family members become more demanding and irrational. Their normal coping mechanisms may be useless if nothing in their past has prepared them to deal with their loved one's illness.

This sense of disorganization or floundering may give way to anger and blame—aimed at you. Try to remember that the anger is displaced and temporary—and has nothing to do with you. As

you acknowledge their feelings, offer family members support and concrete assistance. You might, for instance, suggest that they ask neighbors or friends to help them handle routine chores. (You may even have to remind them to eat.)

Understanding anxiety
For most people, a hospital is an alien environment; its unfamiliar procedures, machines, and terminology intensify the emotional turmoil they're already experiencing. Routines you take for granted can worry the patient's family needlessly. Fortunately, this anxiety generally lasts only until the family develops new ways to cope.

Consider the questions doctors and nurses must sometimes ask family members. To people struggling with anxiety, such questions must seem like assaults: "Have you considered placement for your child?" Or "Would you like us to resuscitate your father in the event that his breathing or heart stops?"

Of course, these questions are important and necessary. But because family members are under a great deal of stress, they might have trouble making decisions. This vacillation may frustrate the health care team, creating tension and misunderstanding.

Remember, though, that the family members may be too overwhelmed to confidently make *any* decisions about their loved one's care. Yet, because decisions need to be made quickly, the family is forced to confront critical questions.

Fostering adjustment

More information, more time, and new ways of coping with the reality of their situation help most families adjust to a loved one's illness. This final stage is a *process* of acceptance—not a single event, but an emotional evolution. How quickly family members reach this final stage of adjustment depends a great deal on their emotional strength as individuals and as a unit.

Even though your time is limited, you can still help a family reach the adjustment stage.

Use your assessment skills

To determine how family members are responding to their loved one's illness, ask yourself these questions:
• How are family members communicating with the health care team? Are they angry, quiet, or aggressive?
• How are family members communicating with each other?
• What are they asking and saying?
• What *aren't* they asking or saying?
• Is there a family spokesperson?

Fine-tune your listening skills. Listen not only to the words spoken but also to the feelings expressed and the behaviors exhibited.

After assessing family members' emotional status, choose your response. Don't take any aggression personally. A conflict with the loved one's nurse will only create more turmoil for the family.

Develop a plan of action

To help the family cope, determine what the family needs from you. Be prepared to give specific

help, such as advice on what procedures mean and which outcomes are possible. And get ready to repeat—often—new and important developments.

The most helpful information you might offer is a realistic orientation to the hospital world. Unmet expectations cause anger and resentment, and family members sometimes have many mistaken ideas about hospital life. They may expect the food to be terrific, the doctors to be easily accessible, and the nurses to be available *immediately* when called.

At times, family members may need more than you can give them with your hectic schedule and workload. One way around this dilemma is to call on the social workers, psychologists, or clergy available at the hospital. Don't overlook community resources, either, such as crisis centers or private therapists.

Family receiving bad news

You probably feel nervous and upset when you have to give a patient's family bad news. That's because you know the news—whether it's a turn for the worse, a longer hospital stay, or the possibility of more surgery—will dash the family's hopes, at least temporarily.

The news might force family members to face a radical change in their lives, and some families can't cope with that possibility. How you communicate bad news can make a big difference in how a patient's family will cope.

Finding a private spot

Knowing where to give family members bad news is almost as big a problem as knowing what to tell them. You've probably been taught that you should tell families bad news in private, but finding a private moment in a private place isn't easy in a busy hospital.

Sometimes, drawing a family away to a private area overdramatizes the situation, making the news seem much worse than it actually is – and upsetting the family unnecessarily.

When you're not sure whether to deliver the news in private or not, ask the family: "I'd like to talk to you about Jeffrey's surgery. Are you comfortable here, or would you like to sit with me in the conference room?"

If you have to give a family very bad or unexpected news, though, privacy's best. In these situations, the family needs to be free to cry, to ask questions, and to adjust to the shock without worrying about other people's reactions. The privacy also protects other patients and families, who might be frightened by the news you're delivering.

Even if the news isn't particularly serious, you'll need to lead a family off to a private room sometimes simply to escape noise and constant interruptions. Freedom from these distractions will help the family concentrate on your news, reducing the likelihood of misunderstandings. And it will show them you care

enough to give their needs and comfort priority.

When you need privacy to escape distractions, put the family at ease by saying something such as "Let's find a quieter place to talk" or "Let's go in the conference room, where we won't be interrupted."

Giving a reason for hope

You and the family members will feel better if you can find some positive aspect in the bad news. Usually you can. That doesn't mean you should minimize the seriousness of the message, but you should try to provide a framework that offers the family some encouragement. Following are five techniques that can help.

Specify "what is"

Too often, people think in terms of what isn't: The patient *isn't* any better. The treatment *isn't* working. The operation *didn't* succeed.

Such a vague, negative response invites the family to speculate on the patient's condition, fuels unnecessary fears, and adds to feelings of helplessness. It's better to be specific about what the patient's condition is – not what it isn't: "Your aunt's condition has worsened in the last hour. She has a fever of 102° F, she's developed pneumonia, and she's quite restless."

Describe the staff's efforts

Don't stop after you've explained "what is." Give the family something to feel hopeful about by describing what the staff has done to counter the setback: "The doctor has started I.V. antibiotics and nasal oxygen to combat the pneumonia. He's started her on a mild tranquilizer to relieve her restlessness. And we're using aspirin and frequent sponge baths to try to bring her fever down."

Don't limit your report to treatment measures aimed at a cure. Even if a patient is beyond hope of cure, you can comfort the family by describing palliative measures: "We're keeping ahead of your father's pain by giving pain medication every 3 hours, and we've been turning him every hour and rubbing his back. He seems much more comfortable than he did last night."

Accentuate the positive
Sometimes you can soften the blow by accentuating positive aspects of the situation. To find something positive in a serious situation, try looking at the long-term effects. For example, if you tell a wife that her husband is unlikely to return to his former job, she may despair and imagine him an invalid. To help her see the positive side, tell her about former patients who've succeeded at less taxing careers and who've learned to appreciate family life and other pleasures they didn't have time for previously.

If you have to tell parents that their child needs more surgery, try to find examples of his improved coping skills. You might say, for example: "Remember how David cried before his surgery last month? Today, he was comforting another boy on the unit. He's really learned to handle the situation well."

Display confidence
One of the greatest tools you have for disarming a family's fear is to display confidence in

the quality of health care at your hospital.

If the patient is on a ventilator, mention the high-quality skills of your respiratory therapy department. If the patient has a serious condition, tell the family how often your unit has successfully cared for others with the same problem.

Get the family involved
Bad news increases a family's feelings of helplessness and powerlessness. Overcome these feelings by encouraging them to redirect their energy from worrying about the patient to contributing to his improvement.

Some family members will be comforted by their ability to give bedside help—giving bed baths, reading to the patient, or feeding him. Other family members may feel uncomfortable providing physical care, but they may be willing to act as liaisons between the family and the doctor or to offer encouragement to other family members.

❖

Family after the patient dies

Each family has its own way of mourning the death of a loved one. Reactions to grief differ, but they fall within a certain range of feelings and symptoms. Yet every family shows some common reactions, which will help you decide what kind of support is needed.

DIFFICULT PERSONS

Symptoms of grief

Families respond to death with both mental and physical grief symptoms. Warn family members that they may experience these symptoms (and watch for them in yourself, too, especially if you were close to the patient):
• anger
• anorexia
• backache
• depression, sadness
• dry mouth
• dyspnea
• exhaustion
• guilt
• headaches
• hollow feeling in the stomach
• inappropriate hostility
• insomnia
• loss of familiar behavior patterns
• lump in the throat
• malaise
• nasal congestion
• nightmares
• preoccupation with images of the dead person
• scratchy eyes
• tears.

Sharing your knowledge
Grief can be best described as a distinct syndrome with predictable psychological and somatic symptoms. You can help grieving families by warning them to expect some of the symptoms after the initial shock of the death. (See *Symptoms of grief*.) Most people have no idea that grief can cause such an array of symptoms, and without your warning, they may feel they're "going crazy." They need your assurance that they're not.

Most people are also unaware of the duration of grief. The acute symptoms associated with the grief syndrome may last for up to a year, with diminishing intensity. But the period of readjusting psychologically to the loss may continue for another year or more. It's complete when the person is able to begin new projects and invest his energy and interest in the community and people around him.

Encouraging good-byes
Many surviving family members have a deep need to say good-bye after a loved one dies. Seeing and touching the body confirms the reality of death and gives the family a feeling of relationship with the body that hospital procedures too often destroy.

Despite this almost desperate need to see and touch the body, many families may be too frightened to ask or to touch without your help. The cultural taboo against touching "death" is that strong.

You can help in several ways:
• Show the family that *you're* comfortable. Put your hand on the bed or on the deceased patient while you're talking to the family; then put your arm around a family member and lead him to the bedside.
• Treat the deceased patient as a *person* in the family's presence. A frightened, grieving family will react to even the most subtle indications that you're indifferent or disrespectful to the dead person.

• Let families decide how much time they need to say good-bye. Many families recognize intuitively that their grief would have been easier to bear if they'd only "had more time to say good-bye."
• Encourage the family to spend some time with the body, but don't insist. A few people will choose not to see the dead person. If that's their preference, show your approval of it.

Showing your emotions

You've been taught professional detachment. But many family members, particularly women, feel comforted when a nurse holds them or cries with them over a patient's death.

They'll be touched by your caring and empathy. Perhaps more important, they'll interpret your expression of loss as permission to show their feelings. Also, by displaying your feelings, you help initiate the grieving process for families who feel such shock over the death that they can't absorb its emotional impact.

Suggesting ongoing support

Many grieving people feel totally alone. Sometimes, doctors and nurses avoid the grieving family or pretend nothing happened after a loved one dies.

Perhaps you think it's not your place to offer this type of support – that family and friends will provide a loving network for the grieving person. All too often, though, relatives and friends avoid the survivor, so it's up to you to offer support. Here's what you can do:
• Encourage families to accept specific offers of help. Many feel

protected when a friend or relative acts as an "alter ego" for the first few days after the death. The friend can perform many functions, such as answering the phone, notifying relatives, helping with funeral arrangements and meal plans, driving and, most important, preventing loneliness.
• If families don't have anyone to help them, suggest that they contact some support networks.

Helping the grieving family may not be easy. But with these techniques and your careful assessment and understanding, you won't have to stand by uncomfortably, not knowing what to do or say.

—————————————❖

Handling coworkers

Because nursing requires you to work closely with other staff members, another person's shortcomings, emotions, or idiosyncrasies can interfere with how you do your job. Any friction between you and your colleagues may be relatively minor and easily resolved through understanding and better communication. Or it may involve a drug-abusing coworker, unsafe practices, or sexual harassment, endangering the welfare of your patients or other staff members or jeopardizing your job. Knowing how to handle yourself can help avert serious problems.

DIFFICULT PERSONS

Rude doctor

A doctor's overbearing behavior can turn your shift into an endurance test. To ensure that it doesn't, you need to take immediate action to get things under control.

You probably know from experience that seething in silence or fighting back doesn't help. Instead, you'll want to calm things down quickly. And because you'll probably have to work with this doctor again, you should develop a long-range plan to head off future disturbances.

Taking immediate action

You might feel embarrassed and angry if a doctor reprimands you—especially in front of a patient and his visitors. But don't strike back with a statement such as "If I changed your patient's dressing and he got an infection, you'd be the first to blame me." He may only become defensive—and more aggressive.

In such a case, you need to confront the situation promptly and deal with the doctor directly. For example, you might say, "Doctor, I'd like to talk with you. Obviously, you were angry when you first came on the floor. But I don't appreciate taking the brunt of your anger when I haven't done anything wrong. The dressing wasn't changed because I'm following hospital policy."

This technique will work because it will call the doctor's attention to a behavior he may not be aware of and point out that his behavior is inappropriate.

Making a long-range plan

When a doctor is rude to everyone, work together to change his behavior. Collaborate with your staff so everyone agrees upon how to handle the situation. For example, you could decide that when the doctor lashes out at a nurse, she'll reply in a matter-of-fact tone, "Excuse me, doctor," then walk away. If he begins the same lecture with another, she should politely excuse herself. And any of you could say, "Doctor, I'll be glad to talk with you when you address me professionally."

❖

Agency nurse

Many staff nurses fall into the trap of stereotyping agency nurses as not being committed to the profession, putting in only the minimum amount of effort, and showing little interest in their work—of being in it only for the money. While this may be true of some agency nurses—and some staff nurses, too—the majority are competent professionals who've simply chosen to work through an agency because they need a flexible schedule. Or perhaps they're new to the area and are trying to decide where to work. (See *Tips for agency nurses.*)

The next time an agency nurse is assigned to your unit, recognize that she's there to help. Here's how you can open the lines of communication.

Tips for agency nurses

Walking into a new environment and trying to function at your maximum capability is difficult. As an agency nurse, you're constantly starting a new job, which means you regularly have to prove your competence. Following these tips can help ensure that your stay is productive and congenial:

• Ask your agency to provide, at the minimum, an environmental orientation.

• Ask your agency to provide the hospital with a profile listing your credentials, strengths, and weaknesses.

• Arrive 15 to 20 minutes before the start of your first shift to acquaint yourself with the hospital and unit.

• Become an effective member of their team by communicating effectively. Begin by introducing yourself to the staff, asking who the charge nurse is, and finding out whether a resource person will be assigned for questions.

• Tell the staff what kind of orientation you've had to the unit. Then say that you're open to their comments and suggestions and want to make yourself as efficient and effective as possible for them.

• Present yourself as a professional. This should help break down any preconceived ideas that the staff has about agency nurses. Be courteous, yet stand firm on issues that may compromise your state's nurse practice act.

• Stay open to questions from staff members; don't alienate them by forcing your opinions on them.

Getting off on the right foot

Start by introducing yourself and the other staff members. Identify the nurse-manager and the charge nurse and tell the agency nurse who will be her resource person. If she hasn't been oriented to the unit, make sure she's shown around.

Encourage the other members of the unit to include the agency nurse in their groups for breaks and dinner. If the agency nurse feels well received, she may be willing to come back, stay extra hours when the staff doesn't want to, or sign up for another time when staffing is low. If staff members keep open minds, they may be able to learn a new way to do a particular procedure or gain a fresh perspective on an old problem.

Enhancing the working relationship

You can go even further to improve the relationship between staff nurses and agency nurses in your hospital. Ask your administration to do the following:

• Require the agency to give nurses an orientation to the unit they'll work on.

• Encourage the agency to develop a core group of people

who return to your health care facility on a regular basis.
• Require the agency to provide the hospital with nurse profiles listing credentials, strengths, and weaknesses.

On your own unit, you can do the following:
• Encourage staff meetings to discuss agency nurses, their role on your unit, and ways to make the most of their abilities and to promote better communication.
• Develop a way to evaluate patient care delivered by agency nurses so that they can receive feedback.
• Realize that if an agency nurse likes your unit, she could become a recruitment candidate for your hospital.

When the staff nurse and the agency nurse work together as colleagues toward a mutual goal, everyone benefits. Because the staff nurse gets the kind of assistance she needs, her morale and overall job satisfaction should be better. The agency nurse, as part of the team, can take more pride in her patient care contributions and her relationship with team members.

❖

Coworker who mistreats AIDS patients

You and your colleagues might prefer *not* to have a patient with acquired immunodeficiency syndrome (AIDS). Perhaps you're anxious about contracting the disease – even though you know that, with proper precautions, you have little to fear. But you're

professionals, so you try not to let your personal feelings affect the care you give. And you realize that AIDS patients often feel scared and vulnerable.

But some of your colleagues may act as though *they're* the vulnerable ones. Sensitive only to their own feelings, they're abrupt and rough with the patients. They may be obsessive about infection control, insisting on double sets of gloves, even performing complete surgical scrubs to check vital or neurologic signs – in full view of the patient.

Getting involved
When you see this happening, you'll need to take action. Follow these steps:
• *Documentation.* Keep a log of every incident of verbal or physical abuse.
• *Education.* Circulate copies of journal articles and epidemiology updates on AIDS to all staff members. This will keep you all informed and reduce fear without singling anyone out.
• *Cooperation.* Arrange for a staff member to be present when the colleague examines the patient. The staff member can hand her extra gloves, help her position the patient, and scrub the sink with disinfectant more calmly than the colleague might on her own. If your manner around AIDS patients is matter-of-fact, perhaps your colleague will relax and treat the patients more gently.
• *Confrontation.* Challenge the colleague whenever she degrades a patient. Ask her how she'd feel if she were treated that way, how she thinks the patient feels, and how you can help her be

more considerate. Your colleague might be shocked, embarrassed, and defensive, but this approach might force her to think about what she's doing.

Planning for the future

To discourage similar problems in the future, develop a plan that includes the following approaches:

• *Staff education.* Hold regular seminars on AIDS with speakers from the Centers for Disease Control and Prevention or local research facilities, and give orientation classes to all new staff members, including doctors. Start a small unit library and stock it with the latest information on AIDS.

• *Staff support group.* Once a month, have all staff members who work with AIDS patients meet for an informal group session to air frustrations, solve problems, and confront fears.

• *Patient education.* Be honest with patients to help reduce feelings of degradation. When you explain isolation rationales, focus on the disease organism, not on the patient. For example, if a patient complains about meal tray precautions, explain, "We don't dislike touching you. But the organisms causing AIDS are carried in saliva, so we must use disposable eating utensils and double-bag them after you use them."

Be honest, too, about other staff members' behavior. If someone is rude, explain that even doctors and nurses act thoughtlessly at times.

• *Interdisciplinary team.* Assemble a psychiatric social worker, a hospital chaplain, a doctor, a nurse and, if appropriate, a member of the local Gay Task Force to monitor AIDS treatment. Have the group meet periodically to discuss such issues as staff and patient education, infection control, psychosocial concerns of patients and staff, treatment protocols, and ethical and privacy concerns.

You may discover that your awareness efforts – and a similar program – could benefit patients with disorders such as hepatitis, tuberculosis, herpes, leprosy, alcoholism, drug addiction, or morbid obesity – and the staff members who care for them.

❖

Alcohol abuser

If you suspect that a coworker has a drinking problem or – worse yet – drinks on the job, you should say something. Her actions may jeopardize patient safety.

First try talking with your colleague about your suspicions. Doing this gives her a chance to admit the problem, discuss the situation on her own with the nurse-manager, and agree to enter a program for substance abusers. If she denies having a problem, you can tell her you're going to talk with the nurse-manager yourself. Then do it.

Checking hospital policy

Perhaps you think you have to catch the coworker in the act before the nurse-manager can take any action. This may not be true. Ask the nurse-manager for a copy of the hospital's policy on suspected alcohol abuse among employees. Double-check whether, in fact, nothing can be done without proof. The policy may distinguish between a "troubled" employee (one who is suspected of having a problem but whose work hasn't been affected) and an "impaired" employee (one whose work has been affected by the suspected problem). See what action the policy requires and whether the hospital will continue employing your coworker if she undergoes treatment and participates in a recovery program.

Maintaining confidentiality
Refrain from sharing with others any information about your coworker's suspected—or actual—problem or the matter's resolution. Remember, her feelings and professional reputation are at stake.

❖

Drug abuser

If you discover a coworker taking drugs, you have several options. But one of them isn't remaining quiet. Like it or not, you have to get involved. Until recently, many people believed that nothing could be done for addicts until they "hit bottom." Today, it's widely recognized that various approaches can motivate a person to get treatment before that happens. One of those treatments is the increasingly popular intervention.

Taking action
Intervention, a precursor to treatment, helps an impaired person acknowledge the problem and seek treatment. It's an organized, nonpunitive effort in which a group of people confronts the impaired person about her behavior and its consequences. The intervention is directed and the group is guided by a facilitator (team leader)—usually an addictions nurse or other professional in the field of chemical dependence.

The intervention team includes 2 to 10 carefully selected people who represent not only the impaired person's professional life but her personal life too—her manager, coworkers, family members, and others who are concerned about her well-being. If possible, someone recovering from chemical dependency should be included. That person's expertise and personal experience can be invaluable.

Planning the intervention
The intervention doesn't have to be scheduled in advance, but a planned intervention works best. Planning allows for organization and rehearsal and gives the team leader time to conduct a thorough investigation, including a review of appropriate records and documentation of incidents. It also gives each team member a chance to thoroughly understand what will occur.

Each team member must accept the person's destructive behavior as part of her illness and understand that her actions don't mean she's a "bad" person. Anyone who can't accept that premise shouldn't take part in the intervention.

That's not to say one or more team members can't feel anger toward the impaired person. For instance, if coworkers discover the impaired person has been volunteering to relieve them of specific tasks just to gain greater access to controlled substances, they have a right to be angry. The impaired person is not only jeopardizing the safety of her own patients but theirs too. However, intervention participants must defuse their anger *before* the intervention takes place. The team leader or another professional should help them to deal with their feelings.

In some cases, an intervention can't be well planned. For instance, when the impaired person's behavior poses an immediate danger to patients or herself, intervention must take place as quickly as possible.

Typically, intervention occurs in three stages: documentation, confrontation, and recommendations.

Document your observations
Documentation is crucial to a successful intervention. Each team member must document her observations. Specific details must be compiled, including the time and date of each incident, where it occurred, what happened, and who witnessed it.

Each participant's account should include objective information as well as feelings about what happened and how the impaired person's behavior affected the participant. The team leader should help the group delete any statements that could be misleading or viewed as judgmental.

While team members are documenting their observations,

the team leader reviews patients' charts, nurses' notes, doctors' orders, and medication (and narcotics) administration records, along with the impaired person's personnel file.

Confront the individual
The meeting room should be private and away from the impaired person's unit. Arrange the chairs in a circle but not around a table, which may give the impression of a court or tribunal. Leave an empty chair for the impaired person opposite the door. The team leader should sit on one side of her; the team member who's emotionally closest to her should sit on the other side.

After explaining why the group has gathered, the team leader should ask the impaired person not to interrupt. Each participant should begin with a positive statement such as "I could always depend on you in the past" or "I really care about you and admire your professional skills." The participant then reads her documentation aloud.

When everyone is finished, give the impaired person a chance to respond. Unfortunately, no matter how thorough the documentation or how compassionately it's shared, some people refuse to admit they have a problem. However, even if an impaired person continues to deny the addiction, the intervention is *never* a failure.

Make recommendations
During the final stage of intervention, the team leader offers the impaired person some options. Basically, the team leader recommends that the person un-

dergo a professional assessment and enter a treatment program, sometimes called a diversion program. If the person refuses, the consequences could include loss of employment and referring the case to the appropriate state board.

Ideally, the impaired person will recognize the problem and agree to enter a treatment program. Sometimes, the person refuses to recognize the problem but agrees to undergo treatment anyway—for the sake of her job.

If the person agrees to treatment, the team leader should ask her to sign a release form permitting the treatment center to let her manager know if she's complying with the program. Finally, the team leader should record what happened during the meeting, including commitments that were made.

❖

Unsafe practices

You know you have a moral obligation to report dangerous, unethical, or illegal practices that may harm your patients. But few situations present a clear, undeniable wrong.

Personal conflicts may add to your uncertainties. You might, for example, feel torn by your loyalty to a colleague or your loyalty to the hospital, if either one is at fault. You might face disapproval from other colleagues. You might endanger your promotion and—in rare circumstances—your job. The threat of legal action could be troubling, too.

The risks are many. Unfortunately, risks are part of your professional responsibilities. There are ways, though, to minimize your risks when you blow the whistle.

Describing the situation
First, write a clear, precise description of the situation. When you finish, your description should answer these questions:
• What, exactly, is the dangerous practice?
• Who, exactly, is endangered, and how?
• How, specifically, would your blowing the whistle be protective?

Make sure you can state in *concrete, specific terms* what's wrong and why it's wrong. A gut feeling isn't enough.

Don't give up too soon. If you're so upset you can't write a clear, precise description, get some help from an uninvolved friend. If your answers seem vague, you either haven't tried hard enough or blowing the whistle is inappropriate.

Don't calculate the risks, and don't evaluate your chances of success. Do one thing at a time.

Maintaining accuracy
Your goal is to stop dangerous, unethical, or illegal behavior. Since this may entail discipline against the person responsible, you must have accurate, detailed, reliable information to back you up.

Remember the keys to accuracy:
• Document everything pertinent.
• Seek verification from others.
• Stick to the facts.

Assessing your motives

Your testimony may be automatically dismissed or discounted if you have self-serving motives. To make sure you're as credible as possible, ask yourself:

• Is my reputation above reproach? If you're considered competent, reliable, honest, and levelheaded by those you work with, you're probably credible.

• What are my motives? Sour grapes, jealousy, or the likelihood of personal gain from your actions will damage your credibility. Genuine concern for your patients or for public health will increase your credibility.

• What codes, rules, regulations, and laws support blowing the whistle in this case? If your case is against a nurse, review the American Nurses' Association's code of ethics. If a doctor is involved, consult the American Medical Association's principles of medical ethics.

Try to find out whether any hospital policies, local and state regulations, or licensing statutes have been violated. The more violations, the more authority and credibility your claim will have. Not only have your personal sensibilities been offended, but the principles of the profession, the rules of the institution, or the laws of the state may have been violated as well.

At this point, you should know whether you have a case for blowing the whistle. If you think you do, proceed.

Getting support

Don't try to be a solitary whistle-blower. If you feel you have to say something, don't make your commitment a matter of record until you've recruited at least one trustworthy confidant and adviser. You need someone who's:

• stable, but willing to take a risk
• open-minded, but decisive
• caring, but clearheaded
• close enough to the situation to understand it, but far enough from it to be objective.

A nurse from another unit, a social worker, or a doctor may come closer to meeting these qualifications than a colleague on your unit.

Following the proper channels

Use the system. You want to get effective action at the lowest possible level. Under most conditions, this means starting with your nurse-manager. (If she's the person you're reporting, go to *her* supervisor.)

If you get no response from your first-line supervisor, go up the ladder. If necessary, go beyond the organization to regulatory agencies, law-enforcement bodies, licensing bureaus, and professional organizations. (See *Going up the ladder*, page 530.)

Standing behind your accusations

Blowing the whistle anonymously has serious drawbacks. Those who review your charges may have trouble evaluating their accuracy and won't know how to get more information. They're likely to suspect the motives of an anonymous tipster, too.

Some won't consider a complaint seriously if the person bringing the charges isn't willing to stand behind them. This is

Going up the ladder

Here's why you should use an "up-the-ladder" approach:
• You want to stop the dangerous practice, not punish someone. By going through channels, you'll minimize damage to personal and hospital reputations.
• If you have to go public later, your credibility will be stronger if you tried to get action on the inside first.
• Going up the ladder will give you a chance to defend your case against managers, department heads, and other organization "rungs." They may identify weak areas in your case that you can strengthen.
• Personal and professional risks are greater if you go outside first. You may be labeled a "traitor" by your colleagues. You might also be disciplined by your organization for not following procedures.

An exception to the rule: If the offensive practice is very dangerous and delay might cause harm or even death to a patient, you're justified in choosing the quickest route. Sometimes this means going outside the institution immediately.

the time to take a risk. You'll enhance the professionalism of nursing – as well as the safety of your patients – by accepting responsibility for any charges you bring.

Being persistent

When you blow the whistle, you're obliged to see the problem through – until the dangerous practice is stopped.

Supervisors who want to cover up the situation may assure you that they'll "take care of the problem." You can show your persistence with some management techniques. For example, follow up your report to a supervisor with one of these comments:
• "When may I expect a result?"
• "Let's look at your calendar...I'll check back with you on Monday morning."
• "I could take this matter to the director. But I'd like to think we can solve the problem at this level."
• "I want you to understand that I think this is a very serious and dangerous problem. I must continue to press for action until it's stopped."

❖

Sexual harassment

Like many nurses, you have had your share of lecherous looks and patronizing pats, but how about real sexual harassment? If a coworker, a doctor, a supervisor, or even a patient makes inappropriate remarks to you, propositions you, or makes you feel that your job is in jeopardy if you don't succumb to his advances, that's serious business.

You can't prevent sexual harassment, but you don't have to be an easy mark, either. Here's what you can do to discourage improper advances and, even more important, what you can do if you're a victim of sexual harassment.

Discouraging sexual harassment
The best course of action is to try to ward off harassment at the outset. Follow these guidelines:
• *Act professionally.* Be friendly, but not too friendly. Don't divulge details of your social life.
• *Differentiate between business and pleasure.* There's a big difference between lunch in the cafeteria and "a drink after work." But if you're uncomfortable about even a lunch date, ask a coworker along.
• *Beware of special favors.* A nurse-manager who asks you to run personal errands is taking liberties. But a nurse who asks a manager for special favors is taking chances. Suppose your boss tries to collect?
• *Ignore advances.* If he says, "How about a drink?" you might say, "That reminds me. Mrs. Baker seems a little dehydrated; could you please check on her?"
• *Confront directly.* Joke or be blunt, but make sure your message is "I'm not interested."
• *Threaten.* Say you'll contact his supervisor, his spouse, your lawyer, or all of them—even if you have no intention of actually doing so.

Reporting sexual harassment
If your attempt to thwart the harassing behavior fails, consider taking these steps:
• *Go over his head.* Take the problem to his supervisor, but lay your groundwork carefully. Keep a written record of your sexual harassment. Include when, where, how, and under what circumstances harassment

took place. Ask coworkers to speak on your behalf. Be prepared, though, for disappointment. Sexual harassment has been in the closet so long that many supervisors (men *and* women) aren't comfortable dealing with it. So your problem might be ignored.
• *Go to the Equal Employment Opportunity Commission (EEOC).* But do this only if you're prepared to quit your job. Even though the EEOC prohibits employer retaliation, working for people you're suing can be awkward.

❖

Complaints

Whenever you have a complaint about your job, you should bring it to your nurse-manager's attention. But make sure you follow your hospital's grievance procedure. If your hospital doesn't have a grievance procedure, then follow the guidelines below.

Taking the first step
Approach your manager and ask to meet privately with her to discuss your complaint. Note the date when you take this step and any subsequent steps.

If your manager puts off your request for a meeting, write up the complaint and submit it to her. Make sure you keep a copy for your records.

Whether you present your complaint orally or in writing, make sure it's factual (don't include opinion or hearsay), to the point (don't ramble), specific (don't generalize), and fair (don't attack others).

Stating your complaint properly

A *properly stated complaint* would be: "I've requested two special days off, at the beginning of October and in the middle of June. You've turned down my requests both times. I haven't received any explanation of why my requests were denied. I'd like to discuss this matter with you."

An *improperly stated complaint* would be: "Why don't you ever grant my requests for days off? I'm constantly amazed at how the rest of the staff always gets what they want. I'd like to know if there's something about me that you don't like. I do my best to please you, but you've obviously chosen to ignore my requests. I demand to know why."

Waiting for a response

Give your nurse-manager time to respond to your complaint. Wait several days before approaching her again.

If your nurse-manager still fails to respond or doesn't give you a satisfactory answer, tell her you intend to go to a higher authority with your complaint.

If your manager *still* doesn't act, make an appointment with a higher authority. This person should review your complaint and the record you've kept of how you've handled the situation. She may invite your manager to come to the meeting with you so the issue is confronted openly.

———————————❖

Handling staff

A nursing unit is like a wheel — if all its parts work together, things roll along smoothly. But if one spoke on the wheel is broken, or one nurse on the unit is impeding others or not doing her share, the ride can get pretty bumpy. Following are some typical problems you may encounter among your staff and ways of getting around them.

Complainer

Almost every unit has a nurse who finds fault with her patients, her supervisors, her peers, her family, her health, even the weather. She thinks her patient loads are too heavy. She thinks her patients are ungrateful. She thinks some of the nurses are lazy.

You're probably tempted to tune out the complainer, but if you listen, you'll realize she's telling you one of three things:
• She doesn't know why her manager has made certain decisions that affect her or even what her manager expects.
• She's frustrated by her lack of control over her job.
• She's getting rewards for complaining.

Making expectations known

Many people don't know what their supervisors want or why. Complaining is their roundabout way of saying "Look, I don't understand what's going on."

Offering explanations – and involving others in your activities – goes a long way toward reducing complaints. For instance, if you need to assign some of your tasks to a licensed practical nurse (LPN) because you're swamped, don't just give the LPN the extra work and assume she'll realize how busy you are. Explain to her *why* you need her help and assure her that you're grateful for it.

If you have to be off the floor all day at meetings, tell your staff where you'll be and what you'll be doing. Afterward, report on the meetings you've attended. Knowing why you have to leave the floor will ease your staff's resentment on a busy day. And sharing information with them later will help them see the value of your meetings.

Even so, explaining *why* isn't enough. You also have to explain *what* – what they expect from the other person's performance. Make clear what results you want. If you don't, you'll hear complaints that are really a demand for structure.

Say, for example, you have a staff nurse who habitually complains about having to stay late to complete her work. She's probably really wondering if you expect her to get all her tasks done on time. You might want to discuss with her how she plans her day to discover if she's overworked or if she needs help setting priorities and managing her time. When you've given her these guidelines, tell her that you expect her to complete her work on time. With that expectation made clear, *you'll* be the one who complains if she doesn't finish on time.

Allowing some control

Many nurses are frustrated by their lack of control over their work situation. And their frustration is a second cause of many chronic complaints.

You can't give everyone complete control over patient care. But you can involve nurses in some decisions by asking them for their suggestions.

By involving the complainer in your decisions, you're rechanneling negative energy. Say, for example, your hospital is switching from team to primary nursing and one team leader is complaining constantly. Instead of ignoring her, offer her a position on the primary-nursing steering committee. She just might become one of the most enthusiastic supporters.

Satisfying the need for attention

A chronic complainer doesn't get traditional rewards like respect and admiration. But she does get attention. If she's a strong personality on the unit, she may be able to create dissatisfaction among the rest of the staff and *that* can be a tremendous reward.

Obviously, you have to be sure you don't take away the rewards of complaining without replacing them. You have to make an effort to compliment the person on her successes during this period. Unfortunately, we all seem to see failures more easily than successes – particularly with regard to a person who has been a disruptive influence on the unit in the past.

To provide effective reinforcement, keep anecdotal notes on the person's performance, and discuss them with her at regular intervals.

For most nurses, the attention given to their efforts – and eventual success – at meeting their problems will satisfy more needs than complaining ever did.

Supporting the rest of the staff

While you're working to turn the complainer into a productive and positive force on the unit, don't forget to continue to give the rest of your team encouragement with your own positive attitudes.

❖

late. Make it clear that lateness is excusable only in exceptional circumstances; reprimand the individual promptly. Remember: Reprimand her for the *behavior* only. Let the staff member know you don't dislike her – just *what she does*.

• Praise your staff occasionally for being on time. Saying at report "It's great to see you all here on time" shows that you appreciate their promptness.

• Be sure to compliment staff members who've overcome their lateness problems. Reward their efforts to change.

❖

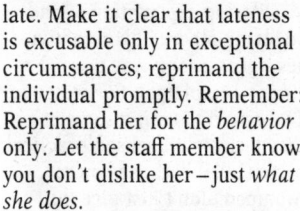

Chronic latecomer

A staff member who is chronically late complicates everyone's schedule. Not showing up on time creates more work for everyone else. A nurse who's late misses report, for one thing. And if she's not there in time to prepare her patient for surgery, someone else will have to pitch in and do it for her. In no time, the whole unit is behind schedule.

If you have a staff member who is a chronic latecomer, try these techniques to get her back on track:

• Set a good example by always being on time yourself.

• Take the change-of-shift report immediately so the previous shift can leave on time and your shift can start on time. This conveys to your staff the importance of punctuality.

• Try to nip the problem in the bud if someone starts coming in

Backstabber

Backstabbing is a classic example of passive-aggressive behavior. A backstabber won't disagree with your new plan to your face, but as soon as you turn your back, she'll sabotage it by complaining to others, breaking promises, or not doing her part to fulfill the plan. Keeping your plans from being sabotaged requires attention to the three steps that follow.

Avoiding jumping to conclusions

If you notice a staff member exhibiting passive-aggressive behavior – such as fidgeting or not looking at you but refusing to express an opinion – don't assume you know why she's upset. Instead, ask her directly what's bothering her.

You might be surprised to discover that she's not concerned about the new scheduling system you're proposing but is worried about learning how to use a new piece of high-tech equipment on the unit.

Analyzing the problem

Getting a passive-aggressive nurse to admit what's upsetting her isn't always easy. And getting her to resolve the problem is even harder. For that reason, you should approach most problems involving passive-aggressive people as long-term management problems, not as short-term interventions. An example:

Suppose you have a nurse on your unit who's strong clinically but who creates problems by criticizing other people behind their backs, particularly nurses who've moved up the clinical ladder to positions of more prestige and a higher salary scale.

By analyzing the whole picture rather than merely reacting to the fact that the nurse criticizes her coworkers, you'll probably discover that the nurse wants to advance up the clinical ladder but is afraid to try. After confirming that theory by talking with the nurse, you can reduce the threat by offering more information, encouraging her, and helping her work on a few requirements at a time.

Making a contract

You may be able to analyze the backstabber's goals by analyzing what she's criticizing. A nurse who complains behind your back about assignments may want more control over assignments. A nurse who complains about scheduling may want more control over scheduling.

When you find out what the person's goals are, offer her a chance to meet those goals. If the person is frustrated by hospital policy, offer her an appointment on one of the policy-making committees. ❖

Workers who don't get along

Personality conflicts are bound to develop on a unit, and when they do, you'll need to act as a mediator. Mediating – rather than resolving – conflicts helps staff members take responsibility for solving their own problems with each other. It also shows the staff that the process is fair and consistent because the mediator doesn't take sides.

Staying out of the fight

As the mediator, your first role is to tell your staff that they have to confront the problem – and the person causing it.

For example, if someone says, "I just can't work with Jane Doe," ask her if she has told Jane that. Most likely, she hasn't, nor does she *want* to. Talk with her a little more to help her analyze what problems she's having with Jane Doe. Then tell her to talk with Jane and report back to you.

You might find that many personality conflicts end when the people involved confront each other. Often, the other person didn't know there was a conflict. Don't be surprised to learn that when Mary tells Jane that she feels as if Jane is always

DIFFICULT PERSONS

putting her down, Jane is astounded and apologetic. Most likely, after Mary gives her a few examples of the behavior she's discussing, Jane will agree not to act that way again.

Arranging a meeting

If the person reports that direct confrontation didn't work, call the two nurses together and tell them you expect them to resolve the problem. Tell them you won't solve the problem for them but that you'll set aside a half hour to try to help them talk the problem through and work out a compromise.

During the discussion, they might need help keeping the conversation on the topic. If so, say something such as "You're talking around the problem now. We need to discuss how the two of you can get along, not how Jane gets along with some other people."

You might also have to remind them to stick to the facts and avoid getting emotional or using excitable language. Finally, you might have to act as a referee by saying, "I think Jane needs a chance to reply to those things before you go on."

Making an unpopular decision

Rarely will your staff members reach the end of an arranged meeting without coming up with a solution. If that does happen, though, it's usually because the conflict is based on deep-seated prejudices rather than personality differences. In those cases, you'll have to intervene.

Simply tell your staff members, "You don't seem able to resolve the conflict, so I'll have to set some ground rules and leave

it at that." Here are some guidelines to impart:
• Don't bicker, quarrel, or make snide remarks; these are unacceptable. You don't have to be friends, but you do have to be professional and work toward the unit's goals.
• The schedule will *not* be rearranged, so learn to work together.
• When you report patient problems to each other, report them fully and on time.
• When you give assignments to each other, give them fairly and clearly.
• Make sure your personal problems don't affect the patients' care or comfort.
• Make sure your personal problems don't affect the unit's morale.

Accepting the realities of leadership

If you handle all disputes this way, your staff will accept such decisions because you've been fair and consistent. That doesn't mean the staff will *like* such decisions. But, hate them or like them, the staff will respond to your fairness by working better together and taking better care of the patients.

❖

10 Sidestepping Charting Pitfalls

RISKS IN CHARTING

Mastering defensive charting

After a patient files a malpractice lawsuit, years can pass before the case goes to court. By that time, your memories of the patient may be faint. You – and others – can only turn to the patient's chart for information.

How you document, what you document, and even what you don't document may heavily influence the outcome of a malpractice case. This section presents a general discussion of the mechanics of protective charting, such as using commonly accepted abbreviations and correcting charting mistakes properly. Note that individual state laws may differ and take precedence. If you have any doubt or question about a specific situation, be sure to consult your own state's laws.

Charting with a jury in mind

In a malpractice case, the patient's chart may offer the best – and perhaps only – defense for your past actions. But if you've charted incorrectly or incompletely, the chart won't come to your defense – it'll work against you. To make sure that you can count on the chart to defend you if you're ever involved in a malpractice suit, follow these critical charting guidelines.

Use appropriate forms

Be sure to use the forms required by your hospital's policy and procedures manual. If, for instance, the manual directs you to use a neurologic flow sheet, you should use it instead of describing a patient's neurologic status in your progress notes. Such a flow sheet helps you document accurately and reminds you to cover all the elements of a complete neurologic assessment.

A jury faced with a properly completed flow sheet will have little doubt that you performed a complete neurologic assessment. But your failure to use an approved form may raise questions as to whether you followed your hospital's policy and met the standards of care.

Write in ink

Because it's a permanent document, the clinical record should be completed in ink (or printed out from a computer). Use only blue or black ink, if possible; green and red ink (the colors traditionally used on evening and night shifts) don't photocopy well. Also, don't use felt-tipped pens on forms with carbons; the pens may not produce sufficient pressure for readable copies.

Write neatly and legibly

Documentation serves as a means of communication among members of the health care team. Effective documentation depends on legible handwriting. Illegible writing hinders communication and can lead to errors in patient care. In a trial, it creates a poor impression, damages your credibility, and can even be interpreted as negligent care. In *Gugino v. Harvard Community*

Health Plan (380 Mass. 464, 403 N.E. 2d 1166 [1980]), an expert witness complained that the progress notes were sketchy. Upon reviewing the material, the judge declared the notes totally illegible and barred their use in court.

Computerized charts help, but what if your hospital doesn't use computers to document nursing care? If your handwriting is sloppy, try printing instead. Then review your notes for legibility before closing the chart.

Note exact times

Be specific about times in the chart. In particular, note the exact time of all sudden changes, significant events, and nursing actions. Avoid block charting such as "7 a.m. to 3 p.m." This sounds vague and implies inattention to the patient. For these reasons, block charting has been prohibited by some state health departments.

Use military time

When you record time, use military time, which is based on a 24-hour clock: for example, 1 p.m. is 1300 hours. Doing this identifies the precise time of day, eliminates the need to note a.m. or p.m., and prevents confusion.

Document accurately

Record the facts—not opinions or assumptions. Never falsify the clinical record to cover up a negligent act. A false record discovered during litigation can destroy the credibility of the entire clinical record. Not only could this influence the verdict, but a falsification could result in the award of punitive damages—

LEGAL LESSON

 Your best defense

The case of *Villeto v. Weilbaecher* (377 So. 2d 132 La. Ct. App. 1979]) illustrates the need for complete documentation. In this case, the nurses noticed that the patient had developed several blisters while recovering from surgery for a fractured kneecap. Each nurse recorded her observations in the nurses' progress notes and reported the blisters to the doctor.

The patient later sued the doctor for failing to treat the blisters. The doctor couldn't defend himself successfully because his record (the doctor's progress notes) didn't mention blisters until 6 days after the nurses documented them.

which may not be covered by your malpractice insurance.

Document completely

Although you don't need to chart routine tasks, such as changing bed linens, you do need to chart all relevant information relating to patient care and reflecting the nursing process. In court, you'll find it difficult to prove that you provided an aspect of patient care if you haven't documented it. For the best legal protection, completely document actual or potential problems, nursing actions taken to resolve or prevent them, and the patient's response to your actions. (See *Your best defense.*)

Use correct spelling and grammar

Misspellings and poor grammar on a chart can cause confusion. They can also convey a sense of unprofessionalism to a jury scrutinizing your charts. To avoid errors, take these steps:
• Keep a dictionary handy where you do the charting.
• Post a list of common misspellings, such as names of commonly used drugs.
• Write brief, clear sentences and avoid using unnecessarily long words.
• Don't avoid using the word "I" when describing your own actions. Saying "I taught the patient how to perform a finger stick" instead of "patient received instruction in performing a finger stick" makes it perfectly clear that you, not another staff member, were the teacher.

Use authorized abbreviations

Standards of the Joint Commission on Accreditation of Healthcare Organizations and many state regulations require health care facilities to use an approved abbreviations list to prevent confusion. Make sure you know and use your hospital's approved abbreviations. (See *Commonly accepted abbreviations*, pages 541 to 559, *Commonly accepted symbols*, pages 560 and 561, and *Dangerous abbreviations*, page 562.)

Using unapproved abbreviations can cause ambiguity, possibly endangering a patient's health. For example, if you use "o.d." for "once a day," another nurse might interpret it as "right eye" and mistakenly instill medication into the patient's right eye instead of giving it once a day.

If an abbreviation has more than one meaning—for example, CVA, which could mean cerebrovascular accident or costovertebral angle—and using the abbreviation might be confusing, take the time to write it out.

Don't sound hesitant

Avoid useless qualifying words such as "appears" when you can clearly state an objective fact. If you write, "patient appears to have bright red fluid coming from incision," a jury might question your intelligence and competence. If you write, "Patient appears restless," the opposing lawyer would surely ask what the patient was doing to make you think he was restless—pacing his room, tossing and turning in bed, fidgeting with his I.V. lines? Years later, you probably wouldn't remember.

Transcribe medication orders carefully

No matter who transcribes doctors' orders, make sure a second person double-checks the transcription for accuracy. Your unit should also have a backup method of checking for transcription errors once every 24 hours. Night-shift nurses usually do this by drawing a line across the order sheet to indicate that all orders above the line have been checked. They also sign and date the sheet to verify that they've done the 24-hour medication check.

If a doctor's order is unclear, ask him for clarification. Don't ask anyone else; they'd be guessing, too. If a doctor is known for his poor handwriting, ask him to read his orders to you before he leaves the unit.

(Text continues on page 559.)

Commonly accepted abbreviations

ABBREVIATION	MEANING
ā	before
āā	of each
AAA	abdominal aortic aneurysm
Ab	antibody
ABC	airway, breathing, circulation
ABG	arterial blood gas
a.c.	before meals
ACE	angiotensin-converting enzyme
ACh	acetylcholine
ACLS	advanced cardiac life support
AD	Alzheimer's disease auris dextra (right ear)
ADH	antidiuretic hormone
ADL	activity of daily living
AER	aldosterone excretion rate
AFIB	atrial fibrillation
AFL	atrial flutter
AFP	alpha-fetoprotein
Ag	antigen
AHD	arteriosclerotic heart disease autoimmune hemolytic disease
AHF	antihemophilic factor (factor VIII)
AICD	automatic implantable cardioverter defibrillator
AIDS	acquired immunodeficiency syndrome
ALL	acute lymphocytic leukemia
ALS	amyotrophic lateral sclerosis
ALT	alanine aminotransferase (formerly serum glutamic pyruvic transaminase [SGPT])

(continued)

Commonly accepted abbreviations *(continued)*

ABBREVIATION	MEANING
a.m.	morning
AMA	against medical advice
AMI	acute myocardial infarction
AML	acute myelocytic leukemia
ANA	antinuclear antibody
AP	anteroposterior apical pulse
APTT	activated partial thromboplastin time
ARDS	acute respiratory distress syndrome adult respiratory distress syndrome
ARF	acute renal failure acute respiratory failure acute rheumatic fever
AS	aortic sounds aqueous solution astigmatism auris sinistra (left ear)
ASA	acetylsalicylic acid (aspirin)
ASD	atrial septal defect
AST	aspartate aminotransferase (formerly serum glutamic oxaloacetic transaminase [SGOT])
ATP	adenosine triphosphate
A.U.	auris utraque (each ear)
AV	arteriovenous atrioventricular
AVM	arteriovenous malformation
BBB	bundle-branch block
BE	barium enema base excess
b.i.d.	twice daily
BLS	basic life support

Commonly accepted abbreviations *(continued)*

ABBREVIATION	MEANING
BMR	basal metabolic rate
BP	blood pressure
BPH	benign prostatic hyperplasia (benign prostatic hypertrophy)
BPM	beats per minute
BRP	bathroom privileges
BSA	body surface area
BUN	blood urea nitrogen
C	Celsius centigrade certified cervical
Ca	calcium
CA	cardiac arrest
CABG	coronary artery bypass grafting
CAD	coronary artery disease
cAMP	cyclic adenosine monophosphate
CAPD	continuous ambulatory peritoneal dialysis
caps	capsules
CBC	complete blood count
cc	cubic centimeter
CC	Caucasian child chief complaint common cold creatinine clearance critical care critical condition
CCU	cardiac care unit critical care unit
CDC	Centers for Disease Control and Prevention

(continued)

Commonly accepted abbreviations (continued)

ABBREVIATION	MEANING
CF	cardiac failure cystic fibrosis
CFS	chronic fatigue syndrome
CGL	chronic granulocytic leukemia
CHB	complete heart block
CHD	childhood disease congenital heart disease congenital hip disease
CHF	congestive heart failure
CK	creatine kinase
CK-BB	creatine kinase, brain
CK-MB	creatine kinase, heart
CK-MM	creatine kinase, skeletal muscle
cm	centimeter
CML	chronic myelogenous leukemia
CMV	continuous mandatory ventilation cytomegalovirus
CNS	central nervous system
CO	carbon monoxide cardiac output
CO_2	carbon dioxide
comp	compound
COPD	chronic obstructive pulmonary disease
CP	capillary pressure cerebral palsy cor pulmonale creatine phosphate
CPAP	continuous positive airway pressure
cpm	counts per minute cycles per minute

Commonly accepted abbreviations *(continued)*

ABBREVIATION	MEANING
CPR	cardiopulmonary resuscitation
CSF	cerebrospinal fluid
CT	clotting time coated tablet compressed tablet computed tomography corneal transplant
CV	cardiovascular central venous
CVA	cerebrovascular accident costovertebral angle
CVP	central venous pressure
d	day
/d	per day
D	dextrose
dB	decibel
D/C	discontinue
D & C	dilatation and curettage
DD	differential diagnosis discharge diagnosis dry dressing
D & E	dilatation and evacuation
DIC	disseminated intravascular coagulation
dil	dilute
disp	dispense
DJD	degenerative joint disease
DKA	diabetic ketoacidosis
dl	deciliter

(continued)

Commonly accepted abbreviations *(continued)*

ABBREVIATION	MEANING
DNA	deoxyribonucleic acid
DNR	do not resuscitate
DOA	date of admission dead on arrival
DS	double strength
DSM-IV	*Diagnostic and Statistical Manual of Mental Disorders,* 4th ed.
DTP	diphtheria and tetanus toxoids and pertussis vaccine
DVT	deep vein thrombosis
D_5W	dextrose 5% in water
EBV	Epstein-Barr virus
EC	enteric-coated
ECF	extended care facility extracellular fluid
ECG	electrocardiogram
ECHO	echocardiogram
ECMO	extracorporeal membrane oxygenator
ECT	electroconvulsive therapy
ED	emergency department
EEG	electroencephalogram
EENT	eyes, ears, nose, throat
EF	ejection fraction
ELISA	enzyme-linked immunosorbent assay
elix	elixir
EMG	electromyography
EOM	extraocular movement

Commonly accepted abbreviations *(continued)*

ABBREVIATION	MEANING
ER	emergency room expiratory reserve
ERCP	endoscopic retrograde cholangiopancrea-tography
ERV	expiratory reserve volume
ESR	erythrocyte sedimentation rate
et	and
ext.	extract
F	Fahrenheit
FDA	Food and Drug Administration
FEF	forced expiratory flow
FEV	forced expiratory volume
FFP	fresh frozen plasma
FHR	fetal heart rate
fl, fld	fluid
FRC	functional residual capacity
FSH	follicle-stimulating hormone
FSP	fibrinogen-split products
FT_3	free triiodothyronine
FT_4	free thyroxine
FUO	fever of undetermined origin
FVC	forced vital capacity
G	gauge
g, gm, GM	gram
GFR	glomerular filtration rate
GI	gastrointestinal
gr	grain

(continued)

Commonly accepted abbreviations (continued)

ABBREVIATION	MEANING
gtt	drop
GU	genitourinary
GVHD	graft-versus-host disease
GYN	gynecologic
h, hr	hour
H	hypodermic injection
HAV	hepatitis A virus
Hb	hemoglobin
HBIG	hepatitis B immunoglobulin
HBsAg	hepatitis B surface antigen
HBV	hepatitis B virus
hCG	human chorionic gonadotropin
Hct	hematocrit
HDL	high-density lipoprotein
hGH	human growth hormone
HIV	human immunodeficiency virus
HLA	human leukocyte antigen
HMO	health maintenance organization
HNKS	hyperosmolar nonketotic syndrome
hPL	human placental lactogen
h.s.	at bedtime
HS	half-strength house surgeon
HSV	herpes simplex virus
HVA	homovanillic acid
HZV	herpes zoster virus
IA	internal auditory intra-arterial intra-articular

Commonly accepted abbreviations *(continued)*

ABBREVIATION	MEANING
IABP	intra-aortic balloon pump
IC	inspiratory capacity
ICF	intracellular fluid
ICHD	Inter-Society Commission for Heart Disease
ICP	intracranial pressure
ICU	intensive care unit
ID	identification initial dose inside diameter intradermal
I&D	incision and drainage
IDDM	insulin-dependent diabetes mellitus
Ig	immunoglobulin
IM	infectious mononucleosis
I.M.	intramuscular
IMV	intermittent mandatory ventilation
in., "	inch
IND	investigational new drug
IRV	inspiratory reserve volume
IU	International Unit
IUD	intrauterine device
I.V.	intravenous
IVGTT	intravenous glucose tolerance test
IVP	intravenous pyelogram
IVPB	intravenous piggyback
J	joule

(continued)

RISKS IN CHARTING

Commonly accepted abbreviations *(continued)*

ABBREVIATION	MEANING
JCAHO	Joint Commission on Accreditation of Healthcare Organizations
JVD	jugular venous distention
JVP	jugular venous pressure
K	potassium
kg	kilogram
17-KGS	17-ketogenic steroids
17-KS	17-ketosteroids
KUB	kidney-ureter-bladder
KVO	keep vein open
L	liter lumbar
LA	left atrium long-acting
LAP	left atrial pressure leucine aminopeptidase
lb., #	pound
LD	lactate dehydrogenase
LDL	low-density lipoproteins
LE	lupus erythematosus
LES	lower esophageal sphincter
LGL	Lown-Ganong-Levine variant syndrome
LH	luteinizing hormone
LLQ	left lower quadrant
LOC	level of consciousness
LR	lactated Ringer's solution
LSB	left scapular border left sternal border
LTC	long-term care

Commonly accepted abbreviations *(continued)*

ABBREVIATION	MEANING
LUQ	left upper quadrant
LV	left ventricle
LVEDP	left ventricular end-diastolic pressure
LVET	left ventricular ejection time
LVF	left ventricular failure
m	meter
M	molar (solution)
m^2	square meter
mm^3	cubic millimeter
MAO	maximal acid output monoamine oxidase inhibitor
MAST	medical antishock trousers (pneumatic antishock garment)
mcg	microgram
MCH	mean corpuscular hemoglobin
MCHC	mean corpuscular hemoglobin concentration
MCV	mean corpuscular volume
MD	manic depressive medical doctor muscular dystrophy
ME	mistaken entry
mg	milligram
mgtt	microdrip or minidrop
mEq	milliequivalent
MI	mental illness mitral insufficiency myocardial infarction myocardial ischemia
ml	milliliter
µg	microgram

(continued)

Commonly accepted abbreviations *(continued)*

ABBREVIATION	MEANING
μl	microliter
MLC	mixed lymphocyte culture
mm	millimeter
MMEF	maximal midexpiratory flow
mmol	millimole
MRI	magnetic resonance imaging
M.R.×1	may repeat once
MS	mitral sounds mitral stenosis morphine sulfate multiple sclerosis musculoskeletal
MUGA scanning	multiple-gated acquisition scanning
MVI	multivitamin infusion
MVP	mitral valve prolapse
MVV	maximal voluntary ventilation
Na	sodium
NA	not applicable
NaCl	sodium chloride
ng	nanogram
NG	nasogastric
NICU	neonatal intensive care unit
NIDDM	non-insulin-dependent diabetes mellitus (Type II diabetes)
NKA	no known allergies
NMR	nuclear magnetic resonance
Noct.	night
NP	nasopharynx nerve palsy new patient not palpable

RISKS IN CHARTING

Commonly accepted abbreviations *(continued)*

ABBREVIATION	MEANING
NPN	nonprotein nitrogen
NPO	nothing by mouth
NR	nerve root nonreactive no refills no report no respirations
N/R	not remarkable
NS, NSS	normal saline solution (0.9% sodium chloride solution)
¼NS	¼ normal saline solution (0.225% sodium chloride solution)
½NS	½ normal saline solution (0.45% sodium chloride solution)
NSAID	nonsteroidal anti-inflammatory drugs
O_2	oxygen
OB	obstetric
OD	occupational disease overdose oculus dexter (right eye)
OGTT	oral glucose tolerance test
OOB	out of bed
OR	operating room
OS	oculus sinister (left eye)
OTC	over-the-counter
OU	oculus uterque (each eye)
oz	ounce
p̄	after
PA	pernicious anemia posteroanterior pulmonary artery
PABA	para-aminobenzoic acid

(continued)

Commonly accepted abbreviations *(continued)*

ABBREVIATION	MEANING
PAC	premature atrial contraction
$PaCO_2$	partial pressure of arterial carbon dioxide
PaO_2	partial pressure of arterial oxygen
PAP	Papanicolaou smear passive-aggressive personality primary atypical pneumonia pulmonary artery pressure
PAT	paroxysmal atrial tachycardia
PAWP	pulmonary artery wedge pressure
p.c.	after meals
PCA	patient-controlled analgesia
PE	pelvic examination physical examination pulmonary embolism pulmonary edema
PEEP	positive end-expiratory pressure
PEFR	peak expiratory flow rate
per	by or through
PET	positron-emission tomography
PID	pelvic inflammatory disease
PKU	phenylketonuria
p.m.	afternoon
PMI	point of maximal impulse
PML	progressive multifocal leukoencephalopathy
PMS	premenstrual syndrome

Commonly accepted abbreviations *(continued)*

ABBREVIATION	MEANING
PND	paroxysmal nocturnal dyspnea postnasal drip
P.O.	by mouth postoperative
PP	partial pressure peripheral pulses postpartum postprandial presenting problem
p.r.n.	as needed
pt.	patient pint
PT	prothrombin time
PTCA	percutaneous transluminal coronary angioplasty
PTH	parathyroid hormone
PTT	partial thromboplastin time
PUD	peptic ulcer disease
PVC	premature ventricular contraction polyvinylchloride
q	every
q a.m.	every morning
q.d.	every day
q.h.	every hour
q.i.d.	four times daily
q.n.	every night
QNS	quantity not sufficient
q.o.d.	every other day
QS	quantity sufficient

RISKS IN CHARTING

(continued)

RISKS IN CHARTING

Commonly accepted abbreviations *(continued)*

ABBREVIATION	MEANING
qt.	quart
R, PR	by rectum
RA	renal artery rheumatoid arthritis right arm right atrium
RAF	rheumatoid arthritis factor
RAP	right atrial pressure
RBB	right bundle-branch
RBC	red blood cell
RDA	recommended daily allowance
RE	rectal examination right ear
REM	rapid eye movement
RES	reticuloendothelial system
Rh	rhesus blood factor
RHD	relative hepatic dullness rheumatic heart disease
RIA	radioimmunoassay
RL	right lateral right leg Ringer's lactate (lactated Ringer's solution)
RLQ	right lower quadrant
RNA	ribonucleic acid
ROM	range of motion right otitis media
RSV	respiratory syncytial virus right subclavian vein Rous sarcoma virus
RUQ	right upper quadrant

Commonly accepted abbreviations *(continued)*

ABBREVIATION	MEANING
RV	residual volume right ventricle
RVEDP	right ventricular end-diastolic pressure
RVEDV	right ventricular end-diastolic volume
RVP	right ventricular pressure
Rx	prescription
SA	sinoatrial
SaO_2	arterial oxygen saturation
sat.	saturated
S.C., SQ	subcutaneous
SCID	severe combined immunodeficiency syndrome
sec	second
SGOT	serum glutamic oxaloacetic transaminase (now called aspartate aminotransferase [AST])
SGPT	serum glutamic pyruvic transaminase (now called alanine aminotransferase [ALT])
SI	International System of Units
SIADH	syndrome of inappropriate antidiuretic hormone
SIDS	sudden infant death syndrome
Sig	write on label
SIMV	synchronized intermittent mandatory ventilation
SL	sublingual
SLE	systemic lupus erythematosus
SOB	shortness of breath
sol., soln.	solution

(continued)

RISKS IN CHARTING

Commonly accepted abbreviations (continued)

ABBREVIATION	MEANING
sp.	spirits
SR	sustained release
SRS-A	slow-reacting substance of anaphylaxis
stat.	immediately
STD	sexually transmitted disease
supp.	suppository
susp.	suspension
$S\bar{v}o_2$	mixed venous oxygen saturation
syr.	syrup
T, Tbs., tbsp.	tablespoon
t, tsp.	teaspoon
tab.	tablet
TBG	thyroxine-binding globulin
TCA	tricyclic antidepressant
TENS	transcutaneous electrical nerve stimulation
TIA	transient ischemic attack
t.i.d.	three times daily
tinct., tr.	tincture
TLC	total lung capacity
TM	temporomandibular tympanic membrane
TMJ	temporomandibular joint
TNF	tumor necrosis factor
t-PA	tissue plasminogen activator

Commonly accepted abbreviations *(continued)*

ABBREVIATION	MEANING
TPN	total parenteral nutrition
TRH	thyrotropin-releasing hormone
TSH	thyroid-stimulating hormone
USP	United States Pharmacopeia
UTI	urinary tract infection
UV	ultraviolet
VAD	vascular access device ventricular assist device
vag., V, PV	vaginal
VDRL	Venereal Disease Research Laboratory (test)
VLDL	very low-density lipoprotein
VMA	vanillylmandelic acid
VO	verbal order
V/Q	ventilation-perfusion ratio
VSD	ventricular septal defect
V_T	tidal volume
WBC	white blood cell
WPW	Wolff-Parkinson-White syndrome
Z/G or ZIG	zoster immune globulin

RISKS IN CHARTING

Avoid taking telephone or other verbal orders whenever possible. If you must take one, repeat the patient's name and the medication order to the doctor, and ask him to verify that it's correct. For example, say "Doctor, you're ordering furosemide 20 mg P.O. q.d. for Anne Richards. Is that correct?"

Document complete information about medications

For each medication you administer, document the date and time of administration, name of the drug, dose, administration route and method, frequency, and your initials. Also document sites for all parenteral injections.

(Text continues on page 563.)

RISKS IN CHARTING

Commonly accepted symbols

SYMBOL	MEANING
Pulses (most commonly used numerical system)	
0	Absent; not palpable
+1	Weak or thready; hard to feel; easily obliterated by slight finger pressure
+2	Normal; easily palpable; obliterated only by strong finger pressure
+3	Bounding; readily palpable; forceful; not easily obliterated
Reflexes	
+ + + +	Very brisk; hyperactive
+ + +	Increased, but not necessarily pathologic
+ +	Average; normal
+	Present, but diminished
0	Absent
Heart murmurs	
1/6 or I/VI	Very faint; barely audible even to the trained ear; may not be heard in all positions
2/6 or II/VI	Soft and low; easily audible to the trained ear
3/6 or III/VI	Moderately loud; approximately equal to the intensity of normal heart sounds
4/6 or IV/VI	Very loud, with a palpable thrill; audible with stethoscope in partial contact with chest
6/6 or VI/VI	Extremely loud, with a palpable thrill; audible with stethoscope over, but not in contact with, chest
Apothecary symbols	
gr.	Grain (about 60 mg)
gtt.	Drop
mx	Minim (about 0.06 ml)
ℨ	Dram
z or ℥	Ounce

Commonly accepted symbols *(continued)*

SYMBOL	MEANING
Other symbols	
c̄	With
Ⓛ	Left
Ⓡ	Right
♂	Male
♀	Female
#	Number; pound
+	Plus, excess
−	Minus, negative, deficiency
±	Plus or minus; either positive or negative; very slight trace
>	Greater than
≥	Greater than or equal to
<	Less than
≤	Less than or equal to
∧	Diastolic blood pressure (commonly used on graphic forms)
∨	Systolic blood pressure
≅	Approximately equal to
≈	Approximately
↑	Increase
↓	Decrease
?	Questionable
0	None; no
1°	Primary; first degree
2°	Secondary; second degree
3°	Tertiary; third degree
1:1	One-to-one
p	After
s̄	Without
ss, s̄s̄, šš	One-half
×	Times

Dangerous abbreviations

PROBLEM TERM	REASON	SUGGESTED TERM
O.D. for "once daily"	Misinterpreted as "right eye"	Write "once daily."
q.o.d. for "every other day"	Misinterpreted as "once daily" or "q.i.d."	Write "every other day."
q.d. for "once daily"	Misinterpreted as "q.i.d."	Write "once daily."
q.n. for "every night"	Misinterpreted as "every hour"	Write "every night," "h.s.," or "nightly."
q h.s. for "every night"	Misinterpreted as "every hour"	Write "h.s.," "every night," or "nightly."
U for unit	Misinterpreted as "0, 4, 6, or cc"	Write "unit."
O.J. for "orange juice."	Misinterpreted as "OD" or "OS"	Write "orange juice."
μg (microgram)	When handwritten, misread as mg	Write "mcg."
sq or sub-q for "subcutaneous"	The q misread as "every"	Write "subcut" or "subcutaneous."
Various chemical symbols	Not understood or misunderstood	Write full name of chemical.
Abbreviations for drug names	Not understood or misunderstood	Use generic or trade name of drug.
Apothecary symbols or terms	Not understood or misunderstood	Use metric system.
per os for "by mouth"	"os" misread as "left eye"	Write "by mouth," "orally," or "P.O."
D/C for discharge	Misinterpreted as "discontinue"	Write "discharge."

When you withhold a medication, document your reasons. If you can't reach the doctor, document your attempts to call him and your reason for withholding the medication.

If the doctor orders a medication or dose you feel is inappropriate, contact him and discuss why you're questioning the order. In your nurses' notes, document when you notified the doctor, what you told him, and how he responded (including any new orders he gave you).

If someone else gives the medication, make sure that this person's name and the time of administration are charted. Document your evaluation of the patient's condition before and after the medication was given.

When charting an incident that involves inappropriate medication administration, clearly document the facts of the situation without defending an action or placing blame. Remember that lawyers usually have access to incident reports.

───────────── ❖

Charting promptly

Try to document pertinent information as soon as possible after an event. That way, you won't be as likely to omit important details, and your charting will be more accurate and clinically useful. If you become involved in litigation, you'll find it easier to defend your actions because prompt charting leaves no question as to when an event occurred. If you can't document at once, note the time when you do

document, explain the delay (for example, "chart not available"), and note the time the event occurred.

Don't wait until the end of your shift to chart the care you give. Your memory for the details will be better if you chart immediately. In court, the opposing lawyer would love to know that you documented his client's care considerably after you provided it because that would allow him to question your memory.

In *Joseph Brant Memorial Hospital v. Koziol* (2 CCLT 170 [S.C.C. 1978]), a nurse failed to chart her observations for 7 hours on a postoperative patient who died during that period. The patient's family sued the hospital, claiming nursing malpractice. The nurse insisted that she had observed the patient and, on the instruction of the assistant director of nursing, added the nursing observations to the patient's medical record after the fact. Citing the altered record, the court ruled that the nurse's failure to chart her observations at the proper time supported the claim that she made no such observations.

If you can't chart immediately, carry a pocket pad for jotting down key phrases and times; then transcribe the information into the chart as soon as possible.

Also, don't be tempted to chart your nursing care or observations ahead of time. If you decide at 5 a.m. to complete your charting for the shift and chart that your terminally ill patient slept through the night, what will you tell a jury if the patient dies before the end of the shift? Charting in advance compromises the entire record's credibility. So always put the correct time in your nurses' notes. That way, the notes will be accurate and they'll also reflect the patient's response to interventions.

the notes, as shown in this example:

Patient ambulated in hallway for 5 minutes, assisted by C. Franklin, NA, who stated that patient complained of right hip pain when bearing weight. D. West, RN.

Charting care given by another

Information in the patient's chart is supposed to reflect the firsthand knowledge of the person writing it. Doctors should regularly document with their own progress notes, as should physical and respiratory therapists and other health care team members. Don't feel responsible for recording routine doctor visits or care provided by other team members.

However, you may sometimes need to chart care that another nurse or nursing assistant gives to one of your patients. If you didn't provide the care directly, your notes should name the person who did and describe the care given. For example, while you're on a break, a fellow nurse may give your patient an analgesic. You might chart this:

1400 hours—Patient states that his pain was relieved after meperidine injection given by M. Medford at 1245 hours. T. Davis, RN.

Similarly, you may need to chart care provided by a nursing assistant if your hospital doesn't permit nursing assistants to make chart entries. Be sure to include the assistant's name in

Filling in blanks

Don't leave blank lines on any chart; fill it in completely. If information requested on the form doesn't apply to your patient, write "NA" for "not applicable" or draw a line through the empty space (depending on hospital policy).

A blank space implies that you failed to give complete care or assess the patient fully. Don't leave room for doubt in a jury's mind. Filling in every space leaves no doubt that you addressed every part of the form. It also prevents others from inserting information that could change the meaning of your original documentation.

Handling late entries

Occasionally, you may find yourself making a late entry in a patient's chart. In some cases, this is legally permissible; in others, it's dangerous.

Late entries are permissible under the following circumstances:
• if the chart was unavailable

when you needed it, such as when the patient was in X-ray or physical therapy
• if you need to add important information after you've completed your nurses' notes
• if you forgot to write notes on a particular chart.

Follow your hospital's procedure for adding late entries. For example, the guidelines probably direct you to write the entry on the first available line, label it "late entry" to show that it's out of sequence, and cross-reference it with the page where it should have appeared. You'll also note the time and date of the entry and, in the body of the entry, the time and date it should have been made.

Here's an example:

Late entry 9/10/94, 0800 hours (chart not available on 9/9/94)

On 9/9 at 1500 hours, patient stated that, while visiting with his family in the lounge at 1300 hours, he tripped and fell to the floor. States he felt pain in his left hip but was afraid to tell anyone about this until his daughter insisted that he report it. No bruises or lacerations noted. Complained of left hip pain when bearing weight. Dr. Krane examined patient at 1515 hours. Patient to X-ray at 1530 hours. A. Hurst, RN.

Above all, don't do anything that might make a jury think you altered or added something to the chart at a later date to cover up an error. If you think you'll need to make a late entry, don't ask other nurses to leave blank lines in the proper spot on the chart; you may need more or fewer lines than they provide. Don't squeeze a late entry into

an existing note or place it in the margins.

If you think a lawsuit might be filed about a particular incident, consult with your nurse-manager and the hospital's lawyer before adding late entries. They'll advise you on what's proper.

❖

Correcting charting mistakes

Occasional charting mistakes are inevitable—and so is the anxious feeling you get when you correct them. Are you doing it properly or in a way that will cast doubt on the chart's accuracy in court?

Never erase an error or cover it up with correction fluid or a black marker. A lawyer will spot the change immediately and question it.

Instead, as hospital policy dictates, use the following procedure to correct mistaken entries:
• Draw a single line through the entry so it remains legible.
• Write "mistaken entry" above or beside the original words. (Don't write "error"—jurors tend to associate the word with a clinical error that harmed the patient.)
• Write the date and your initials next to the words "mistaken entry."
• Then write the correct entry.
• Add "ME" (for "mistaken entry") to your hospital's list of approved abbreviations so you can abbreviate to save time.

Avoiding incomplete records

One of the most serious and frequent charting errors is failing to document aspects of nursing care. When you're busy, getting your work done may seem more important than documenting every detail. But from a jury's viewpoint, an incomplete chart suggests incomplete nursing care. Whether you provided care or not, a jury will most likely see it this way: If you didn't chart it, you didn't do it.

Of course, that's not always true. You may have performed a nursing procedure that you simply forgot to chart. But if the chart doesn't back you up, you'll have a hard time convincing the jury to accept your version of events.

In addition, failing to chart what you consider to be "normal" observations could also get you into trouble in court. In *Collins v. Westlake Community Hospital* (312 N.E. 2d 614 [1974]), a minor patient successfully sued a nurse and hospital for negligence. The determining factor was information missing from the chart.

The boy was hospitalized with a fractured left leg, which was casted and placed in traction. The evening nurse documented the condition of the boy's toes several times during her shift. But the night nurse didn't record the condition of his toes until morning, even though the medical record contained a doctor's order to "Watch condition of toes." At 6 a.m., the nurse documented that the boy's toes were dusky and cold and that the doctor had been contacted.

Ultimately, the boy's leg had to be amputated at the knee because of ischemic necrosis resulting from a blood clot in the femoral artery. The plaintiff claimed the amputation was necessary because the night nurse failed to observe the condition of the boy's toes during the night.

A nurse expert for the defense testified that only abnormal findings needed to be documented, although the progress notes for the same time period the previous night contained circulation checks that didn't reflect abnormal findings. To the jury, the blank chart spoke louder than the expert's words: The jury inferred that no documentation meant no observation, and they found the nurse liable for malpractice.

The appellate court agreed that the absence of entries for a 7-hour period could easily have led the jury to draw the inference that no such observations were made between 11 p.m. and 6 a.m.; therefore, the jury verdict could not be set aside.

Chart omissions, too

Your documentation should demonstrate the implementation of medical and nursing plans of care. If you omit an activity—for example, if you don't give a medication or don't provide a treatment—document the omission and the reason for it. Also document any actions taken to address the omission, if applicable.

Train yourself to anticipate litigation whenever you give patient care. So before you document, assess the situation and decide whether your actions might become significant if a lawsuit arose. If they could, chart them.

❖

Handling replacement copy

Never remove pages from a patient's chart. Regardless of your intentions, you'll invite a jury to question your reliability and your honesty.

If you make a mistake in your charting, never rewrite your notes and discard the original, even for an innocent reason like spilling soda on a page. In a lawsuit, you'd have trouble convincing the opposing lawyer that your actions were so innocent.

If you must rewrite a page, follow this procedure:
• At the top of the page, identify that the page was rewritten—"Notes copied from original of 7/17/94."
• State the reason for the rewrite—"Original illegible due to soda spill." Sign and date the entry.
• Then put the copy *and* the original page back in the chart.

Once something is considered part of the official record, don't discard or destroy it. If you replace an original sheet with a copy, always retain the original in the chart.

❖

Handling countersigning

If you're a registered nurse (RN), your hospital's policy may require you to sign off on chart entries made by LPNs (licensed practical nurses), LVNs (licensed vocational nurses), or nurses' aides. Although legal, this practice, called "countersigning," can still cause a problem in court.

Countersigning doesn't imply that you performed the procedure, but it may represent that you observed the procedure or at least reviewed the entry and approved the care given. To protect yourself, begin by finding out what your hospital's policy says. Does the hospital interpret countersigning to mean that the LPN, LVN, or nurses' aide performed her nursing actions in the countersigning RN's presence? If so, don't countersign unless you were there when the actions occurred.

If your hospital acknowledges that you don't necessarily have time to witness your co-workers' actions, then your countersignature implies that:
• the notes describe care that the LPN, LVN, or nurses' aide had the authority and competence to perform
• you have verified that all required patient care procedures were actually carried out.

To avoid problems, be very careful when countersigning. Review each entry, and make sure that it clearly identifies whoever did the procedure. If you sign off without reviewing an entry or if you negligently overlook a problem the entry raises, you could share liability for any patient injury that results.

———————————————❖

Overcoming specific charting problems

Now that you've learned the general techniques of charting, you also need to learn how to chart specific situations correctly to avoid legal difficulties in the future. For example, how you document a patient's fall, a patient's refusal to comply with treatment, and even what you say about the patient or a coworker could influence the outcome of a medical malpractice lawsuit.

———————————————❖

Criticizing a patient

What you say and how you say it are of utmost importance in documenting defensively. Keeping the patient's chart free of negative, inappropriate information – potential legal bombshells – can be a challenge when you're writing detailed narrative notes. Here are some guidelines to help you sidestep charting pitfalls – and record a more accurate account of your patient's care and status.

If a patient is demanding or abusive, you might be tempted to write this in the chart. Resist the urge. Jurors reading those words may infer that the patient received substandard care because you disliked him.

Avoid negative words

Don't describe the patient in terms that reveal a negative attitude. Instead, get your point across by objectively describing the patient's behavior. For example, instead of charting that he was ranting or out of control, describe specific signs and symptoms: loud voice, abusive language, pounding hand on overbed tray.

Avoid angering patients

Remember, the patient is legally permitted to see his chart if he wants to. Such a request usually occurs after the patient has been discharged. A derogatory reference is likely to make him angry – and an angry patient is more likely to sue.

Also, imagine how your words would sound in a courtroom. The opposing lawyer might say: "It's obvious how this nurse felt about my client – she called him difficult and uncooperative. No wonder she didn't take good care of him – she just didn't like him."

So how do you document a patient's difficult or uncooperative behavior? By describing it objectively – and letting the jurors draw their own subjective conclusions.

———————————————❖

Criticizing coworkers

If you're annoyed at a workload that's oppressive or a coworker who shirks tasks, don't use the clinical record to vent anger or assign blame. For example, don't make an entry like this:

Unable to ambulate patient because there were 2 sick calls this shift and the nurse:patient ratio was 1:18.

Granted, staff shortages may affect patient care or contribute to an incident. But don't refer to staffing problems in a patient's chart. Instead, discuss them in a forum that can help resolve the problem. In a confidential memo or an incident report, call the situation to the attention of the appropriate personnel, such as your nurse-manager. Also, review your policy and procedures manual to determine how you're expected to handle this situation.

In court, a comment about workload could be misconstrued as having a bearing on a patient's condition. Such a shortage may or may not have had a direct effect on a patient – but a jury will believe it did.

Don't air staff conflicts

Entries about disputes with nursing colleagues (including characterization and criticism of care provided), questions about a doctor's treatment decisions, or reports of a colleague's rude or abusive behavior reflect personality clashes and don't belong in the medical record. Here's an example:

Patient noted to have sacral decubitus approximately 3 cm wide and 1 cm deep. Day shift apparently never turned the patient to provide skin care.

Comments like this aren't legitimate concerns about patient care. Worse, such entries may trigger further investigation by the opposing lawyer, who is likely to exploit any conflict among codefendants.

As you would with staffing problems, address concerns about a colleague's judgment or competence in the appropriate setting. Talk with your nurse-manager or nursing supervisor (just make sure that you have the facts). Consult with the doctor directly if an order puzzles you. Share your opinions, observations, or reservations about colleagues with your nurse-manager or nursing supervisor only; avoid mentioning them in a patient's chart.

If you discover personal accusations or charges of incompetence in a chart, speak with the writer of the criticisms and point out the implications of including such conflicts in the medical record.

Charting the use of restraints

Once restraints have been ordered and applied, you need to document carefully. Your charting should show that the restraints are clinically necessary; otherwise, you could be accused of false imprisonment.

Here's what you need to document:
• the reason for the restraints or a description of the behavior that necessitated them; for example, you might write: *Patient repeatedly trying to climb over side rails*
• interventions that were used before applying restraints and why they were ineffective; for example, you might record: *Patient instructed to remain in bed and*

use call button—patient disoriented to time and place
• the type of restraint, the date and time of application, and the patient's response to the restraints.

Also make sure that the record clearly shows ongoing monitoring of the restrained patient. You should record the following:
• assessment of the skin and the respiratory and circulatory systems for any injuries or impediments caused by the restraints
• symptoms that justify the continued use of the restraints
• temporary release of the restraints every 2 hours with performance of range-of-motion exercises before reapplying
• change of patient position at frequent intervals.

Patient refusal of restraints
Suppose the doctor orders restraints or side rails, but the patient or his family are against their use. Make sure that your documentation clearly shows that this puts the patient at risk for a fall and that you informed the patient or family of the risk. Record your assessment of the patient and why you feel he needs restraints or side rails; discussions or conversations with the patient, family, and doctor regarding the use of restraints or side rails; and alternative interventions being used to prevent patient injury.

Some hospitals also require the patient to sign a refusal of treatment release form. This form protects you, the patient's doctors, and the hospital from liability. You should also document that the patient was competent to sign such a release form.

———————————————— ❖

Taking verbal orders

Another area of legal concern is taking and documenting doctors' verbal orders. Errors made in interpreting or documenting verbal orders can lead to mistakes in patient care and liability problems for you.

Clearly, verbal orders can be a necessity—especially if you're providing home care. But in a hospital, you should take verbal orders only in an emergency when the doctor can't immediately attend to the patient.

Documenting verbal orders
Carefully follow your hospital's policy for documenting a verbal order, using a special form if one exists. Generally, you'll follow this procedure:
• If time and circumstances allow, have another nurse read the order back to the doctor.
• Record the order on the doctor's order sheet as soon as possible. Note the date, and then record the order verbatim.
• On the following line, write "v.o." for verbal order or "t.o." for telephone order. Then write the doctor's name and the name of the nurse who read the order back to the doctor.
• Sign your name and write the time.
• Draw lines through any spaces between the order and your verification of the order.

Have the doctor countersign
Make sure that the doctor countersigns the order within the time limits set by your hospital's policy. Without this countersignature, you may be held liable

Don't fail to document

Failing to chart a patient's fall can actually lead to—not avoid—a lawsuit. Consider this example.

The doctor's orders for Mrs. Cauthen state: "Out of bed for 20 minutes, three times daily, as tolerated."

After explaining the doctor's plan to Mrs. Cauthen, a nurse helps her out of bed. But, as soon as the nurse helps her to her feet, Mrs. Cauthen drops to her knees. She's not hurt but appears angry. She says she fell because the nurse made her get out of bed. The nurse gets Mrs. Cauthen back in bed, assesses her for injuries, and hears her say she's not hurt. Then, without charting the incident, notifying the doctor, or completing an incident report, the nurse leaves to care for another patient.

Two hours later, a different nurse reads Mrs. Cauthen's chart and assumes she hasn't been out of bed. Again, as soon as Mrs. Cauthen tries to stand, she collapses. But this time, she fractures her hip.

Mrs. Cauthen complains to the doctor about her two falls, and the doctor immediately notifies the nursing supervisor about the undocumented incident. The hospital places the first nurse on probation for something she considered a minor charting omission. However, had Mrs. Cauthen sued the hospital, the nurse would have been facing a malpractice charge.

for practicing medicine without a license.

❖

Documenting a patient's fall

Two percent of all hospitalized patients fall, and 75% to 85% of all incidents in hospitals are due to patient falls. Your nursing documentation will be an important factor in your defense if you're sued because a patient of yours falls and harms himself. (See *Don't fail to document.*)

Almost anything can cause a patient to fall. Elderly patients may be confused, disoriented, and weak. Postoperative patients may also be weak and unsteady. And any patient can become disoriented from medications so that he can't react quickly enough to save himself from falling.

When documenting a fall, record not just the fall itself but also measures you took to prevent a fall. Regardless of preventive measures, you must document the fall on the nurses' notes and also complete an incident report. Your notes should contain descriptive, objective in-

PREVENTIVE PRACTICE

 Preventing falls

You have a responsibility to protect your patient from falls. To do this, take the precautions listed below, especially when caring for a high-risk patient. Be sure to document each precaution taken.
• Keep the bed's side rails up when indicated.
• Orient the patient to time and place, especially if he's elderly.
• Monitor the patient regularly or continually, depending on his condition.
• Provide adequate lighting and a clean, clutter-free environment.
• Make sure that someone helps the patient whenever he gets out of bed, and that he wears proper shoes when walking.
• If you feel the patient needs restraints, call the doctor for an order before applying them.
• Be sure that the call button is within the patient's reach and that he knows how to operate it.

formation supported by facts. (See *Preventing falls*.)

Completing an incident report

Despite the best training and intentions, "incidents" occur in the hospital. You have a legal duty to report any incidents of which you have firsthand knowledge. If you don't, you could be fired and also charged with malpractice, especially if a patient was injured.

The incidents you report are certain events inconsistent with the hospital's ordinary routine. These include patient injuries, patient complaints, medication errors, and injuries to employees and visitors.

An incident report serves two main purposes. First, it informs the hospital's administrators of the incident so they can consider changes to help prevent similar incidents. This is known as "risk management." Second, it alerts the administrators and the hospital's insurance company to the possibility of a liability claim and the need for further investigation. This is known as "claims management."

Filing a report

Only a person with firsthand knowledge of an incident should file an incident report, and only the person making the report should sign it. Never sign a report describing circumstances or events that you didn't witness personally. Each person with firsthand knowledge should fill out and sign a separate report.

Your report should:
• identify the person involved in the incident
• document accurately and truthfully any unusual occurrences that you witnessed
• record details of what happened and the consequences for the person. Include sufficient information so that the administra-

tors can decide whether the matter requires further investigation.
• not contain opinions, judgments, conclusions, or assumptions about who or what caused the incident
• not contain suggestions on how to prevent the incident from happening again. (See *Completing an incident report*, pages 574 to 576.)

Don't chart incident reports
The incident report isn't part of the patient's clinical record. However, it may be used in litigation. Many states now consider it "discoverable evidence"; if the opposing lawyer learns of its existence, he can subpoena it and use it as evidence.

Never note in the clinical record that an incident report was filed or attach a copy to the chart (unless law or hospital policy specifically requires you to do so). Don't use the words "incident report" in your charting. Do, however, include the clinical details of the incident in your nurses' notes; for example:

Found patient lying on the floor at 1250 hours. Vital signs were stable. Notified Dr. Gary Dietrich at 1253 hours, and he saw patient at 1300 hours.

This is a sufficient statement of the facts. Make sure that the descriptions in the incident report and the nurses' notes mirror each other.

❖

Documenting noncompliance

Suppose a patient won't comply with nursing or medical interventions. Do you know how to document his noncompliance so you're legally protected?

Don't hesitate to indicate if the patient is noncompliant in his behavior and words. Noncompliance—and your chart notes to support it—may actually prevent a lawsuit, as few lawyers want to take clients who are partially, if not completely, responsible for their own poor response to treatment.

In your nurses' notes, clearly document your instructions and anything the patient does despite them. Describe his behavior and use his actual words. Then report the problem to your nurse-manager, the doctor, and any other appropriate staff person. This shows that you recognized the potential for harm to the patient and tried to prevent it. If the patient's care is later questioned, you'll have important documentation to defend yourself.

Noncompliance takes several forms. Patients typically ignore instructions regarding diet, getting out of bed, hospital discharge, follow-up appointments, and medications.

Refusal to observe diet restrictions
Nurses often discover unauthorized food or drinks at the patient's bedside. One nurse discovered that a diabetic patient's friends were sneaking beer and sugary foods to his hospital

(Text continues on page 577.)

RISKS IN CHARTING

Completing an incident report

When you witness a reportable event, you must fill out an incident report. Forms vary among health care facilities, but most include the information in this chart.

INCIDENT REPORT

Name of person _____

Address _____

Date of report	Date of incident	Time of incident	If ED patient, give unit number

LOCATION OF INCIDENT
- ☐ Patient room
- ☐ Patient bathroom
- ☐ OR
- ☐ ED
- ☐ Hospital grounds
- ☐ Nurses' station
- ☐ Other _____

IDENTIFICATION
- ☐ Inpatient
- ☐ ED patient
- ☐ Outpatient
- ☐ Employee
- ☐ Volunteer
- ☐ Visitor
- ☐ Other _____

☐ Admitting diagnosis of patient _____

CONDITION BEFORE INCIDENT

Level of consciousness (previous 4 hours)
- ☐ Alert
- ☐ Confused, disoriented
- ☐ Uncooperative
- ☐ Sedated (drug: _____)
- ☐ Unconscious

Call system within reach
- ☐ Yes ☐ No

Ambulation
- ☐ OOB
- ☐ OOB with assistance
- ☐ Bed rest with BRP
- ☐ Complete bed rest
- ☐ Not specified
- ☐ Other (specify) _____

Side rails
- ☐ Up
- ☐ Partially up
- ☐ Down

Restraints present
- ☐ Yes ☐ No
Ordered
- ☐ Yes ☐ No

Bed height
- ☐ High
- ☐ Low

NATURE OF INCIDENT

Fall
- ☐ While ambulatory
- ☐ While sitting
  - ☐ Chair
  - ☐ Commode
- ☐ From bed
- ☐ Off table, stretcher, or equipment
- ☐ Found on floor
- ☐ Other _____

Medication
- ☐ Error in patient identification
- ☐ Incorrect drug
- ☐ Incorrect dosage
- ☐ Incorrect route
- ☐ Timing
- ☐ Duplication
- ☐ Omission
- ☐ Incorrect I.V. solution hung
- ☐ Incorrect I.V. rate
- ☐ Other _____

Completing an incident report *(continued)*

NATURE OF INCIDENT *(continued)*

Surgical
☐ Consent problem
☐ Incorrect sponge and instrument count
☐ Foreign object left in patient
☐ Other _____

Equipment
Type _____
Control and serial number ___
_____
☐ Malfunction
☐ Shock
☐ Burn
☐ Other _____

Date of last maintenance _____
BioMed notified
☐ Yes ☐ No
Risk Management notified
☐ Yes ☐ No

Describe the incident.
_____

Burn
☐ Chemical
☐ Cigarette
☐ Treatment
☐ Hot liquid
☐ Other _____

Miscellaneous
☐ Patient refuses treatment
☐ Needle stick
☐ Injuries in treatment
☐ Infection
☐ Discharge against medical advice
☐ Struck by door
☐ Other _____

Personal property
☐ Damaged ☐ Lost
☐ Other _____
Describe items.
_____
_____

Witnesses: ☐ Yes ☐ No
If yes, note names, addresses, and phone numbers, and indicate if they're employees, visitors, etc.

1. _____ 2. _____

DISPOSITION
Seen by
☐ Attending doctor
☐ ED doctor

Treatment
☐ Not indicated
☐ Treatment given
☐ Treatment refused
☐ X-ray ordered
☐ Admitted to hospital
☐ Follow-up care indicated

Examination findings
_____

Doctor's signature
_____

NOTIFICATION
(include your name, the date, and the time)
Attending doctor notified
☐ Yes ☐ No _____
Supervisor notified
☐ Yes ☐ No _____
Noted in chart
☐ Yes ☐ No

Sick call request completed
☐ Yes ☐ No

Patient or family notified
☐ Yes ☐ No

☐ Documented in progress notes

(continued)

RISKS IN CHARTING

Completing an incident report *(continued)*

GENERAL DATA
Attending doctor _____

| Room number | Bed number | Shift ☐ 1 ☐ 2 ☐ 3 |

Additional details of incident

_____

_____

_____

_____

_____

_____

_____

_____

_____

_____

_____

_____

_____

| Signature | Title | Date |

Director's summary (detail follow-up to above incident and action taken)

_____

_____

_____

_____

_____

_____

_____

_____

_____

| Signature | Title | Date |

room. She also had to remind the patient repeatedly that he wasn't permitted to smoke. After the patient decided to transfer to another hospital, one of his legs had to be amputated. He wanted to sue the first hospital for negligence that had necessitated the amputation. But when his lawyer found the nurses' complete documentation of the patient's noncompliance, he refused to accept the patient as a client. A lawsuit was never filed.

Getting out of bed

You may tell a patient that he must stay in bed or that he must call you for help if he wants to get up, but still find him climbing over the bed rails. Or you may discover well-meaning relatives helping him up because they don't want to trouble you. Any of these actions puts the patient at risk for a fall—and you at risk for a lawsuit. You can protect yourself by carefully documenting your instructions and any act of the patient's that violates them.

0900 hours—Assisted patient to bedside chair. Patient complained of feeling light-headed when standing. Noted to have an unsteady gait. Instructed patient to call for assistance to get OOB. All side rails up when patient in bed. Call light within reach. J. Daly, RN

1030 hours—Found patient on the floor at bedside. Patient stated she put the side rails down and got OOB by herself. Assisted back to bed. Vital signs stable. No bruises or lacerations noted. No complaints of pain. Dr. Connely notified. Patient reminded to call for assistance. Stated she understood. J. Daly, RN

Leaving against medical advice

If a patient tells you he's planning to leave the hospital, you should find out why he wants to leave, and then tell your nurse-manager and the patient's doctor. The doctor should talk with the patient about the risks of refusing further treatment, and then ask him to sign a release form indicating that he understands the risks. If the doctor is unavailable, you can do this; just make sure that you document the points you discussed with the patient. Whether or not you handle this, you're expected to document the patient's decision to leave against medical advice, the reasons he gives for leaving, the actions that were taken, and the time the patient left.

A patient may not tell you he's planning to leave; you may just discover him missing. Naturally, you should first try to find him within the hospital. If you can't find him, notify your nurse-manager, his doctor, and the police (if necessary). Usually, you'll call the police if the patient is at risk for harming himself or others or if he has left the hospital with a medical device (such as a heparin lock) in place.

In your nurses' notes, you should note the time that you discovered the patient missing, your attempts to find him, and the people you notified. Also document any other pertinent information. Here's an example:

2300 hours—Patient's vital signs stable, no complaints of pain. H. Carey, RN

2330 hours—Called to patient's room by his roommate. Roommate stated that patient got dressed and said he was leaving the hospital. Roommate stated

*that patient left 5 minutes ago.
T. Worley, nursing supervisor;
M. Schwartz, security officer; and
Dr. Fallon notified of patient's
disappearance. Calls placed to
other units describing patient so
staff could look for him.
H. Carey, RN*

*2345 hours – Attempted to
contact patient's wife without
success. Stafford Township police
notified of patient's disappearance. Officer Bagley said an officer would go to the patient's
home to look for him. H. Carey,
RN*

Missing follow-up appointments

Many patients fail to show up for
scheduled follow-up appointments at the clinic, emergency
department, or doctor's office.
Therefore, always document the
date of the patient's scheduled
return visit for further care. Also
document that you discussed the
scheduled appointment with
him, so he can't say later that
you didn't tell him when to return. If the patient misses an appointment, consider sending him
a certified letter – return receipt
requested – as proof that you followed up on the matter. In some
states, you're also required to
make and document a phone
call, noting whether the patient
was at home or not, to whom
you spoke, or whether the call
went unanswered.

Medication refusal or abuse

If your patient fails to adhere to
his medication schedule or adds
other drugs to his regimen, you
should describe the incidents in
your nurses' notes. Perhaps you
find illegal or unprescribed
drugs at the patient's bedside or
see evidence that he's been

hoarding his pain medication.
Perhaps his behavior suddenly
changes after he's had visitors,
and you suspect the visitors of
providing narcotics or other
drugs. Or perhaps the patient
flatly refuses to take a prescribed
medication. Document every incident, and include the patient's
reasons, if he tells you.

Here's how you would document one such incident:

*1400 hours – Patient's wife
present at bedside. Patient awake,
alert, and oriented × 3. No complaints of pain or discomfort at
this time. C. Pace, RN*

*1500 hours – Patient found to
be lethargic and disoriented to
time and place. Pupils equal,
constricted. BP – 98/60, P – 72,
R – 10. Patient stated, "My wife
gave me some of her Demerol
pills because I had back pain. I
didn't want to bother you." Dr.
Jones notified. C. Pace, RN*

*1510 hours – Dr. Jones in to
examine patient. BP – 100/68, P –
76, R – 12. Neurologic status unchanged. C. Pace, RN* ❖

When a patient contributes to his injury

One of your patients may do
something that keeps him from
responding well to nursing and
medical care or that contributes
to his injury. Or he may not do
something that might have
helped him. These behaviors are
called "potentially contributing
patient acts." Handling this
problem correctly when you
chart can reinforce your defense
in a malpractice lawsuit. Usu-

ally, jurors are unsympathetic to patients who don't cooperate with health care team members.

Behaviors that constitute potentially contributing patient acts—and the reasons behind them—vary. A patient may provide only partial details of his health history, current medications, or previous treatments. Or he may refuse to answer questions on these topics at all. Perhaps he's tired of answering the "same" questions from so many different people. Perhaps he doesn't understand why staff members need the information. Or perhaps he considers the information too personal and suspects staff motives.

The following is an example of what to chart when the patient refuses to answer questions:

1300 hours—While obtaining information for patient's admission data base, I asked him how much regular insulin he takes in the morning. Patient said, "I'm sick and tired of answering all these questions. Why do you need to know that, anyway? Leave me alone so I can get some rest." I explained to the patient that information about his insulin is very important in planning his care and in making sure he receives the correct dose. He continued to refuse to provide the information. Dr. Perry notified. D. Raymond, RN

Perhaps a patient *can't* give you important information. An altered level of consciousness, severe pain, fear, a psychiatric problem, a language barrier, or disorientation may prevent him. If so, clearly document the reason for your difficulty communicating with the patient. Then try

to get the information you need from a relative, friend, personal doctor, or other source.

When a patient threatens a lawsuit

If a patient or family member ever threatens to sue you or the hospital—or any other health care professionals or facilities—take the threat seriously. Such comments may be important evidence in a subsequent lawsuit. (See *Why nurses are sued*, page 580.)

Carefully document the comments in your nurses' notes. Then report the information to the appropriate people, such as your nurse-manager, the hospital's risk manager, and the patient's doctor. Your chart entry might sound like this:

1200 hours—Patient's wife angry and stated that she is going to sue the hospital because her husband is not getting good nursing care. Attempted to comfort wife. While I was trying to elicit more information from patient's wife, she became more angry and agitated, continuing to state that she is going to sue the hospital. K. Meyer, nurse-manager, and Dr. Holmes notified. L. Howard, RN

Why nurses are sued

The list below shows the most common reasons that malpractice cases are brought against nurses. For various reasons, the mishaps that provoke a malpractice suit may be out of your control. What remains in your control, however, is your timely and accurate documentation of the patient's condition and situations, your nursing interventions, and other relevant data.

By documenting that you provided appropriate care and charted it, the record should protect you and your employer and may go a long way to avert a malpractice suit.

Medication administration
• Incorrect medications and dosages
• Incorrect injection site
• Injury from injection

Obstetric and related care
• Nursing error or negligence causing injury during delivery
• Delay in notifying doctor, causing injury
• Failure to monitor neonate's condition
• Failure to provide proper neonatal care

Patient falls
• Side rails left down
• Medicated patient left unattended
• Injury caused when moving or turning patient
• Patient left unattended on stretcher or examination table

Surgery and related care
• Foreign object left in patient
• Failure to monitor patient in postanesthesia room
• Negligent postoperative care

Care involving I.V. lines, catheters, and tubes
• Infiltration
• Negligence causing emboli
• Improper insertion causing injury
• Injection of improper solution
• Improper inflation of catheter bulbs

Record keeping
• Inaccuracy, or failure to record information
• Failure to use standard abbreviations
• Failure to communicate with doctor
• Breach of confidentiality

Personal liability
• Damage to insured's property
• Malicious acts
• Intentional tortious conduct

When a medical record is subpoenaed

If you learn that you're being sued, your first impulse might be to review the patient's chart and fill in any missing information. Don't—it's illegal and you'll probably get caught. By the time a lawsuit has been filed, the opposing lawyer has already seen a copy of the chart. He'll notice any subsequent changes you make and won't hesitate to accuse you in court. He may even introduce experts who can date the ink samples on individual entries. The jury won't forget that you tampered with the evidence.

Compromising credibility

Any instance of tampering can create additional problems. Trying to cover up minor errors that weren't negligent makes every entry seem questionable. If the jury feels the chart's accuracy is unreliable, you could lose a case you should have won.

For example, suppose you gave hydromorphone instead of morphine to your postoperative patient. That fact might have no bearing on his malpractice lawsuit for a postoperative pulmonary embolism. But if you tamper with the chart, your entire case becomes suspect. So you might face an expensive out-of-court settlement.

If the opposing lawyer can prove that someone tampered with the chart, the patient might at least have more time to file a claim. Tampering is fraud, and fraud has a longer statute of limitations than malpractice. (See *Applying the statute*, and *What

Applying the statute

The statute of limitations, which sets a time period for enforcing a person's rights, varies widely among states. The following rules help determine the limits:

• *Occurrence*. The statute begins on the day of the patient's injury.

• *Termination of treatment*. If an injury results from a treatment series, the statute begins on the final treatment date.

• *Constructive continuing-treatment*. If a patient is injured after leaving your care because subsequent health care providers relied on your previous care decisions, the statute begins on the last day of treatment by the other providers.

• *Discovery*. The statute begins when an injury is discovered.

• *Fraud*. If a nurse or doctor willfully concealed information, the statute may extend indefinitely.

• *Minor patient*. The statute may not begin until the patient reaches the age of majority.

constitutes tampering? page 582.) Worse, the charges against you could multiply. And the judge could allow the jury to award punitive damages, which aren't covered by malpractice insurance. And if any records have been destroyed, the hospital *and you* could face fines for failing to produce documents the court demanded to see.

❖

RISKS IN CHARTING

LEGAL LESSON

 # What constitutes tampering?

Of course you know that tampering with a medical record is unethical and illegal. But exactly what constitutes tampering? The following actions can put you in legal jeopardy:

• *Filing an incident report after the fact.* If your employer asks you to fill out an incident report long after the fact (or in response to a lawsuit), talk to your lawyer. Incident reports should be filed at the time of the incident.

• *Adding to an existing record.* Occasionally you may be asked to fill in the blanks on your charts because the medical records department needs to obtain a complete patient record.

Be careful about what you add after the fact. It's probably safe to sign an entry that you know you wrote. But adding assessment findings, times, or other details is risky. Relying on your memory may make the added information inaccurate. And a jury would see this as tampering, not just completing the record.

• *Omitting significant information from a record.* Don't let anyone pressure you into omitting or concealing information. If you're asked to omit something crucial, take your concerns up the chain of command as far as the hospital's administrator and lawyer, if necessary. If your hospital doesn't have nurse-managers, consult your state nursing board for guidance.

Bowing to pressure puts you at risk for charges of concealing information. And most malpractice insurance doesn't cover illegal acts.

• *Rewriting the record.* If you make a mistake in charting, never rewrite your notes and discard the original. The court would assume the evidence on the missing page was so damaging that you had to destroy it.

If you must copy an unreadable page, retain the original page and file both pages in the chart.

• *Adding to someone else's notes.* Never alter another person's documentation, even if you think it contains a simple error or an obvious omission. In court, the other person may deny making the entry that you changed, leading the jury to question the validity of the entire chart.

For the same reason, never let anyone else try to fix a charting error you've made. If you discover someone has altered your notes, talk with your nurse-manager and follow through until the problem is corrected. The person who made the change may simply be unaware of the legal risk of tampering.

As a precaution, date every entry, record the time, write in ink on consecutive lines, and sign each entry. Don't leave any space between the entry and your signature.

11 Preventing legal liability

LEGAL LIABILITY

Your rights as an employee

Your legal risks off duty

Your risks in malpractice lawsuits

Your risks in specialty areas

Working on specialty units offers exciting challenges and increased responsibilities – and extra risks of liability. This section will help you learn how to cope with the legal risks inherent in various hospital units.

Emergency department

Emergency departments (EDs) are the most hectic areas of a hospital. Nurses are expected to assess all kinds of patients, comfort distraught relatives, respond to orders, answer the phone... without knowing what the next minute will bring. The stress, chaos, excitement, and frustration can be overwhelming – and, if you're not careful, legally perilous.

Protecting yourself from liability while providing safe patient care requires attention to certain guidelines.

Listen to parents

Although a child may appear healthy, always pay attention to parents who tell you he's just not acting right. After all, they know their child better than anyone. No matter what the facts, if the child is injured because of your inattention to a parent's remarks and the case goes to court, the jury's sympathy will probably be with the parent – not with the hospital or you.

Don't give advice over the telephone

Never give telephone advice unless you're following a specific protocol under the direction of a designated medical director. The protocol should include documentation of the caller's complaint and the specific advice given. EDs without a formal protocol should have a written policy directing employees to tell callers, "It's against our policy to give medical advice. Please call your personal doctor or come to the emergency department."

Take verbal orders only in emergencies

Verbal orders are legal if they're written on the patient's chart as soon as possible. But getting some doctors to document their verbal orders can be an uphill battle. Your best protection is to ask your nurse-manager, the ED's medical director, or the hospital administrator to inform doctors that ED nurses won't carry out verbal orders except in emergencies.

Reassess patients after treatment

Not only is this good nursing care, but the guidelines from the Joint Commission on Accreditation of Healthcare Organizations require you to document a patient's response to treatment. If your patient doesn't respond as expected, you'll have a record of the interventions you took to ensure his comfort and well-being.

Never assume intoxication

Don't jump to conclusions – just because a patient is behaving erratically doesn't mean that he's intoxicated. First, you should rule out head injury, hypoglycemia or hyperglycemia, electrolyte imbalances, and other physiologic reasons.

Heed your gut feelings

A well-developed "sixth sense" is one of the most important qualities of an ED nurse. When all else indicates your patient is stable but inside you know something isn't right, listen to that inner voice. Reassess your patient, ask for a second opinion from another nurse, or share your concerns with the ED doctor.

Report suspected abuse

Legally, you're obligated to report suspected child or adult abuse. The law provides protection for reporting suspected abuse, even if it proves to be unfounded.

Record unstable vital signs

If other patients need your attention, you might not be able to stay with an unstable patient constantly. But you must record his vital signs regularly as required by policy and protocol—otherwise, you could be found negligent and liable if he later develops a serious complication.

Perform triage correctly

Patient care is ultimately the ED doctor's responsibility. But if you're a triage or charge nurse (rather than a staff nurse), you can be held liable for a patient's injury that results from incorrect triage. If you work in a very busy ED or if you're often short-handed, ask the admissions clerk to perform initial assessments and recognize emergency conditions.

Report substandard care. If you believe that patients in your ED aren't receiving treatment quickly enough from appropriate medical personnel, document your concerns by writing a memo. Then give copies to your nurse-manager, the medical director of the ED, and the hospital administrator, and keep a copy for your personal files. ❖

Operating and postanesthesia rooms

Patients in the operating room (OR) and postanesthesia care unit (PACU) need constant, specialized care. But this kind of care presents particular legal risks.

Knowing the most common causes of malpractice suits arising from these areas will help you protect yourself. They are:
• failure to check the patient's chart for a consent form, a preoperative laboratory form, electrocardiogram or X-ray results, or allergy warnings before surgery
• failure to perform a sponge and instrument count after surgery or performing it incorrectly
• inadequate postoperative observation of the patient in the OR or PACU, in transit between these two places (where most malpractice lawsuits arise), or in transit to the medical-surgical unit
• anesthesia errors by anesthetists (more commonly anesthesiologists).

Taking precautions

Here's some advice for avoiding legal errors in the OR and PACU:

• If you're a PACU nurse, accompany all postoperative patients to the medical-surgical unit. If this is impossible because of tight staffing, at least accompany high-risk patients – those with chest tubes, for example.

• If you're a nurse-anesthetist, remember that, in most states, the medical standards for anesthesiologists apply to your performance. If you don't meet them and you harm a patient, you're liable.

• Familiarize yourself with your state's nurse practice act, the nurse practice standards of the Association of Operating Room Nurses, and your hospital's written policy on OR emergencies.

• Carry adequate malpractice insurance. Generally, a hospital's malpractice insurance policy covers both OR and PACU nurses, but in the rare case that your hospital's policy is inadequate or the hospital refuses to defend you, you may need your own professional liability insurance.

❖

Pediatric unit

Children can be injured on pediatric units just as easily as they can at home. When injuries occur, nursing negligence is commonly the cause.

To avoid patient injury and possible malpractice lawsuits, be sure to follow your hospital's policy regarding the appropriate patient ages for cribs and youth beds, and check that each bed works properly. Childproof each room by covering unused electrical outlets with protectors and locking away all medications, disinfectants, and equipment. Also, supervise hospitalized children when they're playing together. You can be held liable if one child hurts another while they're under your care.

Listed below are other precautions to reduce your legal risks:

• Establish rapport with both the child and his family. Building trust may help prevent a future lawsuit.

• Keep up-to-date with the latest developments in pediatrics. Even if your state doesn't require you to take continuing education courses, keep current by reading professional literature and by attending seminars given by your hospital as well as by other agencies and organizations.

❖

Short procedure unit

Because their patients are in and out the same day, nurses who work on short procedure units face major legal risks in all phases of patient care, from assessment to discharge teaching.

Assessment

Despite the thoroughness of early screening tests, you should still perform your own nursing assessment when the patient is admitted. To determine whether he really is ready for surgery that day, find the answers to these questions: If he was told to fast after midnight, did he follow these instructions? Does he have a cold, fever, suspicious rash, or any other signs or symptoms that might affect his reaction to anesthesia and surgery? If he takes morning medications, did he take them today?

Informed consent

Obtaining informed consent is the doctor's responsibility, but many hospitals require nurses to clarify the doctor's explanation and answer any patient questions. So, if a patient is confused about the procedure he consented to, you can provide more information. If he remains confused, or if you don't feel qualified to give him the information, document your observations on his chart and make sure that the doctor answers his questions. Whatever the outcome, document the entire conversation between you and the patient as well as your conversation with the doctor.

Never prepare a patient for surgery unless you have his signed consent form in hand. If consent forms at your hospital are often missing or are consistently late, encourage your hospital administration to implement this policy: Every patient's consent form must be attached to his chart 24 hours before surgery or his surgery will be rescheduled.

Observing and reporting

Because many short procedures are performed under general anesthesia, you'll need to watch for adverse reactions to the anesthetic and report them to the anesthesiologist and surgeon.

Discharge assessment

Short procedure unit patients are typically discharged the same day they're admitted. So be especially alert when assessing for postoperative problems.

If the patient was sedated for the procedure and hasn't made arrangements for a ride home, call a taxi for him or help him contact a friend or relative. Most hospitals have a written policy that the procedure won't be started unless the patient has someone with him who'll take him home upon discharge. Don't let the patient drive himself home or take public transportation. He could have an accident while still under the effects of sedation, and you could be held liable if he or someone else is injured.

Patient teaching

In the short procedure unit, patient teaching is mostly discharge teaching. The doctor should give the patient discharge instructions before surgery, but don't assume he did this. If the patient got instructions, don't assume he understands them. To protect yourself from liability, take the following steps:

• If your hospital doesn't have a policy on discharge teaching, try to establish one. It should require that patients receive discharge instructions before admission.

• Make sure your short procedure unit has preprinted discharge teaching instructions, especially for frequently performed procedures. Individualize your teaching with specific written instructions whenever necessary. If preprinted instructions aren't available, write the instructions yourself.

• If possible, teach both the patient and his partner about discharge orders to reinforce the probability of compliance after discharge.

• Have your patient repeat the instructions to you to make sure he understands them.

• Determine whether the patient is capable of following the instructions; if he isn't, contact the appropriate support services and the doctor.

• Document painstakingly what you taught the patient, including what written instructions you gave him, if any; how he responded to those instructions; and what other actions you took, such as contacting a support person or agency.

——————————————— ❖

Obstetric unit

Obstetrics involves some of the greatest legal risks for doctors and nurses, although doctors receive a far higher number of claims. An obstetric nurse has a responsibility to both the patient and her unborn child. Their survival can depend on her judgment and her appropriate and effective action. When a birth doesn't turn out as expected, families often sue for malpractice.

Malpractice claims against obstetric nurses usually contend that the nurse failed to adequately assess and monitor a pregnant patient. (See *Failure to monitor.*) Another risk occurs if nurses don't relay significant

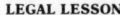

LEGAL LESSON

 Failure to monitor

Failure to adequately assess and monitor a pregnant patient is the number one cause of malpractice lawsuits against obstetric nurses. For example, in one case, a mother entered an Indiana hospital to give birth to her 13th child. A nurse examined her, prepared her for delivery, and hung an oxytocin drip. Although the mother's other children had all been born without complications, this child had cerebral palsy. In the subsequent lawsuit, the mother testified that no one monitored her contractions for 2 hours after the nurse hung the oxytocin drip. The jury awarded her $350,000.

findings to the doctor. So, to avoid liability, closely monitor a patient in labor, especially if she's receiving oxytocin or another I.V. medication, and keep the doctor up-to-date on her condition. Also, pay attention to what the patient tells you during labor, especially if she's had other children. She may be the first to recognize a problem.

By the way, the courts have maintained that the father's presence in the delivery room is a privilege, not a right. However, many hospitals allow fathers to participate in the birth. If your hospital allows this, make sure that both the patient and the father have given the doctor their consent, and that the doctor has agreed.

❖

Psychiatric unit

Because psychiatric patients are usually ambulatory, are often heavily medicated, and may be uncooperative, their nurses may end up in touchy legal situations. One such situation is when a patient commits or attempts suicide. Both psychiatric and non-psychiatric hospitals have been sued because of this.

A hospital isn't automatically liable because a patient commits suicide on its premises. However, when caring for a suicidal patient, nurses and other hospital personnel must carry out the doctor's orders and the hospital's policies regarding suicide precautions. If a patient talks about committing suicide, tell the doctor immediately and document that you did so in the patient's medical record.

❖

Your patient's rights

The law protects a patient's basic human rights while he's receiving health care. These rights include the right to informed consent, the right to refuse treatment, and the right to control access to his records.

Ensuring informed consent

Has this ever happened to you? An hour before a patient is scheduled for surgery, you discover that he never signed his consent form. You may think about obtaining the consent yourself, rather than taking the time to contact the doctor. But don't – this could be illegal.

Obtaining informed consent is clearly the doctor's legal duty, not the nurse's. What you can do is remind the doctor that the consent form must be signed – in fact, many hospitals require their nurses to do this.

All competent adults have the right to make decisions about their own health care. To make an informed decision, the patient must have sufficient information, such as the nature of the procedure, its benefits and risks, and alternatives. By signing the consent form, the patient affirms that he's received an explanation of the procedure and has had an opportunity to ask questions. While you have no direct responsibility for explaining the procedure to the patient, you should still clarify the doctor's explanation and answer any questions. However, always refer specific informed consent questions to the doctor.

How to witness a consent

While a witness may be optional, many doctors prefer you to be present because a witness may help in defending a lawsuit. If you do sign as a witness, then you should actually see the doctor obtaining the patient's signature. Be aware that you're witnessing only the fact that the patient signed the form voluntarily; the doctor must decide whether the patient is competent and understands the explanation.

When the patient is incompetent

If the patient isn't competent, his next of kin (determined by state laws) may give consent. The next of kin is usually the patient's spouse; if he has no spouse, then it would be his adult children, followed by his parents, and then his adult siblings. The doctor needs the consent of only one of the responsible parties.

State laws prevail on issues of incompetent patients. Many times, hospitals request signatures of next of kin on informed consent forms, even though the document isn't legal. This practice is followed because it ensures that someone on the patient's behalf is aware of the need for the procedure or surgery.

When the patient is a minor

Although minors usually may not legally consent to their own medical care, every state has enacted some legislation to allow minors to consult for specific medical conditions and needs, such as venereal diseases, alcohol and drug abuse, birth control information, pregnancy care, and communicable diseases. An emancipated minor may consent to all of his own medical treatment. In most states, an emancipated minor is one who is married, in the military, or lives away from home and is finan-

cially independent. Some states allow emancipation for the non-married minor parent of a child. Make sure that you know your state's law on the issue of minors and informed consent.

In emergencies, the law doesn't require informed consent, although it's always preferable to obtain it if time allows. (See *Can consent be implied?* page 592.)

When a companion wants to give consent

You've probably cared for patients who weren't legally married or who had live-in lovers of the same sex. But can a companion give consent to a patient's treatment, and what are your liabilities in this situation?

A live-in companion can give consent under two conditions: if the patient signed a durable power of attorney for health care designating the companion as the surrogate decision maker or if the patient and companion have a legally recognized common-law marriage (although many states don't recognize such a marriage). Otherwise, if you allow a companion to make these decisions, you could be held liable if the patient is harmed.

Durable power of attorney for health care

The provisions in a durable power of attorney for health care go into effect when the patient becomes incompetent. Look for a signed copy of the form on the patient's chart. If it's not there, don't let the companion make treatment decisions until you obtain it.

Can consent be implied?

If a patient is unconscious or incompetent, a doctor may be able to perform an emergency procedure under the theory of "implied consent." But first, the doctor should make every effort to contact a family member. Most states have a consent statute that delineates the hierarchy of family members who may consent for a patient's treatment in these situations.

Suppose the doctor tries but can't reach the family? The law presumes that people want to live, so if waiting for someone to give consent would endanger the patient, the doctor can treat him under the theory of implied consent. Then he should document reasons for the emergency procedure in the patient's chart.

Common-law marriage

In the case of common-law marriage, some states consider a man and woman married if they've lived together for 7 years and meet other criteria, such as representing themselves as married. But don't take the patient's or companion's word for this. The court has to verify the marriage before you can legally let the companion make treatment decisions.

Not all states recognize common-law marriages. Among those that do, most do not recognize same-sex couples.

Protecting yourself

If neither of the above conditions is met, a relative (parent or sibling, for example) or a court-appointed guardian must take responsibility for giving consent for treatment and for withholding treatment. The patient's companion may also request the court's permission to act as a guardian.

To avoid legal problems, always ask about the person's relationship to the patient. If the patient is incompetent and hasn't designated a surrogate decision maker, try to find out who his next of kin is. If he is competent and says he doesn't have a family, suggest that he grant durable power of attorney to someone he trusts – such as his companion. If you believe something isn't right, consult with your nurse-manager about the appropriate action to take.

❖

Ensuring the right to refuse treatment

We've all had patients refuse treatment. For example, an elderly diabetic patient may refuse to have a leg amputated, or another patient may wish to discontinue dialysis. When this happens, we're torn between wanting to protect the patient's health and defend his legal rights. How can we avoid liability?

Competent adults have a right to refuse treatment, even if it's lifesaving. Legally, their wishes must be respected as long as they understand that they could die as a result of their decision.

This same legal principle applies when a patient refuses care because of religious or personal beliefs. However, the courts occasionally limit this right, such as in cases involving pregnant patients, when the decision affects the fetus's life, or in cases involving blood transfusions. Also, parents may not be allowed to impose their religious beliefs on their children when those beliefs could cause the child's death. This last situation depends on state law and whether or not the hospital seeks legal guidance through a court-appointed guardian.

If the patient is incompetent, the family assumes responsibility for expressing his wishes, which he may have documented through an advance directive, such as a living will.

Dealing with advance directives

Suppose you're caring for a 65-year-old man who's unconscious from a major stroke. He doesn't have an advance directive, and his family is virtually paralyzed by shock, grief, and indecision. Do you know how to help them make a decision without breaking the law?

The Patient Self-Determination Act, passed by the U.S. Congress in 1990, requires hospitals and other health care facilities, including managed care organizations that receive Medicare or Medicaid funds, to advise all patients of their right to refuse treatment and to inform them of any relevant state law dealing with advance directives. Most institutions ask the patient if he knows his rights in this area, request a copy of his advance directive if he has one, and offer help to complete one if he doesn't. Under this federal law, a patient can't be forced to sign an advance directive as a condition of care, nor can he be discriminated against if he chooses not to sign.

Following life-support guidelines

Because nursing assessments are part of the admissions procedure, you may be expected to explain about advance directives to your patients. You also must make sure you understand your hospital's policies on life-support issues. They should be consistent with these guidelines:

• Don't call a code if the doctor has written a do-not-resuscitate (DNR) order. Reviving a patient could expose you to charges of assault and battery or even criminal negligence.

• Unless your hospital has a policy to the contrary, never accept an oral DNR order. In most hospitals, it's not valid unless the doctor writes it in the patient's chart.

• Don't accept a "slow code" order – an informal, oral instruction that nurses not promptly call codes on certain patients or that they respond slowly or incompletely. Participating in a slow code could result in criminal charges as well as in civil charges of negligent care.

• In the absence of a written DNR order, always call a code –

even if the patient is terminally ill.

• If a competent, terminally ill patient asks for DNR status, notify the doctor so he can write an order. Legally, you can't honor the patient's wishes without an order – that would amount to practicing medicine.

• Likewise, don't accept DNR instructions from a patient's family without a written doctor's order.

• If a patient presents a living will, alert the doctor – even if state law doesn't require him to honor it. Most doctors will abide by a living will even when not required to do so by law. (In states with living will statutes and natural death acts, a doctor could be prosecuted for ignoring an advance directive.)

• If the doctor writes a DNR order for a patient who's not terminally ill, alert your nurse-manager so the order can be reassessed. Depending on the circumstances, you may want to talk with a representative of the hospital's ethics committee for clarification.

• If the patient is incompetent and the doctor and family are making care decisions in the absence of a durable power of attorney for health care or another advance directive, alert your nurse-manager and the hospital's ethics committee to make sure that the patient's rights are protected.

• If a patient makes a dying declaration – a statement in anticipation of immediate death – record the statement verbatim in his chart. Such a declaration can be significant (especially if it's an admission of criminal behavior). Also, in states that honor

oral wills, a patient may actually give away some of his property in a dying declaration if his statement is witnessed by two people and documented immediately. The limited number of states that allow oral wills usually allow personal property only up to a certain dollar amount to be given away by this means. ❖

Admitting a psychiatric patient against his will

Patients are sometimes admitted to psychiatric hospitals or units against their will. If taking part in this procedure makes you uncomfortable, you have good reason. It's a legal gray area that must be handled carefully.

Under some circumstances, a patient who needs psychiatric help but who refuses to be admitted voluntarily can be legally admitted against his will. But you must follow your hospital's policy – and your state's laws – exactly, or you may risk legal repercussions.

If the patient is competent, all you can legally do is try to talk him out of leaving. But suppose he has a history of violence or poses a threat to himself? If such a patient refuses admission, notify hospital and nursing administrators immediately. If state law allows it, they may get police assistance to restrain the patient.

Most state laws require that a doctor then assess the patient to determine his mental competence. They also require a hearing – either before or after involuntary commitment, depending on how severe the patient's problem is and how immediate the danger.

If your hospital has a policy on managing patients who refuse treatment, follow it exactly. It should reflect state laws and specifically answer such questions as: How long and for what reasons may a patient be detained? When can you use forcible restraints? Who may order the use of restraints? Who may apply the restraints?

❖

Avoiding breach of confidentiality

With the growing number of patients who are positive for the human immunodeficiency virus (HIV), nurses are faced with issues of confidentiality every day. But even if your patient doesn't have a communicable disease, he may want his records kept private. Does the law say that you must always honor his wishes? If not, who decides?

Typically, you shouldn't disclose confidential information about a patient, such as his diagnosis or medical record, to a third party who doesn't need to know. People who need to know are hospital personnel directly involved in the patient's care and anyone else the patient gives you permission to tell.

But, in a few instances, you may have a legal duty to disclose such information. For example, most states require health care professionals to report cases of suspected child abuse. The state provides immunity for anyone disclosing this information, even if it turns out to be incorrect. The only requirement is that the person doing the reporting not be maliciously motivated. As a rule, you have a duty to disclose confidential information when a third party may suffer harm if you don't. (See *Divulging HIV status*, page 596.)

Informing nurses of a patient's HIV status

If a patient doesn't know or doesn't tell you that he's HIV-positive, you could care for him without ever knowing his status. But if the hospital realizes that a patient is infected with HIV, do you have a legal right to know?

You have the right to know, but only if you're directly involved in the patient's care. At the same time, though, the patient has a right to expect confidentiality. To balance these seemingly conflicting rights, legislatures in most states exempt health care workers from strict confidentiality in this type of situation.

Information about a patient's HIV status should be shared on a need-to-know basis only. So before you divulge this sensitive information to a coworker, be absolutely certain that the person really needs it to do her job. Of course, a nurse can't disclose information about a patient's care, including HIV status, to a family member (or health care professionals not involved in his care) without the patient's permission.

For more information about specific laws in your state, contact the board of nursing or the

LEGAL LIABILITY

LEGAL LESSON

Divulging HIV status

Mr. Harvey is admitted to your unit in critical condition with *Pneumocystis carinii* pneumonia and a diagnosis of acquired immunodeficiency syndrome (AIDS). He's comatose and not expected to live.

Ms. Carter, Mr. Harvey's girlfriend, tells you that she and her three young children have lived with the patient for 5 years. She obviously doesn't know that he has AIDS because she keeps asking you what's wrong with him. You feel that she has a right to know the truth, but the doctor disagrees. Can you legally divulge this information?

Unfortunately, you can't. Only the doctor can tell Ms. Carter about Mr. Harvey's diagnosis, and he can decide not to.

As a rule, a doctor can't discuss a patient's diagnosis with a relative or friend without the patient's permission. However, in many states, the law allows—but doesn't require—the patient's doctor to divulge information to someone who may be at risk for human immunodeficiency virus (HIV). If the patient refuses to admit his diagnosis to someone he may have infected (or if he can't, as in this case), the doctor may inform that person. But it's the doctor's decision, and he can decide against it.

If you find yourself in a similar position, discuss your concerns with the doctor, inform your nurse-manager, and take the problem to your hospital's ethics committee, if necessary.

---

office of the state legislator for your district.

Giving information to the police

Let's say the police ask you for a patient's name, phone number, address, employer, or other information. Would disclosing these facts violate the patient's right to privacy and confidentiality? Or should you be a good citizen and tell?

The answer is surprisingly direct: Don't give out any information about a patient, including the fact that he's been treated, unless the police produce a warrant. Your professional responsi-

bilities outweigh your civic duties.

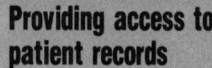

Providing access to patient records

Besides the medical personnel providing care for a patient, other people often express an interest in reading the patient's record. For example, the patient himself, his family members, or even a lawyer may wish to see the record. To whom should you permit access?

When a patient wants to read his record

One day, when you're recording a patient's vital signs, he asks to read his chart. Without thinking, you hand it over. Now you're wondering: Was my action legal?

Although records are the hospital's physical property, their content belongs to the patient. State law or hospital policy usually gives patients the right to review their own records. However, for the utmost legal protection, refer the patient to your nurse-manager. She can ask him to make a written request to see his record, which you can then put in his chart.

When family members ask to read records

What should you do if a family member asks to read a patient's chart? Can you give permission without being accused of breach of confidentiality and invasion of privacy?

Because medical records belong to the hospital, hospital policy, not the doctor or nurse, determines who can see the chart. Family members need a signed and dated permission letter from the patient before they can read his chart. So, the next time a family member asks to see a patient's chart, refer him to your nurse-manager. She can ask the patient to sign a permission letter, which should protect you legally.

When a lawyer asks to read records

Suppose you're an occupational health nurse for a corporation, and one of the company's lawyers requests the medical records of a former employee. This employee is suing the corporation for mental stress and other illnesses he claims resulted from working there. The lawyer says the records belong to the corporation so he's entitled to have them to defend the corporation. Would handing them over be a breach of patient confidentiality?

In this case, the lawyer is right. This former employee made his physical and psychological health an issue, so his records are an open book. In other words, he can't sue the corporation over mental and physical ailments brought on by his job and expect to maintain his privacy or right to confidentiality.

❖
_____

Your legal risks on the job

As a nurse, your chances of being named a defendant or co-defendant in a malpractice lawsuit are growing. One reason is today's litigious climate. Another reason is that nurses are taking on expanded responsibilities that inevitably lead to increased legal accountability. This means that you need to thoroughly understand your basic legal rights, responsibilities, and risks in everyday nursing practice. If you don't, you may be setting yourself up for a lawsuit.

This section describes your legal risks and responsibilities in several everyday situations.

Avoiding assessment, planning, and intervention errors

Most lawsuits against nurses don't arise from highly technical, sophisticated care. They arise from errors you make in basic care, such as in assessment, planning, and intervention. (See *Failure to complete drain removal.*)

Assessment errors
These typically include:
• failing to adequately gather and chart information about the patient
• failing to recognize the significance of certain information, such as laboratory values, intake and output measurements, vital signs, and complaints of pain that require immediate action.

To avoid assessment errors, your initial assessment should include the patient's chief complaint; his personal and family health history; known and suspected allergies and drug reactions; any prescription, over-the-counter, or illicit drugs he's taking; physical assessment data; his mental and emotional state; and relevant lifestyle habits (such as diet, alcohol use, smoking, and exercise). Check your policy and procedure manuals for anything more that your hospital requires. Document this initial assessment as soon as possible.

If the patient can't provide all the information you need, mark his chart accordingly. Don't leave any blanks – this implies that you didn't assess him thoroughly. If appropriate, ask the patient's relatives to supply missing information. Just make sure that you talk with him again if anything they tell you is confusing or incomplete or contradicts something that he said.

Errors in planning
These typically include:
• failing to chart each problem you discover during the assessment and include it in your plan of care
• failing to use language in your plan of care that other nurses will understand
• failing to ensure continuity of care from shift to shift by ignoring the initial plan of care or by drifting away from the intended goals
• failing to give discharge instructions that the patient understands.

How can you avoid these planning errors? By planning your care, communicating clearly, and then carefully explaining discharge instructions.

Planning
Don't underestimate the value of a well-thought-out plan of care. It'll give you a clear approach to the patient's problems. Phrase each patient-problem statement clearly, and modify statements as you gather new assessment data. Also state the plan of care for solving each problem, and then identify the actions you intend to take.

If you're working from a computer-generated, standardized plan of care, individualize it for each patient. The plan and solutions should be realistic because they could become the standard of care you must measure up to in court. You won't fare well if the plan was ignored for most of the patient's stay or if the goals were unrealistic to start with.

Communication

Always communicate clearly in the chart and when giving a verbal report. When charting, use only hospital-approved abbreviations, and try to express your observations in quantifiable terms. For example, "output adequate" isn't as helpful as an exact measurement.

Teaching

Follow your plan through by carefully explaining discharge instructions. If possible, include the patient's spouse or other relative (with the patient's permission). Ask the patient to demonstrate what you just taught him or to repeat your instructions. Record how well he understood—for example, "patient able to demonstrate insulin injection" or "patient verbalizes understanding by rephrasing the instructions." Also chart the instructions you gave him. A copy of written instructions is the best evidence of what you reviewed.

Don't assume you can skip basic instructions. Even intelligent, cooperative patients make mistakes—inserting birth-control pills vaginally, for example, or failing to dilute baby formula.

Failure to complete drain removal

Failure to remove a drain after surgery was the allegation in *Guilbeaux v. Lafayette General Hospital* (589 So.2d 629 [La. App. 3 Cir. 1991]). After back surgery, a wound drain was placed in Roy Guilbeaux's back to drain excess blood. Several days later, the surgeon asked the nurse on duty to remove the drain, which she did.

After discharge, Mr. Guilbeaux continued to have pain in his back, leg, and hip, so he went to another doctor for a second opinion. New X-rays revealed a 3½" (1 m) strip of the drain tube in his back, approximately ¼" (.6 cm) from the nerve root.

Mr. Guilbeaux needed additional surgery to remove the drain tube. He was left with back problems, continual pain, and exacerbated impotence.

Both the nurse and the hospital were named as defendants in the lawsuit—for which Mr. Guilbeaux was awarded considerable damages.

The lesson? Before you remove a drain, check the operating room report or the packaging for the drain length; after removal, make sure that you have the entire piece.

Intervention errors

These typically include:
• failing to interpret and carry out a doctor's orders
• failing to perform nursing tasks correctly
• failing to pursue the doctor if he doesn't respond to telephone calls or to notify your nurse-manager if he's unavailable.

Classic intervention errors involve nursing tasks you learned early in your education, such as reading a written order; transcribing a telephone order; identifying a patient before performing a nursing procedure; positioning patients; administering medications; counting sponges, needles, or instruments; and applying restraints. If you make a mistake and a patient is injured because of it, you could become the target of a negligence lawsuit.

Continuing education can help you avoid intervention errors, so keep up-to-date on the latest treatments and medications. Also, question any orders that don't seem appropriate. ❖

Coping with understaffing

Understaffing can cause substandard patient care, increased errors, and careless documentation. In lawsuits where understaffing is the key issue, the courts generally hold hospitals primarily responsible. But they may find charge nurses liable as well because they're responsible for making work assignments.

One way hospitals remedy staffing problems is by floating nurses from well-staffed units to understaffed units. Unfortunately, floating can also increase nurses' legal risks, especially if they float to unfamiliar areas.

Cutting the risk

Most understaffing-related malpractice lawsuits involve nurses who fail to continually monitor a patient or to report any significant changes in the patient's condition to the doctor. Here's how to reduce your risk of legal problems stemming from understaffing:
• Become familiar with your state's nurse practice act so you know what extra responsibilities you can legally take on when you float to other units.
• Know your hospital's policies on floating. For example, if your employment contract says you aren't required to float, you can refuse; otherwise, you can't. If you feel uncomfortable with a floating assignment, voice your concerns to your supervisor and document them.
• Push for continuing education programs if you work in a small hospital where staff is floated freely. These programs will help you maintain and broaden your clinical skills. (See *When staffing policy compromises patient safety.*)
• Inform your supervisor and request more help if you notice a staffing problem that could seriously compromise patient care. If help isn't available, after your shift is over, file a documented report and send it up through channels or to your risk manager. This won't necessarily protect you if a patient is injured while in your care, but it will show that you made a sincere at-

When staffing policy compromises patient safety

Imagine yourself in this situation: Two critical care nurses usually work on your four-bed intensive care unit (ICU), even when there's only one patient. But now nursing administration wants to change the policy. When only one patient is on the unit, it'll be staffed with one registered nurse (RN) and one monitor technician (an emergency medical technician [EMT]). The other RN will be floated, but she'll be available for immediate recall to the unit. The nurse-manager, who isn't a critical care nurse, will fill in when the ICU nurse takes a break.

If you think this proposed policy is legally dangerous, you're right. Having only one experienced nurse on the unit is risky enough, but leaving the unit in the hands of the nurse-manager and the EMT is irresponsible and negligent.

Not the best solution

Another issue involves using EMTs as monitor technicians. It's not the best solution for staffing shortages, but the laws in some states are so vague that ancillary personnel are being used in this manner. However, if they're working as monitor technicians, they're under the direction of the hospital—which is expected to prepare them for the tasks they'll undertake.

To ensure patient safety, monitor technicians must be competent, and a policy must be in place to measure their competence on an ongoing basis. If you're a nurse in the above situation, contact your local chapter of the American Association of Critical-Care Nurses for feedback on what other hospitals are doing.

You should also talk with your nurse-manager immediately—the stakes are just too high. If you're at an impasse with her, you should document your concerns in a memo and send it through administrative channels. And continue to send memos until things change. Make sure you keep copies for your own files.

empt to protect your patients. Remember to keep a copy for your personal files.

If you're a director of nursing or a charge nurse, assign your staff properly, make sure that they're competent to perform their tasks, and supervise them continually.

Delegating to unlicensed personnel

One consequence of understaffing is the need to delegate nursing duties to nonnursing staff such as nursing assistants. What are the legal ramifications for nurses who delegate the responsibilities?

Unless forbidden by state law, hospitals may allow unlicensed nursing assistants to catheterize and suction patients, remove arterial lines, and even help a doctor insert a pulmonary artery catheter. However, the hospital should provide a course to prepare them for tasks allowed by state law and hospital policy. It should also set up a system to check the credentials of those assistants certified at other hospitals and require them to pass a written examination.

Once the nursing assistants have been properly certified, nurses can then delegate appropriate tasks to them. Just make sure that you know what they're allowed to do and how skillful they are. As you would when delegating to any other staff member, assign only tasks that fit the person's demonstrated abilities. ❖

Using restraints legally

The use of restraints has become a controversial issue. Activists claim that restraints improperly limit personal freedom, and some patients have actually choked to death trying to escape from them. However, failing to protect an agitated patient from injury by using restraints could expose you to negligence charges.

Federal regulations now mandate strict procedures for using restraints in long-term-care facilities, and many are adopting restraint-free policies. But most hospitals still use safety devices and medications

to limit patient movement under certain circumstances.

Guidelines for restraints
To protect your patients and avoid legal problems, follow the guidelines for applying restraints in your hospital's policy and procedure manuals. They should cover all types of physical and chemical restraints, including bed rails, vest restraints, wrist restraints, and tranquilizers.

Also follow this general advice:
• When weighing the need for restraints, assess the underlying medical or psychological reasons for the patient's agitation or confusion. Restraints should be applied only for the patient's health and safety – not for the staff's convenience or to cope with understaffing. (See *Liability for not restraining*.)
• If you apply restraints, document the specific behavior that makes them necessary.
• Get a doctor's order before applying restraints – unless you feel the patient should be restrained immediately. Then take appropriate action and notify the doctor as soon as possible.
• Make sure that physical restraints fit properly; remove them and check the patient's circulation at least once every hour. Document this in your nurses' notes.
• When feeding a restrained patient, make sure that he's sitting upright to reduce the risk of choking.
• Don't let a family member tell you whether the patient should or shouldn't be restrained. Use your own judgment. Remember, you can't legally delegate responsibility to a family member,

LEGAL LESSON

 Liability for not restraining

Ronald Brookover, who is mentally retarded, was injured in a car accident at age 9. Afterward, he periodically suffered both generalized motor and akinetic epileptic seizures. As he grew older, the seizures became more severe.

When Ronald was age 36, he was admitted to the hospital for a corpus callosotomy—a two-phase procedure that separates the brain's left and right hemispheres and helps control seizures. Three days after the first surgery, Ronald—who wasn't restrained—called for assistance to go to the bathroom. When no one responded, he climbed out of bed, fell, and fractured his hip. His parents sued the hospital because he hadn't been restrained.

At the end of trial, the jury found the hospital negligent (*Brookover v. Mary Hitchcock Memorial Hospital*, 893 F.2d 411 [1st Cir. 1990]). The real issue, said the court, involved the hospital's failure to restrain Ronald—"a mentally retarded [patient] who had just been in the hospital for an operation that cut his brain in two. In our judgment, the evidence of negligence on the part of the hospital...was so overwhelming that it completely eradicates the question of whether the hospital was negligent in failing to respond to Ronald's call with reasonable alacrity."

even if he offers to sit with the patient. However, you can delegate responsibility to other registered nurses (including private-duty nurses), licensed practical nurses, and professional sitters and other nonlicensed personnel who, in your judgment, are competent and properly prepared.

Restraining a patient against his wishes

Suppose an elderly but lucid patient who's been pulling at his I.V. tubing refuses to let you apply restraints? Can you restrain him anyway without legal consequences?

Because a competent patient has the right to refuse care, you could face charges of battery if you restrain this patient against his wishes. However, if a doctor orders restraints, you're obligated to carry out that order or inform him and your nurse-manager why you can't. Otherwise, you could be liable for negligence if the patient is harmed.

Your best course of action is to immediately assess the patient's mental status, document your assessment and the patient's reason for refusing the restraints, and report your findings to the doctor. Then he can decide whether or not to change his order.

Preventing patient falls

Patient falls are responsible for more lawsuits alleging negligence on the part of hospitals and nurses than any other kind of injury. How can you protect your patient from harm and yourself from liability?

Nurses and doctors aren't automatically liable for patient falls. The courts expect you to continually evaluate your patients' needs and take proper precautions, so you may be held liable if a patient falls because you neglected to do this. But if he falls despite your having taken all proper precautions to protect him – and you can produce documented evidence of the quality of your care – your risk of liability is much less.

Why patients fall

Elderly, infirm, sedated, or mentally incapacitated patients are most apt to fall, although any patient can fall when the circumstances are right. Once you know which patients are most apt to fall, you can help protect them. To determine who they are, consider why they fall. For example:
• The patient's illness and medications may make him less aware of his surroundings.
• The complex diagnostic and therapeutic procedures the patient is undergoing may make him less aware of his surroundings.
• The unfamiliar environment, without the usual protection of family and friends, may confuse the patient or put unexpected stumbling blocks in his path.

Add to these problems the crucial factor of the patient's age. In or out of the hospital, elderly people are most likely to fall, and when they do, they're apt to suffer serious injury. Most falls occur in people ages 60 to 69 due to changes resulting from the aging process. For instance, decreased visual acuity and difficulty in distinguishing color can compound the problem of being in an unfamiliar environment. Even if an elderly patient's proprioception is only slightly affected, he may stumble getting out of bed.

Time of day also may be significant. Many falls result when the patient gets out of bed at night to use the bathroom. Sleepiness, darkness, and an unfamiliar environment can lead to poor footing and a fall. ❖

Handling equipment malfunctions

Sophisticated equipment can be a lifesaver for the patient – or a source of liability for you. Although most hospitals do routine safety checks, equipment can still fail at the worst possible moment, leaving you and the hospital at risk for a lawsuit.

If you know a piece of equipment isn't functioning properly, you're legally obligated to take steps to resolve the problem, and then to document what you did. Most often, this means calling the maintenance department and asking them to replace or repair malfunctioning equipment.

But if the defect isn't readily apparent, are you still liable if something goes wrong? Not if adequate checks were made. Unless the equipment is obviously defective and you use it anyway, neither you nor the hospital is liable for the patient injury it may cause. Who is liable? Usually, liability rests with the manufacturer.

Risk-reduction tips
To reduce your risk of liability, follow these guidelines:
• Follow the manufacturer's instructions for operation and maintenance of all equipment.
• Know what equipment you're responsible for checking and whom to call if it malfunctions or needs servicing. Nurses routinely check some equipment (for example, intubation equipment, monitors, and defibrillators); the maintenance department or a biomedical specialist checks the rest.
• Fix or report any defective equipment immediately. Ask that it be removed from the unit before someone else tries to use it.
• When equipment fails during use, document the entire incident, including the actions you took, and advise your hospital's risk manager.
• Urge your hospital to hold continuing education classes (if it's not already doing so) to review proper use of new equipment and equipment already in use. ❖

Letting family members help with patient care

If family members ask to help care for a loved one, be very cautious about what you let them do. Something as innocent as walking an unsteady patient to the bathroom could result in an injury to the patient or family member and a negligence lawsuit against you and the hospital.

Remember the hospital's liability
The hospital is legally responsible for every patient's safety, and family members don't have the preparation that you do to fulfill this obligation. So never allow them to give even routine care to a recent postoperative patient or to perform any other tasks that could endanger the patient's health or safety.

This doesn't mean you should exclude family members from a loved one's care. They can safely give back rubs, assist with meals and bathing, and walk up and down the hall with ambulatory patients.

Check hospital policy
Help protect yourself by checking your hospital's policy and procedure manuals for information about involving family members in a patient's care. If you don't find anything, talk with your nurse-manager or the hospital's risk manager. Try to get specific guidelines so you can tell family members exactly what they can and can't do.

If a family member ignores your instructions, reinforce them and document your conversation in the nurses' notes. Your notes could be important evidence if the family member continues to ignore your warning, the patient is injured, and you wind up in court.

❖

Signing a prescription for a doctor

Nurses – especially those in office practices – are sometimes asked by doctors to write prescriptions for patients and then sign the doctor's name. Is this legal?

Nurses should never follow a doctor's order to write a prescription and sign his name. Doing so is legally considered prescribing drugs, which is a medical practice. Of course, many states do allow nurse practitioners to write prescriptions, but they sign their own name, not the doctor's.

If a doctor ever asks you to write a prescription and sign his name, try one of these legal alternatives: If your hospital policy allows, take a verbal or telephone order from the doctor, who would then have to countersign it later according to protocol. Or (even safer) ask the doctor to have standing orders typed up for his signature. Then you can distribute the orders to his patients. Some units have used this practice with discharge orders for years. Not only is this system efficient, but it could also save you from charges of practicing beyond the scope of your license.

❖

Handling medication orders from nonphysicians

If a nurse practitioner or a physician's assistant writes medication orders in your hospital, are you legally bound to obey them?

In some states, nurse practitioners and physician's assistants are allowed to write medication orders. But before you follow such an order, protect yourself from liability by taking these measures:
• Order a copy of your nurse practice act from your state nurses' association to see what's permitted in your state. In most states, a physician's assistant must be directly supervised by a doctor in all duties, including writing medication orders. Also, many states prohibit nurses from following a physician's assistant's order if it isn't authorized by the supervising doctor.
• Check your hospital's policy; it may not conform to your nurse practice act. If the policy says you can't take orders directly from nurse practitioners or physician's assistants, refuse to follow any such order until the attending doctor countersigns it. If the situation is life-threatening, don't wait for his signature. But even then, you could be liable for practicing outside the scope of your nurse practice act or for violating hospital policy.
• No matter what your state law or hospital policy, if you question a nurse practitioner's or physician's assistant's actions, contact the supervising doctor before carrying out the order. If state law permits autonomous nurse practitioner practice and

doesn't require a supervising doctor, then follow the procedure for questioning a doctor's medication order.

• Discuss your concerns with your nurse-manager, director of nursing, or hospital administrator.

• Ask for assignment to your hospital's policy and procedure committee. Then help make sure that hospital policy conforms with your state's nurse practice act – and work to change the policy if it doesn't.

• Become involved in your state nursing association so you can have some say about whose orders you should follow. ❖

Avoiding drug dispensing

Dispensing is selecting a medication, then labeling or packaging it and giving it to someone else to administer. Administering is giving a single dose of a prescribed medication to a patient. A nurse who dispenses drugs can be charged with practicing pharmacy without a license.

Typically, state laws allow nurses to administer drugs and pharmacists to dispense them. One exception may be if a patient needs a medication that isn't stocked on your unit and a pharmacist isn't on duty. Then you're probably legally safe if you take a single dose from the hospital pharmacy and give it yourself. That's administering, not dispensing.

Helpful hints

Follow the guidelines below to keep from dispensing drugs:

• Never take a container of medication from the pharmacy after hours for use on a unit.

• Never refill empty containers.

• If you work in a facility that allows patients to go on weekend and day trips, never place medication in a container you've labeled so the patient can take it while he's away. (This may be common practice in many hospitals, but you're on shaky legal ground if you do it.) Instead, plan ahead so the pharmacist can fill the medication order before the patient leaves.

• To avoid having to refill stock medication containers, make sure you order adequate supplies during pharmacy hours.

• If you or your supervisor must frequently enter the pharmacy after hours to fill new drug orders or refill stock orders, discuss your concerns with your director of nursing. Then, ask her to meet with the hospital's pharmacy director to try to improve pharmacy staffing – or at least to arrange to have a pharmacist on call for emergency drug orders. ❖

Delegating drug administration

When units are understaffed, nurses run the risk of delegating medication administration and other tasks to subordinates who aren't qualified to perform them. This can lead to negligence lawsuits if a patient is harmed.

LEGAL LIABILITY

You're responsible for delegating medication administration only to qualified nurses. So when you delegate, make sure that the person is permitted to administer medications under your state law and hospital policy and that she's competent to do so. If she's not, you could be legally liable.

Imagine if you assigned I.V. lidocaine administration to a pediatric nurse unfamiliar with cardiac care unit routine. You could both be liable for negligence, especially if she administered the medication improperly and injured the patient. Also, some hospitals don't allow noncritical care nurses to administer I.V. medications.

Or suppose you asked a licensed practical nurse (LPN) to administer medications, and your state law doesn't authorize LPNs to do this. The LPN could be charged with practicing outside the scope of her nurse practice act, and you and your employer could be charged with aiding and abetting that unauthorized practice.

Tips for safe delegating

Here are some additional suggestions for avoiding liability when delegating medication administration:
• After you've delegated the task, make sure that the drug was actually given. If it wasn't, and the patient is harmed, both you and the nurse you delegated to could be held liable.
• Ask your nurse-manager for periodic updating and posting of the skills and judgments nurses need for all types of medication administration.

• Ask for posted lists of who can administer medications together with reminders of related hospital policies and procedures. This list may one day help you defend a charge of negligent delegation if the name of a nurse you've delegated to is on it.

❖

Managing a patient who won't take medication

Have you ever forced a patient to take a medication because he really needed it? If so, you may have left yourself open to assault and battery charges.

In the last few years, many medical experts, legislators, and lawyers have debated this issue. As a result, some state laws now address the patient's right to refuse "excessive or unnecessary" medications. However, they don't define "excessive" or "unnecessary."

You may administer medication against a patient's will if he's in danger of harming himself or others. But if he isn't, forcing drugs probably violates his rights. Most likely he'd be successful if he filed assault and battery charges.

One more issue bears examining – that of patient advocacy. Some patients – such as those on psychiatric units – may be so severely impaired that they can't seek counsel to protect their rights. If that's the case, you and other nurses on the unit need to be their advocates. When you believe a patient is being excessively or unnecessarily medicated, you might discuss the situation with other members of the health care team, including the unit manager.

❖

Questioning a doctor's order

Do you always assume the doctor is right and follow his orders even if they seem vague or medically inappropriate? If you do, you could be jeopardizing your nursing career.

You're responsible for questioning any dubious order you receive. Some orders may actually be detrimental to your patient's health and legally dangerous for you. Here are four types of orders you must always question.

Ambiguous orders
Follow your hospital's policy for clarifying any orders that are vague or have more than one possible interpretation, and make sure that you document your actions. If your hospital doesn't have such a policy, contact the prescribing doctor, ask him to clarify the orders, and document the conversation and your actions. Then ask your nursing administration for a step-by-step policy to follow if this occurs again.

Inappropriate orders
A change in your patient's condition may mean that a standing order is no longer appropriate. If so, delay treatment until you can contact the doctor and clarify the situation. Follow your

hospital's policy for clarifying the order.

If you're an inexperienced nurse, clarify all standing orders with the prescribing doctor. Or tell your supervisor that you're uncertain about following the order, and let her decide whether to delegate the responsibility to someone more experienced.

If you carry out the order and the treatment affects the patient adversely, discontinue it and report all unfavorable signs and symptoms to the doctor. Resume treatment only after you've discussed the situation with the doctor and clarified his orders. Then document meticulously.

Any order a patient questions
If the doctor changes his orders when you're off duty, the patient may know something about his prescribed care that no one has told you. So if a patient protests a procedure, medication dosage, or medication route, claiming that it's different from the usual or that it's been changed, give him the benefit of the doubt. Question the doctor's orders, following your hospital's policy if one exists.

Telephone orders
Whenever a doctor gives you an order by telephone, document all the details. Follow your hospital's policy to the letter. If your hospital doesn't have a formal policy, document your conversation and subsequent actions as follows:
• Write down the date and time of the call, the doctor's name, and the patient's condition and other circumstances that prompted the call.

LEGAL LIABILITY

• Review the patient's condition in detail with the doctor.
• Write down his orders as you listen.
• Read the orders back to him to make sure that you've recorded them accurately.
• Document that you read the orders back to the doctor and that he confirmed them.

———————————————❖

Taking telephone orders from a doctor's staff

You've probably called a doctor's office for orders and had his nurse relay them to you–then felt uneasy afterward. This common practice could put you in legal hot water.

Ideally, a verbal order should come directly from the doctor's mouth. In many states, a nurse practitioner, clinical nurse specialist, or nurse-midwife may also give–and a staff nurse may accept–orders based on nursing assessment and nursing diagnosis.

If an office nurse relays the doctor's orders, carefully follow your hospital's policy on verbal orders. It should spell out whether you can accept an order from anyone besides a doctor. You might also ask your director of nursing to write a memo to those doctors who frequently let their staff relay orders. The memo should request that the doctors review with their office staff the proper procedure for communicating a nurse's request and their prescribed treatment.

———————————————❖

Handling a patient who wants to leave

You could be faced with a patient who threatens to leave the hospital against medical advice. Should you try to detain him, or would this be violating his rights?

A competent patient's right to refuse treatment generally includes the right to leave the hospital against medical advice. But it's a no-win situation. If a patient leaves and something happens to him, you and the hospital can be held liable. However, the patient would also be held accountable because he contributed to his injury. You probably wouldn't have to pay damages–or, if you did, the amount would be reduced by the percentage of blame assessed against the patient. In some states, the patient's contribution to his injury negates all damages he might have received.

Usually, all you can do is try to talk the patient out of leaving; detaining him could result in charges of unlawful restraint or false imprisonment.

Exception to the rule

One exception is if the patient could endanger himself or others by leaving. For example, suppose he had a capped central venous line that he refused to let you remove. The line could clot, cause an embolus, and open the door to sepsis, or the catheter could shear and migrate or cause bleeding. In this case, if the patient still refuses to let you remove the line after you explain these possible consequences, he can be detained until he agrees to have it removed, without legal repercussions.

Always get help

If a patient ever threatens to leave against medical advice, don't try to handle the situation alone. Call in the doctor, your nurse-manager, and security (if needed). Ask a psychiatric clinical nurse specialist to talk with the patient if psychosocial factors are affecting his judgment.

Also, carefully follow your hospital's policy. Document what you did (such as calling the patient's family and providing routine discharge care) and what you said (such as explaining the medical risks of leaving). ❖

Coping with premature discharge

The introduction of the diagnosis-related groups system into health care has created financial pressure on hospitals to release patients as early as possible. Unfortunately, some patients are being released too early (or think they are). If you fail to actively oppose the discharge of a patient who you think isn't ready to leave the hospital and he suffers harm later because he wasn't ready, you may eventually be charged with nursing negligence.

Protect yourself by telling your nurse-manager and the doctor that you think a patient isn't ready for discharge. If necessary, send your objection through administrative channels up to your hospital's medical director. Document your objections, too. ❖

Handling a doctor who won't write a DNR order

Some doctors aren't comfortable writing do-not-resuscitate (DNR) orders, even if the patient requests it. This puts you in a difficult legal position if the patient has a cardiac or respiratory arrest.

Even if a patient requests not to be resuscitated, most states require you to resuscitate him if there's no DNR order. This law seems to contradict the Patient Self-Determination Act (1990), which affirms a patient's right to choose the type of treatment he would accept or reject and to indicate these choices in an advance directive.

Your hospital's policy and procedure manuals should reflect your state law and should also include a process for ensuring that doctors expeditiously write DNR orders for patients who want them. If this provision isn't in your manuals, speak with your nurse-manager about updating them.

If you're having this problem right now, continue pressing the doctor for a DNR order. If he resists, consult with your nurse-manager, who'll most likely talk with the doctor herself. If she doesn't get anywhere, she should consult with the director of nursing and the doctor's superior. ❖

Medicolegal deaths

Did you know that all of these scenarios involve medicolegal deaths?

• Morton Steele, 59, an insulin-dependent diabetic, regularly ignored his diet and foot care. When he developed raging cellulitis over his ankle, he was admitted to the hospital for treatment. To help bring Mr. Steele's blood glucose level under control, the doctor ordered a stat dose of 20 units of regular insulin. Misreading the order, an inexperienced nurse gave 2 ml (200 units) of regular insulin by I.V. push. Mr. Steele went into insulin shock and died the next day.

• Laura Davis, 44, had a long history of depression. After a fight with her husband, she took an overdose of acetaminophen. By the time she was found and rushed to the hospital, she'd suffered severe, irreversible liver damage. She died 4 days later.

• Artemis Hewitt attributed his longevity to a nightly glass of Irish whiskey. At age 90, he walked to the neighborhood grocery store nearly every day. When he didn't show up for 3 days in a row, the shopkeeper asked the sheriff to check on him. Mr. Hewitt was found slumped over in his favorite rocker, an empty whiskey glass by his side. Apparently he'd died peacefully in his sleep.

Not all cases are so clear-cut, and you may occasionally question whether a death really requires an investigation. For example, if a chronically ill patient dies of complications, should you notify the medical examiner? As a rule of thumb, the answer is yes – when in doubt, call and ask. It's much better to make a few unnecessary calls than to miss even one case that should be investigated.

Reporting a death

You've undoubtedly cared for many patients who've died violently or unexpectedly – from suicide, murder, accident, an unusual postoperative complication, or some unknown cause. But did you know that many other types of deaths must be reported either to the coroner or medical examiner (depending on locale), and that not reporting them is negligent?

Criteria for investigation

Any death that must be investigated is called a medicolegal death. (See *Medicolegal deaths*.) Although laws vary among jurisdictions, the following situations always require a thorough investigation:

• Death by suicide or homicide, regardless of the weapon or method involved.

• Death of an infant or a child, even if it's clearly accidental or from apparently natural causes. Infants who die from sudden infant death syndrome must undergo autopsy to rule out other possible causes, including child abuse, infection (such as interstitial pneumonitis), or a congenital defect. (An expected death from a terminal natural disease is sometimes an exception to this rule.)
• Death involving negligence or damaged or improperly used equipment. These types of deaths, which could involve medical malpractice or nursing negligence, often generate lawsuits. A thorough, objective investigation helps establish the facts.
• Death occurring less than 24 hours after admission to a hospital. Some jurisdictions exclude hospices from this rule.
• Death occurring within 24 hours of surgery or another invasive procedure.
• Death involving poisoning, illicit drugs, or any type of drug overdose. An autopsy helps rule out other possible causes of death; a complete toxicologic evaluation identifies the specific drugs involved.
• Death by motor vehicle accident, including cars, motorcycles, boats, airplanes, and recreational vehicles. In some cases, only a thorough investigation can establish whether the victim was the driver or a passenger.
• Death by other types of accidents, such as falls, drownings, or electrocution.
• Death by fire or smoke inhalation because fires can be set to cover up homicides.

• Death occurring on the job, to help determine if work conditions contributed to the death.
• Death from natural causes when no doctor is in attendance. This holds true even if the deceased was elderly and his death isn't suspicious. Similarly, any unexpected death of a previously healthy person must be examined, even if he regularly saw a doctor for routine care.
• Death involving firearms or other mortal weapons. Whether the death was accidental or deliberate is irrelevant.
• Death of a prominent person, even if no foul play is involved. An investigation will satisfy the press and end unfounded rumors.
• Death of an unidentified person. Identifying unknown remains is one of a medical examiner's primary responsibilities.
• Death involving a public health hazard, such as toxic spills and epidemics of reportable contagious diseases.
• Death of anyone in police custody, regardless of the circumstances.

❖

Providing postmortem care in a medicolegal death

When a medicolegal death occurs, you must know how to handle the victim's body. If you're careless or uninformed, you could destroy evidence and hinder the investigation.

Whenever you anticipate an investigation, take special precautions with the victim's body.

Don't touch, clean, or alter it in any way without the medical examiner's consent. If the room must be used for another emergency, move the body and the stretcher it's on to another room within the suite, but don't allow it to be taken to the morgue without permission.

Leave all tubes and catheters in the body, along with any drainage they contain. This includes nasogastric and endotracheal tubes and any drainage, indwelling urinary catheters with drainage bags and any urine, and all I.V. lines and fluid containers.

Hospital policy may allow you to cap I.V. tubing at the hub and discard the I.V. container and remaining tubing. If so, carefully document the amount of fluid infused. The medical examiner will need this information to determine how diluted the blood in the heart and extremities may have been. Then he'll decide where to take blood and tissue specimens for toxicologic study.

Getting ready for the family

If the family wants to see the body, don't clean it up as you normally would. Don't clean or pack wounds or clean up blood flow or splatters. Leave any jewelry or clothing on the victim as it is.

Explain the circumstances to the family before they see the victim. Describe his appearance and give them the option of viewing him as he is or waiting until after the medical examiner's initial examination. Make sure that a nurse, chaplain, or other caregiver is available to

accompany and support them if they wish.

❖

Your rights as an employee

As a nurse, you're an advocate for patients' rights. But you also need to safeguard your own rights. This section looks at the right to refuse an assignment, the question of abandoning patients, and the issue of required testing for human immunodeficiency virus.

Refusing a work assignment

If you're temporarily assigned to an unfamiliar unit and feel you aren't qualified to care for patients there, can you legally refuse the assignment?

Refusing for lack of qualifications

As a general rule, nurses can't refuse patient care assignments. However, if you feel that you aren't qualified to perform a particular assignment, document your concerns in writing and submit the note to your nurse-manager, while keeping a copy for yourself. Emphasize your belief that you might harm patients. If your nurse-manager still insists that you accept the assignment because no alternative exists, then accept it.

In *Francis v. Memorial Hospital* (1986), a New Mexico intensive care unit nurse refused to take temporary charge of an orthopedic unit, even though the hospital had a policy of floating nurses to other areas. He stated that he wasn't familiar with orthopedic procedures and might jeopardize patient safety. After refusing to be oriented to the other unit, he was suspended indefinitely. He subsequently filed suit against the hospital, but the court ruled against him, saying that the hospital's floating policy was valid.

Refusing on ethical grounds

Under most circumstances, you aren't allowed to refuse an assignment because of ethical or personal beliefs. For example, in *Warthen v. Toms River Community Memorial Hospital* (1985), a New Jersey nurse refused to dialyze a terminally ill patient for moral and ethical reasons. She was fired, after which she sued for reinstatement. During the trial, she supported her position with guidelines from the American Nurses' Association's Code of Ethics. The court rejected her argument, claiming that if individual health care providers asserted their own values, then the health care delivery system would be in chaos.

However, many states do allow nurses to refuse to participate in abortions and even sterilization procedures. But no court has upheld a nurse's right to refuse to care for a patient with acquired immunodeficiency syndrome.

Facing the issue of abandonment

Let's say that your unit is chronically understaffed and you're often asked to work multiple shifts. If you've ever been tempted to just walk out rather than work an extra shift, don't. You could be sued for abandonment.

You can face negligence charges for abandonment if a patient suffers after you leave the scene. But even if no one is hurt, you could still be charged with insubordination and fired on the spot.

Theoretically, leaving a patient during a code—even if you have a legitimate reason—could also be considered abandonment. But proving such a charge in court would probably be difficult, especially if many professionals were involved in the code. You'd still be open to a charge of insubordination, though, as you would if you refused to float to an unfamiliar unit. To fully protect yourself from such charges, be aware of labor issues as well as your patient responsibilities. (See *A question of abandonment*, page 616.)

Refusing employer demands for HIV testing

You've just applied for a job as a staff nurse at a local hospital. You're surprised when the human resources director says that

LEGAL LIABILITY

A question of abandonment

Suppose a doctor at your hospital routinely sends his patients off the unit for studies at his nearby office. Because these patients have I.V. lines, a nurse from the unit accompanies them in the ambulance, stays at the office during the procedure, and escorts them back.

You've done this several times, but it worries you. Could you be accused of abandoning your other patients?

The answer is maybe. You're still responsible for your patients on the unit – unless you delegate their care to another nurse. Of course, your nurse-manager shares responsibility because she made the assignment and she's letting you transport a patient to an off-site location.

If the doctor wants patients transported to his office, he should hire qualified personnel to transport them, supervise the procedure, and return them to the hospital. Even so, you probably can't refuse to accept this assignment from the doctor. Unless you're working under a collective-bargaining agreement

that prohibits this kind of assignment, you could be reprimanded or even fired for refusing to go.

Before this happens again, talk with your nurse-manager. Show her documentation of specific instances when patient safety was compromised because you or one of your colleagues had to leave the hospital. (Ask for their input, too.) Make sure that you keep copies of the documentation, along with notes of your conversation with the nurse-manager, for your personal records.

Then ask her to approach nursing and hospital administrators with your concerns. They should be looking at both the legal and financial ramifications of this situation. If a patient is harmed, they'd share liability because they're primarily responsible for providing adequate staffing. Plus, they're losing money. The tests aren't being done in-house, yet the hospital is paying a nurse to accompany patients. The doctor, meanwhile, is making money.

you'll have to have a human immunodeficiency virus (HIV) antibody test as a condition for employment. Is this legal?

Preemployment HIV antibody testing is legal as long as you give written, voluntary consent

and all potential employees are treated equally. But you can't be denied employment if you test positive – or if you refuse to be tested. An employer who discriminates based on HIV status violates two federal laws: the Rehabilitation Act and the Americans with Disabilities Act (being HIV-positive is considered a disability under these laws). Violations carry stiff fines; the employer could lose federal funding.

To avoid being caught in a catch-22, this employer should consider dropping preemployment HIV-antibody testing. Instead, employees should be urged to know their HIV status and to stringently follow universal precautions outlined by the Centers for Disease Control and Prevention and the Occupational Safety and Health Administration. People who test HIV-positive should consult with appropriate authorities to determine which procedures they can perform safely.

_____❖

Your legal risks off duty

When you're on duty, written guidelines, policies, and laws dictate what you can do legally. But when you're off duty, few professional and legal guidelines exist, so the legal limits of your actions aren't clear-cut. Although relatively few lawsuits are brought against nurses for off-duty actions, you do run some legal risks. This section covers three key areas: giving health care advice to friends, providing health care to friends, and giving off-duty emergency care.

Giving health care advice to friends

We've all had friends ask for our professional advice – and we've probably all given it. But suppose your advice is wrong? Could you get into legal trouble?

You assume legal risks whenever you give health care advice to friends. In the courts' view, even a casual conversation can sometimes establish a nurse-patient relationship, making you liable for the consequences of your advice. To minimize your legal risks, follow these guidelines:

• Find out if your professional liability insurance, or your employer's, provides you with off-duty coverage.

• Know whether your state's nurse practice act discusses giving advice to friends.

• Give advice only within the confines of your nurse practice act, education, and experience.

• Make sure that the advice you give is up-to-date. You'll be judged on current nursing standards if your advice results in a lawsuit.

• Never speculate about your friends' illnesses or ailments.

• Don't suggest that friends change or ignore their doctors' orders.

• Don't give your friends any advice about medical care.

• Never offer any advice that, if wrong, could result in serious or permanent injury.

_____❖

PREVENTING LEGAL LIABILITY

The woman next door asks you to administer her allergy injections.

Providing health care to friends

The woman next door asks you to administer her allergy injections. Should you be a good neighbor and say yes, or is this legally reckless?

The law says that a registered nurse may administer injections only if she has written approval from the patient's doctor; both the doctor and the nurse must be licensed in the state where the injections will be given.

But you should also consider other factors. First, providing professional help to a friend creates a nurse-patient relationship that makes you legally responsible for any outcome of your actions. So, you must administer care the same way any reasonable, prudent nurse would in similar circumstances. If you fail to meet that standard and your neighbor is injured, he could successfully sue you.

Second, you must also meet the standards required of any professional who's currently capable of performing the same task. So, if your skills are rusty or outdated, your nursing care might not meet current standards. And that might place you in legal jeopardy.

It's best, then, not to get involved in giving injections or any other care that isn't simple first aid. Instead, tell your neighbor to contact her doctor or a local hospital, where a qualified person will surely be able to help out.

Handling an emergency when you're off duty

If you witness an accident or see someone in trouble, your first impulse is to help out when you're off duty. But even though you're acting out of compassion, you may still feel vulnerable to a malpractice lawsuit.

The law recognizes this dilemma and says that most people don't have a "duty to rescue." (People who do have a legal duty are those who perform rescues as a regular part of their job, such as firemen and emergency medical technicians.) This means you don't have to offer assistance to victims in emergencies unless:

• you're responsible for the victim's condition (for example, you're involved in an automobile accident)

• your state has a statutory mandate (such as the "duty to rescue" law in Vermont or the "right to assistance" law in the province of Quebec, Canada, under which anyone [not just a nurse] must help victims in emergencies).

So, unless either of those two exceptions applies, you can offer to help in an emergency or decide not to help. Either way, you're protected by law.

Obligations if you help

Although the decision to help an accident victim is voluntary in most states and Canadian provinces, once you decide to help, you immediately incur an obligation to live up to the standards of the average, reasonably prudent nurse in a similar situation. Failure to meet these standards can result in a lawsuit—although the law grants you more leeway in what's expected when you're off duty.

If you voluntarily aid an accident victim while you're off duty and injure him through your negligence, you can't be sued for the injury, unless the court decides you were grossly negligent. Gross negligence is defined as care that is reckless and falls well below the reasonable standard.

Good Samaritan laws

In deciding negligence cases for off-duty emergency care, courts ask: "Has the nurse's action caused the victim to be measurably worse?" To win a malpractice lawsuit, the victim must prove that your imprudent care caused measurable damage. Because he already was injured in the accident, he'll probably have difficulty proving your error caused or worsened his injuries, especially if the court feels you performed within the standards of good nursing care.

All states have Good Samaritan laws to strengthen your legal position in off-duty emergencies. By limiting your liability, these laws encourage you to give assistance. They offer you immunity from lawsuits when you help an accident victim, as long as you don't intentionally or recklessly cause injury.

Unfortunately, Good Samaritan laws vary among states, and not all laws protect out-of-state nurses.

❖

Your risks in malpractice lawsuits

In the last 25 years, the number of malpractice lawsuits filed against nurses has risen dramatically. Why? Because patients are increasingly aware of their right to receive quality health care—and increasingly willing to fight for it.

Even so, you can still protect yourself from lawsuits. The best way is by giving your patients top-quality nursing care, according to the highest professional standards. You should also know your patients' rights and do your best to uphold them, and know your own rights and how to safeguard them.

This section deals with four malpractice issues: getting sued, giving a deposition, settling out of court, and buying your own liability insurance.

Strengthening your defense

Every nurse worries about being sued for malpractice someday. But how many of us know what to do and what not to do to defend our care and keep from harming our own defense?

First of all, being sued for malpractice doesn't mean you've actually committed malpractice—most of these lawsuits ultimately fail. The guidelines that follow can help you survive litigation.

Hiring a lawyer

If a patient sues you and the hospital where you work, then the hospital's insurance company will handle the case, supplying a lawyer to defend you as the hospital's employee. You should verify this with your hospital's risk manager.

If the patient sues only you, then you're on your own. The first thing you should do is see your professional liability agent. Most often your insurance company will appoint a lawyer to defend you.

If you don't have insurance, you're not satisfied with the lawyer the insurance company provides, or the company won't cover you because you failed to pay a premium on time or committed some other violation, find a

lawyer using the following methods:

• If you work in a hospital with a legal services department, find out if the hospital will provide you with a lawyer or refer you to one.
• If you have a relative or a friend who's a lawyer or a judge, ask him for a referral.
• If you're a member of a professional association, see if they can refer you to a lawyer.
• If none of these situations applies to you, contact your local bar association, listed in the business phone directory, for a referral. Find a lawyer who's experienced in medical malpractice cases.
• Before you hire a lawyer, ask other health care professionals if they've heard of him, and go by his reputation.

Tell your lawyer everything
Don't withhold information—you could harm your own defense. Tell your lawyer as much about your case as possible, including its strengths and weaknesses. Don't be afraid to be honest; your conversations are privileged. (See *Hiring a lawyer*.)

Don't speak directly with the plaintiff's lawyer
Don't bother giving the plaintiff's lawyer a piece of your mind—he already knows how you feel and probably doesn't care. Ethically, he shouldn't speak directly with you anyway, unless your own lawyer consents

to the conversation (which he probably won't). The plaintiff's lawyer might let you talk in the hope that you'll say something to help his client's case.

The only times you should speak with the plaintiff's lawyer are at your deposition and at the trial, if it gets that far. Your lawyer will be with you then, and he'll object to inappropriate questions.

Don't speak directly with the plaintiff
After the lawsuit is filed, anything you say to the plaintiff that even remotely suggests you did something wrong will come back

to haunt you at the trial. You'll have the chance later to express your thoughts.

Don't talk with reporters

If you receive phone calls or visits from local reporters, don't denounce the plaintiff, his lawyer, or the legal profession in general. Bad-mouthing the opposition may make you feel better, but it won't help your case.

Don't alter the patient's records

By the time the lawsuit is filed, the plaintiff's lawyer already has a copy of the original chart. He'll be quick to detect any changes you make later and just as quick to point them out in court. He might even bolster a weak case by persuading the jury that you tried to cover up important, potentially damaging evidence.

If you're aware of an error in the patient's chart, notify the hospital's risk manager and your lawyer.

❖

Giving a deposition

If a lawyer wants your deposition for an upcoming medical malpractice lawsuit, do you know what to expect? If not, you could be in for an unpleasant surprise. A deposition is more than a simple exchange of information. It's a sworn testimony given under an oath to tell the truth. And it can be an ordeal if you don't know how to handle yourself.

A deposition is part of the discovery process, which takes place before a case goes to trial. It gives opposing parties a chance to obtain information from one another so neither has an unfair advantage at trial. Based on this information, they may decide to settle the case out of court, drop the suit entirely, or continue with the previously filed suit.

You may be asked to give a deposition even if you haven't been named in the suit, if a lawyer thinks you may have information that could help settle the case. You'll definitely have to give one if a malpractice suit has been filed against you.

Typically, during a deposition, the opposing lawyer will ask you questions. Your own lawyer is there to protect you from unnecessary harassment and from questions you aren't obliged to answer.

Your rights

Understanding your rights as a witness will help you get through a deposition. You should hire your own lawyer; don't use the hospital lawyer because his duty is first to protect the interests of the hospital. Your lawyer will discuss these points with you.

You can demand a subpoena

Insist on receiving a subpoena; it's the only way the opposing side can force you to give a deposition. And usually it's accompanied by a small fee. If you're entitled to the fee and don't receive it before the scheduled deposition, ignore the subpoena.

You don't have to travel far

You can't be forced to appear at a deposition outside your county or outside the jurisdictional boundaries of the U.S. District Court where you live (depending on whether the case was filed in state or federal court). If the opposing lawyer wants your testimony, he'll travel to you.

Your lawyer can be present
You can—and should—have your own lawyer present during the deposition. In fact, you can refuse to give your deposition at the scheduled time if your lawyer isn't present. The deposition can be rescheduled.

You can take aids with you
When you go to the deposition, you can carry anything that might help you—notes you've jotted down, a calendar for remembering dates, publications you may want to quote from, such as hospital policies and procedures, the American Nurses' Association's Standards of Care, and nursing journals. But any of these items may be designated as exhibits, and you'll have to leave them with the court reporter. So, before the deposition, make copies for the court and plan to leave the originals at home.

You can take your time
Don't rush to answer a question. You can take all the time you need to check the papers or manuals you've brought with you and to compose your answer. When replying, stick to the facts as you know them firsthand; don't offer secondhand information or opinions unless the opposing lawyer specifically asks for them.

You can take a break
The opposing lawyer may wait until you seem tired before he asks you the hardest or trickiest

questions. To avoid tiring or appearing tired, get up and stretch frequently, and ask for a break whenever you need one. You can also insist on a specific time limit, such as no more than 3 hours per session.

You can be brief
Answer the opposing lawyer's questions as briefly and simply as you can. Don't volunteer extra information, and don't try to answer the question you think he'll ask next. You're not there to educate him. And if he tries to cut short your reply, you can say that you haven't finished. Your own lawyer may then ask that you be allowed to finish, or he may give you time to do so during his examination.

You can ask for clarification
If you don't understand a question or if it makes no sense, don't try to guess what the examining lawyer means. Ask him to repeat or rephrase it.

You don't have to answer every question
If the opposing lawyer asks you for an opinion about something you feel unqualified to address, you can refuse to answer and give your reason.

If the opposing lawyer asks a question that seems to have nothing to do with the case, such as a question about your personal life, you don't have to answer. Just explain why.

The judge may still require you to answer a question, but wait for his ruling. The opposing lawyer can't force you to answer; only the judge can. But be careful; you could be held in

Resisting pressure tactics

During the deposition, a lawyer may try to confuse you or get you to change your answer. Here's how you can defeat his tactics.

Silence. After your answer, the lawyer may wait silently, hoping you'll become flustered and keep talking. Resist the urge to say more; force him to speak.

The incomplete question. The lawyer may ask you a hypothetical question that leaves out key information. If it's incomplete or makes no sense, say so. If you don't feel you can answer it, don't even try.

The yes-or-no demand. The lawyer may insist that you answer a question either "yes" or "no." Don't let him intimidate you. You can answer any way

you wish: "Maybe" or "I don't remember" or "yes, but..." with an explanation added. Otherwise, you risk having an incomplete or misleading answer entered into the record.

The challenge. Don't let the lawyer bait you with a leading question such as, "Do you mean to tell me...?" Stand by what you said originally, if you said what you meant. You don't have to justify your actions or beliefs.

The off-the-record ploy. Don't let the lawyer lure you into divulging information by telling you that what you say is off the record. Nothing is off the record, not even what you say during breaks. If it would help the lawyer's case, he'd use it at the trial.

contempt for repeated refusals without a good reason.

Always refuse to answer a question if that's what your lawyer advises. Before answering any question, wait at least 5 seconds. Not only does this give you time to think what you're going to say but it also gives your lawyer time to object to the question. (See *Resisting pressure tactics*.)

You don't have to incriminate yourself

If you believe the answer to a question would hurt your reputation, you can claim your Fifth

Amendment right to avoid self-incrimination. You can say, "I refuse to answer that question because it might tend to incriminate me." But beware: If you've already answered a question on the same subject, you no longer have a Fifth Amendment right to remain silent on that subject; you'll have to answer.

Don't use your Fifth Amendment right without a very good reason. If the case goes to trial, the opposing lawyer could use your silence on a subject to discredit you.

You can claim lawyer-client privilege

Any conversation with your lawyer is privileged (unless it takes place in the presence of a third party). You may say something like this: "That question pertains to conversations between my lawyer and me; I invoke the lawyer-client privilege in not answering it." Again, beware: You waive that right if you start talking about anything you and your lawyer discussed. So be alert for any apparently harmless questions that might make you mention a privileged conversation. Also, your conversations with the hospital lawyer may not be covered by the lawyer-client privilege because he might not be considered your personal lawyer—another reason to hire your own lawyer.

During the deposition, if you're unsure about whether you should invoke this privilege, ask your lawyer.

You can review the deposition

Once you give a deposition, your answers stand as stated. You have a right to read the transcript and to correct typographic errors or misspellings or make other nonsubstantive changes before signing it. But you may not change an answer that you feel is wrong or incomplete. To do that would be perjury and would lose the trial for you before it began. That's why it's crucial to consult with your own lawyer before the deposition and to think before speaking during the deposition.

Settling out of court

Very few malpractice lawsuits actually go to court. If you're ever involved in a malpractice lawsuit, chances are that your lawyer will settle out of court. But he'll need your help to make this settlement, and you'll need to know your rights.

When you discuss settlement with your lawyer, remember these points.

Know the terms of your policy

If you're covered by professional liability insurance, the terms of your policy will determine whether you, your lawyer, or the insurance company can control the settlement. Most policies don't permit the nurse to settle a case without the consent of the insurance company.

In fact, policies, especially those provided by hospitals, permit the insurance company to settle without the consent of the individual nurse involved.

Review your policy to determine your settlement rights. If the policy isn't clear on this point, call your hospital's insurance administrator or the insurance company and ask for clarification.

Provide information

Offer your insurance company's representative and your lawyer all the information you can about the case. They will then be able to evaluate your liabilities and the plaintiff's liabilities, and determine the best settlement with the plaintiff.

As an attending nurse, you may be in the best position to

provide crucial observations concerning the patient's state of mind – often the basis of a successful settlement.

Avoid further expenses

If you settle your case out of court, it doesn't mean that you're admitting any wrongdoing. The law regards settlement as a compromise between two parties to end a lawsuit and avoid further expense. In other words, you may choose to pay a settlement rather than incur possibly greater expenses (both financial and emotional) by defending your innocence at a trial.

———————————————❖

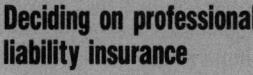

Deciding on professional liability insurance

In any work setting, you're at risk for malpractice suits, and the risk increases if you work in a specialized setting such as the intensive care unit. Professional liability insurance can protect you financially. Without it, you'd probably have to pay any judgment out of your own pocket. To satisfy a judgment in many states, the courts can take almost everything you own, except for a limited amount of your equity in your home and the clothes on your back. This includes your salary and any future inheritance.

You may think that, as a hospital employee, you're protected by the hospital's policy. This might be true at work if you carry out only the duties outlined in your specific job description. However,

the policy might not cover you for any duties that go beyond your job description. And, if the policy hasn't been updated to reflect current nursing practice, you might not be covered for duties such as performing physical examinations; assessing, treating, and prescribing under standing orders; and assuming administrative roles. What's more, anything you do on your own time – such as tending sports injuries at a local school or giving health advice to a neighbor – wouldn't be covered.

Types of policies

Professional liability insurance may cover either the time the malpractice occurred (occurrence-based policy) or when a lawsuit is filed (claims-made policy).

An *occurrence-based policy* protects you against any incidents occurring during a policy period, regardless of when the patient files a claim against you – even if that comes after the policy ends. The important date is the date the incident occurred, not the date the claim is made.

A *claims-made policy* protects you only against claims made against you during the policy period. The important date is the date the claim is filed, not the date the incident occurred. In addition, a lawsuit doesn't have to be filed for an incident to be covered. A "claim" can also be allegations by a patient or lawyer, a letter received from a dissatisfied patient, or your awareness of potential harm to a patient because of personal negligence.

A claims-made policy is less expensive than an occurrence-based policy because the insurance company is at risk only for the duration of the policy. However, you can purchase an extended-reporting endorsement, or tail coverage, which in effect turns your claims-made policy into an occurrence-based policy.

Either type of policy will provide maximum dollar amounts to cover claims. Usually, this figure is expressed as a double amount, such as $300,000/$500,000. The smaller number is the maximum amount the insurer will pay to protect you from any one injury arising out of a single nursing malpractice occurrence. The larger number is the maximum amount the insurer will pay for all claims under that policy in the policy period. There's no limit to the number of lawsuits the insurer will defend you against.

Policy components

An insurance policy has three parts:
• *agreement* – the insurance company's promise to protect you if a claim that's covered by the policy is made
• *contract conditions* – your rights and obligations and the insurance company's; any failure to fulfill an obligation or to protect a right could breach the contract
• *exclusions* – the acts that aren't covered by the policy; make sure you fully understand these exclusions.

Coverage limits

All malpractice insurance policies cover professional liability. Some also cover personal liability, medical payments, assault-related bodily injury, and all property damage.

However, coverage is limited to the acts and practice settings specified in the policy. Make sure that your policy covers your specific nursing role and normal duties. Check whether the policy also provides coverage for the following incidents:
• misuse of equipment
• errors in reporting or recording care
• failure to properly teach patients
• errors in administering medication
• mistakes made while providing care in an emergency, outside your employment setting
• mistakes made while providing advice or care in nonemergency situations, such as offering diabetes counseling or hypertension screening at a health fair.

Also ask if the policy provides protection if your employer (the hospital) sues you. And, because a policy usually covers only the person named on the policy, ask specifically if it covers you for negligence on the part of nurses under your supervision.

Policy limitations

A professional liability policy won't cover every situation. For example, it won't cover acts outside the scope of the state nurse practice act or license, criminal acts, or punitive damages. And it may specifically exclude certain types of nurses such as nurse-anesthetists.

❖

Index

INDEX

---

i refers to an illustration; t refers to a table

INDEX

i refers to an illustration; t refers to a table

i refers to an illustration; t refers to a table

i refers to an illustration; t refers to a table